American Nursing Review for

NCLEX RN

Fourth Edition

American Nursing Review for

NCLEX RN

Fourth Edition

Carol J. Bininger, RN, PhD
Phyllis F. Healy, RN,C, PhD
Jane M. Lamp, RN,C, MS
Marianne W. Rodgers, RN, EdD, PNP

SPRINGHOUSE CORPORATION
SPRINGHOUSE, PENNSYLVANIA

STAFF

Senior Publisher
Matthew Cahill

Art Director
John Hubbard

Managing Editor
David Moreau

Acquisitions Editors
Patricia Kardish Fischer, RN, BSN; Louise Quinn

Senior Editor
Karen Diamond

Clinical Consultants
Collette Bishop Hendler, RN, CCRN; Lori Musolf Neri, RN, MSN

Copy Editors
Cynthia C. Breuninger (manager), Karen C. Comerford, Brenna H. Mayer, Pamela Wingrod

Designers
Arlene Putterman (associate art director), Cindy Marczuk

Production Coordinator
Margaret A. Rastiello

Editorial Assistants
Beverly Lane, Mary Madden

Manufacturing
Deborah Meiris (director), T.A. Landis, Otto Mezei

Printed in the United States of America.

℞ A member of the Reed Elsevier plc group

Library of Congress Cataloging-in-Publication Data

American nursing review for NCLEX-RN/Carol J. Bininger... [et al.].—4th ed.
   p.cm.
   Includes bibliographical references and index.
   1. Nursing—Examinations, questions, etc. 2. Nursing—Outlines,syllabi, etc. I. Bininger, Carol J.
   [DNLM: 1. Nursing—examination questions.
WY 18.2 A512 1998]
Rt42.A43 1998
610.73'076—dc21
DNLM/DLC   97-17857
ISBN 0-87434-905-2 (alk. paper)   CIP

CONTENTS

Part IV: Maintaining homeostasis

Part V: Review of clinical nursing

Perioperative nursing

Mental health nursing

Maternal-newborn nursing

Part VI: ANR Post-Test

Part VII: Appendices, references, and index

Contributors

Clinical coordinators

Carol J. Bininger, RN, PhD
Mental health nursing

Phyllis F. Healy, RN,C, PhD
Adult nursing

Jane M. Lamp, RN,C, MS
Maternal-Newborn nursing

Marianne W. Rodgers, RN, EdD,
PNP
Child nursing

Contributing authors

Carol J. Bininger, RN, PhD
Assistant Professor
Ohio State University

**Kathleen C. Blanchfield, RN,
MS**
Consultant
Evangelical Hospital Systems
Illinois

Janet Z. Burson, EdD, RD, LD
Associate Professor
University of Southern Maine

Doris W. Campbell, RN, PhD
Assistant Professor
University of Florida

Margery G. Garbin, RN, PhD
President
C-NET
New Jersey

Phyllis F. Healy, RN,C, PhD
Associate Professor
University of Southern Maine

Patricia Ann Howard, RN, MS
Clinical Associate
Ohio State University

Carole M. Kingsbury, RN, EdD
Vice President, Testing
C-NET
New Jersey

Ann W. Kurtz, RN, MSN
Assistant Professor
University of South Florida

Jane M. Lamp, RN,C, MS
Clinical Associate
Ohio State University

Barbara A. Lee, RN, MS, CRNA
Staff Anesthetist
Austin Anesthesia Group
Texas

Elizabeth J. Mason, RN, PhD
President
EXCELCARE, Inc.
Pennsylvania

Leona A. Mourad, RN, MSN, ONC
Associate Professor Emeritus
Ohio State University

Nancy L. Potts, RN, MSN
Instructor
St. Petersburg Junior College
Florida

Marianne W. Rodgers, RN, EdD,
PNP
Associate Professor
Chairperson, Undergraduate
Program
University of Southern Maine

Carol L. Schaffer, RN, JD
Director
Cleveland Clinic Home Care
Services
Ohio

Noreen B. Vincent, RN, MS
Instructor
University of Southern Maine

Patty J. Walden, RN, MS
Director, Staff Development
Augustana Hospital
Illinois

Doris E. Wilson, RN, MA
Consultant
Private Practice
Florida

Elaine A. Zimbler, RN, MS
Consultant
Private Practice
New York

John Zunino, BA
Vice President, Information
Systems
C-NET
New Jersey

Consultants

F. William Balkie, RN, MBA, CRNA
President
American Nursing Review
New Jersey

Jenkin Vaughn Williams
Executive Vice President
American Nursing Review
New Jersey

x

Preface

The introduction of managed care as the predominant health care delivery system in the United States has led to major changes in how professional nursing is practiced. The entry-level nurse today is expected to possess greater clinical knowledge and skills and the ability to practice in a wider variety of health care delivery settings, from the traditional hospital-based practice to the more autonomous home health nursing practice. The earlier discharge of acutely ill clients from hospitals has required nurses to expand their knowledge of complex technical equipment and develop new insights into how clients and their families respond to the presence of this equipment in the home. The increased nursing competencies required for professional nursing practice and the responsibility for ensuring that you have them has never been greater.

How this book can help

To enter the practice of professional nursing, a nurse is required to pass the National Council Licensure Examination for Registered Nurses (NCLEX-RN). The sole purpose of the examination, often referred to as the "State Boards," is to assure the public of a nurse's competence to practice entry-level nursing safely and effectively. Passing the NCLEX-RN is crucial to a nurse's career. Nurses know they must be fully prepared, both educationally and psychologically. To achieve this level of preparation requires a well-planned study of nursing basics and a keen understanding of test-taking strategies, with particular awareness of what to expect in test questions on the NCLEX-RN. Nurses seeking licensure in the United States take the examination by the computerized adaptive testing (CAT) method. Learning how this testing method works is an important part of the study process.

Now in its fourth edition, *American Nursing Review for NCLEX-RN* has been updated to help nurses pass the computerized licensure examination; it reviews all the essential nursing information likely to appear on the test. To prepare for the NCLEX-RN, most nurse educators recommend the following:
• Establish a baseline of current knowledge.
• Understand how the NCLEX-RN is constructed and scored.
• Master successful test-taking skills and strategies.
• Pursue a general review of basic nursing content, concentrating on weak areas that require further study.
• Use a measuring tool, such as a post-test, to evaluate study results and final preparedness for the examination.

American Nursing Review for NCLEX-RN contains all the elements needed to accomplish these objectives. Written by clinical experts and test development specialists, the book offers a pretest to evaluate your current knowledge, insights on how the NCLEX-RN is constructed, valuable test-taking tips, a comprehensive review of nursing essentials, and a post-test that identifies knowledge strengths and deficiencies *before* you take the actual examination. In addition, the book includes a computer disk with two more tests containing 150 new questions not duplicated in the book.

Organization and content

Divided into seven parts, the book provides a progressive framework for effective study. Part I, "Pretest," poses 60 questions covering all areas of professional nursing to help establish a baseline of your current knowledge. Correct answers with rationales and a useful diagnostic scoring device follow the test. When used conscientiously, the diagnostic profile will accurately pinpoint weak areas to focus on as you proceed through the book.

Part II, "Taking NCLEX-RN," explains the computerized test and the plan from which it is derived, reveals how test questions are constructed, and presents well-documented strategies for passing the exam. Knowing what the test is all about will give you confidence and a decided psychological uplift. The section also includes information of special interest to Canadian nursing graduates, who continue to take the paper-and-pencil examination.

Part III, "Fundamental nursing concepts and skills," consists of two sections that review essential information applicable to any nursing setting. The first section, *Nursing concepts,* covers a wide spectrum, ranging from legal issues and rehabilitation to human growth and development. It begins with the book's unifying theme—the nursing process—and examines how client needs are resolved through assessment, diagnosis, planning, implementation, and evaluation (or client outcomes). Special attention is devoted to the nursing diagnosis (or analysis) phase, tracing the historical development of the uniform nursing diagnosis nomenclature and explaining how nursing diagnoses assist in planning client care. Topics have been revised for the fourth edition to reflect changes in the profession (and hence, on the exam). New material on case management, home health care, and gerontologic nursing have been added to prepare you for nursing realities in the current health care delivery system.

The second section, *Nursing skills,* covers procedural skills common to all areas of clinical practice, such as blood transfusion, anticipatory guidance, and discharge planning. This information is important to nurses who are beginning practice in mental health, maternal-infant, child, and adult nursing. The discussion of arrhythmia interpretation will enhance your ability to recognize life-threatening arrhythmias and to intervene as necessary. Questions on arrhythmias regularly appear on the NCLEX-RN. The principles of cardiopulmonary resuscitation (CPR) have been updated to conform with American Heart Association guidelines as of 1993. Because these guidelines are updated frequently, you should confirm the latest guidelines before taking the examination.

Part IV, "Maintaining homeostasis," examines client problems that threaten any body system: inflammation, shock, pain, acid-base disturbances, fluid and electrolyte imbalances, and immobility.

Part V, "Review of clinical nursing," is organized around the nursing process and introduces clinical situations (case studies), a format that has proven highly successful for NCLEX-RN preparation.

Each clinical situation is preceded with an overview of the health problem. The client's problems are solved using the five steps of the nursing process. Rationales for each assessment and implementation are given alongside each nursing behavior.

The CAT exam incorporates case studies in the test items. In this book, nursing diagnoses provided for each case are those you would likely establish after analyzing the assessment findings. By no means are the diagnoses meant to be all-inclusive for any client who may have the health condition being reviewed; for this reason, you may find it useful to consider additional nursing diagnoses for some of the conditions, particularly if you do not feel completely comfortable in developing nursing care plans.

The five clinical areas covered in Part V— perioperative, mental health, maternal-infant, child, and adult nursing—also encompass specialty areas (for example, community health nursing and gerontologic nursing). *Perioperative nursing* examines routine preoperative and postoperative nursing care applicable to all clients undergoing surgery; consequently, it does not employ a case-study approach. It does, however, apply the nursing process to perioperative nursing.

Mental health nursing covers the psychodynamic responses and psychological defenses of people facing severe anxiety and stress. The text presents important therapeutic communication and mental health nursing principles in carefully designed clinical situations. Among this section's 11 featured topics are anxiety disorders, substance abuse, Alzheimer's disease, and borderline personality disorder. The fourth edition also has the latest drugs used in treating mental disorders.

Maternal-newborn nursing reviews 17 health problems associated with the maternity cycle, beginning with family planning. Still controversial to some, family planning has important implications for health teaching for all nurses, and test items on this topic may appear on the NCLEX-RN. The section provides information on a normal pregnancy from conception through postpartum, complications of pregnancy (including new material on preterm labor), high-risk conditions, complications of labor and delivery, nursing care of the newborn, and health care teaching of new parents, among other topics. The adolescent parent is of particular interest because of the increasing prevalence of teenage parenthood and the important role nurses play in teaching adolescents about the psychological and physiologic changes associated with pregnancy.

Child nursing is organized developmentally by age-group (infants, toddlers, preschoolers, school-age children, and adolescents). Clinical situations describe 22 health problems, ranging from tracheo-esophageal fistula, pyloric stenosis, and acute acetaminophen poisoning to leukemia, sickle cell anemia, and cystic fibrosis. This section includes a new entry on asthma, a common health problem among pediatric clients.

Adult nursing is organized primarily by body system, concluding with sections devoted to communicable diseases and oncology nursing. The text reviews more than 50 health problems, including myocardial infarction, Parkinson's disease, pulmonary tuberculosis, hip fracture, burns, cataract extraction, diabetes mellitus, gastric ulcer, acute and chronic renal failure, AIDS, and breast cancer. For each health problem, the text also provides relevant laboratory studies and abnormal findings. (NCLEX-RN includes test items on laboratory studies and the nurse's role in ordering them.)

Part VI, "ANR Post-Test," consists of a sample

test designed to mirror the current NCLEX-RN test plan. Comprising 105 test items (the same number of items received by the average nurse taking the NCLEX-RN over the past 2 years), the test covers all clinical areas, all phases of the nursing process, and all categories of client needs. After carefully reviewing this book, take the post-test to evaluate your study effectiveness and your readiness for the NCLEX-RN. Following the test are correct answers, along with rationales for both correct and incorrect answers and codes for the phase of the nursing process and client needs category. To identify possible weaknesses in your knowledge and test-taking skills, complete the self-graded performance profile that follows the post-test.

Part VII, "Appendices, references, and index," offers more useful information to round out your study program: normal laboratory values, this year's official list of NANDA-approved nursing diagnoses, formulas and equivalent measures for safe and accurate dosage calculation and drug administration, U.S. and Canadian licensing bodies, the American Nurses Association Code for Nurses, selected references to inspire further reading and study, and a comprehensive index for locating topics quickly.

Special features
Numerous tables, flowcharts, and illustrations appear throughout the book to enhance recall, clarify complex topics, or expand on concepts presented in the main text. Glossaries accompanying each clinical study area in Part V define significant or easily misunderstood terms.

Additionally, each study area concludes with a "Selected drugs" table specifically created for that section; information presented in the table highlights possible testing items on the NCLEX-RN. In each drug chart, the side effects listed are those that are most common or potentially life-threatening.

NCLEX-RN practice disk
The new practice disk included with this edition (see inside back cover) offers limitless opportunities for further review of NCLEX-RN content in the new computerized format. The disk contains 150 questions in two tests that cover all areas of the NCLEX-RN test plan; these questions do not duplicate test items in the book. Complete with step-by-step operating instructions, the program uses the same screen layout and keyboard functions as those you will see and use on the actual NCLEX-RN CAT. You can take the tests repeatedly, with a random selection of questions each time; choose questions by clinical study area, nursing process step, or client needs category; review the correct answers and rationales after each question (learning mode); and obtain a performance appraisal at the end of the test (proficiency mode). No previous computer knowledge is needed.

A highly effective study tool for more than 15 years, *American Nursing Review for NCLEX-RN* contains all the information you need to prepare for the State Boards. This fourth edition includes many improvements and new material to keep it abreast of the ever-evolving NCLEX test plan. We are confident you will continue to use the book as a reference even after the NCLEX-RN is only a memory. Good luck on the test, and congratulations on choosing nursing as a career.

— F. WILLIAM BALKIE, RN, MBA, CRNA
President
American Nursing Review

— JENKIN VAUGHN WILLIAMS
Executive Vice President
American Nursing Review

Part I

Pretest

Part I

Pretest

Instructions

This pretest has been designed to determine your current knowledge base before you begin your study program for the NCLEX-RN. By analyzing the results, you can identify the areas in which you may wish to do more comprehensive study.

The pretest contains 60 questions, written in the format used in the computerized examination (given to U.S. examinees only). There are four possible answers for each question. Read each question and all possible answers carefully; then select the best answer.

Take no more than 60 minutes to complete this pretest. If you have difficulty understanding a question or are not sure of the answer, place a small mark next to the question number—but still select an answer, even if you have to guess. The mark will help you recall that you had trouble with that question. However, be aware that on the computerized examination, you will not be able to go back to a question or go on to the next question without selecting an answer choice. (Examinees taking NCLEX-RN in Canada still have this option, however.)

In this pretest, possible answers are numbered 1, 2, 3, and 4 to help identify the correct answer and the rationale. These numbers will not appear in the actual computerized NCLEX-RN.

This test	NCLEX-RN
○ 1. Atonic	Atonic
○ 2. Dystonic	Dystonic
○ 3. Hypotonic	Hypotonic
○ 4. Hypertonic	Hypertonic

After you have completed the pretest or the 60-minute time limit expires, check your responses against the correct answers provided on pages 11 to 16. Then complete the diagnostic profile on page 17.

Now, select a quiet room where you will be undisturbed, set a timer for 60 minutes, and begin.

Questions

1. A 60-year-old male client with a history of angina has been taking nitroglycerin. He states that "everything is fine, except that I get chest pain while having sex with my wife." Which of these responses by the nurse would be best?
   ○ 1. "Have you thought of seeing a sexual therapist for counseling?"
   ○ 2. "You'll have to limit your sexual activity."
   ○ 3. "You should expect that intercourse at your age may pose some problems."
   ○ 4. "You may be helped by taking a nitroglycerin tablet just before intercourse."

2. A client has been placed on a low-cholesterol diet. The nurse should advise the client to reduce intake of which of these foods?
   ○ 1. Cottage cheese.
   ○ 2. Eggs.
   ○ 3. Veal.
   ○ 4. Chicken.

3. A client is admitted to a psychiatric hospital for treatment of agoraphobia. For the past 3 months, she has been afraid to leave her home, and she and her husband have agreed that hospitalization is necessary. When the staff nurse introduces herself, the client starts to cry and says, "I'm so afraid to be here. I'm not crazy. I just want to go home." Which response by the nurse would be most appropriate?
   ○ 1. "Try not to be so upset now. Let's get busy helping you."
   ○ 2. "You seem upset. I will sit here with you."
   ○ 3. "You can't go home until we've helped you with your fears."
   ○ 4. "Is there some way I can help you?"

4. A nursing assistant asks the nurse why a client's physician doesn't just force an agoraphobic client to get out of the house to help her get over her fears. Which understanding of the treatment of phobias should the nurse's response include?
   ○ 1. People must gain a sense of control over the feared object—they cannot be forced when they're not ready.
   ○ 2. People use their fears to consciously avoid taking responsibility for their lives.

3. The treatment approach is intentionally slow to help lull the client into a sense of fearlessness.

4. Forcing people into fearful situations can cause acute psychosis.

5. The nurse finds an agoraphobic client standing in front of a sign-up sheet for a field trip to a shopping mall. The client says, "If I had any guts, I'd sign up for this trip. What do you think I should do?" Which comment by the nurse would help the client make an appropriate decision?

   1. "You have plenty of guts! Why not sign up now?"
   2. "I'm not here to tell you what to do, but if I were you, I'd go."
   3. "It sure is a great trip. I think you'd enjoy it."
   4. "Let's discuss what you're thinking about this trip."

6. A 15-year-old female client with bulimia nervosa tells the nurse she does not like the other teenagers on the ward. The nurse senses the client's disdain toward her peers. Which nursing action would best help the teenager with peer relationships?

   1. Point out to the client how she affects others.
   2. Ask the client why she doesn't like her peers.
   3. Carefully select same-age peers to include in an activity with the client.
   4. Have the client choose an activity that would include herself, the nurse, and some peers as participants.

7. A client is diagnosed with prostate cancer. Initial treatment will include diethylstilbestrol. When teaching the client about the medication, the nurse should tell him he probably will experience which side effects?

   1. Priapism and increased libido.
   2. Hoarseness and muscular hypertrophy.
   3. Hirsutism and increased abdominal girth.
   4. Gynecomastia and a high-pitched voice.

8. Which is the best way to deal with a toddler who is having a temper tantrum?

   1. Reason with the child.
   2. Threaten the child.
   3. Spank the child.
   4. Ignore the child's outburst.

9. A client visits the prenatal clinic for the first time after missing two menstrual periods. She suspects she may be pregnant, and tells the nurse that the first day of her last menstrual period was June 30, 1997. According to Nagele's rule, which of these dates is the client's expected date of confinement?

   1. March 14, 1998.
   2. March 30, 1998.
   3. April 6, 1998.
   4. April 13, 1998.

10. A client has a positive pregnancy test. Which hormone is related to this finding?

    1. Luteinizing hormone (LH).
    2. Follicle-stimulating hormone (FSH).
    3. Human chorionic somatomammotropin (hCS).
    4. Human chorionic gonadotropin (hCG).

11. Besides the hormonal changes indicated by a positive pregnancy test, which physiologic change would have occurred by the time a client had missed two menstrual periods?

    1. Diastasis recti.
    2. Decreased glomerular filtration rate.
    3. Bluish discoloration of the vaginal vault.
    4. 50% increase in blood volume.

12. A pregnant client who received dietary instructions during her first visit to the prenatal clinic returns for a follow-up. The nurse asks her what she had for lunch that day. Which response would indicate that the client followed the dietary instructions?

    1. Cheeseburger, salad, fruit, and milk.
    2. Bouillon, crackers, fruit, and milk.
    3. Ham sandwich, pickles, pie, and iced tea.
    4. Cottage cheese, tomatoes, crackers, and coffee with cream.

13. A client has questions about exercise during pregnancy. Which approach would be the most appropriate for the nurse to take?

    1. Recommend that the client follow an exercise routine.
    2. Assure the client that her pregnancy is normal and she need not adjust her usual activities.
    3. Give the client a pamphlet explaining recommended exercises.
    4. Explore the amount and type of exercise the client is doing.

14. The physician has ordered ferrous sulfate 100 mg t.i.d. for a pregnant client. Which instruction should the client be given?
    ○ 1. Take the medication just before meals and with plenty of fluid.
    ○ 2. Take the medication with milk at mealtimes.
    ○ 3. Take the medication with an antacid after meals.
    ○ 4. Take the medication with orange juice between meals.

15. At 28 weeks' gestation, a pregnant client's laboratory values include the following:
    Blood: hemoglobin, 11 g/dl; hematocrit, 36%.
    Urine: glucose, trace; acetone, negative; albumin, negative. These results probably indicate which of the following?
    ○ 1. Anemia.
    ○ 2. Preeclampsia.
    ○ 3. Diabetes mellitus.
    ○ 4. Pseudoanemia of pregnancy.

16. A male client is receiving an antihypertensive agent. Which of these potential side effects would be *most* important for the nurse to discuss with him?
    ○ 1. Impotence.
    ○ 2. Nausea and vomiting.
    ○ 3. Nasal stuffiness.
    ○ 4. Postural hypotension.

17. Infants achieve structural control of the head before the trunk and extremities. Which of these universal principles of development does this reflect?
    ○ 1. Development proceeds in a cephalocaudal direction.
    ○ 2. Development proceeds in a proximal-distal fashion.
    ○ 3. The sequence of development is from simple to complex.
    ○ 4. The sequence of development is from general to specific.

18. A male client has been on glucocorticoid therapy for the past year. He calls the nurse to report that he has been vomiting for the past 2 days and has not taken his "hormone" pills. The nurse should plan the client's care based on which potential effect of glucocorticoids?
    ○ 1. The client may develop adrenal insufficiency.
    ○ 2. The client is at risk for developing pituitary syndrome.
    ○ 3. The client's own adrenal glands will start to produce more glucocorticoids immediately.
    ○ 4. The client's pituitary gland will increase production of corticotropin immediately.

19. A divorced computer programmer is admitted after taking 15 secobarbital sodium (Seconal) capsules. Three days later, the client is transferred from the intensive care unit to the psychiatric unit. Quiet and withdrawn, the client refuses to get out of bed for breakfast. Which response by the nurse would be *most* appropriate?
    ○ 1. "It's a beautiful day today. Time to get up."
    ○ 2. "It's time to get up. I'll help you get ready for breakfast."
    ○ 3. "It's time to get up for breakfast. Let's get ready."
    ○ 4. "It's the policy on this unit to be up and dressed for breakfast."

20. The nurse has been working with a depressed male client for 1 week. This morning, the client comes to the dining room with hair uncombed and shirt unbuttoned. Which of these actions should the nurse take *first*?
    ○ 1. Approach the client and offer to help him finish getting dressed.
    ○ 2. Ignore the client's appearance and help him find his place at the table.
    ○ 3. Sit with the client and help him eat the food.
    ○ 4. Walk with the client until he notices that his shirt is unbuttoned.

21. Which statement by a depressed client most clearly indicates a high suicide potential?
    ○ 1. "The future looks bleak for me."
    ○ 2. "Don't worry about me. I'll be all right."
    ○ 3. "A handful of my red pills will cure me."
    ○ 4. "Life's a drag. I'm thinking about curing this."

22. A depressed client participates in unit activities and meets regularly with a nurse. One morning, the client asks the nurse to get the comb from the bedside table. Next to the comb, the nurse finds 10 secobarbital capsules. After confiscating the capsules, what should the nurse do next?
    ○ 1. Report the finding to the other team members.
    ○ 2. Tell the client about finding the capsules and ask if the client was planning to commit suicide.
    ○ 3. Sit with the client for the rest of the day and increase suicide precautions.
    ○ 4. Give the client the comb; then suggest that the client and nurse go for a walk.

23. Which measure should the nurse take when providing care to a client in Buck's traction?
    ○ 1. Maintain the head of the bed at a 45-degree angle.
    ○ 2. Ensure that the client's right heel touches the bed.
    ○ 3. Remove the weights when bathing the client's lower extremities.
    ○ 4. Allow the weights to hang freely at the foot of the bed.

24. A client admitted with pulmonary edema improves. The physician's current orders include digoxin 0.25 mg daily, furosemide 40 mg daily, and nasal oxygen at 2 liters/minute. To evaluate the effectiveness of digoxin, the nurse should observe for:
    ○ 1. increased urine output.
    ○ 2. increased pulse rate.
    ○ 3. decreased respiratory rate.
    ○ 4. lowered blood pressure.

25. A client with pulmonary edema is receiving digoxin and furosemide. When planning the client's care, the nurse would include three of the following observations. Which observation is *not* indicated?
    ○ 1. Note changes in appetite.
    ○ 2. Note changes in the respiratory rate.
    ○ 3. Observe urine output.
    ○ 4. Assess for neurologic intention tremor.

26. A client with pulmonary edema is receiving continuous oxygen therapy and daily doses of furosemide and digoxin. When the client complains of no appetite and asks to have the food tray removed, the nurse's best action should be based on knowledge that:
    ○ 1. many clients dislike hospital food.
    ○ 2. anorexia is common in clients receiving oxygen.
    ○ 3. furosemide causes decreased appetite in many clients.
    ○ 4. anorexia may be an early sign of digoxin toxicity.

27. A boy, age 7, recently was diagnosed with juvenile-onset diabetes mellitus. He takes NPH and regular insulin. His mother asks the nurse if he can go on an afternoon hike during an upcoming weekend camp-out. Which response by the nurse would be the best?
    ○ 1. "He should have a snack, such as a cheese sandwich and a glass of milk, an hour before the hike and should carry a fast-acting source of glucose."
    ○ 2. "He should not go on the hike. The possible effects of extraordinary activities are just too unpredictable."
    ○ 3. "He should increase his morning dosage of NPH insulin by approximately one-third to cover his increased metabolic rate during the hike."
    ○ 4. "Do you feel it's really appropriate for him to participate in a weekend camp-out when he has physical limitations?"

28. A client with hypertension is receiving chlorothiazide (Diuril) to reduce blood pressure. The nurse should instruct the client to eat which of these foods regularly?
    ○ 1. Apples.
    ○ 2. Liver.
    ○ 3. Low-fat milk.
    ○ 4. Dried fruits.

29. A client visits the company nurse for treatment of a minor paper cut on her right arm. The nurse is aware that the client had a right mastectomy 5 years ago. Further action by the nurse should be based on which understanding?
   - ○ 1. Previous removal of lymph nodes places the client at increased risk for complications.
   - ○ 2. After 5 years, the client is no longer at risk for complications.
   - ○ 3. Only underlying psychological problems could cause someone to be concerned with a minor paper cut.
   - ○ 4. On-the-job stress is probably the real cause of the client's visit.

30. Laboratory results for a client who is receiving chemotherapy include the following: hematocrit, 34%; hemoglobin, 11 g/dl; platelet count, 48,000/mm³; and white blood cell count, 4,000/mm³. All of the following goals are indicated in the care plan. Which one should take priority?
   - ○ 1. To prevent infection.
   - ○ 2. To prevent bleeding.
   - ○ 3. To prevent anemia.
   - ○ 4. To prevent alopecia.

31. A client is told that a tuberculin skin test is positive. Which statement would indicate that the client understands the test results?
   - ○ 1. "I have had previous exposure to tuberculosis."
   - ○ 2. "I have immunity and cannot develop the disease."
   - ○ 3. "I currently have active tuberculosis."
   - ○ 4. "I have a reactivation of a healed primary lesion."

32. A client, age 14, has been sexually abused by her father for the past 2 years. Now she is 8 weeks pregnant, and asks the nurse what she should do about the pregnancy. Which reply would be *best*?
   - ○ 1. "Because you are so young, you stand a good chance of having a miscarriage."
   - ○ 2. "That's a decision only you and your mother can make."
   - ○ 3. "I think it would be all right for you to have an abortion. Is that what you'd like to do?"
   - ○ 4. "Making a sound decision is not always easy. What are your thoughts about the pregnancy?"

33. A 15-month-old boy is admitted to the pediatric unit with a diagnosis of bilateral serous otitis media and bacterial meningitis. All of the following rooms are available on the pediatric unit. The nurse should plan to put the client in which one?
   - ○ 1. An isolation room off the main hallway.
   - ○ 2. A private room two doors away from the nurses' station.
   - ○ 3. A semiprivate room with a 15-month-old child who has meningitis.
   - ○ 4. A four-bed room with two toddlers who have croup.

34. To best meet the developmental needs of a 15-month-old hospitalized boy, the nurse should take which measure?
   - ○ 1. Ask his mother to room in with him.
   - ○ 2. Turn the television to his favorite cartoons.
   - ○ 3. Arrange for other staff to visit him at regular intervals throughout the day.
   - ○ 4. Tape a bright red punching balloon onto the side of his crib.

35. Which of these statements by the mother of a 15-month-old boy with bacterial meningitis would indicate that she understands the nurse's discharge teaching?
   - ○ 1. "I wish I had brought my child to the doctor sooner. The next time, I'll be more careful."
   - ○ 2. "We'll need to see the doctor every week or so until we're sure everything is all right."
   - ○ 3. "Next time he pulls on his ears or won't lie down, I'll take him to the doctor right away."
   - ○ 4. "I'm glad we'll be going home soon and that all of this business with infections and meningitis is behind us."

36. A client who has been diagnosed with conductive deafness is scheduled for a stapedectomy and has been taught about the condition. Which statement by the client would indicate a need for further instruction?
   - ○ 1. "Bone conduction of sound is still effective."
   - ○ 2. "My acoustic nerve is injured."
   - ○ 3. "Otosclerosis is a cause of my condition."
   - ○ 4. "Air conduction of sound is impaired."

37. After a stapedectomy, a client complains of fluctuations in hearing ability. The nurse should suspect which complication?
    - ○ **1.** Injury to the cochlea.
    - ○ **2.** Injury to the facial nerve.
    - ○ **3.** Labyrinthitis.
    - ○ **4.** Closure of the oval window.

38. After an above-the-knee amputation, a client returns to the unit from the recovery room. The nurse helps transfer the client from the stretcher to the bed. Before leaving the bedside, the nurse should make sure the client and the stump are in which positions?
    - ○ **1.** The client should be lying prone, and the stump should not be elevated.
    - ○ **2.** The stump should be abducted with a pillow between the client's legs.
    - ○ **3.** The client should be in a side-lying position, with the stump externally rotated.
    - ○ **4.** The client should be lying on the back, with the stump elevated slightly on a pillow.

39. After an amputation, which item is essential to keep at the client's bedside?
    - ○ **1.** Elastic bandages.
    - ○ **2.** Suture set.
    - ○ **3.** Dressings.
    - ○ **4.** Tourniquet.

40. The physician asks the nurse to change the dressing of a client who has had an above-the-knee amputation. When rewrapping the elastic bandage on the stump, the nurse should wrap it in which direction?
    - ○ **1.** From the groin to the stump.
    - ○ **2.** From the stump to the groin.
    - ○ **3.** From the waist to the thigh to the stump.
    - ○ **4.** From the waist to the stump, then up the thigh to the groin.

41. A client who has undergone an above-the-knee amputation has been in a wheelchair for 3 hours. The nurse assists him to bed, placing him in the prone position. Why is this position most appropriate?
    - ○ **1.** It decreases edema of the stump.
    - ○ **2.** It strengthens the abdominal muscles.
    - ○ **3.** It extends the affected hip joint.
    - ○ **4.** It prevents pressure ulcer formation.

42. Several hours after a leg amputation, a client complains of cramping pain in the toes of the amputated foot. When discussing this pain with the client, which approach would be best for the nurse to take?
    - ○ **1.** Mention that the client will receive pain medication in 30 minutes.
    - ○ **2.** Tell the client that the phantom pain will lessen in 2 to 3 days.
    - ○ **3.** Review the reasons for phantom pain with the client.
    - ○ **4.** Mention that phantom pain is a common occurrence.

43. A client sees a physician, complaining he has no energy and fears he has a terrible disease. He reports he has had trouble sleeping and completing his normal daily work for the past 3 months. The physical examination is normal. The client denies any recent losses. He seeks psychiatric care and is admitted to a psychiatric hospital. After meeting with the nurse for 3 weeks, the client starts the one-on-one session again by saying, "I'm such a failure. I can't earn a living. I'm never successful." Which response by the nurse would be most therapeutic?
    - ○ **1.** "We all feel discouraged at times."
    - ○ **2.** "I'd like to discuss your plans for today."
    - ○ **3.** "You're not a failure. Look at what a successful salesman you've been."
    - ○ **4.** "It's hard to feel like you're a failure. Let's talk about your plans for the future."

44. A depressed client is sitting in the activities room, staring at the wall. Which nursing intervention would be the *most* appropriate?
    - ○ **1.** Give the client free access to the activities materials, and ask what she wants to do.
    - ○ **2.** Give the client time to select an activity, and sit with her until she gets busy.
    - ○ **3.** Give the client equipment for making a collage, and show her how to do it.
    - ○ **4.** Give the client a 500-piece jigsaw puzzle, and tell her to do the best she can.

45. A client on the psychiatric unit slams down the phone after talking to his wife. He says, "She's the reason why I'm here." Which response by the nurse would be most appropriate?
    ○ 1. Tell him he has a lovely wife.
    ○ 2. Tell him we all get angry with our loved ones at times.
    ○ 3. Say nothing and show interest in his further comments.
    ○ 4. Suggest that they take a walk to work off some of his anger.

46. A client with insulin-dependent diabetes mellitus is admitted to the hospital for reevaluation. Approximately 3 hours after the client receives 20 units of regular insulin, the nurse assists with morning care. Which assessment findings would lead the nurse to suspect the client is having an insulin reaction?
    ○ 1. Air hunger and acetone breath.
    ○ 2. Vomiting and flushed skin.
    ○ 3. Nausea and headache.
    ○ 4. Confusion and diaphoresis.

47. During a hypoglycemic (insulin) reaction, a client is alert but cannot swallow. Which would be the *best* nursing action to take?
    ○ 1. Administer orange juice.
    ○ 2. Administer 50% glucose intravenously.
    ○ 3. Administer epinephrine subcutaneously.
    ○ 4. Administer glucagon intramuscularly.

48. A client is admitted to the nursing unit in acute abdominal pain. The physician diagnoses peritonitis. Abdominal assessment reveals three of the following findings. Which one would *not* occur with peritonitis?
    ○ 1. High-pitched bowel sounds.
    ○ 2. Abdominal distention.
    ○ 3. Diffuse abdominal pain.
    ○ 4. Constipation.

49. A client with peritonitis has a Salem sump that is connected to low wall suction. Which strategy should the nurse include in the plan of care?
    ○ 1. Turn the client from side to side every 4 hours.
    ○ 2. Irrigate the nasogastric tube through the blue opening.
    ○ 3. Measure nasogastric drainage every 24 hours.
    ○ 4. Increase the amount of suction if no drainage appears.

50. A newborn, 1 hour old, is admitted to the newborn nursery from the delivery room. The mother had polyhydramnios, and the health care team suspects the newborn has a tracheoesophageal fistula (TEF). The nurse should assess the newborn for all of the following *except:*
    ○ 1. abdominal distention.
    ○ 2. bile-stained vomitus.
    ○ 3. coughing, cyanosis, and choking.
    ○ 4. excessive drooling.

51. A newborn undergoes surgery that consists of repair of a TEF and a gastrostomy. Between the 3rd and 14th postoperative days, the newborn receives feedings through the gastrostomy tube. Which action should the nurse perform as part of the gastrostomy feeding?
    ○ 1. Inject 3 to 5 cc of air through the tube and listen over the stomach with a stethoscope.
    ○ 2. Feed through the gastrostomy tube with the newborn positioned on the left side.
    ○ 3. After the feeding, leave the gastrostomy tube unplugged and elevated above the level of the stomach.
    ○ 4. Immediately after the feeding, turn the newborn onto the right side and plug the gastrostomy tube.

52. When assessing a client with chronic obstructive pulmonary disease, the nurse would expect which laboratory finding?
    ○ 1. Elevated red blood cell count.
    ○ 2. Decreased platelet count.
    ○ 3. Increased PaO_2 and decreased $PaCO_2$ levels.
    ○ 4. Elevated serum cholesterol.

53. A pediatric client is about to have skin traction applied. The client's mother says, "I thought everyone who needed traction had to have skeletal traction." When discussing traction with her, the nurse can mention that skin traction has which advantage over skeletal traction?
    ○ 1. It is easier to apply.
    ○ 2. It causes fewer complications.
    ○ 3. It prevents rotation of the extremity.
    ○ 4. It can be maintained for longer periods.

54. A client with rheumatoid arthritis is receiving ibuprofen (Motrin). Which statement would indicate that the client has a correct understanding of ibuprofen?
- ○ **1.** "I should take the medicine between meals."
- ○ **2.** "The medicine will increase my appetite."
- ○ **3.** "The medicine may cause diarrhea."
- ○ **4.** "I should stop the medicine if my joints start to swell."

55. A child, age 2, is brought to the emergency department (ED) by her parents, who state that she refuses to move her right arm. X-rays reveal a dislocated right shoulder and a simple fracture of the right humerus. During the child's stay in the ED, the nurse observes all of the following behaviors by the child. Which behavior most strongly suggests the child has been abused and should be carefully documented by the nurse?
- ○ **1.** The child tries to sit up on the stretcher.
- ○ **2.** The child tries to move away from the nurse.
- ○ **3.** The child does not answer the nurse's questions.
- ○ **4.** The child does not cry when she is being moved.

56. A hospitalized toddler, age 2 ½, has not tried to feed himself. The primary nurse notes a poor nutritional intake. To increase the child's food intake, the nurse should attempt all of the following measures *except:*
- ○ **1.** giving the child finger foods.
- ○ **2.** setting the child in a high chair for meals.
- ○ **3.** providing nutritious snacks between meals.
- ○ **4.** keeping a 6-oz bottle of milk in the crib between feedings.

57. During a team meeting to discuss a pediatric client suspected of having been abused, a nursing assistant says, "We shouldn't let that child's parents visit her at all. After all, they put her here in the first place!" The nurse's response to the assistant should be based on which understanding about abusive parents?
- ○ **1.** They should not visit their child in the hospital.
- ○ **2.** They should not visit until the child is ready for discharge.
- ○ **3.** They should visit on a limited schedule set up by the health team and should be supervised during all visits.
- ○ **4.** They should be encouraged to visit frequently and should be welcomed by the staff.

58. During a visit to the pediatric out-patient clinic, a mother says her 3-year-old son has not yet received any "shots." The nurse's response should be based on which understanding?
- ○ **1.** The child will need double the number of immunizations now because he is no longer an infant.
- ○ **2.** Immunizations can safely be delayed until the child enters nursery school.
- ○ **3.** At his age, immunizations are contraindicated.
- ○ **4.** Up to age 6, the same immunizations are given.

59. In a client with a spinal cord injury, which clinical finding would indicate spinal shock?
- ○ **1.** Loss of sweating.
- ○ **2.** Urinary incontinence.
- ○ **3.** Hypertension.
- ○ **4.** Muscle spasticity.

60. A client with a spinal cord injury has autonomic dysreflexia. Which action should the nurse take *first*?
- ○ **1.** Call the physician.
- ○ **2.** Place the client in reverse Trendelenburg's position.
- ○ **3.** Administer a sedative on a standing order.
- ○ **4.** Check the client for a fecal impaction.

STOP. THIS IS THE END OF THE PRETEST.

Answers and rationales

In the pretest answers below, the question number appears in boldface type, followed by the number of the correct answer. Rationales for correct answers and, where appropriate, for incorrect options follow. To help you evaluate your knowledge base and application of nursing behaviors, each question is classified as follows:
NP = Phase of the nursing process
CN = Client need

1. Correct answer—4
Clients with angina commonly are taught to take a nitroglycerin tablet before intercourse to prevent anginal pain caused by an increased cardiac workload. Nitroglycerin dilates the coronary arteries, increasing circulation to the myocardium.
NP: Implementing
CN: Physiologic integrity

2. Correct answer—2
The nurse should advise the client to limit intake of eggs, which are high in cholesterol. The other foods would be recommended on this client's diet.
NP: Implementing
CN: Physiologic integrity

3. Correct answer—2
The most appropriate response would be to acknowledge the client's feelings and offer support. Options 1 and 3 slight the client's feelings. Option 4 is unrealistic; a client experiencing high anxiety would have trouble giving a specific response.
NP: Implementing
CN: Psychosocial integrity

4. Correct answer—1
A client can best deal with a phobia by gaining a sense of control over the feared object. People do not consciously use phobias. Instilling a sense of fearlessness is an unrealistic expectation. People experience high anxiety, not acute psychosis, when forced into fearful situations.
NP: Implementing
CN: Psychosocial integrity

5. Correct answer—4
Encouraging the client to discuss feelings would help the nurse elicit more information. Giving advice (op-

tions 1 and 2) or false reassurance (option 3) would be inappropriate.
NP: Implementing
CN: Psychosocial integrity

6. Correct answer—4
Allowing the client to select the activity would give her some control over the situation. Because clients with eating disorders struggle with issues of control, they can benefit when given the chance to have input in their treatment program. Options 1 and 2 would put the client on the defensive. Option 3 would take control away from her.
NP: Implementing
CN: Psychosocial integrity

7. Correct answer—4
Diethylstilbestrol, an estrogen, causes feminizing side effects. Therefore, the client probably will experience gynecomastia and a high-pitched voice.
NP: Implementing
CN: Physiologic integrity

8. Correct answer—4
Ignoring the child's outburst (while reducing external stimulation and removing objects that could cause injury) is the most appropriate management technique. During a tantrum, an upset toddler is incapable of dealing with reason or threats (options 1 and 2). The tantrum results from loss of control; spanking the child (option 3) would increase insecurity, which already is present.
NP: Implementing
CN: Health promotion and maintenance

9. Correct answer—3
Using Nagele's rule (the most common method for estimating the date of confinement), the nurse would take the first day of the last normal menstrual period (June 30), subtract 3 months (March 30), and add 7 days (April 6).
NP: Analyzing
CN: Health promotion and maintenance

10. Correct answer—4
Human chorionic gonadotropin is produced by the trophoblastic tissue of the placenta and secreted into the urine and serum of a pregnant woman shortly after the onset of pregnancy. Luteinizing hormone (option 1) and follicle-stimulating hormone (option 2) are anterior pituitary hormones necessary for developing and releasing the mature ovum and for synthesizing estrogen and progesterone. Human chorionic

somatomammotropin (option 3) is a placental hormone that acts similarly to the pituitary growth hormone. It produces a diabetogenic effect in pregnant women and is not diagnostic of pregnancy.
NP: Analyzing
CN: Health promotion and maintenance

11. Correct answer—3
Chadwick's sign, a bluish discoloration of the vaginal vault, occurs from increased vascularity and would be evident by the time a client had missed two menstrual periods. Diastasis recti (option 1) occurs late in pregnancy. The glomerular filtration rate (option 2) increases by approximately 50%. Blood volume (option 4) peaks at 30% to 50% above normal during the second trimester.
NP: Assessing
CN: Health promotion and maintenance

12. Correct answer—1
A nutritionally sound lunch includes two servings of a grain and one serving each of fruit, vegetable, and milk or a milk product. The cheeseburger, salad, fruit, and milk contain sufficient protein, minerals, and vitamins to meet the pregnant client's nutritional needs. The other options are nutritionally inadequate. Additionally, options 2 and 3 are high in sodium.
NP: Evaluating
CN: Health promotion and maintenance

13. Correct answer—4
Because moderate exercise is encouraged during pregnancy, the best approach is to assess the amount and type of exercise in which the client currently engages. Options 1, 2, and 3 do not provide for assessment of the client's individual needs, nor do they explore possible client concerns.
NP: Planning
CN: Health promotion and maintenance

14. Correct answer—4
The client should be told to take ferrous sulfate between meals with orange juice. Food and antacids inhibit absorption of iron.
NP: Implementing
CN: Physiologic integrity

15. Correct answer—4
Hemoglobin and hematocrit levels may decline slightly from hemodilution, resulting in the pseudoanemia of pregnancy. This is most noticeable during the second and third trimesters. In true anemia (option 1), caused by inadequate iron intake, hemoglobin and hematocrit levels are lower than the values given. The given laboratory values do not indicate preeclampsia (option 2). During pregnancy, the renal threshold decreases, allowing glucose to spill into the urine. Lactosuria also may occur as the breasts prepare for lactation. Thus, a small amount of glucose in a pregnant woman's urine is not unusual and does not indicate diabetes (option 3), although it should be reported.
NP: Analyzing
CN: Health promotion and maintenance

16. Correct answer—4
Potential side effects of antihypertensive agents include postural hypotension, impotence, nausea, vomiting, and nasal stuffiness. Of these, postural hypotension is the most hazardous because the client could fall and suffer a serious injury.
NP: Implementing
CN: Physiologic integrity

17. Correct answer—1
Control of the head before the trunk and extremities is best described as cephalocaudal, or development from head to tail.
NP: Assessing
CN: Health promotion and maintenance

18. Correct answer—1
Glucocorticoid therapy will have caused the client's adrenal glands to have atrophied. If the client suddenly stops this therapy, acute adrenal insufficiency (Addison's crisis) may occur.
NP: Planning
CN: Physiologic integrity

19. Correct answer—2
This response gives the client direction and support. Option 1 is incorrect because of the client's depression—the client does not care if it is a beautiful day. Saying "let's" (option 3) implies fusing between client and nurse. Option 4 offers no support.
NP: Implementing
CN: Psychosocial integrity

20. Correct answer—1
A depressed client may find it difficult to do even the simplest things, such as combing the hair, and may need direction and support in performing these tasks. Options 2 and 3 ignore the fact that the client's personal grooming has not been performed. Option 4 is wrong because the client may not notice that his shirt is unbuttoned; this offers no help with personal grooming needs.

NP: Implementing
CN: Psychosocial integrity

21. Correct answer—3
This remark not only indicates the client's seriousness about suicide but also reveals a specific plan. Options 1, 2, and 4 do not include a specific plan.
NP: Analyzing
CN: Psychosocial integrity

22. Correct answer—2
By telling the client that the nurse found the pills and then asking about the client's intentions, the nurse provides for the client's safety needs and directly addresses the issue of suicide with the client. The other options only remove a source of danger; they do not directly address the issue of suicide with the client.
NP: Implementing
CN: Safe, effective care environment

23. Correct answer—4
Weights on a traction apparatus should hang freely and unobstructed. Option 1 is incorrect because the head of the bed should be elevated no more than 30 degrees. Option 2 is incorrect because the affected heel should be raised off the bed. Option 3 is incorrect because the weights should not be removed from traction.
NP: Planning
CN: Physiologic integrity

24. Correct answer—1
Increased urine output indicates greater cardiac output. The pulse rate decreases as digoxin (Lanoxin) slows the rate of conduction through the heart. Digoxin would not significantly alter blood pressure or respirations.
NP: Evaluating
CN: Physiologic integrity

25. Correct answer—4
Changes in appetite, respiratory rate, and urine output may indicate improvement in the client's condition or may occur as side effects of the medication. Intention tremor, a symptom of multiple sclerosis, is irrelevant to the client's condition.
NP: Planning
CN: Physiologic integrity

26. Correct answer—4
Anorexia and gastric irritation are early—and sometimes overlooked—signs of digoxin toxicity. A client

who dislikes hospital food (option 1) would say so. Oxygen administration and furosemide (Lasix) therapy (options 2 and 3) do not cause anorexia.
NP: Analyzing
CN: Physiologic integrity

27. Correct answer—1
A snack with intermediate-acting sugars (such as lactose in milk) ensures adequate blood glucose levels during the expected peak action of NPH insulin taken in the morning. Increasing the morning NPH insulin dosage (option 3) increases the risk for a hypoglycemic reaction. Options 2 and 4 discourage the mother from promoting a normal life for her diabetic child.
NP: Implementing
CN: Physiologic integrity

28. Correct answer—4
A client who is receiving chlorothiazide (Diuril) should be instructed to increase potassium intake, because thiazide diuretics cause potassium and sodium excretion during diuresis. Dried fruits are the only high-potassium item among the options listed.
NP: Implementing
CN: Physiologic integrity

29. Correct answer—1
Removal of axillary lymph nodes places the postmastectomy client at increased risk for infection for the rest of her life. All mastectomy clients are taught to prevent injury, to avoid blood pressure checks and venipunctures on the arm on the side of surgery, and to seek prompt treatment if a problem results.
NP: Analyzing
CN: Physiologic integrity

30. Correct answer—2
The primary goal should be to prevent bleeding. A platelet count below 50,000/mm^3 indicates a severe platelet deficiency. The client is at great risk for bleeding and probably requires a platelet transfusion. The other laboratory values are only slightly below normal and do not place the client at great risk.
NP: Analyzing
CN: Physiologic integrity

31. Correct answer—1
A positive reaction indicates a person has been exposed to tuberculosis in the past. Although this person may be at increased risk for developing active tuberculosis, a positive skin test does not indicate active tuberculosis.

NP: Analyzing
CN: Physiologic integrity

32. Correct answer—4
Asking the client to discuss how she feels about her pregnancy enables the nurse to elicit more information and provides an opportunity to explore all possible alternatives before any decision is made. Options 1 and 2 evade the issue. Option 3 puts the nurse in charge; the client may feel coerced into making a decision to please the nurse.
NP: Implementing
CN: Psychosocial integrity

33. Correct answer—2
The best room for this client is a private room two doors away from the nurses' station. With bacterial meningitis, he should be in isolation for at least the first 24 hours after admission. In addition, during the initial acute phase, he should be as close as possible to the nurses' station for maximum observation.
NP: Planning
CN: Safe, effective care environment

34. Correct answer—1
The child's developmental needs would best be met by having his mother room in with him. At 15 months, he is at maximum risk for experiencing separation anxiety.
NP: Implementing
CN: Health promotion and maintenance

35. Correct answer—3
His mother shows full understanding of discharge teaching when she repeats the specific signs to watch for. Pulling on the ears, refusing to lie down, and shaking the head back and forth are common signs of otitis in toddlers. If they occur, the child should be checked promptly by a physician. Option 1 expresses guilt. Option 2 indicates only understanding of the need for follow-up care. Option 4 does not indicate a realistic understanding of the condition.
NP: Evaluating
CN: Health promotion and maintenance

36. Correct answer—2
In conductive deafness, the acoustic nerve is not damaged. Although air conduction of sound waves is impaired, bone conduction is not. Otosclerosis can cause conductive deafness.
NP: Evaluating
CN: Physiologic integrity

37. Correct answer—4
During stapedectomy, the diseased stapes is removed from the oval window and replaced with a prosthesis. Fluctuation in hearing results from closure of the oval window caused by trauma or separation of the prosthesis.
NP: Analyzing
CN: Physiologic integrity

38. Correct answer—4
Stump elevation increases venous return and decreases edema. Abduction and external rotation should be avoided.
NP: Evaluating
CN: Physiologic integrity

39. Correct answer—4
Hemorrhage is the most common complication after an amputation. Thus, a tourniquet should be kept at the bedside in case of hemorrhage.
NP: Planning
CN: Physiologic integrity

40. Correct answer—2
Wrapping the bandage from the stump to the groin will aid venous return and help shape the stump into a cone. Options 1, 3, and 4 encourage either venous stasis or engorgement and should be avoided.
NP: Implementing
CN: Physiologic integrity

41. Correct answer—3
If the client doesn't spend some time each day in the prone position, which extends the stump, a flexion contracture may develop.
NP: Analyzing
CN: Physiologic integrity

42. Correct answer—3
To learn to cope with the phantom pain, the client first needs to understand the reasons for the pain.
NP: Implementing
CN: Physiologic integrity

43. Correct answer—2
The most therapeutic response would be to focus the client's thoughts on the present. Option 1 diminishes the client's feelings by giving the impression that everyone feels this way. Option 3 refutes the client's feelings and calls attention to something the client currently doesn't believe. Option 4 does not address the client's present needs.
NP: Implementing
CN: Psychosocial integrity

44. Correct answer—3
Making a collage is easy and does not require great concentration. Options 1 and 2 call for the client to make a decision, and option 4 demands that she concentrate carefully, both of which would be difficult in her depressed state.
NP: Implementing
CN: Psychosocial integrity

45. Correct answer—3
Maintaining interest encourages the client to discuss his feelings further. Options 1 and 2 minimize or ignore his feelings. Option 4 implies that he needs to work off his anger without talking about it.
NP: Implementing
CN: Psychosocial integrity

46. Correct answer—4
Confusion occurs when the brain is deprived of needed glucose, and diaphoresis results from the developing shocklike state. Nausea, vomiting, flushed skin, air hunger, and acetone breath are signs and symptoms of ketoacidosis.
NP: Analyzing
CN: Physiologic integrity

47. Correct answer—2
The nurse should administer an I.V. bolus of 50% glucose to a hospitalized client who is having a hypoglycemic reaction and cannot swallow. Glucagon, a substance produced by the pancreas to increase the blood glucose level, could be administered intramuscularly by a caregiver at home if the client cannot swallow but remains conscious. Epinephrine, an adrenergic agent, would stimulate the pancreas to increase insulin in the blood, further decreasing the blood glucose level.
NP: Implementing
CN: Physiologic integrity

48. Correct answer—1
Bowel sounds are absent in peritonitis. Abdominal distention and pain are classic signs of peritonitis; constipation also may occur.
NP: Assessing
CN: Physiologic integrity

49. Correct answer—1
Turning the client will aid suctioning. For the nasogastric tube to be effective, the blue opening should remain open and clear of solution or secretions. Drainage is measured every 8 hours, and suction should not be increased without an order.

NP: Planning
CN: Physiologic integrity

50. Correct answer—2
Tracheoesophageal fistula (TEF) does not cause bile-stained vomitus. In the most common type of TEF, the distal esophagus is attached to the trachea and cannot receive food or fluid; therefore, vomiting should not occur. Abdominal distention (option 1) is significant with the most common type of TEF. Coughing, choking, cyanosis, and drooling (options 3 and 4) are classic signs of TEF.
NP: Assessing
CN: Physiologic integrity

51. Correct answer—3
After the gastrostomy tube feeding, the nurse should elevate the tube and leave it unplugged to allow reflux of stomach contents through the tube instead of through the newly repaired esophagus. The gastrostomy tube is kept in place in the stomach with an inflated bulb at the end of the catheter. The newborn should be placed on the right side, with the head of the bed slightly elevated, to provide for gravity drainage. The gastrostomy tube should not be plugged after feeding because gastric reflux may occur over the fresh operative site or be aspirated.
NP: Implementing
CN: Physiologic integrity

52. Correct answer—1
The red blood cell count increases to help carry hemoglobin to offset chronic hypoxia, which is common in clients with chronic obstructive pulmonary disease.
NP: Assessing
CN: Physiologic integrity

53. Correct answer—1
Of all traction types, skin traction is easiest to apply because no pins are inserted into bones. Specially prepared nurses can apply skin traction but not skeletal traction.
NP: Implementing
CN: Physiologic integrity

54. Correct answer—3
Common gastrointestinal side effects of ibuprofen (Motrin) include anorexia, nausea, and diarrhea.
NP: Evaluating
CN: Physiologic integrity

55. Correct answer—4
The behavior that most strongly suggests child abuse is not crying when moved. A victim of child abuse typically does not complain of pain, even with obvious injuries, for fear of further displeasing the abuser.
NP: Assessing
CN: Safe, effective care environment

56. Correct answer—4
The only technique the nurse should not try is leaving a bottle in the crib. At age 2 , the child should not need or get a bottle. The child is capable of drinking from a cup and should be encouraged to do so. Toddlers left with bottles in their cribs may develop nursing bottle syndrome.
NP: Planning
CN: Health promotion and maintenance

57. Correct answer—4
The nurse working with abusive families needs to understand that abusive parents should be encouraged to visit their child and should be welcomed to the unit by the staff. Many abusive parents love their children but lack effective parenting skills. During the child's hospitalization, the staff has the opportunity to model appropriate parenting behaviors for the parents.
NP: Analyzing
CN: Health promotion and maintenance

58. Correct answer—4
According to the recommended schedule of immunizations from the American Academy of Pediatrics, the same immunizations are given up to age 6.
NP: Analyzing
CN: Health promotion and maintenance

59. Correct answer—1
Loss of sweating occurs below the level of the cord lesion. Spinal shock also causes urine retention, a marked reduction in blood pressure, and motor paralysis.
NP: Assessing
CN: Physiologic integrity

60. Correct answer—4
Autonomic dysreflexia can be caused by a full bowel or bladder or by a urinary infection. Removing the cause of the dysreflexia will relieve symptoms.
NP: Implementing
CN: Physiologic integrity

Analyzing the pretest

Total the number of incorrect responses on the pretest. A score of 1 to 10 indicates that you have an excellent knowledge base; 11 to 15, good; 16 to 20, fair. If your incorrect responses total 21 or more, you'll need intensive study; a review course is recommended.

For a more detailed analysis of your performance, complete the *Pretest self-diagnostic profile* worksheet on page 17. First, in the top row of boxes next to "QUESTION NUMBER," record the number of each question you answered incorrectly. Then, beneath each question number, check the box that corresponds to the reason you answered incorrectly, along with the category of client need and nursing process for that question. Finally, tabulate the number of check marks on each line in the right-hand column marked "TOTALS." This will provide an individualized profile of weak areas that you should study further before taking NCLEX-RN.

Pretest self-diagnostic profile

QUESTION NUMBER																								TOTALS
Test-taking skills																								
1. Misread question																								
2. Missed important point																								
3. Forgot fact or concept																								
4. Applied wrong fact or concept																								
5. Drew wrong conclusion																								
6. Incorrectly evaluated distractors																								
7. Mistakenly indicated wrong answer																								
8. Read into question																								
9. Guessed wrong																								
10. Misunderstood question																								
Client need																								
1. Safe, effective care environment																								
2. Physiologic integrity																								
3. Psychosocial integrity																								
4. Health promotion and maintenance																								
Nursing process																								
1. Assessing																								
2. Analyzing																								
3. Planning																								
4. Implementing																								
5. Evaluating																								

Part II

Taking NCLEX-RN

Taking NCLEX-RN

Introduction

Anyone who wants to practice as a registered nurse in the United States must be licensed by the nursing licensure authority in the state or territory in which he or she intends to practice. To obtain this license, one must pass the National Council Licensure Examination for Registered Nurses (NCLEX-RN).

Your success on NCLEX-RN depends on your nursing knowledge base, your study program for the test, and your confidence level. If you plan to take the exam in the United States, you also must understand the computerized adaptive testing (CAT) method. (In Canada, NCLEX-RN still is being given by the paper-and-pencil method. See *Taking NCLEX-RN in Canada*.)

Understandably, you may feel anxious about taking the exam on a computer, especially if you haven't had much practice with one. This chapter provides helpful information about the test, acquaints you with the new computerized format, and offers effective strategies for passing NCLEX-RN.

To become even better acquainted with taking a computerized exam and to obtain additional experience with NCLEX-RN questions, be sure to take the two tests on the computer disk included with this book. The tests use the same keyboard functions and screen layout as those used on the actual exam, and they offer 150 new questions not found in the book.

Taking NCLEX-RN in Canada

If you plan to take NCLEX-RN in Canada, be aware that the Canadian exam is still given the traditional way—by paper and pencil. Does this mean your test-taking strategies will differ from those of U.S. examinees, who now take NCLEX-RN by computer? Yes and no.

Like all NCLEX-RN candidates, you'll need to be thoroughly prepared—intellectually, emotionally, and physically. But unlike U.S. examinees, you can change an answer or return to a question later if you develop a mental block or forget the nursing knowledge or principle.

Your test is timed. Pace yourself accordingly, using your wristwatch. Allot an average of 1 minute to answer each question. Some questions will take only a few seconds to read and answer; others will take longer.

Be sure to use all the allotted time. Don't be distracted by examinees around you who finish the test and leave the room ahead of you. Remember, finishing early does *not* mean the questions were answered correctly.

If you have time remaining at the end of the test, go back and reexamine any unanswered questions. If you really can't decide on a response, read the stem and then the first answer option; repeat this process with each remaining option. This allows you to evaluate each option specifically by formulating a complete statement from the stem and the options. If you still can't decide which answer option is best, make an educated guess from the two most likely choices. You will not lose points for guessing.

If you decide to change an answer, be sure to erase carefully, because the test will be scored with an electronic scanning machine that can't determine the intended answer when erasures show.

Registration, test sites, and schedules

Once you have met all eligibility requirements to be a professional nurse, you must apply to take NCLEX-RN through your state board of nursing. Shortly after your application is approved, you will receive an "Authorization to Test" from the Educational Testing Service (ETS) Data Center, which will instruct you to make an appointment to take the exam at a Sylvan Technology Center of your choosing. There are more than 200 of these centers throughout the United States, with at least one in each state or territory. Each center has up to 10 computer terminals available for candidates. A proctor will help you get started and will monitor security during the test.

The computerized NCLEX-RN, which lasts a maximum of 5 hours, is offered 15 hours every day, Monday through Saturday, throughout the year (on Sundays by special arrangement). Make sure you are thoroughly prepared by the time you call to schedule an exam date—you will take the test no later than 30 days from the day you call to schedule. If you wish to schedule a retest after previously failing the exam, your test date will be within 45 days of your call. You may reschedule your appointment, without charge, by telephoning the test center at least 3 days before your test date.

Computerized adaptive testing

Since 1994, the NCLEX-RN has been a computerized test in which a candidate must answer enough questions of varying levels of difficulty to demonstrate minimum competence as an entry-level nurse. The computerized adaptive test (CAT) differs from the standard paper-and-pencil test in other ways as well. The most obvious difference is that instead of sitting at a table with a test book and a pencil, you will sit in front of a computer terminal, interacting with it as you take the exam.

The adaptive test chooses test items based on your response to the previous question; the computer will "adapt" to your answers, correct or incorrect, by selecting harder or easier items for the next question. For example, at the start of the exam, a question of medium-level difficulty may appear on the screen. If you answer this question correctly, the computer then will ask a more difficult question; if you answer incorrectly, the computer will ask an easier question.

The test bank contains thousands of questions, each categorized according to the NCLEX-RN test plan and assigned a level of difficulty using a complex statistical formula. Every time you answer a question, the computer will search the test bank for the next appropriate question based on the difficulty level of the previous question and the accuracy of your response. This process continues until the computer can determine your competence in all areas of the test plan. Because each test is individualized, the number of questions can range from 75 to 265 (15 of these will be practice questions).

Viewing questions on the computer screen

These illustrations show the two types of questions you will see on the computer screen when taking the computerized NCLEX-RN. The left illustration shows a stand-alone question (one with no case study). The right illustration shows a question that includes a case study.

Which of these behaviors most strongly indicates that a client who has recently delivered a baby is bonding with her newborn?

A. She changes the baby's diaper when wet.
B. She holds the baby close during and after breast-feeding.
C. She gives the baby her mother's name.
D. She is always talking to her friends about the baby.

A 64-year-old client is admitted to the medical unit with a myocardial infarction. A stat dose of morphine SO_4 10 mg was given for chest pain. Orders include bed rest, morphine SO_4 for pain, and oxygen by nasal cannula.

Besides controlling pain, which of these goals should take priority in planning the client's care at the time of admission?

A. Minimize energy expenditure.
B. Increase urine output.
C. Decrease cholesterol level.
D. Teach about the disease.

The computerized test begins with brief instructions on using the computer and then provides a short practice session. Previous computer experience is *not* necessary. You will use only two keys on the keyboard: the *space bar* and the *enter key*. All other keys will be inoperable. You will use the space bar to move the cursor among four possible options; you will press the enter key to select your answer. To make sure you don't select an answer unintentionally, the computer will ask you to confirm your choice by pressing the enter key a second time.

One question at a time will appear on the computer screen. Some questions are stand-alone items; others are based on brief case studies, which will appear to the left of the question. (See *Viewing questions on the computer screen*.)

After carefully reading the question, press the space bar to move among the four possible answer options. Analyze each option, and then select the one that best answers the question. Press the enter key twice to record your choice. You must answer every question until the test ends; unlike the paper-and-pencil testing method, the computer will not let you skip an item or go back to a previous question. The test will end when the computer has determined your competence level in all test areas. The test center will transmit your results electronically to the Educational Testing Service. Your state board of nursing will notify you of the results in 4 to 6 weeks. No test results will be released over the telephone.

NCLEX-RN test categories

Each NCLEX-RN test question is coded by one nursing process and one client needs category, as described below.

NURSING PROCESS

Assessment
Establishing a data base (20% of test).

Analysis (or Diagnosis)
Identifying actual or potential health care needs and problems (establishing nursing diagnoses) on the basis of assessment (20%).

Planning
Setting goals to meet client needs and designing strategies to achieve those goals (20%).

Implementation
Initiating and completing actions necessary to accomplish the defined goals (20%).

Evaluation
Determining the extent of success in achieving health care goals (20%).

CLIENT NEEDS
• Safe, effective care environment: 15% to 21%
• Physiologic integrity: 46% to 54%
• Psychosocial integrity: 8% to 16%
• Health promotion and maintenance: 17% to 23%

NCLEX-RN test plan

All questions on the computerized NCLEX-RN adhere to a test plan, or blueprint, that organizes questions according to various test categories (see *NCLEX-RN test categories*). The two major components of the test plan are the *nursing process* (consisting of five steps) and *client needs* (consisting of four categories). Each test question relates to one nursing process step and one client need category.

Nursing process

The nursing process is a scientific method of applying nursing principles to client care. Each of the five steps of the nursing process carries equal weight on the test. Specific nursing actions for each step are listed on pages 24 and 25.

1. Assessment: Gathering subjective and objective information about a client
• Collect information by reading hospital records and by observing verbal and nonverbal interactions among the client, family, friends, hospital staff, and other reliable sources.
• Examine common data sources for information.
• Recognize symptoms and findings.
• Assess the client's ability to perform activities of daily living.
• Assess the client's environment.
• Assess the nurse's reaction to the client.
• Confirm all observations and perceptions by gathering additional data.
• Monitor the client personally rather than rely solely on machines.
• Challenge orders and decisions by health team members, as appropriate.
• Communicate information gathered to other team members.

2. Analysis (Nursing Diagnosis): Identifying real or potential risks for health care needs and problems based on assessment findings
• Organize, interpret, and validate assessment data.
• Gather additional data when necessary.
• Identify and communicate nursing diagnoses to the health care team.
• Determine the client's needs and the staff's ability to meet them.

3. Planning: Establishing goals to meet client needs
• Include the client, family, friends, and other health team members in setting goals.
• Mutually establish goal priorities.
• Anticipate the client's needs.
• Involve the client, family, friends, and other health team members in developing care strategies.
• Document all information needed to manage the client's needs.
• Plan for the client's comfort and the maintenance of optimum functioning.
• Select the best nursing measures to deliver effective care.
• Identify community resources to assist the client and family.
• Coordinate the client's care with other providers.
• Delegate care responsibilities to other providers.
• Formulate outcomes of nursing interventions.

4. Implementation: Carrying out actions that accomplish established goals
• Organize and manage the client's care.
• Perform or aid the client in performing activities of daily living.
• Provide comfort to the client.
• Help the client maintain optimum functioning.
• Teach the client and family.
• Apply proper technique in giving client care.
• Initiate lifesaving measures in life-threatening emergencies.
• Provide care that enables the client to achieve self-care and optimum independence.
• Supervise and validate the activities of other health team members.
• Record all appropriate information, orally and in written reports.

5. Evaluation: Measuring the success of goal achievement
• Compare actual outcomes with expected outcomes.
• Evaluate client compliance with prescribed therapy.
• Record the client's response to care.
• Change the plan of care and reorder priorities as needed.

Client needs

The client's health needs constitute the second major part of the NCLEX-RN test plan. The four categories of client needs (listed below) are established from analysis of a large-scale nursing job survey conducted every 3 years.

1. Safe, effective care environment: The nurse meets the client's needs while promoting environmental safety and providing coordinated and goal-oriented care, quality assurance, and safe and effective treatments and procedures.

2. Physiologic integrity: The nurse meets the physiologic needs of the client with a potentially life-threatening or chronically recurring condition, and of the client at risk for development of complications or untoward effects of treatments, by providing basic care, by reducing risk potential, and by promoting physiologic adaptation and comfort.

3. Psychosocial integrity: In stress-related or crisis-related situations, the nurse meets the client's needs for psychosocial integrity throughout the life cycle by promoting coping skills and psychosocial adaptation.

4. Health promotion and maintenance: The nurse meets the client's needs throughout the life cycle by promoting continued growth and development, self-care, integrity of support systems, and prevention and early treatment of disease.

Preparing for the examination

To prepare for the exam, you must study thoroughly, plan carefully, and master test-taking strategies. The following tips can help ensure your success on NCLEX-RN.

Study thoroughly
• Become well versed in all topics that the exam is likely to cover, and answer as many practice questions as you can. After answering the questions in each clinical area of this book, take the sample tests in Part VI, which will ensure that you've been exposed to all areas of the test plan.
• Complete the self-evaluation form after the sample tests to help you determine why you may have answered a question incorrectly. This analysis will enable you to pinpoint topics that may require further study.
• Become familiar with all parts of a test question (see *Parts of a test question,* page 26).
• Take a review course or organize a study group with others planning to take the exam.
• Ask a nursing instructor or colleague for help or clarification if you encounter material that is unfamiliar or difficult to understand.

Parts of a test question

Multiple-choice test questions on the examination are constructed according to strict psychometric standards. As shown below, each question has a stem, four options, a key (correct answer), and three distractors (incorrect answers). A brief clinical situation, or case study, often precedes the question.

Stem ——————— 1. A 55-year-old client is taking digoxin and furosemide. Which of the following foods should you instruct him to include in his daily diet?

Options ———————
○ tomato juice ——————————— Key (Correct answer)
○ low-fat yogurt ——————————— Distractor
○ dried fruit ——————————— Distractor
○ organ meats ——————————— Distractor

Plan carefully
• Schedule your examination at a test site near your residence, if possible, so you can familiarize yourself with parking facilities and travel time before the test date.
• If you must travel far and stay overnight, make hotel arrangements well before the test date to make sure you have a convenient place to stay.
• Schedule your examination for the time of day when your performance peaks. Some people work best in the early morning; others, in the late afternoon or early evening.
• Get a good night's sleep the night before the test. Staying up late for last-minute cramming probably will hurt rather than help your performance.
• Eat a nutritious breakfast on the day of the test.
• Wear layered clothing so you can easily adapt to the room temperature at the test center.
• Keep your admission ticket and identification where you can easily retrieve them when you leave for the test site. You must present your "Authorization to Test" from the ETS Data Center, along with two forms of identification with your signature, including one photo ID. Without them, you will not be permitted to take the test.
• Try to avoid last-minute anxiety that could sap your energy or disturb your concentration. Although mild anxiety is normal and can heighten your awareness, too much anxiety can impair your performance. If test anxiety has been a problem in the past, practice relaxation techniques (such as guided imagery) as you study, and be ready to use them during the actual test.

Apply test-taking strategies
• Read case studies carefully. They contain information you will need to answer the question correctly.
• Pay special attention to such words as *best, most, first,* and *not* when reading the question (stem). These words, which may be italicized, capitalized, or otherwise highlighted in some way, usually provide clues to the correct response. For example, consider the question, "What should the nurse do *first?*" All of the listed options may be appropriate nursing actions for the given circumstances, but only *one* action can take top priority.

• Try to predict the correct answer as you read the stem. If your predicted answer is among the four options, it is probably the correct response.

• Read each question and all options carefully before making your selection.

• If two options seem equally correct, reread them; they must differ in some way. Also reread the stem. You may notice something you missed before that will aid your selection. If you still are unsure, make an educated guess. The computer will not let you skip a question.

• Remain calm if a question focuses on an unfamiliar topic. Try to recall clients who have had problems similar to those in the question. Determine the nursing principles involved in your clients' care and how they may apply to the test question. This may help you eliminate some options and increase your chances of choosing the right answer.

• Take the necessary time for each question without spending excessive time on any one item. You will have up to 5 hours to take the test. Pace yourself accordingly.

• Pay no attention to other candidates or the time they need to complete their tests. Because each test is individualized, some tests contain more questions than others.

• Take advantage of breaks during the test to give your mind and body a needed rest. The first mandatory break is given after 2 hours of testing and lasts 10 minutes. Candidates may take an optional break 90 minutes after testing resumes. If you tend to get hungry, bring a small snack with you to eat during the breaks. Do some stretching exercises, too, during breaks to help you relax.

Developing and following an organized study plan will provide the best assurance that you are fully prepared to succeed on the NCLEX-RN. Approach the test with confidence. Good luck, and congratulations on choosing nursing as a career.

Part III

Fundamental nursing concepts and skills

Fundamental nursing concepts and skills

Introduction

Nursing has evolved from a task-oriented occupation to a recognized professional discipline with its own theories and concepts of health care. Applying these theories and concepts to the biological and social sciences is the hallmark of current professional nursing practice. Part III reviews fundamental nursing concepts and skills common to the care of all clients, incorporating essential scientific principles that beginning nurses are expected to know when they take the NCLEX-RN.

The first group of entries focuses on nursing concepts essential to effective nursing practice. "The nursing process" reviews the foundation of modern nursing—assessment, diagnosis, planning, implementation, and evaluation. "Nursing diagnosis: A critical part of the nursing process" takes a closer look at how the nurse's diagnostic skills play such a crucial role in planning, implementing, and evaluating client care. "Leadership and management" uses role theory as a springboard for discussing the manager-worker relationship and the characteristics and skills that each can contribute to ensure group effectiveness—a noteworthy topic for nurses at every level. "Legal principles and nursing practice" examines origins and types of law, the nurse's legal responsibilities in various situations, and important client rights, such as informed consent, privacy, and the right to refuse treatment. "Therapeutic communication" reveals how the nurse can enhance the client's self-esteem and ability to function by effectively using verbal and nonverbal communication. "Growth and development" explores human psychosocial, cognitive, physical-motor, and social behavior patterns throughout the life span. "Nutrition" offers a review of food selection guidelines, human energy requirements, and essential vitamins, minerals, and other nutrients. "Family: The primary unit of health care" examines both traditional and contemporary concepts of *family*, highlighting its characteristics, functions, and developmental tasks and stages. "Rehabilitation" explores factors, goals, treatments, aids, and the client's psychological responses. "Grieving" reviews the major phases of grieving and describes nursing interventions to help the client cope with an impending death or a significant loss. The last four entries in this group review principles of gerontologic nursing, case management, home health care, and infection control.

The second collection of entries emphasizes basic nursing skills needed to provide quality care for clients in any setting. "Physical assessment" covers the essential client data all nurses must record when taking a health history and performing a physical examination. "Blood transfusion" reviews measures the nurse must take to promote the client's safety and prevent complications. "Arrhythmia interpretation" presents information the nurse needs in order to recognize life-threatening arrhythmias. "Cardiopulmonary resuscitation" outlines what the nurse should do when an unresponsive client requires immediate life support. "Anticipatory guidance" reveals the essentials of client teaching. Finally, "Discharge planning" examines the numerous ways in which the nurse can help ensure continuity of client care.

NURSING CONCEPTS

The nursing process

Introduction

The nursing process—a scientific, systematic method of problem solving--forms the organizing framework for effective nursing practice. Using the nursing process in an ongoing, dynamic, and interactive manner with the client assures the client of a scientific approach to, and continuous monitoring of, all the nursing care received (see *Steps of the nursing process*).

The following five steps make up the nursing process.

Assessment

This initial phase of the nursing process involves collecting data and establishing a comprehensive data base. The nurse records subjective and objective data, including diagnostic test results.

Identification of a nursing diagnosis

The next step in the nursing process begins with data analysis, which leads to identifying specific client needs and establishing nursing diagnoses according to a prescribed format and nomenclature. For a more detailed review of nursing diagnoses, see the next entry, "Nursing diagnosis: A critical part of the nursing process." Additionally, refer to Appendix 3, which contains the most current list of nursing diagnoses approved by the North American Nursing Diagnosis Association (NANDA).

Planning and goal setting

After analyzing data and establishing nursing diagnoses, the nurse plans how to solve client problems according to their priority, identifying goals or client outcomes to measure the effectiveness of nursing actions. Goal setting ideally is a mutual activity performed by the nurse and the client.

Steps of the nursing process

The nurse proceeds through the five steps of the nursing process, moving from assessment to evaluation. Depending on the evaluation findings, the nurse may update or change any of the previous steps.

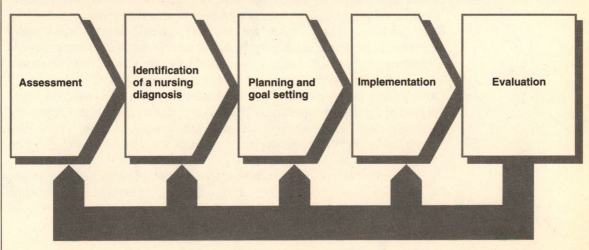

Assessment → Identification of a nursing diagnosis → Planning and goal setting → Implementation → Evaluation

Implementation

This fourth phase involves nursing actions based on the plans that have been established to achieve the desired client outcomes. Implementation includes everything a nurse does to meet client needs, such as health teaching, administering treatments and medications, providing support and comfort to the client and family, documenting all client care and, as necessary, compensating for the client's inability to perform certain activities. Implementation implies that the nurse understands the rationale for all nursing actions.

Evaluation

The last phase of the nursing process, evaluation, focuses on the effectiveness of care the client receives, with a review of the extent to which the nursing process has met its goals. For goals achieved, no further action is necessary. For unmet goals, the nurse adjusts strategies at the appropriate phase to meet client needs.

Nursing diagnosis: A critical part of the nursing process

The nursing diagnoses derived from the physical assessment and history data collected during the assessment phase of the nursing process provide the basis for all subsequent nursing care.

A nursing diagnosis includes a clinical judgment about an individual, family, or community that has been reached through a deliberate, systematic process of data collection and analysis. The diagnosis provides the basis for prescribed, definitive therapy (for which the nurse is accountable) and concisely states the cause of the client's condition if the cause is known. A nursing diagnosis has the following components:
• a word or phrase about the degree or amount of change noted, indicated by such words as *altered, impaired, ineffective, intolerance,* or *dysfunctional*
• the immediacy of the problem, commonly indicated by *actual* or *risk*
• the tissue or system involved, such as skin, bowel, bladder, pulmonary, or cardiac
• the type of problem, such as injury, fracture, or rape
• the activity affected, such as mobility, coping, interaction, or home maintenance
• the cause or etiology, indicated by *related to* or *due to.*

A well-constructed nursing diagnosis, therefore, sets the direction for the client's care plans and goals. The words *actual* and *risk* help the nurse and the client prioritize goals. For example, "actual impairment of skin integrity related to open sacral pressure ulcer" indicates the need to set an immediate goal that "the pressure ulcer will heal" or that "the client will regain skin integrity with a healed pressure ulcer." The initial nursing diagnosis should refer to the tissue or system most in need of corrective care. Thus, a client with a myocardial infarction warrants an initial nursing diagnosis related to the cardiac and circulatory systems. Another high-priority nursing diagnosis concerns the client's knowledge deficits related to the diagnosis, treatment regimen (including its benefits and risks), and self-care needs. Teaching related to these factors is an initial and ongoing nursing activity as the client's treatment regimen proceeds, the condition changes, and the client regains independence.

The efforts of many individuals produced the current nursing diagnoses. Some of the first articles using the words "nursing diagnosis" were written by Chambers and Komorita and appeared in the early 1960s in the *American Journal of Nursing*. Others associated with nursing diagnoses include Yura, Walsh, Carpenito, Kim, McFarland, McLane, Gordon, and Campbell, each of whom has published textbooks on nursing diagnoses.

The leading force in reviewing and developing new nursing diagnoses is the North American Nursing Diagnosis Association (NANDA), whose membership includes nursing experts from the various nursing disciplines. Members meet yearly to review and refine established nursing diagnoses and develop new ones. NANDA bases its diagnoses on human response patterns of exchanging, communicating, relating, valuing, choosing, moving, perceiving, knowing, and feeling. Other nursing diagnoses derive from functional health patterns, such as activity and exercise, elimination, nutrition and metabolism, sleep and rest, cognition, perception, and coping and stress tolerance. The categories of nursing diagnoses consider the physical, social, emotional, cognitive, spiritual, cultural, and environmental sources of disequilibrium experienced by each client. A nursing diagnosis focuses on the client's *health* care needs, whereas a medical diagnosis focuses on disease.

The nursing process offers a way of thinking related to nursing care. The nursing diagnosis forms a vital and integral part of that process to make each client's care specific and individualized (see Appendix 3, "NANDA-approved nursing diagnoses," for a current listing).

Leadership and management

I.   **Introduction**
A. *Leadership* is the capacity to influence the activities of one or more individuals or groups to achieve established goals
B. A leader's primary functions include *communicating* the goals clearly to the group, *motivating* the group to excel, *initiating* new procedures and methods, *facilitating* task accomplishment by considering the group's needs and goals, and *integrating* all parts into a whole (for example, coordinating all aspects of client care both within the nursing unit and among other departments in the hospital)
C. *Management* is a form of leadership that focuses on achievement of organizational goals
D. A manager's primary functions include *planning* the methods used to achieve goals, *organizing* the structure in which plans are carried out, *hiring and scheduling* staff to help carry out the plans, *delegating* tasks to the staff members, and *controlling* staff performance by measuring it against established standards
E. Goal attainment in the workplace depends on several factors, including the workers' perceptions of their roles, the leaders' skills and management style, and the structure of the work environment

II. **Role theory**
A. Role theory is a theoretical framework for describing, analyzing, and understanding social interaction
B. Four fundamental concepts form the basis of role theory
1. *Role* refers to the behavior patterns ideally enacted by an incumbent of a position in a social system (for example, the role of nurse educator should involve such behaviors as motivating students, evaluating the curriculum, and diagnosing students' learning difficulties, among others)
2. *Role expectations* are the behavior patterns that the incumbent and others expect of the incumbent

a. Role expectations for a given position such as staff nurse evolve from various sources, including standards of professional nursing practice, legal and ethical standards, work settings (through job descriptions and types of nursing care delivery system), clients, physicians, and other professionals

b. Other influences on role expectations include one's personality, needs, beliefs, and value system

3. *Role enactment* or *role performance* refers to the incumbent's actual behavior

4. A *role conflict* occurs when an incumbent must conform to mutually exclusive, contradictory, or inconsistent expectations

a. A person's behavior may differ from how others uniformly perceive that the person should behave in a given role

b. Others may disagree about how a person should behave in a given role

c. One person may perform multiple roles that compete for the person's time and energy

d. A person may have mixed feelings about a chosen role

e. A person may be uncertain about which role to choose

f. How the role conflict is resolved can either benefit or harm the social system and the individuals working within it

(1) In nursing, a role conflict may lead to better client care or improved morale among the staff (for instance, staff complaints of insufficient time for client teaching may compel administrators to reduce staff workload)

(2) On the other hand, a role conflict can strain relations among different departments in a hospital or instill anger and frustration among staff members (for example, a nurse's request for a transfer may be denied, possibly leading to job dissatisfaction, diminished performance, and resignation)

C. Leaders and managers use principles of role theory to resolve conflicts

1. When people in various positions within a group are dissatisfied, angry, or stressed, a leader or manager can analyze their roles by asking several pertinent questions

a. What are the sources of conflict?

b. Has the conflict developed because the role for a position has not been clearly defined?

c. Do the people in the group have differing expectations for the role?

2. Depending on the results of the analysis, the leader may use one or more strategies to resolve the conflict

a. Ask the group members to describe their role expectations

b. Clarify for the group what their expectations should be

c. Help the group to set priorities

d. Identify measures they can take to diffuse anger or relieve stress

III. Primary roles of leaders and managers

A. To achieve organizational goals, leaders and managers must clearly *communicate* them to the staff, using one of two forms of communication

1. *Interpersonal communication* refers to the transmission of a message from one person to another, or to a small group, with the intention that the message will be received and understood

2. *Organizational communication* refers to the formal or informal system an organization uses to communicate with its members
   a. *Formal* communication refers to the established system for receiving information from and relaying information to people within or outside the organization
   b. *Informal* communication refers to messages sent and received through social interaction that occurs outside formal channels (for example, "the grapevine")
   c. Organizational communication may flow downward (from management to staff), upward (from staff to lower and middle management to senior management), or horizontally (from one person or group to another at the same organizational level)
3. Communication is a six-step process
   a. The sender formulates a message, which should be clear and complete
   b. The sender encodes the message with verbal and nonverbal information (for instance, the tone of a message about an emergency situation may include a sense of urgency)
   c. The sender transmits the message (such as through a speech or memo)
   d. The receiver decodes the message, interpreting it into meaningful information
   e. The receiver takes action as a result of receiving and interpreting the message
   f. The sender and the receiver of the message provide feedback, continually exchanging and clarifying information
      (1) Feedback to subordinates about job performance serves as a control measure for managers
      (2) Feedback about job performance should be:
         (a) helpful to the worker
         (b) objective rather than judgmental
         (c) specific rather than general
         (d) timely
4. Communication can dramatically influence the nurse's role and job performance
   a. Effective change-of-shift communications between nurses can improve continuity of care and promote individualized care planning
   b. Accurate and thorough documentation creates a permanent record of care delivered and communicates information about the care to other health care providers
   c. Confidential communications between a client and a nurse should not be shared with other caregivers unless the information is vital to the client's well-being

B. To accomplish their objectives, leaders and managers *delegate* tasks, assigning responsibility for completing the tasks to subordinates
   1. Delegation has several benefits
      a. It allows the manager to devote more time and attention to higher priorities
      b. It boosts workers' confidence and increases their ability to perform tasks
      c. It promotes cooperation and cohesiveness in the group
   2. To delegate effectively, leaders and managers must consider the nature of the task and the characteristics of the worker

     a. Does the task fall within the worker's role expectations?

     b. Is the task congruent with legal requirements (such as nurse practice acts), professional standards, and institutional policies (such as job descriptions)?

     c. Can the task be matched to the worker's personal preferences?

     d. Does the worker have the time and resources to accomplish the task?

3. When delegating, a seasoned leader or manager tries to follow these principles:

     a. Give clear, specific instructions about the task, including objectives, a time frame for completion, and results expected

     b. Be familiar enough with the task to be able to advise the worker of any anticipated problems in its completion and to discuss possible solutions

     c. Be available to provide guidance if unexpected problems occur or if the worker needs help in completing the task

     d. Allow the worker some latitude on how to complete the task

     e. Instill confidence in the worker's ability to perform well, especially on a new task

     f. Provide appropriate feedback—either positive reinforcement for a job well done or constructive and specific suggestions for improvement when a task is not completed as expected

     g. Expect occasional errors, and try to arrange another opportunity for the worker to perform the task

     h. Remember that the final responsibility for any delegated task remains with the leader or manager

C. Leaders and managers *teach* staff members to ensure efficiency and safety in the workplace and to help staff members acquire new knowledge, skills, and abilities

1. Effective teaching is most likely to occur when the teacher follows these learning principles:

     a. Feedback strengthens learning

     b. Learner satisfaction increases learning potential

     c. Personal learning styles require individualized approaches to teaching

     d. Learning is enhanced by the learner's active participation

     e. Motivation increases learning

     f. Mutual goal setting produces meaningful learning

     g. Relevant learning experiences motivate the learner

     h. Mild anxiety may benefit the learner

2. After completing a teaching session, the leader or manager should evaluate what the workers have learned

     a. An accurate evaluation cannot take place unless the leader has established measurable objectives

     b. The leader should use evaluation techniques that are appropriate to what is being learned

     c. The leader should provide prompt feedback on the results of the evaluation

3. If several staff members have the same task to learn, the leader should consider referring them to a staff education department

D. Acting as agents of change, leaders and managers may *innovate* a new task, goal, method, or perspective to subordinates

1. To initiate change successfully, the agent must be willing to take risks and must plan changes that are appropriate to the group

2. The agent exhibits one of two behaviors to effect change
   a. Exhibiting *directive behavior,* the agent uses one-way communication to explain what subordinates should do and when, where, and how they should do it
   b. Exhibiting *supportive behavior,* the agent uses two-way communication to provide emotional support to subordinates and to facilitate task accomplishment
3. Leaders and managers—and their subordinates—experience three phases of change
   a. During the first phase, *unfreezing,* the leader or manager begins to challenge and perhaps prohibit customary or traditional behaviors in order to introduce new alternatives
   b. During the second phase, *changing,* subordinates begin to accept the alternative behavior patterns in one of two ways
      (1) They identify with and emulate new models provided by the environment
      (2) They internalize new models when success depends on it
   c. During the third phase, *refreezing,* subordinates integrate the new behaviors into their personalities (maintaining the new behavior requires reinforcement from the leader or manager)
E. To ensure the safety and efficacy of products made or services rendered, leaders and managers *control* quality by regularly reviewing departmental operations, standards, and procedures
   1. In nursing, *quality assurance* refers to the systems used to monitor the outcomes of nursing interventions and departmental activities by comparing them with established standards
      a. The level of nursing care provided and its effects on clients are assessed by examining the nursing process and client outcomes
         (1) The nursing process is the scientifically organized sequence of activities undertaken by nurses in caring for clients
         (2) Client outcomes are the end result of nursing care
      b. Methods of assessment include audits of open and closed records, peer review, rating scales or questionnaires filled out by clients and families, and direct observation by the nurse
      c. Sources of nursing care standards include state nurse practice acts and other rules and regulations that legally define nursing, the Standards of Practice promulgated by the American Nurses' Association, the Standards for Nursing Services of the Joint Commission on Accreditation of Health Care Organizations, and state and federal government agencies
      d. Nursing leaders and managers regularly perform quality assurance procedures
         (1) They identify standards, goals, and methods of performing quality assurance activities
         (2) They measure actual performance
         (3) They compare results of performance with standards and goals
         (4) They take action to correct weaknesses and to reinforce strengths
   2. Ensuring quality control also involves *risk management*—a system for anticipating, acquiring, and maintaining the skills and resources needed to prevent mishaps and to respond effectively when a mishap occurs
   3. Numerous risk factors can be found in the nursing setting

      a. An institutional procedure may not comply with standards (for instance, if a nurse's job description falls outside the scope of nursing practice)

      b. A nurse may injure a client through an act of commission or omission (for example, administration of the wrong drug or failure to obtain the client's informed consent)

      c. A nurse manager may ignore a potentially damaging problem (such as failure to take corrective action when documentation proves the existence of ineffective care or unusual occurrences on a nursing unit)

      d. An institution may lack a system to resolve problems effectively (for example, when poor communication between departments or between middle and upper management prevents the prompt reporting and correcting of errors)

4. The staff nurse plays a valuable role in quality assurance and risk management; specific tasks include the following:

      a. Define individual performance goals to improve care and to reduce risks to clients

      b. Assist in defining the goals for quality assurance and risk management on the nursing unit

      c. Participate in nursing unit meetings to identify problems that need further evaluation

      d. Suggest methods for attaining standards when monitoring reveals problems

      e. Assist in planning changes in nursing unit practices to correct deficiencies

IV. Leadership and management styles

A. An *authoritarian* style is characterized by structure, order, and a much greater emphasis on task accomplishment than on the people who perform the tasks (a useful style in a crisis such as a code blue)

B. A *permissive* or *laissez-faire* style is characterized by minimal, if any, direction or control (a useful style when leading highly motivated professional groups such as a research project team)

C. A *democratic* style is characterized by group participation and collaboration in decision making and by high productivity (the preferred management style in most work settings, because people usually perform more effectively when they have an equal voice in decision making)

V. The nurse's role in various work settings

A. The structure of the work environment can significantly influence the nurse's role

B. An efficient structure enables nursing staff to achieve the goals set for client care

C. Common structural patterns in nursing settings include functional nursing, team nursing, and primary nursing

1. In *functional nursing,* nurses are assigned to specific tasks

      a. They may administer medications, make rounds with physicians, or provide direct client care

      b. Accountability rests primarily with the nurse-manager

2. In *team nursing,* nurses share responsibility for a group of clients

      a. The team usually includes RNs, LPNs, and nursing assistants

      b. Accountability rests with the team leaders and the nurse-manager

3. In *primary nursing,* each nurse is assigned a caseload of clients in the nurse's "district" (nursing unit), beginning with the client's admission and continuing through discharge
   a. The primary nurse is responsible for all aspects of nursing care
   b. An associate nurse cares for the client in the primary nurse's absence

VI. Leadership and management of nursing groups
A. A nursing group consists of two or more nursing personnel (RN, LPN, LVN, nursing assistant) brought together to carry out the goals of nursing, such as providing client care, solving client care problems, and solving staff problems (stress, demanding workload) that interfere with client care)
B. Primary roles of the group leader include learning to know and accept other group members, securing agreement from members on the group's purpose, and establishing structures, rules, and procedures for accomplishing group goals
C. Primary roles of group members include relating well to others (known as the interpersonal role), providing clear directions and information (informational role), and making sound decisions after using effective problem-solving techniques (decisional role)
D. All nursing groups share certain characteristics
   1. *Group norm* refers to the group's standard of performance or behavior
   2. *Group conformity* refers to the group's adherence to established norms
   3. *Group cohesiveness* refers to a collective desire to participate in the group despite forces acting on the members to leave it
E. Effective group performance is more likely when certain conditions apply
   1. Goals are clearly defined
   2. Members agree to goals and are committed to them
   3. Goal achievement is clearly measurable
   4. Group goals are congruent with broader organizational goals and with personal goals of group members
   5. Group expectations are clearly defined and communicated (low role ambiguity)
   6. Group expectations are compatible with those of the organization (low role conflict)
   7. Members are usually able to meet group expectations (low role overload)

Legal principles and nursing practice

I. Definition of law
A. Law is a set of rules and principles derived from several sources and enforceable by legal processes
B. Laws provide a means of settling disputes, compensating for injuries caused by another, and disciplining and isolating individuals for wrong doing as defined by society
C. Essential to any society's progress and survival, laws form an important basis for nursing practice

II.   Sources of law

A. Four sources of law—constitutions, judicial opinions, legislation, and regulations—form the legal basis of nursing practice

B. A *constitution* is a document that incorporates the basic principles by which an organization governs itself

1.   The federal government and each state have a written constitution

2.   The U.S. Constitution contains the fundamental laws of the nation

    a. It defines the branches of government: legislative, executive, and judicial

    b. It specifies a division of powers between the federal government and the states

    c. It sets forth each citizen's basic rights; for example, the right to privacy, guaranteed to all citizens by the Fourteenth Amendment, supports a client's right to consent to or refuse treatment, even life-sustaining treatment

C. A *judicial opinion* is the court's official position on a legal dispute, written by the judge who presides over the court case

1.   Usually, judicial opinions emanate from appeals or higher courts in the state or federal court system as a result of disputes brought before lower courts by the litigants (those who bring the lawsuit or are otherwise involved in it)

2.   These opinions, published in what is usually called the legal reporter system, are also referred to as case law or case decisions

3.   Judicial opinions form precedent—a body of law that is often the basis for future decisions

4.   Judicial opinions address nursing practice in such areas as employment, licensure, malpractice and negligence, and crimes

D. *Legislation* is the set of rules created by the legislative branch of government at the federal, state, or local (city or county) level

1.   The legislative branch of government, which meets periodically, is elected by the people

2.   Also called statutes or statutory law, legislation is published and made available to the public; some states publish legislation in a book called a code or an annotated code

3.   Nursing practice is shaped by many pieces of legislation, particularly the state nurse practice act and state and federal public health laws

4.   Legislation results from the legislative process, which involves the study of issues, drafting of a bill, discussion, compromise, redrafting, and voting for or against the bill's passage

5.   A bill—the proposed law—usually becomes law when more votes are for passage than against, and after the governor (in state legislation) or the president (in federal legislation) signs the bill (in some circumstances, legislation can become law without the governor's or the president's approval)

E. *Regulations* are the rules created by the executive branch of government

1.   The executive branch is headed by the governor of a state or the president of the United States

2.   The legislative branch enacts laws granting the executive branch the authority to write regulations

3.   Regulations are created through the regulatory process, which involves the study of issues, publication of the proposed rule, a period of public input (through written opinions or testimony at hearings), possible redrafting, and publication of the final regulation

    4.   Federal regulations are found in the *Code of Federal Regulations,* and state regulations are usually found in the state's *Code of Regulations*

    5.   The government agency created by the state nurse practice act, usually called the state board of nursing, has the power to write specific rules that govern and control nursing practice within its jurisdiction

III. Types of law

A. *Civil law* refers to a wide range of legal issues that are unrelated to criminal acts

    1.   Usually, civil law involves disputes between two or more individuals or entities

    2.   Civil disputes related to safe nursing practice may involve an employment contract, a tort, or a violation of a client's rights (see Sections IV, V, and VI, pages 41 to 48)

B. *Administrative law* deals with enforcement of government agencies' rules and regulations

    1.   Licensure and the state's power to discipline nurses involve the administrative law and process

    2.   A state can make rules that govern nursing based on its "police power," the power to act to protect public health, safety, and welfare; for instance, a state can prohibit a nurse from practicing nursing if the nurse is found guilty of unprofessional conduct (see Section VII, pages 48 and 49)

C. *Criminal law* refers to a set of laws that define offenses against society

    1.   Crimes involve public wrongs (wrongs against society)

    2.   The criminal justice and law enforcement systems exist to investigate, prosecute, and (if the accused is found guilty) punish the offender (see Section VIII, page 49)

IV. Civil disputes and nursing practice: Contracts

A. The law of the nurse's workplace is derived from federal and state statutes and judicial opinions, employer personnel handbooks, civil service rules, employer practice, collective bargaining agreements, and employment contracts

B. A *contract* is a written or oral agreement between two or more individuals that has several elements to its formation, interpretation, and enforcement

    1.   A contract can be individual or collective (such as a union contract)

    2.   A contract specifies the time period within which the conditions of the agreement must be met

    3.   Contract elements include offer, acceptance, and consideration (usually monetary compensation)

V. Civil disputes and nursing practice: Torts

A. A *tort* is a private wrong or a breach of a legal duty to the rights and interests of others

B. An injured litigant (usually called a *plaintiff*) can receive remedy for a tort, commonly in the form of damages, if the litigant presents adequate evidence to prove that an injury occurred

C. Courts recognize three types of torts: unintentional, intentional, and quasi-intentional

1. An *unintentional tort* is an act that fails to meet a duty owed to an-
    other person (the plaintiff) and leads to the person's injury
    a. In nursing, the two most common types of unintentional tort are
        negligence and malpractice
    b. *Negligence* is an unintentional tort involving four elements: duty,
        breach of duty, proximate cause, and damages
        (1) *Duty* refers to the nurse's legal obligation to provide nursing
            care to a client
            (a) The nurse has the duty to meet a reasonable and prudent
                standard of care under the circumstances
            (b) The nurse must deliver care as any other reasonable and
                prudent nurse would under similar circumstances
            (c) Standards of care are found in policy and procedure
                manuals, nursing education, experience, and publica-
                tions of professional associations and accreditation
                groups
        (2) *Breach of duty*—failure to provide the expected reasonable
            standard of care under the circumstances—can take two
            forms:
            (a) The nurse may fail to provide care (breach by omission
                of the duty)
            (b) The nurse may provide care in an unreasonable manner
                (breach by commission of the duty)
        (3) *Proximate cause* refers to the causal connection between the
            breach of duty and the resulting injury
            (a) Proximate cause does not necessarily involve a direct
                cause-and-effect relationship, but the plaintiff must pro-
                duce evidence that the nurse's action or inaction led to
                the plaintiff's injury
            (b) State laws vary in the language used to define proximate
                cause
            (c) If the definition uses the term "but for," the plaintiff must
                prove that the injury would not have occurred but for the
                nurse's breach of duty
            (d) If the definition uses the term "substantial factor," the
                plaintiff must prove that the nurse's breach of duty was a
                substantial factor in the injury
            (e) If the definition uses the term "foreseeability," the plain-
                tiff must prove that the nurse's breach of duty foreseeably
                led to the plaintiff's injury; that is, that the nurse should
                have known what would happen
        (4) *Damages* refers both to the physical or psychological injury
            and to monetary compensation awarded to the plaintiff for in-
            curring the injury
            (a) The plaintiff must prove that an injury occurred and
                present evidence showing its monetary value
            (b) The plaintiff can request compensatory, nominal, or pu-
                nitive damages
            (c) *Compensatory damages* are awarded to reimburse the
                plaintiff for the expenses, rehabilitation, and pain and
                suffering related to the injury
            (d) *Nominal damages* are awarded to indicate a defendant's
                wrongdoing when little if any injury occurred

        (e) *Punitive damages* are awarded to the plaintiff in special circumstances, usually to punish the defendant for an especially egregious or outrageous act

  c. *Malpractice* is negligence by a member of a profession (such as nursing), differing from negligence only in that the standard or duty owed is a professional one, based on special knowledge and skills

    (1) The plaintiff in a malpractice action must prove all the elements of negligence, usually with expert witnesses to testify about the professional duty owed and whether it was breached

    (2) Not all states automatically apply a professional standard to nurses; some states still apply a nonprofessional one, and other states apply a professional standard only when the nurse's act required special knowledge and skill

  d. Negligence and malpractice lawsuits also involve legal principles about who bears *liability* (responsibility) for resulting injuries

    (1) *Personal liability* refers to responsibility for one's acts (for example, if a client sustains injuries because a staff nurse administers the wrong drug or fails to monitor the client properly, the nurse can be found liable for those acts)

    (2) *Vicarious liability* refers to responsibility for another person's acts; such liability can take one of two forms

        (a) The principle of *respondeat superior* addresses an employer's responsibility for injuries caused by an employee's negligent acts, if those acts were performed within the scope of employment and when an employment relationship existed (for example, if a hospital-employed nurse fails to detect a hematoma under the blood pressure cuff of a heavily heparinized ICU client, the hospital and the nurse are both liable)

        (b) *Corporate liability* refers to an employer's responsibility for injury caused by an employee who acted according to the employer's decisions (for example, because a hospital determines its budget, staff, and client population, the hospital—not the nurse—is liable for injury that results from understaffing)

  e. Nurses can avoid or defend negligence and malpractice lawsuits by following these principles:

    (1) Know the standard of care—the duty owed the client—before delivering care

    (2) Deliver care that meets the standard

    (3) Document care accurately and concisely, following the health care facility's policies and procedures (documentation reflecting that a standard of care was met can serve as a nurse's best defense; the adage "if it wasn't charted, it wasn't done" receives credence in most jurisdictions)

  f. Other defenses may apply to a nursing negligence case, depending on the facts presented

    (1) Federally employed nurses hold personal immunity from liability (under federal legislation known as the Federal Tort Claims Act)

    (2) All nurses hold immunity from liability for making a good faith report of child abuse, which all states require of nurses

(3) A case can be dismissed if the plaintiff does not file the lawsuit within a legislature-specified time, known as a statute of limitation

2. An *intentional tort* is a willful act that injures another person or the person's property

   a. *Assault* is the threat of imminent harmful or offensive bodily contact

   b. *Battery* is bodily contact with another person without the person's permission or consent

   c. *False imprisonment* is unlawful restraint of a person against the person's will

   d. *Intentional infliction of emotional distress* is extreme, outrageous, or intolerable conduct toward another, causing emotional harm

3. A *quasi-intentional tort* is an act that interferes with a person's intangible interests, such as privacy or reputation

   a. A nurse may be charged with *invasion of privacy* and *breach of confidentiality* for revealing personal information about a client to an unauthorized person

   b. A nurse may be charged with *defamation* for injuring the plaintiff's reputation in the community as the result of a false statement, either spoken (slander) or written (libel)

     (1) Truth is a viable defense against a defamation charge

     (2) False statements about another person's professional competence can lead to a defamation lawsuit

VI. Civil disputes and nursing practice: Client rights

A. *A Patient's Bill of Rights* (see pages 46 and 47), written by the American Hospital Association, contains a sample list of patient (client) rights

B. Although not law, this code lists many rights of clients legally recognized through sources of law mentioned above

C. Client rights include informed consent, freedom from unreasonable restraint, the right to refuse treatment, and the right to privacy and confidentiality

1. *Informed consent* refers to the client's involvement in and agreement with treatment decisions based on careful consideration of all information pertinent to the client's condition

   a. For informed consent to be recognized by the court, several conditions must be met

     (1) The consent must be voluntary

     (2) The information given to the client must include the nature of the proposed treatment, its foreseeable risks and benefits, any alternatives to the proposed treatment, and the consequences of choosing to do nothing

     (3) The consent must be given by a person who is legally competent to do so

   b. The physician has the legal obligation to obtain a client's informed consent to medical treatment

   c. Nurses are commonly assigned the task of obtaining a signed consent form and witnessing the client's signature; doing so legally obligates the nurse, if called later, to testify about anything relating to what the nurse saw, heard, or knew about the consent

d. A nurse who is concerned about the validity of an informed consent has a legal obligation to tell the physician and the nursing supervisor about the concerns and to document their having been so informed

e. Legal competence differs from medical or mental competence
  (1) Legal competence is a presumption established by the state legislatures (usually a chronological age, such as 18 years); thus, everyone over age 18 is presumed legally competent, and everyone under age 18 is presumed legally incompetent
  (2) For those under age 18 (known as minors), legislatures have established exceptions to the rule of presumed incompetency; unless one of these exceptions applies, informed consent for treatment of a minor must be obtained from the minor's parent or legal guardian
  (3) Consent from a parent or legal guardian usually is not required if the minor is married, has a child, lives independently, or seeks certain types of health care services (such as for pregnancy, substance abuse, or a mental health problem)

f. After reaching the legal age, one can lose the legal capacity to consent only through a formal judicial process
  (1) In this proceeding, a court determines, usually on the basis of medical and psychiatric testimony, whether the person is incompetent; if the court finds the person incompetent, the court appoints a guardian (who becomes the person who gives the informed consent)
  (2) In some situations, the court must not only rule on incompetency but also determine whether the individual needs involuntary commitment to an institution for treatment
  (3) Before it orders involuntary commitment, the court must receive clear and convincing evidence that the individual poses a danger to self or to others with no other less restrictive treatment available
  (4) The rules to make these determinations vary among the states

g. Informed consent may not be required under certain circumstances
  (1) In life-threatening emergencies, client consent is implied
  (2) A client may tell the physician that he or she does not want to know the appropriate information (known as waiver)
  (3) The physician's professional judgment may dictate that fully informing a client would act as a substantial detriment to the client and cause harm (known as the physician's therapeutic privilege)

2. *Freedom from unreasonable restraint* recognizes the client's autonomy and freedom of movement
  a. The client must receive care in a safe, prudent manner
  b. Health care providers can legally restrain a client under certain conditions previously defined by law and by the health care facility's policies and procedures
    (1) The restraints must be necessary to meet the client's therapeutic needs or to ensure the safety of the client or others
    (2) The least restrictive type of restraint must be used first
    (3) Use of restraints must be accompanied by the physician's orders except in an emergency

A Patient's Bill of Rights

Effective health care requires collaboration between patients and physicians and other health care professionals. Open and honest communication, respect for personal and professional values, and sensitivity to differences are integral to optimal patient care. As the setting for the provision of health services, hospitals must provide a foundation for understanding and respecting the rights and responsibilities of patients, their families, physicians, and other caregivers. Hospitals must ensure a health care ethic that respects the role of patients in decision making about treatment choices and other aspects of their care. Hospitals must be sensitive to cultural, racial, linguistic, religious, age, gender, and other differences as well as the needs of persons with disabilities.

The American Hospital Association presents *A Patient's Bill of Rights* with the expectation that it will contribute to more effective patient care and be supported by the hospital on behalf of the institution, its medical staff, employees, and patients. The American Hospital Association encourages health care institutions to tailor this bill of rights to their patient community by translating and/or simplifying the language of this bill of rights as may be necessary to ensure that patients and their families understand their rights and responsibilities.

BILL OF RIGHTS*

1. The patient has the right to considerate and respectful care.

2. The patient has the right to and is encouraged to obtain from physicians and other direct caregivers relevant, current, and understandable information concerning diagnosis, treatment, and prognosis.

Except in emergencies when the patient lacks decision-making capacity and the need for treatment is urgent, the patient is entitled to the opportunity to discuss and request information related to the specific procedures and/or treatments, the risks involved, the possible length of recuperation, and the medically reasonable alternatives and their accompanying risks and benefits.

Patients have the right to know the identity of physicians, nurses, and others involved in their care, as well as when those involved are students, residents, or other trainees. The patient also has the right to know the immediate and long-term financial implications of treatment choices, insofar as they are known.

3. The patient has the right to make decisions about the plan of care prior to and during the course of treatment and to refuse a recommended treatment or plan of care to the extent permitted by law and hospital policy and to be informed of the medical consequences of this action. In case of such refusal, the patient is entitled to other appropriate care and services that the hospital provides or transfer to another hospital. The hospital should notify patients of any policy that might affect patient choice within the institution.

4. The patient has the right to have an advance directive (such as a living will, health care proxy, or durable power of attorney for health care) concerning treatment or designating a surrogate decision maker with the expectation that the hospital will honor the intent of that directive to the extent permitted by law and hospital policy.

Health care institutions must advise patients of their rights under state law and hospital policy to make informed medical choices, ask if the patient has an advance directive, and include that information in patient records. The patient has the right to timely information about hospital policy that may limit its ability to implement fully a legally valid advance directive.

5. The patient has the right to every consideration of privacy. Case discussion, consultation, examination, and treatment should be conducted so as to protect each patient's privacy.

6. The patient has the right to expect that all communications and records pertaining to his/her care will be treated as confidential by the hospital, except in cases such as suspected abuse and public health hazards when reporting is permitted or required by law. The patient has the right to expect that the hospital will emphasize the confidentiality of this information when it releases it to any other parties entitled to review information in these records.

7. The patient has the right to review the records pertaining to his/her medical care and to have the information explained or interpreted as necessary, except when restricted by law.

8. The patient has the right to expect that, within its capacity and policies, a hospital will make reasonable response to the request of a patient for appropriate and medically indicated care and services. The hospital must provide evaluation, service, and/or referral as indicated by the urgency of the case. When medically appropriate and legally permissible, or when a patient has so requested, a patient may be transferred to another facility. The institution to which the patient is to be transferred must first have accepted the patient for transfer. The patient must also have the benefit of complete information and explanation concerning the need for, risks, benefits, and alternatives to such a transfer.

A Patient's Bill of Rights *(continued)*

9. The patient has the right to ask and be informed of the existence of business relationships among the hospital, educational institutions, other health care providers, or payers that may influence the patient's treatment and care.

10. The patient has the right to consent to or decline to participate in proposed research studies or human experimentation affecting care and treatment or requiring direct patient involvement, and to have those studies fully explained prior to consent. A patient who declines to participate in research or experimentation is entitled to the most effective care that the hospital can otherwise provide.

11. The patient has the right to expect reasonable continuity of care when appropriate and to be informed by physicians and other caregivers of available and realistic patient care options when hospital care is no longer appropriate.

12. The patient has the right to be informed of hospital policies and practices that relate to patient care, treatment, and responsibilities. The patient has the right to be informed of available resources for resolving disputes, grievances, and conflicts, such as ethics committees, patient representatives, or other mechanisms available in the institution. The patient has the right to be informed of the hospital's charges for services and available payment methods.

The collaborative nature of health care requires that patients, or their families/surrogates, participate in their care. The effectiveness of care and patient satisfaction with the course of treatment depend, in part, on the patient fulfilling certain responsibilities. Patients are responsible for providing information about past illnesses, hospitalizations, medications, and other matters related to health status. To participate effectively in decision making, patients must be encouraged to take responsibility for requesting additional information or clarification about their health status or treatment when they do not fully understand information and instructions. Patients are also responsible for ensuring that the health care institution has a copy of their written advance directive if they have one. Patients are responsible for informing their physicians and other caregivers if they anticipate problems in following prescribed treatment.

Patients should also be aware of the hospital's obligation to be reasonably efficient and equitable in providing care to other patients and the community. The hospital's rules and regulations are designed to help the hospital meet this obligation. Patients and their families are responsible for making reasonable accommodations to the needs of the hospital, other patients, medical staff, and hospital employees. Patients are responsible for providing necessary information for insurance claims and for working with the hospital to make payment arrangements, when necessary.

A person's health depends on much more than health care services. Patients are responsible for recognizing the impact of their lifestyle on their personal health.

CONCLUSION
Hospitals have many functions to perform, including the enhancement of health status, health promotion, and the prevention and treatment of injury and disease; the immediate and ongoing care and rehabilitation of patients; the education of health professionals, patients, and the community; and research. All these activities must be conducted with an overriding concern for the values and dignity of patients.

*These rights can be exercised on the patient's behalf by a designated surrogate or proxy decision maker if the patient lacks decision-making capacity, is legally incompetent, or is a minor.

    (4) Health care providers must closely monitor the client, release the restraints periodically, and remove them when the client's condition no longer warrants their use

    (5) Accurate and thorough documentation must reveal all pertinent details of the care given to the client, including how and why restraints were applied and removed

3. The *right to refuse treatment* provides that every competent adult may refuse treatment, even life-sustaining treatment

    a. Also known as the right to withhold consent, this right and all the requirements of informed consent apply to a client's decision to refuse treatment

    b. Like other client rights, the right to refuse treatment is not absolute and must be considered by the court in relation to the interests of society; thus, the client's right to refuse may be outweighed by the court's responsibility to preserve human life, protect innocent third parties, prevent suicide, or maintain the ethical integrity of the medical profession

    c. Many states have enacted legislation that permits a client to make health care decisions in advance

       (1) A *living will* is a document in which a client instructs family and health care professionals about medical care that should or should not be provided if the client becomes incapacitated; a living will should become part of the client's medical record

       (2) *Durable power of attorney* is a legal document in which a client identifies a proxy, or surrogate, decision maker in case the client becomes incapacitated; this document should also be included in the client's medical record

    d. State laws vary on the issue of substituted consent; if the client lacks the capacity to make informed decisions, health care professionals usually turn to the client's family members and close friends, and the court may or may not formally appoint these surrogate decision makers

  4. The *right to privacy and confidentiality* recognizes a client's autonomy and right to be left alone

    a. Because the client and the health care provider have a relationship based on trust, the client may reveal private information that will enhance treatment; in return, the health care provider must keep the information confidential

    b. The client has the right to access personal health records and to obtain a copy of the records

    c. Health care providers have the responsibility to maintain health records in a secure, controlled manner

    d. Information can be revealed only with the client's permission or when required by law; for instance, physicians must report acquired immunodeficiency syndrome (AIDS) and other communicable diseases to the federal and state governments, but they must still keep such reports confidential

VII. Administrative disputes and nursing practice

  A. State governments regulate nursing practice through an executive branch office, usually called a state board of nursing

  B. Legislation known as the state nurse practice act creates the state board

  C. Each state typically regulates several areas of nursing practice

    1. The state regulates the nursing profession's *licensure examination* by determining the rules and requirements for admission or entry into nursing practice

    2. In most states, the nurse practice act defines the legal *scope of nursing practice*; the state can discipline, fine, censure, or take other appropriate steps against one who practices nursing without meeting the state requirements

3. The state regulates the *professional conduct* of licensed nurses by defining unprofessional conduct
   a. The state has the power to initiate investigations, bring charges of misconduct, and levy disciplinary measures
   b. Chemical impairment (drug or alcohol abuse) is the most common reason for disciplinary action against a nurse
   c. A nurse charged with unprofessional conduct has the right to due process, including notice of the specific charges, an opportunity to present evidence to counter the charge, and representation by an attorney hired by the nurse
4. Each state regulates *nursing education* by establishing the requirements of and approving the educational programs for nurse preparation

VIII. Criminal disputes and nursing practice

A. Most states recognize two types of crime: *felonies* and *misdemeanors* (some states use the generic term *offenses,* categorizing these as *crimes*—felonies and misdemeanors—or *violations*)

B. The primary difference between the types lies in the crime's degree of severity—and thus in the length and type of sentence or penalty imposed on the convicted criminal
   1. Felonies entail more serious offenses and warrant lengthy prison sentences
   2. Misdemeanors, which are less serious, usually result in a short prison sentence, a fine, or both

C. Criminal codes or statutes define the elements of each crime; the prosecutor must prove the existence of these elements beyond a reasonable doubt

D. A defendant in a criminal case has constitutionally provided rights, such as the right to legal counsel

E. For an act to be considered criminal, the prosecutor must prove the defendant's *culpability*; that is, the defendant committed the act intentionally, knowingly, recklessly, or in a criminally negligent manner

F. Mental impairment precludes the possibility of culpability; thus, the law does not support convicting a person who was affected by mental disease or a mental defect when committing the act
   1. A person who is found not guilty by reason of insanity is committed to a treatment facility and released after recovery
   2. Definitions of mental impairment differ among jurisdictions

G. Nurses have been convicted of such crimes as murder, fraud, patient abuse, and illegal use of controlled substances

Therapeutic communication

I. Characteristics

A. Has a purpose and is goal directed
B. Enhances the client's self-esteem and ability to function
C. Can be verbal or nonverbal
D. Promotes the client's spiritual healing

Characteristics of social and therapeutic relationships

In an effective nurse-client relationship, the nurse uses therapeutic communication to shed light on and promote healthy changes in the client's behavior. The following chart contrasts important differences between a therapeutic relationship and a purely social one.

SOCIAL RELATIONSHIP
- Focuses on mutual sharing, with each participant giving and receiving
- Promotes mutual pleasure
- Has no time constraints
- Does not involve a contract
- Does not require the participants to examine their behavior or possess a specialized knowledge base

THERAPEUTIC RELATIONSHIP
- Focuses on the client, with the nurse giving and the client receiving
- Promotes client healing
- Is time-limited
- Involves a contract between nurse and client
- Requires the nurse to have a sound understanding of human behavior and to examine the nurse's and the client's behaviors from a theoretical perspective

---

II.   **Goals**
    A. Self-discovery
    B. Clarification of thoughts, feelings, and actions
    C. Exploration of new coping skills or behavior patterns

III.   **Nursing actions that impede therapeutic communication**
    A. Giving advice to the client
    B. Changing the subject
    C. Confronting the client prematurely
    D. Ignoring the client's message
    E. Stating or implying that the client is wrong
    F. Using clichés that raise false hopes or do not address the problem (for example, "Everything will work out")
    G. Dominating the session by talking excessively
    H. Asking "why" questions

IV.   **Nursing actions that promote therapeutic communication**
    A. Assessing the client's behavioral patterns
    B. Diagnosing the client's underlying needs
    C. Developing goals with the client (if the client's anxiety level permits)
    D. Responding in a way that enhances the client's self-esteem and functioning
    E. Avoiding role conflicts
    F. Evaluating the outcome

V.   **Focus of nursing interventions**
    A. Individual
       1. Emphasizes the client
       2. Is particularly helpful when the client is highly anxious or disorganized
       3. Affords the nurse greater control than in group or family settings
    B. Group
       1. Emphasizes group work and group processes

Techniques that facilitate communication

TECHNIQUE	DESCRIPTION	EXAMPLE
Silence	Refraining from speech to give the client (and the nurse) time to sort out thoughts and feelings	*Client:* "I hate you and everyone else." *Nurse:* Remains silent, with the body in an open position, and observes the client.
Self-disclosure	Sharing personal information at an opportune moment to convey understanding	*Client:* "My husband's death was like losing a major part of my life." *Nurse:* "I had a similar feeling when my husband died."
Suggestion	Posing alternatives for client consideration	*Client:* "I won't see a shrink!" *Nurse:* "Have you ever thought about...?" *Client:* "I don't like that, either." *Nurse:* "What would happen if you...?"
Confrontation	Acknowledging discrepancies in the client's verbal and nonverbal behaviors; calling attention to evasions, distortions, smoke screens, and game playing	*Client:* "I don't have a problem with alcohol." *Nurse:* "You say that alcohol has not created any problems for you, yet you have had two DWIs [driving while intoxicated] and your wife nags you about your drinking."
Concreteness	Clarifying the meaning of the client's communication; being clear, direct, and to the point	*Client:* "They said...." *Nurse:* "Who said that?"
Genuineness	Giving honest feedback when the client is ready; acting in a congruent manner with the client	*Client:* "You look bored." *Nurse:* "I'm not bored, but I do feel very tired." *Client:* "Do you think I'm weird?" *Nurse:* "Sometimes."
Immediacy	Acknowledging what is occurring between the nurse and the client as it happens	*Client:* "I think I have the right to know as much about you as you know about me." *Nurse:* "Sounds like you may not be too sure that I'll be able to understand what you are experiencing."
Empathy	Experiencing another's feelings temporarily	*Client:* "This whole thing is a mistake. I shouldn't even be here." *Nurse:* "Sounds like it's difficult for you to be here."
Respect	Conveying openness, a nonjudgmental attitude, and a desire to hear what the client has to say	*Client:* "What difference does it make? You just think I'm wrong, anyway." *Nurse:* "Try me. I'd like to hear about what's been happening."
Reflection	Paraphrasing what the client has said	*Client:* "The cop was out to get me. He had no reason to pull me over. It was a real set-up." *Nurse:* "You believe that it was unfair for the police to pull you over."
Broad opening	Using a general statement or question to encourage the client to set the direction for the session	*Client:* Enters room, takes a seat, and looks expectantly at the nurse. *Nurse:* "What's up?" or "How has it gone since we last met?" or "How are you today?"
Restating	Repeating what the client has said to indicate that the nurse is listening and interested; may encourage the client to elaborate	*Client:* "I don't belong here." *Nurse:* "You don't belong here?" *Client:* "Of course not. I'm not like the others here. I'm educated and have a good job."
Focusing	Assisting the client to explore a specific topic	*Client:* "I don't know where to begin." *Nurse:* "What's your biggest problem now?" *Client:* "I can't decide about..." *Nurse:* "Let's talk about that. Perhaps more discussion will help you decide."

The communication continuum

Words can help the nurse create a healing atmosphere. But when chosen poorly, they can jeopardize nurse-client rapport and even harm the client's emotional well-being. Think of verbal communication as a continuum from destructive to constructive. Destructive communication can damage a client's self-esteem; constructive communication builds and preserves it.

DESTRUCTIVE COMMUNICATION
• Erodes self-esteem
• Conveys disrespect

CONSTRUCTIVE COMMUNICATION
• Promotes self-esteem
• Aids self-discovery
• Conveys respect

---

    2. Provides a supportive environment for group members to interact, share feelings and information, make decisions, develop socializing skills, and learn to do likewise in all interpersonal relationships

C. Family
    1. Emphasizes the client's family or significant other
    2. Is based on the concept that the client's identified psychological or physical problems affect the family or express family dysfunction
    3. Provides opportunities for the client's family members or significant other to alter and improve their communication patterns, define their desired relationships, and clarify their roles

D. Milieu (applicable in residential hospital settings)
    1. Recognizes that clients and staff members influence each other as they are influenced by others
    2. Promotes collaboration of staff and clients to achieve goals
    3. Encourages clients to participate actively in recovery by solving problems arising from group living, developing rules for living, learning to manage conflict, and dealing effectively with relationships

---

Growth and development

Introduction

A vital aspect of the nursing role is to understand the client's physical, cognitive, and psychosocial levels of growth and development. This entry reviews psychosocial and cognitive development together with physical-motor and social-play development throughout the life span. Ages listed are approximate.

Overview of psychosocial development

Erik Erikson postulated a theory of personality development that begins with Freudian theory but emphasizes the *healthy* aspects of personality development rather than the pathologic ones, building from predictable, age-related stages. Erikson describes key conflicts or core problems from which, after successful completion or mastery of one problem, the individual moves on to the next problem. Each conflict has a favorable and unfavorable component. No core problem is ever solved in its entirety. With each new situation, the core problem demands another resolution.

Sense of trust versus mistrust: Birth to age 1

Development of basic trust is the most important aspect of a healthy personality. The infant, through the relationship with a primary caregiver (usually the mother), learns that basic needs will be met. Consistent, loving care by a caregiver who touches, holds, caresses, feeds, and cleans the infant builds this sense of trust. When care is inconsistent, deficient, or lacking, or when basic needs remain unmet, the infant learns mistrust.

Implications for nursing include parent education on infant care techniques that promote the infant's sense of trust. From a basic trusting relationship with primary caregivers, the infant develops self-trust and trust in others. This stage corresponds to the *oral* stage described by Sigmund Freud.

Sense of autonomy versus shame and doubt: Age 1 to 3

The infant who has developed basic trust can then proceed to autonomy (independence) and body control (trust). The child now has the physical and motor ability to get around independently, together with an increasing ability to manipulate the environment and other people. The child can hold on or let go. One obvious example of this is sphincter control—the child can dominate a household with toileting! The child wants to use these new powers and skills to do things independently. Rituals, negativism, and temper tantrums reflect uncertainties associated with gaining mastery and control. Lingering feelings of shame and doubt will result if the child is made to feel small, shamed, or unnecessarily dependent. This stage corresponds to Freud's *anal* stage.

Application of nursing knowledge during this stage focuses first on assessing, via family history, the child's usual routine, use of physical security objects, and sensorimotor independence, and then on facilitating maximal consistency in these areas. The skillful nurse will assist caregivers in offering choices to the child and in not chastising or shaming the child in response to negative behaviors. Accepting and explaining the child's regressive behaviors in response to illness and stress are important nursing activities.

Sense of initiative versus guilt: Age 3 to 6

Vivid imagination, magical thinking, a budding sense of right and wrong, and increased awareness of body parts characterize this period of personality development. The child's imagination engenders fantasies and stories that the child believes. Anxiety may give rise to night terrors, fears of bodily mutilation, physical aggression, and "acting out" behaviors. This stage corresponds to Freud's *phallic stage*.

Nursing planning and interventions for the preschooler include providing concrete explanation and demonstration of treatments and procedures and opportunity for acting-out participatory play. Avoid threatening terminology, such as "cutting off" a body part when explaining a surgical procedure; encourage outward expression of fear, anxiety, anger, and pain; and shun labeling behavior as "good" or "bad."

Sense of industry versus inferiority: Age 6 to 12

During this stage, the child becomes a success-oriented worker and producer. Aspiring to be best in everything—games, school, making friends, building models, and completing projects—the child begins tasks and activities that can be seen through to conclusion and gradually learns the social skills of cooperation, compromise, negotiation, completion, and achievement. The child learns to play and live by rules. Because winning and being successful are so important, the child does not like to fail or to get behind in schoolwork. The child is very sensitive. Feeling wronged, having failed in some way, or having not met someone's expectations at school, the child will avoid going to school. Feelings of inadequacy may lead to feelings of inferiority. This stage corresponds to Freud's *latent* stage.

Nursing interventions during this phase include promoting activities that the child can complete independently and fostering the child's self-esteem by praising achievements and appropriate behavior.

Sense of identity versus role diffusion: Age 12 to 19

Similar to the toddler searching for autonomy, the adolescent, in seeking to gain personal identity, often demonstrates negativism (resistance to parental authority and values), ritualism (for example, a desire for brand-name clothing, stereotyped vocabulary, peer social activities), and emotional lability—all reflecting the emotional turmoil involved in the uncertain outcome of dramatic body image changes and the question "Who am I?" Peers significantly influence adolescent values and decision making. Unresolved answers to the complex questions of adolescence may lead to role diffusion. This stage corresponds to Freud's *puberty* stage.

Nursing care during this period should focus on involving the adolescent in decision making as much as possible, mutually setting goals, and encouraging the adolescent's active participation in implementing a care plan. Supplies needed to enhance body image (for example, shampoo or a hair dryer) should be made readily available to the hospitalized adolescent. The nurse should impose as few limits as possible—and expect even those to be challenged. Awareness of the potential impact of any threat to body image, whether temporary (pimple) or permanent (amputation), also mandates the nurse's use of therapeutic communication skills.

Sense of intimacy versus isolation: Age 20 to 40

During this stage, developmental tasks involve the ability to share and to form commitments with other persons without fearing the loss of one's own identity. When they do not achieve intimacy, individuals focus on their own needs to the exclusion of all other interests.

The nurse assesses the stresses and changes experienced during this period and provides teaching and resources to help the client maintain health. A client who requires hospitalization, especially prolonged hospitalization, may face lost employment benefits, a disrupted lifestyle, and decreased self-esteem. The nurse must not be judgmental of the client's needs and lifestyle and must refrain from imposing personal attitudes.

Sense of generativity versus stagnation: Age 40 to 65

Generativity means helping the next generation become adults. During this stage of life, the individual assumes work, family, and community responsibility. Individuals who fail to develop responsibilities become egocentric, care only about themselves, and do not develop further.

The nurse should consider the many responsibilities and stresses affecting the client during this period, assessing the client in relation to these stresses and providing resources and emotional support not only to the client but also to the client's family and friends.

Sense of integrity versus despair: Age 65 years and older

During this period, people review their life events. If those events satisfy them, they are content. If not, they become hopeless and desperate.

The nurse should recognize the physical and social changes occurring during this period and the limitations they may place on an individual. At the same time, the nurse should promote independence and the use of skills that the client retains. The nurse needs to encourage each client to perform self-care at the client's own pace. Stimulation of functioning senses becomes highly important. The nurse must treat each client as an adult even if the client behaves like an adolescent or child. The elderly client whose friends, relatives, and contemporaries die will need emotional support when evaluating life's events.

Overview of cognitive development

Jean Piaget developed the best known and most comprehensive theory regarding children's thinking, or *cognition*. The development of cognition represents a continuous and orderly process. Piaget postulated four major stages, each derived from and based on accomplishments of the previous stage.

Sensorimotor: Birth to age 2
In this stage of simple learning, the child progresses from reflex activity to repetitive behavior and then to imitative behavior. Displaying a high level of curiosity, the child begins to develop a sense of self as different and separate from the environment.

The child learns that objects have permanence and existence even if they are not visible. Examples of this development are the emerging social smile and differentiated cry of the infant, progressing to the self-exploration of hands, then feet. The infant imitates pattycake and then peek-a-boo, finally realizing that the hidden object is still there. (See "Physical-motor and social-play development" for other examples of this progression.)

Preoperational: Age 2 to 7
The inability of the young child to empathize characterizes this stage, in which the child interprets objects and events solely in relationship to self.

The child cannot make deductions or generalizations. Learning and thinking embrace only what the child sees, hears, feels, or experiences. With increasing language skills, imaginative play, questioning, and interacting, the child begins to elaborate concepts and "correct" experiences. Near the end of this stage, reasoning becomes intuitive and the child begins to work with problems of weight, length, size, and time.

Concrete operations: Age 7 to 11
As a result of increasingly logical and coherent thought, the child can now sort, classify, order, and organize facts about the world. The child collects and saves everything from stamps to crickets and toads. Although containers may differ, the child realizes that weight, volume, and number may be the same; problem solving proceeds in a concrete manner.

Although the child can deal with several aspects of a situation at one time, abstractions remain incomprehensible. The child can now recognize other points of view, however, as evidenced by a stronger desire for companionship and teamwork.

Formal operations: Age 12 to 15
During this period, characterized by flexibility, the adolescent learns to deal with abstractions and abstract symbols. Arriving at answers, the adolescent may confuse the ideal world with the real world but can nevertheless solve problems, develop

Physical-motor and social-play development

hypotheses, test them, and reach conclusions. The adolescent, working through moral, ethical, religious, and social issues, begins to achieve an adult identity.

Normal physical and motor development is usually categorized by age level, although each person's development is ongoing and unique, and progress in one level may overlap into another. Such overlap is also true of social or play behaviors, which correspond with physical-motor developmental levels. The following discussion presents behaviors of special interest when providing nursing care.

Birth to 3 months

The infant's physical-motor skills develop quickly. At 1 month, the infant's eyes will follow bright, moving objects; at 2 months, the crossed-eye reflex disappears; at 3 months, a stimulus evokes a social smile response. Also at 3 months, the infant can rest on the forearms, keeping the head in midline, and discovers hands and stares at them. Stepping reflex disappears and Landau reflex appears. Now able to lift the head and chest, the infant holds a rattle and stares at it and can follow any moving object with the eyes.

Social-play skills also emerge. The infant responds when a caregiver shakes a rattle or dangles a bright, moving object (such as a mobile). The infant also responds favorably to the caregiver's smiles, caresses, and speech. When the infant is awake, the caregiver should rock, pat, and play with the infant and change his or her position regularly. During this time, the infant usually reacts positively to a busy box and enjoys the freedom to kick. The caregiver should put the infant in a prone position on the floor. The infant expresses demands by crying, enjoys sucking, and reacts affectionately to all who approach. By the third month, the infant coos, babbles, gurgles, and laughs aloud; responds to his or her name; shows pleasure; and makes sounds and faces in reaction to the social play of others.

4 to 6 months

During this time, the infant holds the head up for longer periods, displays improved eye coordination, and turns from the back to the side. At 5 months the infant can sit with support and at 6 months can turn over completely. By the 5th or 6th month, birth weight doubles, and the infant begins to turn the head toward familiar sounds.

The 4-month-old infant recognizes his or her parents, demands attention by fussing, grasps objects with both hands, and shows excitement with the whole body. By 5 months, the infant is playing with the toes and smiling at a mirror image. At 6 months, the infant holds out arms to be picked up and shows definite likes and dislikes.

6 months

The 6-month-old infant can raise the chest and upper abdomen, keeping the weight on the hands, and can sit in a high chair with a straight back. Now able to turn from the back to the abdomen, the infant can hold a bottle or eat a cracker independently and can grasp the feet and pull them to the mouth. Teething may begin at this time.

Social development is characterized by loud laughter, the ability to distinguish familiar and strange faces, and the desire to be picked up and held. The infant enjoys rattles and stuffed toys, displays frequent mood swings, and begins imitating others (for instance, by coughing or sticking out the tongue).

7 months

The infant can sit and lean forward on the hands and can transfer objects from one hand to the other. Upper central incisors typically erupt during this period. Socially, the infant begins to display a fear of strangers. Oral aggressiveness (biting) is evident, and the infant will reject disliked foods by keeping the mouth closed.

8 months

The infant shows increased bowel and bladder regularity, sits steadily, releases objects at will, and exhibits a beginning pincer grasp. Social development during this time is primarily characterized by the infant's dislikes, such as for getting dressed or having a diaper changed.

9 months

By this time, the infant can typically pull to a standing position, and upper lateral incisors may erupt. Socially, the infant begins to exhibit a fear of being left alone.

10 months

Although crawling most of the time, the infant can step with one foot if supported by a person or an object. The infant by now has a neat pincer grasp but a crude release. New social-play behavior patterns emerge and others continue. Fear of strangers increases, and scolding elicits a strong reaction. The infant continues to imitate others (as when waving "bye-bye") and looks at and follows pictures in a book.

11 months

By now the child is creeping, with the abdomen off the floor, and can stroll while holding on to a person or an object. Able to put objects into a container and remove them, the child also begins to drop objects deliberately—either to marvel at their sound or to gain the attention of others. During this period the child begins to learn self-feeding and will help with dressing. Playing games such as peek-a-boo and shaking the head "no" are common.

12 months

Having tripled in weight, the 1-year-old child can sit alone and can roll over. The child usually has eight teeth by the end of the 1st year.

If not already evident, the child develops a fear of strangers and clings to the mother. Able to understand simple commands, the child can also help with dressing and points to indicate desired objects. As social-play skills become more sophisticated, the child discriminates in giving affection and shows fear, anxiety, and sympathy. Having learned to repeat behaviors that elicit laughter, the child continues to imitate, wave "bye-bye," and shake the head "no."

10 to 14 months

Creeping and crawling for locomotion, the child can pull up to a standing position independently and can stand for extended periods with support. By the end of this stage, the child is walking with a broad, stiff-legged gait. The stage is also characterized by attempts at self-feeding with a spoon, poking and probing with the index finger, and a fondness for finger foods.

13 to 15 months

The child likes to empty containers and fill boxes, drops objects intentionally, can put a spoon to the mouth and drink from a cup, and hands objects to people. Able to creep upstairs, the child cannot come down; attempts to back downstairs begin at 15 to 16 months. The child can build two-block towers and put a round peg in a round hole.

Socially, the child wants to be with adults but also enjoys playing alone, exploring kitchen cupboards, and imitating housekeeping duties. At this time the child does not differentiate sex roles. Displaying a fondness for kissing pictures and mirrored reflections, the child asks for things by pointing and grunting. He can remove shoes and perform self-feeding. By now the child wants and enjoys an audience and is capable of affection and sympathy, especially in the form of sympathetic crying.

16 to 24 months

With physical-motor skills blossoming, the child explores the physical world widely and is all over the house. Falling less frequently now, the child walks backward with a broad-based gait; walks forward and runs with a stiff, wide-based gait; and stoops to pick up toys. The child can throw a ball and unzip zippers; loves to push, pull, tug, bang, carry, and hug toys; and manages a spoon without rotation. By 15 to 18 months, the anterior fontanel closes.

The child continues to play solitarily, is profoundly ritualistic, and exerts control with temper tantrums. At 18 months, sphincter control begins (the child controls adults through toileting). The child likes to clean up messes, flush the toilet, run water, and put things in their place; uses push-pull, noisy toys; points to body parts on request; shows sustained interest; imitates others; finds security in thumb sucking or in a favorite blanket or toy; and becomes easily frustrated and angry. Personal identity begins, with differentiation between "you" and "me."

Age 2

The child can put on shoes and pants, wash and dry hands, begin to use scissors and string large beads, and undress. The 2-year-old child tries to dance; pinches, kicks, hits, and bites; goes up and down steps one at a time; and can turn pages. Still ritualistic, the child engages in solitary and some parallel play; imitates older children; uses three-word phrases; is shy with strangers (negativism peaks at 2 years); develops fears of bed-wetting, animals, and being deserted; may become a fussy eater; and displays slower growth.

Age 3

The child can ascend steps with alternating feet, ride a tricycle, copy a circle, build a nine- to ten-cube tower, and perform self-feeding completely. The child's pulse rate is about 95 beats/minute; respiratory rate, about 24 breaths/minute; and blood pressure, 100/67 (±25) mm Hg.

By this time, the child has developed a vocabulary of about 900 words, displays telegraphic speech, and is constantly asking questions. The child knows his or her own sex and identifies with it, engages in parallel and associative play, and can better tolerate brief separation from the parents or the primary caregiver.

Age 4

The child hops on one foot, skips, catches a ball, throws overhand, uses scissors, and can lace (but not tie) shoes.

Questioning reaches a peak during this time, and exaggerated stories and mild profanity are typical. The child cannot conceive that, although an object's shape may change, its mass remains the same; judges by one dimension (centering); has developing sense of right and wrong; identifies strongly with parent of opposite sex; and still experiences many fears.

Age 5

Eruption of permanent teeth may begin. The child jumps rope and can tie shoelaces.

Social development also continues. The child can now identify coins and name at least four colors, knows the days of the week, engages in cooperative play, attempts to resolve fears and anxieties through play, tries to be brave, and is independent in self-care activities, such as bathing and dressing.

Age 6

With increased activity, the child's appetite increases; plain food, snacking, and eating on the run become favored by the 6 year old, who begins to dislike bathing. Possessing more poise and greater control of motor abilities, the child is in constant motion, practicing coordination of large and fine motor groups.

Temper tantrums reappear at age 6. Becoming more self-centered, boastful, and bossy, the child enjoys dramatic play to enact feelings and often is "fresh," rude, and ready to fight. During this stage, fears develop concerning the supernatural, unusual noises, the mother's death, and any self-injury, and persistent night terrors are common.

Age 7 to 9

The child begins to lose baby teeth at age 6 to 7, with first molars coming in at about age 7. Physical-motor changes at ages 7, 8, and 9 are subtle, but the child develops better coordination of physical and motor skills and practices to achieve perfection. Less brisk and wiggly than at age 6, the child's movements are more fluid and graceful.

During this time, the child is more likely to shout than act out; resists bathing less and shows little interest in clothes; prefers to play with the same sex; competes but does not like to lose; and withdraws from situations rather than resist. More contemplative than before, the child can be moved by sad stories and is becoming a real family member with chores and responsibilities. The gang stage begins; close relationships with peers begin to take shape. The child begins to collaborate and compromise; the major fear is failure.

Age 10 to 12

Rapid changes in height, weight, body contour, and physiology typically coincide with an increased appetite and an awkwardness in motor ability. With such rapid growth, the child begins to envision adulthood. Onset of secondary sex characteristics occurs in some boys, and girls can no longer compete with boys in physical strength. At this stage, the child requires an adequate explanation of body changes, and one who lags behind in physical development needs special understanding as he or she compares body changes with those of classmates and friends.

During this stage, girls usually seem wiser and more poised than boys. For both sexes, companionship becomes more important than play as a social behavior. Club membership and teamwork play increasingly significant roles, although the sexes tend to remain apart. The child likes to run errands, enjoys crafts and music, and seeks others' ideas and opinions.

CONCEPTS AND SKILLS

Age 13 to 16

The early teenager may be awkward and uncoordinated, with poor posture, and may tire easily because heart and lung growth does not keep pace with that of the rest of the body. Although the adolescent has a large appetite, a preference for fast foods and fad diets can lead to poor nutrition and lethargy. Physiologic problems that concern the teenager include acne, increased perspiration, and a propensity to blush easily. The teenager develops a full growth of pubic and axillary hair.

The adolescent likes parties, dances, movies, daydreaming, telephone conversations, books, and hobbies. The peer group becomes extremely important. While beginning to become emancipated from the parents, the adolescent develops crushes on or attachments to neighbors or teachers. During this stage, the adolescent typically shows increased interest in the opposite sex, and strong friendships develop with one or two friends. Concerns embrace morality, ethics, religion, and social customs. The adolescent requires help in adjusting to and accepting body changes.

Age 17 to 19

A young man has a beginning beard, his structural growth is near completion, and his physique is that of a mature male, including genital size and pubic hair. A young woman may grow 2 to 4 inches taller after menarche; breasts and pubic hair have reached adult development, and she is capable of reproduction about 1 year after menses begins. Both the young man and the young woman have more energy as the growth spurt slows.

The young adult is more mature and begins to enjoy an interdependent relationship with the parents while finding increasingly less satisfaction from the peer group. Learning to balance pleasure and responsibility, the young adult engages in romantic love affairs and may still daydream about adult life but also begins to establish career goals and plan how to achieve them. Parents may need assistance facing the loss of their dependent child.

Age 20 to 30

Physical strength and physiologic reserve are at a maximum, and the person's health needs usually are not significant.

Body image and sexuality are extremely important during this time. Selection of a marriage partner—and perhaps the decision to have children—commonly occurs. Marriage and parenthood necessarily entail periods of adjustment fraught with increased stresses, such as changing one's lifestyle to accommodate children and socializing the children into the family. Optional lifestyles (celibacy, childless marriage, single parenthood, homosexuality, communal living) may also develop, each of which has inherent stresses and periods of adjustment, compromise, and change.

Age 30 to 40

As physical strength, physiologic reserve, and systemic functioning begin to diminish, proper nutrition becomes more important. The person requires fewer fats and calories in the diet and may require more vitamins and iron. Exercise is essential to regulate appetite, release tension, enhance rest and sleep, increase muscle tone, and improve the person's well-being.

Choice of vocation and career successes and failures largely determine the person's social status and roles. Unemployment or unsatisfying employment may lower self-esteem. Hectic schedules and limited income during this phase may contribute to an unhealthful diet. To attain career goals, the person may work or worry excessively, at the expense of needed sleep and relaxation.

Age 40 to 65

Physical strength, physiologic reserve, and systemic functioning continue to diminish, mandating a low-calorie, high-vitamin diet with limited saturated fat. Exercise is still important but should be less strenuous. During this stage, the person may have concerns about stiff joints, wrinkles, gray hair, baldness, dentures, poor hearing or vision, menopause, osteoporosis, nervousness, or depression. Angina and coronary occlusion, cancer, hypertension, peptic ulcer, and (if the person smokes) respiratory disease are common. Stresses during this phase may lead to substance abuse or insomnia. Sexual problems may also develop; mutilating surgery, chronic disease, or menopause can dramatically lower the person's self-esteem, particularly if the sexual partner does not provide emotional support.

Assuming more significant and varied roles at this stage than at any other stage in the life span, the adult is now responsible not only for the self, spouse, and children but for parents, co-workers, and community members. As children grow up and begin their own families, the adult in this stage may need to rethink goals and consider lifestyle changes. The empty nest syndrome may occur, causing depression. A woman sometimes sees this period as an opportunity to continue education and enter or resume a career; a man may need to prepare for a second vocation.

Age 65 and over

Physical strength, physiologic reserve, and systemic functioning decline. Hearing and vision loss may be more pronounced, and cataracts may require surgery. Other common geriatric problems include immobility, constipation, indigestion, arteriosclerosis, stroke, peripheral vascular disease, hypertension, coronary occlusions, and cancer. A man may have benign prostatic hypertrophy or experience the climacteric. A woman may have osteoporosis, resulting in bone fractures. The elderly person may have multiple chronic illnesses, with accompanying exacerbations and remissions. Prolonged bed rest proves highly detrimental during this stage— lack of exercise can impair digestion, circulation, muscle and joint function, and mental alertness. Decreased sensitivity of taste buds and olfactory receptors typically causes the elderly adult to overseason foods. Exercise, though important, must be tailored to individual needs.

Having worked hard to achieve career goals, the elderly adult wants to enjoy the carefree leisure of retirement. Pursuing hobbies, spending time with family and friends, and participating in community events can provide enjoyment and satisfaction. The new lifestyle usually means living on a fixed income, however; thus, the person with an inadequate income worries about the present and the future and may live with other persons on fixed incomes simply to make ends meet. Declining health and the loss of family and friends can result in grieving, loneliness, and depression during this stage, and some persons withdraw from society (disengagement). Because reconciliation is important to many elderly adults, misunderstandings may be forgotten and relationships improved.

Nutrition

I. Introduction

A. Nutrition is the process by which foods are selected and ingested and their nutrients are absorbed and used by the human body

B. The essential nutrients are carbohydrates, fats, protein, vitamins, and minerals (Water, essential to sustain life, transports nutrients throughout the body and may contribute minerals when consumed)

C. Foods contain the nutrients and energy that the body requires for growth, activity, and health maintenance

D. All people require the same nutrients, but the amounts needed vary according to sex, age, size, activity level, and state of health

II. Food selection guidelines

A. Individual food preferences are influenced not only by the taste and odor of specific foods but also by the availability of foods, family economic status, cultural and religious preferences and restrictions, and the food purchaser's knowledge of nutrition

B. Several guidelines have been developed to help individuals plan and evaluate food intake

C. Recommended dietary allowances (RDAs), intended for use primarily by health care professionals, are levels of essential nutrients considered adequate for meeting the nutritional needs of 97.5% of the healthy population

   1. Daily consumption of various foods from different food groups provides the best means of meeting RDAs

   2. RDAs are not to be confused with the U.S. Recommended Daily Allowances (USRDAs), separate standards used by the Food and Drug Administration for nutrition labeling purposes

D. Recommended daily servings from the basic food groups constitute a nutritious daily food plan (see *Food Guide Pyramid*)

E. Dietary Guidelines for Americans, most recently revised in 1990 by the U.S. Department of Agriculture and the Department of Health and Human Services, emphasize health improvement by reducing the intake of harmful foods and stressing moderation in eating habits

   1. Eat a variety of foods

   2. Maintain a healthy weight

   3. Avoid excessive fat (especially saturated fat) and cholesterol

   4. Eat plenty of vegetables, fruits, and grain products

   5. Avoid excessive sugar

   6. Avoid excessive sodium

   7. Drink alcohol in moderation, if at all

III. Energy needs and balance

A. Energy is required for basal metabolism—ongoing internal processes such as respiration, heartbeat, and glandular activity

B. The rate of this metabolism, the basal metabolic rate (BMR), is influenced by sex, age, body composition, and physiologic status

C. The energy value of foods is measured in kilocalories, commonly known as calories

   1. Carbohydrates, fats, and protein are the only nutrients that supply calories

Food guide pyramid

Each of these food groups provides some, but not all, of the nutrients you need. No one food group is more important than another—for good health you need them all. Go easy on fats, oils, and sweets, the foods in the small tip of the pyramid.

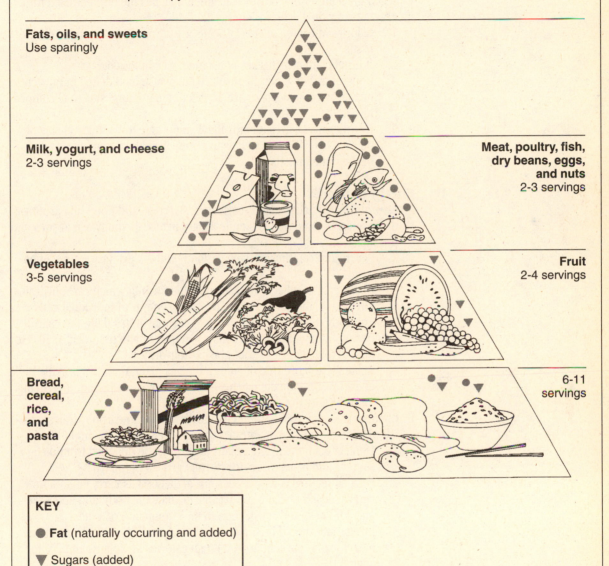

Fats, oils, and sweets
Use sparingly

Milk, yogurt, and cheese
2-3 servings

Meat, poultry, fish, dry beans, eggs, and nuts
2-3 servings

Vegetables
3-5 servings

Fruit
2-4 servings

Bread, cereal, rice, and pasta

6-11 servings

KEY

● **Fat** (naturally occurring and added)

▼ Sugars (added)

These symbols show that fat and added sugars come mostly from fats, oils, and sweets, but can be part of or added to foods from the other food groups as well.

Source: U.S. Department of Agriculture, Human Nutrition Information Service, August 1992, Leaflet No. 572.

2. Carbohydrates and protein each provide 4 calories/g; fats provide 9 calories/g
3. Carbohydrates and fats are the preferred energy sources, leaving protein for its important role in tissue maintenance
4. Besides basal metabolism, calories are needed for physical activity and for the 10% increase in BMR that occurs after eating

D. When the number of calories consumed matches the number used for energy, an individual achieves energy balance
   1. Calories in excess of energy needs are stored as fat in body adipose tissue
   2. If insufficient calories are consumed, weight loss occurs
   3. Undernutrition generally results from a sustained deficit in nutrient intake; as protein stores are depleted, the immune system is compromised
   4. Overnutrition leaves an individual vulnerable to the toxic effects of nutrient overdoses as well as to excess weight gain and associated health impediments

IV. Energy nutrients

A. *Carbohydrates* occur mainly as sugars, starches, and fiber; all carbohydrates must be modified to simple sugars before the body can absorb and use them
   1. Sugars and starches provide the body with its primary source of energy
   2. Glucose, also called blood sugar, is the form in which carbohydrates circulate in the bloodstream, providing energy to individual cells
   3. The body requires at least 100 g of carbohydrates daily, the central nervous system needing a constant supply of glucose; ideally, 50% to 60% of total calories should be carbohydrates
   4. Although not a source of energy, fibrous plant materials provide bulk, and a low fiber intake has been linked with constipation, diverticulitis, and cancer of the colon

B. Commonly known as fats (and chemically similar to carbohydrates), *lipids* provide the most concentrated source of energy to the body
   1. Linoleic acid, the essential fatty acid, must be obtained from dietary sources and is necessary for normal growth of infants
   2. Besides serving as an energy source, dietary fats carry fat-soluble vitamins, cushion vital body organs, insulate the body, and add a feeling of fullness and satisfaction to the completion of a meal
   3. Ideally, fats should be limited to 30% of total calories; the requirement for linoleic acid is 3% of total calories for infants and 2% for adults
   4. In choosing dietary fats, consider the benefits of fish (such as mackerel or tuna), which contain omega-three fatty acids, and oils (such as peanut, canola, or olive oil), which contain monounsaturated fatty acids; both groups of fatty acids help reduce the risk of coronary heart disease

C. *Protein* provides the foundation for all body cells
   1. Protein is broken down by the body into its individual components, the amino acids
   2. Eight essential amino acids cannot be made by the body and must be obtained from food
   3. The principal function of protein is to provide the amino acids needed for growth and the formation of enzymes, hormones, antibodies, muscles, hemoglobin, and other body tissues

Reviewing selected vitamins

	MAJOR FUNCTIONS	PRIMARY SOURCES	CLINICAL DEFICIENCIES	TOXICITIES
Water-soluble vitamins				
Vitamin C	Collagen formation, wound healing, resistance to stress and infection, blood vessel elasticity	Citrus fruit, strawberries, broccoli, cabbage, green peppers	Easy bruising, bleeding gums, delayed wound healing, scurvy	Gastrointestinal upset, diarrhea, kidney stones
Thiamine (B_1)	Carbohydrate metabolism, nerve transmission	Pork, peanuts, whole grains	Poor appetite, leg cramps, depression	None
Riboflavin (B_2)	Carbohydrate, protein, and fat metabolism; normal appetite	Milk, meat, wheat germ	Mouth lesions, scaly skin, glossitis	None
Niacin	Carbohydrate, protein, and fat metabolism; healthy skin	Meat, peanuts, whole grains	Pellagra, dermatitis, diarrhea, depression	Flushing, tingling, vision disturbances
Pyridoxine (B_6)	Amino acid synthesis, fatty acid metabolism	Meat, whole grains, nuts	Skin lesions, depression, seizures	None
Folic acid	Nucleic acid synthesis, amino acid breakdown, red blood cell formation	Green, leafy vegetables; asparagus; broccoli	Slow growth, megaloblastic anemia	None
Cyanocobalamin (B_{12})	Formation of nucleic acids, bone marrow, and red blood cells	Meat, eggs, fish	Pernicious anemia, nervousness, weakness	None
Fat-soluble vitamins				
A (retinol)	Normal vision and growth, healthy epithelium, aid to reproduction	Dark green and yellow fruits and vegetables, margarine and butter, whole milk and cheeses	Night blindness, thickened cracked skin, poor growth, reduced resistance to infection	Skin rashes, hair loss, vomiting, abnormal bone growth, increased intracranial pressure
D (cholecalciferol)	Absorption and utilization of calcium and phosphorus, bone matrix formation	Sunlight, fortified milk	Rickets (in children), osteomalacia (in adults)	Elevated serum calcium, kidney damage, growth retardation, vomiting, diarrhea
E (tocopherol)	Antioxidant (protects cell membrane)	Vegetable oils, margarine, nuts, whole grains	None	Headache, nausea, fatigue, dizziness, blurred vision
K (menadione)	Blood clotting (prothrombin formation)	Intestinal bacteria (synthesize adequate vitamin K)	Hemorrhage	Excessive breakdown of red blood cells (synthetic form)

CONCEPTS AND SKILLS

Reviewing selected minerals

	MAJOR FUNCTIONS	PRIMARY SOURCES	CLINICAL DEFICIENCIES
Calcium	Bone and tooth formation, blood clotting, muscle contraction, transmission of nerve impulses, normal heart rhythm	Milk, cheese, yogurt, broccoli, collards, kale, greens, canned salmon with bones	Osteoporosis, slow blood clotting, tetany, poor tooth formation
Phosphorus	Bone and tooth formation, carbohydrate and fat metabolism, pH buffer systems	Cheese, meat, milk and milk products, carbonated beverages	Osteoporosis, slow blood clotting, tetany, poor tooth formation
Magnesium	Carbohydrate, fat, and protein metabolism, adenosine triphosphate formation, nerve transmission, muscle contraction	Grains, green vegetables, milk, meat	Fluid and electrolyte imbalance, skin breakdown
Sodium	Fluid balance, nerve transmission, muscle contraction	Table salt, processed and preserved foods, milk and dairy products, protein foods	Headache, nausea, muscle spasm, mental confusion, fluid and electrolyte imbalance, cardiac disturbances, hypertension, edema
Potassium	Fluid balance, muscle activity	Widespread in all food groups, especially fruits and vegetables	Fluid and electrolyte imbalance, muscle weakness, tachycardia, cardiac arrhythmia, renal failure, severe dehydration

Trace elements

Iron	Hemoglobin formation (as component of myoglobin)	Meats, whole grains, dried fruit, legumes	Iron deficiency anemia
Iodine	Regulation of basal metabolic rate (as component of thyroxin)	Iodized salt, saltwater fish	Goiter
Zinc	Protein synthesis, normal growth and sexual maturation, wound healing, normal senses of taste and smell, enzyme formation	Meats, legumes, nuts	Slow wound healing, altered senses of taste and smell, poor growth, delayed sexual development
Fluoride	Strengthening of tooth enamel	Fluoridated drinking water, fluoride supplementation	50% to 70% increase in tooth decay

4. The adult requirement for protein is 0.8 g/kg of ideal body weight
5. Protein is 16% nitrogen
   a. In a healthy adult (except one who is pregnant or lactating), nitrogen intake equals nitrogen output
   b. With disease, tissue wasting occurs, and nitrogen losses exceed nitrogen intake; this negative nitrogen balance ceases when tissue repair begins
6. Insufficient protein intake can compromise the immune system, impairing the body's response to stress and infection

V. Vitamins and minerals
   A. Vitamins are needed daily in small quantities to sustain growth and health; they are classified as water-soluble or fat-soluble (for detailed information, see *Reviewing selected vitamins,* page 65)

B. Minerals are inorganic elements that help with many vital body functions and give the body its structural strength and rigidity (for detailed information, see *Reviewing selected minerals*)

VI. Nutrition requirements through the life cycle

A. The infant's nutritional needs are greater than those of any other age-group
   1. Protein and fluid needs are two to three times greater than those of an adult
   2. Breast milk or formula alone is satisfactory for the first 5 to 6 months of life, at which time solid foods should be incorporated into the daily diet

B. Childhood and adolescence are characterized by growth spurts that demand a gradually increasing intake of all nutrients; snacking, often thought a bane, can contribute significantly to nutritional quality, particularly in adolescent years

C. Nutritional needs of most adults under age 65 remain largely unchanged, with two exceptions
   1. Caloric and iron requirements generally decrease
   2. Pregnancy and lactation warrant special attention
      a. Sound nutritional practices during pregnancy usually lead to a higher birth weight
      b. Daily nutritional needs include increases in calories (+300) and iron (+15 mg); protein intake increases to 60 g/day and calcium to 1,200 mg/day
      c. The need for folic acid doubles during pregnancy and usually requires a vitamin supplement
      d. A weight gain of 24 to 30 lb (11 to 14 kg) is recommended, although a gradual gain over the last two trimesters is more important than the total amount gained
      e. Lactation requires even more calories than does pregnancy
         (1) Body fat reserves accumulated during pregnancy supplement the additional 500 dietary calories needed daily for lactation
         (2) An additional 2 quarts of fluid are needed daily to prevent dehydration and to produce an adequate milk supply

D. For those over age 65, adequate protein to maintain the immune system and muscle strength becomes increasingly important

Family: The primary unit of health care

I. Definitions of family

A. Basic social unit; the primary unit of health care

B. Traditional definitions
   1. Group of people united by blood, marriage, or adoption who live in the same household and share a common culture
   2. Traditional nuclear American family consisting of husband, wife, and children

C. Newer concepts
   1. One or more people who live together fulfilling certain roles and functions defined by the individual and the group
   2. Those bound by blood, love, or both
   3. Family unit without an adult

II. **Characteristics of families**
  A. Loving and affectionate relationships (usually)
  B. Long-term associations
  C. Consideration of members as unique individuals

III. **Functions of families**
  A. Care and rearing of children
  B. Transmission of cultural values, traits, and rituals from one generation to another
  C. Socialization
  D. Provision of food, shelter, clothing, safety, and comfort
  E. Communication and decision making

IV. **Types of families**
  A. Single adult living alone
  B. Beginning nuclear (husband and wife)
  C. Single parent
  D. Nuclear (husband, wife, and minor children; the most common family type in American society)
  E. Extended (three or more generations forming a kinship network)
  F. Expanded (various age or kinship groups or unrelated family members)
  G. Communal (formed for specific ideologic or societal purposes; may comprise nuclear, extended, or expanded family units)

V. **Developmental tasks and stages (Duvall, 1977)**
  A. Tasks
    1. Physical maintenance of the family unit
    2. Allocation of resources
    3. Division of labor
    4. Socialization of family members
    5. Reproduction or recruitment and release of family members
    6. Maintenance of order
    7. Placement of members into the larger society
    8. Maintenance of motivation and morale
  B. Stages in family life cycle
    1. Expanding families (from marriage and parenthood until children leave home)
      a. Childless couple establishing first home
      b. Expectant family or childbearing family (from first pregnancy through the first 30 months of the child's life)
      c. Family with preschool children
      d. Family with school-age children
      e. Family with teenagers
    2. Contracting families
      a. Family with young adults
      b. Middle-age parent family
      c. Aging family

VI. **Family assessment data**
   A. Family constellation (names, relationships, ages, sexes)
   B. Education levels
   C. Occupations
   D. Communication patterns
   E. Finances
   F. Residences
   G. Transportation needs
   H. Family goals and functioning
   I. Typical daily activities
   J. Religious preferences
   K. Avocation and recreational interests
   L. Health resources
   M. Strengths and coping mechanisms
   N. Weaknesses and problems
   O. Goals

Rehabilitation

I. **Definitions**
   A. Adaptation to living with a disability or handicap
   B. Activities that facilitate this adaptation

II. **Factors affecting rehabilitation**
   A. Severity or extent of injury (loss of some or all nerve pathways, muscles, bones, or circulation to a portion of the body)
   B. Treatment and facilities (immediacy, adequacy, and continuity of medical, surgical, nutritional, and pharmacologic treatments)
   C. The client's age, education, and psychological response to injury (all of which influence the client's ability to understand and participate in rehabilitative efforts)
   D. Health care personnel (those skilled in various disciplines to develop and administer a rehabilitation program)
   E. Financial resources (to pay for the facilities, treatments, and personnel services required for rehabilitation)
   F. Legislation (to protect the rights of clients requiring rehabilitation)

III. **Goals of rehabilitation**
   A. Short-term: to regain mobility, retain remaining abilities and, when possible, prevent further incapacity or disability
   B. Long-term: to return the functioning client to a normal environment

IV. **Activities and rehabilitation aids**
   A. Activities of daily living, including the ability to breathe; to dress, feed, bathe, move, and transfer oneself; to eliminate; and to communicate
   B. Exercises
      1. Use time and repetition to help a client regain or increase muscle tone, strength, and precision
      2. May involve therapists, family members, nurses, or other persons, depending on the client's needs or the expertise required

CONCEPTS AND
SKILLS

3. May be of several types
    a. Active (performed by the client)
    b. Active-assisted (performed by the client with therapist assistance)
    c. Resistive-active (performed by the client with resistance provided by weights or devices)
    d. Passive (performed without the client's active participation)
    e. Selective or special (individualized to meet a client's needs to exercise a particular group of muscles for particular activities; for example, breathing exercises)

C. Heat or cold therapy
    1. May be moist or dry
    2. May involve short-term or long-term application for vasoconstriction or vasodilation
    3. Must be intermittent to allow for tissue recovery (clients with impaired circulation have decreased tolerance for heat or cold therapy)

D. Ambulatory aids
    1. Walkers (lightweight, foldable, height-adjustable devices for assistance with weightbearing or mobility; the client must be cautioned about the safe degree of weightbearing and must be taught to turn, sit, or stand to prevent falls and injury)
    2. Crutches (wood or aluminum, axillary-supported or forearm-supported, with two-, three-, or four-point gaits; the client must learn to walk, sit, rise, and go up and down stairs with one or both crutches)
    3. Canes (wood or metallic supports with one-, three-, or four-point bottoms; if using only one cane, the client holds it in the hand *opposite* the affected leg)
    4. Wheelchairs (metal or wood and metal, with detachable arm or leg rests, straps, and other supports; may be battery operated or manually pushed; the client must learn to transfer correctly from the chair to a bed, car, and home)
    5. Braces (cloth, foam, or metallic supports for one or more joints; may be worn continuously or intermittently)
    6. Utensils (aid use by the handicapped; handles may be lengthened, enlarged, swiveled, hinged, or otherwise adapted for individual need)

E. Agencies for rehabilitative aid
    1. Bureau of Vocational Rehabilitation (for assistance in determining vocational interests, skills, and abilities and in finding aid for education and placement)
    2. Social Security Administration (for disability aid and services)
    3. Medicare and Medicaid (for primary or supplemental aid)
    4. Insurance companies (for individualized coverage)

F. Respiratory aids
    1. Postural drainage (to increase excretion of respiratory secretions)
    2. Incentive spirometry (to improve respiratory ventilation)
    3. Machine-assisted breathing apparatus (to increase respiratory depth and prevent atelectasis)

G. Genitourinary rehabilitation
    1. Continuous bladder catheterization
    2. Self-catheterization and bladder training
    3. Bowel-training programs
    4. Penile prosthesis (to help maintain an erection)
    5. Sexual counseling (to help the client cope with necessary adjustments)

H. Speech rehabilitation
   1. Speech therapy (to relearn the language or alternate speech methods)
   2. Mechanical speech-amplifying aids
I. Occupational therapy
   1. Home management—preparation, assistance, and learning
   2. Craft preparation and education for muscle use
   3. Occupational retraining of muscles, joints, and the entire body
J. Physical therapy
   1. Specialized retraining for muscle use or muscle substitution to regain or maintain muscle strength
   2. Assistance in any of the above rehabilitation techniques
K. Nutritional therapy
   1. Individualized dietary teaching for a client with a modified diet (high- or low-calorie, high-vitamin, high- or low-protein, acid ash, or low-sodium regimens or modifications, as needed)
   2. Modifications for home cooking and other food preparation and eating.

V.   Psychological responses to rehabilitation
A. Factors that influence the client's response
   1. Age and personality
   2. Severity or extent of injuries
   3. Potential for partial or full recovery
   4. The client's stress response pattern
   5. Initial and continued medical, nursing, and rehabilitative care
B. Common response pattern to rehabilitation
   1. First phase (disbelief)
      a. Primary behaviors: anger, hostility, withdrawal, apathy, denial
      b. Other symptoms: irritability, sleeplessness, tension, numbness, fears, and vague pains (some of these behaviors may reflect the "alarm" reaction of Selye's stress response from the "onset" or "stressful event" stage of crisis intervention models)
      c. Nursing considerations
         (1) Allow the client to express feelings
         (2) Accept dependency behaviors and provide care as needed
         (3) Encourage participation by the client and family, if appropriate
         (4) Refer the client for vocational rehabilitation, if appropriate
   2. Second phase (awareness, transition, impact, and perception of the event)
      a. Gradual realization of the extent of injury or disability
      b. Possible behaviors: depression, anxiety, anger, silence, sadness, and grief (grief, sadness, and crying may or may not directly correlate to the injury or disability, but they represent the client's personal responses to developing awareness)
      c. Nursing considerations
         (1) Keep the lines of communication open
         (2) Accept the client's outward expressions of grief, sadness, anger, and guilt
         (3) Encourage and teach self-care as the client becomes able
         (4) Seek a psychiatric consultation if the client prolongs reactions
         (5) Refer the client for vocational rehabilitation, if appropriate

CONCEPTS AND SKILLS

3. Third phase (use of coping mechanisms—resistance, reorganization, disequilibrium, and retreat)
   a. Gradual realization of the disability's permanence, wavering between acceptance and rejection
   b. Possible behaviors: self-pity (even while actively participating in care), bargaining (for relief from pain, physical therapy, and so forth), and extreme dependence on others for detailed care
   c. Nursing considerations
      (1) Continue to accept the client's expressions and behaviors
      (2) Encourage active participation in physical therapy, occupational therapy, hydrotherapy, and so forth, as the client's condition dictates
      (3) Teach the client and family self-care techniques
4. Fourth phase (resolution, convalescence, acknowledgment)
   a. Certainty of the disability's permanence, characterized by vacillation between rejection and acquiescence (the client gradually leans more toward tolerance and acceptance if reactions are "normal" or "healthy")
   b. Nursing considerations
      (1) Accept the client's vacillations while preparing and teaching self-care
      (2) Allow sufficient time and opportunities for the client and family to become confident and proficient in care procedures
      (3) Follow up on vocational rehabilitation referrals
5. Fifth phase (identity change, restoration of equilibrium, recovery, or exhaustion; regaining as much health as possible)
   a. Active participation of the client in self-care and preparation for discharge
   b. Preparation of the family for the client's return home or transfer to a rehabilitation unit
   c. Nursing considerations
      (1) Ensure that the client and family can perform self-care
      (2) Complete continuity-of-care referrals as needed

Grieving

I. **Grieving**
   A. Psychological process that allows one to cope with a loss and accept it as a reality; may last from 2 months to 1 year or longer
   B. Phases stated by Kübler-Ross
      1. Denial and isolation
      2. Anger
      3. Bargaining
      4. Depression
      5. Acceptance
   C. Phases stated by Engel
      1. Shock and disbelief, characterized by rejection or denial
      2. Developing awareness, characterized by weeping and lashing out at loved ones and others
      3. Restitution or resolution, characterized by integration of negative and positive aspects of the lost person or object so that the individual can confront the loss comfortably

---

Comparing grief and clinical depression

A client who appears to be suffering from clinical depression may actually be experiencing a phase of grieving. This chart shows the major distinctions between the two conditions.

Characteristics of grief	Characteristics of clinical depression
• Healthy response	• Unhealthy response
• Self-resolution	• Self-resolution unlikely
• Little if any guilt	• Overwhelming guilt
• Self-esteem intact	• Loss of self-esteem
• Sadness	• Hopelessness, despair, and helplessness
• Ability to meet life's demands intact	• Impaired ability to meet life's demands
• No biochemical imbalance	• Possible biochemical imbalance
• Temporary loss of interest in pleasurable activities (anhedonia)	• Pervasive anhedonia

---

II.   Significant losses that cause grief

    A. The client's impending death

    B. Loss of health, such as in cancer or another debilitating disease

    C. Loss of a body organ or part

    D. Loss or impending loss of a loved one (family member, friend, or pet)

    E. Loss of a treasured object (such as one's home)

III.   Goals of nursing interventions

    A. To help the client accept feelings and express concerns

    B. To help the client resolve anger and guilt

    C. To help the client "give up" the lost person or object

    D. To help the client remember comfortably both negative and positive aspects of the lost person or object

Principles of gerontologic nursing

I.   Introduction

    A. Since the early 1970s, the number of Americans over age 65 has been increasing dramatically; the U.S. government projects that there will be 70 million Americans over age 65 by 2030

    B. As the population ages, more demands are put on the health care delivery system by the elderly, forcing greater focus on their special needs

    C. The normal aging process leads to a steady deterioration in physical strength and to the development of chronic illnesses that threaten an older person's quality of life and independence

    D. Gerontologic nursing, conceived in the 1960s, concerns itself with the care of elderly clients and the development of processes that meet older adults' special needs

    E. Gerontologic nursing practice focuses on helping elderly clients maintain optimum autonomy despite physiologic, pathological, and psychosocial changes that occur during aging

II. Theories of the aging process

A. Developmental theories

1. In 1963, E. Erikson postulated that the major developmental task of the elderly was to choose between ego integrity and despair
   a. *Ego integrity* refers to accepting one's lifestyle and the choices made during life
   b. *Despair* refers to being dissatisfied with one's life and wishing for another chance to make different choices about how to live it
2. In 1972, R. Havighurst identified tasks that need to be completed during one's life
   a. Completion leads to contentment
   b. Unfulfillment leads to dejection and failure

B. Social theories

1. According to the *activity theory,* satisfaction with becoming older means living a middle-age lifestyle
2. According to the *continuity theory,* adjusting successfully to the aging process requires continuing the patterns of living that have been established over one's lifetime; old habits and ethical values provide continuity as one moves from one age phase to another

III. Changes associated with aging

A. Physiologic changes

1. Skin: becomes wrinkled, dry, thin, and pale; tends to sunburn and bruise easily
2. Cardiovascular: cardiac output and stroke volume decrease, pulse rate slows, blood pressure increases, peripheral pulses become weaker, especially in the legs
3. Respiratory: respiratory rate increases and lung expansion decreases, effective coughing is diminished
4. Musculoskeletal: diminished muscle mass and strength, trunk shortening, decreased joint mobility, bone demineralization
5. Nervous: slowed reflexes, reduced ability to respond to multiple stimuli, reduced cerebral circulation
6. Gastrointestinal: dry mouth, swallowing difficulties, decreased production of digestive enzymes and peristalsis, increased flatulence and constipation
7. Genitourinary: decreased kidney efficiency, voiding difficulties, urine retention, nocturia, incontinence
8. Reproductive: dyspareunia in females, vaginal itching and irritation, decreased estrogen, decreased size of penis and testes, delayed erection, decreased sperm count
9. Senses: diminished hearing, taste, smell, and vision; reduced ability to adapt to darkness and increased sensitivity to glare

B. Psychosocial changes

1. Stress about retirement and reduced income
2. Development of feelings of unworthiness because of perceived loss of productivity
3. Potential for social isolation
   a. Attitudinal isolation results from societal rejection because of age bias
   b. Presentational isolation results from social withdrawal because of changes in body image, mental or physical functional loss, or self-consciousness

        c. Behavioral isolation results from social withdrawal because of unacceptable social behavior, such as confusion, incontinence, or erratic behavior

   4. Reduced memory retention

   5. Changes to the environment

        a. Moving from a house or an apartment to a retirement community

        b. Reorganization of one's living environment to prevent falls

   6. Fear of dying

        a. Death to an elderly person is not always a "blessing"

        b. Elderly people still have goals they want to achieve and are not necessarily prepared to die until these goals are fulfilled

   7. Stress from loss of a significant other

IV. Gerontologic nursing process

A. Assessment

   1. Assess the client's developmental level to identify how he feels about aging

   2. Assess the client's functional level so appropriate goals and outcomes can be developed

   3. Assess the client's living environment to determine if adjustments are needed

   4. Determine if the client has health complaints that may need immediate attention to ensure optimum health

   5. Note financial and support resources available to assist the client in maintaining an optimum level of independent function

   6. Evaluate the client's coping skills so a realistic care plan can be developed

B. Nursing diagnoses

   1. Nursing diagnoses are developed from data obtained during the nursing history and physical examination

   2. Frequently expressed concerns by the older adult that may warrant a nursing diagnosis include:

        a. Sexual functioning difficulties

        b. Changes in physical appearance and function

        c. Concerns about social interaction

        d. Problems with grieving over loss of spouse

        e. Specific physical complaints

C. Planning and goals

   1. Goals should focus on assessment data

   2. Goals should be prioritized according to the nature of the problem

   3. Priority should be given to the client's perception of the problem's importance

   4. Goals should always be realistic and set to achieve the client's optimum level of independent function

D. Interventions

   1. Promote socialization to help the client build secondary social relationships

   2. Use therapeutic communication to build a trusting nurse-client relationship

   3. Use reality orientation to maintain or restore the client's sense of awareness

   4. Promote positive body image to build the client's self-confidence and to foster the willingness of others to interact with the client

5. Inform the client and family of the availability of health care services to ensure that health problems are adequately treated
6. Teach family members about respite care (short-term care given to a dependent client so that the permanent caregivers may have a break from the stress of continual-care responsibility)
7. Teach the client and family how to make their home safe and comfortable; this will minimize the risk of injury from falls and maximize the client's comfort at home
8. Promote ambulation and range-of-motion exercises to maintain muscle strength, stimulate circulation, and reduce the risk of pressure ulcers
9. Promote urinary and bowel continence to foster self-esteem and minimize the risk of institutionalization

E. Evaluations
   1. The client's response to the interventions is measured against the goals set in the care plan
   2. When outcomes do not match established goals, a revised care plan is developed
   3. Desired outcomes in a gerontologic nursing care plan include:
      a. Client maintains proper body alignment when sitting and walking
      b. Client actively engages in a planned activity program with others
      c. Client seeks out and maintains social contacts
      d. Client maintains urinary and bowel continence
      e. Client is oriented to person, place, and time
      f. Client is free of bodily injury
      g. Client knows how to seek health care and does so when needed

Principles of case management

I. Background information

A. Over the past decade, major changes within the U.S. health care delivery system have led to the proliferation of health maintenance organizations (HMOs), preferred provider organizations (PPOs), and managed care
B. The concept of managed care has dominated health care delivery in the 1990s and is expected to do so well into the 21st century
C. With this domination, the distinctions between delivery systems (for example, HMOs vs. PPOs) have become unclear; the systems share the common features of prenegotiated payment for services, precertification for care, utilization review, and limited choices in selecting a health care provider
D. Managed care has its roots in the public health nursing model, which provided for one nurse to assume responsibility for meeting (managing) the health care needs of a number of clients and families
E. The managed care delivery system has created the need for a specialized health delivery practitioner: the case manager
F. Professional nurses, by virtue of the breadth of their education and experience, are ideal case managers

II. The case management model

A. Definition and description

    1. Case management is a systematic approach to delivering total client care within specified time frames and economic resources

    2. Case management includes the client's entire illness episode, crosses all care settings in which care is received, and involves collaborating with all health personnel who care for the client

    3. Case managers focus on coordinating care for a client group with complex care requirements; the clients usually have similar diagnoses and needs, and they require common therapies

B. Goals of case management

    1. Case management attempts to direct client care to ensure:

        a. Quality of care

        b. Appropriateness of care

        c. Timeliness of services rendered

        d. Cost-effectiveness of care given

    2. The goals of case management remain the same regardless of the care setting

C. Critical pathways in case management

    1. Critical pathways are interdisciplinary care plans that must be carried out for a group of clients (caseload)

    2. Critical pathways are the tools for monitoring caseloads to ensure that clients reach desired outcomes

    3. Critical pathways can fall into one of two groups

        a. Medical-drug orders, diagnostic procedures, prescriptions for therapies

        b. Nursing comfort interventions, client-teaching activities, self-care activities

    4. Critical pathways are followed regardless of the health care setting

D. Roles of case managers

    1. Case managers are accountable for the appropriate delivery of health care services in a timely and cost-effective manner

    2. They use critical pathways to ensure that desired client outcomes are achieved

    3. They facilitate referrals to the multidisciplinary care team

    4. They supervise discharge planning

    5. They provide the client with appropriate resources to meet the care plan and troubleshoot for the client if problems occur

    6. They use quality assurance programs to evaluate the quality, timeliness, and cost-effectiveness of client care

E. Characteristics of case managers

    1. According to current guidelines established by the American Nurses Association, nurse case managers should:

        a. Hold a baccalaureate degree in nursing and a master's degree and certification as a clinical nurse specialist in the client's disease area

        b. Have 3 years of clinical nursing experience

    2. Case managers must possess expert knowledge to set client goals and outcomes, must clearly understand and be willing to work within the financial constraints of current health care systems, and must be skilled at developing strategies for quality improvement

    3. They must have highly developed skills of communication, negotiation, and collaboration with other health care providers

4. They must know which resources are available in health care facilities and the client's community

Principles of home health care

I. Introduction

A. The introduction of managed care to the U.S. health care delivery system has accelerated the need for providing more health care in the home

B. Clients with chronic health problems who used to receive periodic care in a hospital now are cared for exclusively at home

C. Early discharge of clients who have had surgery or an acute illness has raised the acuity level of clients in home care

D. Elderly clients with chronic illnesses are being treated at home with greater frequency, thereby raising the level of skills required by the caregivers

E. Nurses, the traditional providers of community-based care, are being called upon by the federal government, through Medicare regulations, home health agencies, and insurance providers, to direct the delivery of home health care, both skilled and unskilled

F. Providing effective home health care requires enhanced clinical skills and an understanding of home care rules and regulations

II. Home health care services

A. Home health care is the delivery of multidisciplinary health services to clients and their families wherever they live

B. The focus of home health care service is to restore the optimum level of client and family independence

C. Professional home health services include:
1. Skilled nursing care
2. Teaching health care
3. Interdisciplinary collaboration among professional health care providers to ensure cooperation, continuity of care, and compliance with government eligibility requirements
4. Identification and communication of community resources to help the client and family achieve care plan outcomes

D. Ancillary home health services include:
1. Home health aides
2. Housekeepers
3. Companions

E. Home health care equipment services include:
1. Beds and ambulatory aids
2. Portable dialysis units
3. Ventilators and infusion pumps

III. Factors that influence effective home care

A. Thorough family education about the health problem

B. Educated professionals trained in the relevant skills to deal with the health problem

C. Effective social support services

D. Appropriate living environment

E. Reliable transportation and local emergency health facility
F. Competent care managers

IV. Home health nursing

A. Clinical responsibilities
   1. Wound care: debriding and irrigating wounds, assessing wound healing, teaching wound care
   2. Drug therapy compliance: teaching drug actions, side effects, and administration schedules; monitoring drug therapy effectiveness and client compliance
   3. Nutrition: assessing the client's nutritional status, administering tube and parenteral feedings, teaching proper nutrition habits, monitoring diet compliance
   4. Elimination: providing enterostomal care, teaching the client and family the correct use of irrigation catheters and proper skin care, monitoring the client for infection
   5. Mobility: demonstrating use of assistive devices, performing range-of-motion exercises
   6. Infection control: teaching the family universal precautions, monitoring the home environment to identify areas that promote infection

B. Psychosocial responsibilities
   1. Being aware of socioeconomic factors and cultural and family dynamics in the client's home
   2. Recognizing that the home health nurse is a guest in the client's home
   3. Remaining nonjudgmental about the client's beliefs
   4. Accepting the client's ability to learn and willingness to follow directions

C. Legal and ethical responsibilities
   1. Complying with the laws and regulations regarding home care
   2. Working within an approved care plan
   3. Ensuring that physician collaboration on the treatment plan has been obtained
   4. Ensuring that the client's or family's written permission to enter the home has been obtained
   5. Maintaining confidentiality about the client's condition and treatment when asked by family, friends, or neighbors
   6. Providing documentation of care to ensure continued and optimum reimbursement for the client
   7. Understanding when and how to withdraw services when reimbursement authorization expires

D. Personal safety precautions
   1. Know the neighborhood and the safest route into and out of it
   2. Carry agency, police, and emergency facility phone numbers
   3. Inform the agency of daily visit schedule, with phone numbers of each client
   4. Report in to the agency by phone after each visit
   5. Do not drive an expensive automobile, wear expensive jewelry, or show a lot of money
   6. Do not enter the home if anyone is intoxicated, hostile, or demonstrating obnoxious behavior
   7. Never enter a home until invited, and leave if feeling unsafe

Principles of infection control

I. Introduction
A. For infection to occur, a series of events must be completed
   1. A causative organism must be present
   2. A reservoir host for the organism must exist
   3. A transmission route from the reservoir host to a susceptible host must be present
   4. A means of entry into the new host must exist
B. Preventing and controlling the spread of infection requires eliminating or blocking one or more of these events
C. As primary caregivers, nurses play a major role in preventing the onset and spread of infection
D. Well-established and proven interventions can prevent and control infection

II. Interventions for controlling infection
A. Prevent transmission
   1. Wash hands thoroughly before and after each client contact, after handling body fluids and wastes, and after handling contaminated equipment
   2. Use protective barriers
      a. Use gloves when handling open wounds, dressings, or contaminated equipment
      b. Wear a mask or respirator when caring for clients with airborne infections
      c. Wear a gown, goggles, and hair and shoe covers during potential exposure to sprayed body fluid
   3. Use isolation techniques
      a. Isolate a client with a communicable disease or one who could endanger the immediate environment with body fluids
      b. Place body substances in a leakproof or puncture-proof container, and bag soiled linen
B. Ensure proper teaching on infection
   1. Engage in client and family teaching
      a. Assess the client's knowledge level about infection
      b. Teach control measures to use in the home to prevent transmission
         (1) Frequent hand washing
         (2) Using separate dishes and utensils
         (3) Maintaining clean environment
         (4) Keeping vaccinations current
   2. Update staff teaching as needed
      a. Maintain immunizations
      b. Use universal precautions in client care (see *Universal precautions for health care workers*)
      c. Review the infection process with staff members
C. Maintain the client's protective defense mechanisms
   1. Ensure intact, healthy skin
      a. Promote regular bathing to remove organisms
      b. Suggest use of lubricants to keep skin hydrated and prevent cracking

Universal precautions for health care workers

Universal precautions are designed to protect health workers from infection by communicable diseases. They should be used in all health care settings.

I. Definitions
  A. Occupational exposure to blood and other materials
    1. Exposure: the reasonably anticipated skin, eye, mucous membrane, or parenteral contact with blood or other potentially infectious materials that may result from the performance of duties
    2. Parenteral: the piercing of mucous membranes or the skin barrier through such events as needlesticks, human bites, cuts, and abrasions
  B. Potentially infectious materials
    1. Human body fluids: semen, vaginal secretions, cerebrospinal fluid, synovial fluid, pleural fluid, pericardial fluid, peritoneal fluid, amniotic fluid, saliva, any body fluid that is visibly contaminated with blood, and all body fluids in situations in which it is difficult or impossible to differentiate one body fluid from another
    2. Any unfixed tissues or organ (other than intact skin) from a living or dead human
    3. HIV-containing cell or tissue cultures, organ cultures, and HIV- or HBV-containing culture medium or other solutions
II. Protection techniques
  A. Personal protective equipment
    1. Health care personnel at risk for exposure to potentially infectious materials must use protective equipment, such as gloves, gowns, face shields, resuscitation bags, pocket masks, or other ventilation devices
    2. Personal protective equipment is considered protective if it does not permit blood or other potentially infectious materials to pass through clothes, undergarments, skin, eyes, mouth, or other mucous membranes
    3. Masks, eye protection (such as goggles or glasses with solid side shields), and face shields must be worn whenever there is risk of splashes, spray, spatter, or droplets of blood or other infectious materials
  B. Hand washing
    1. Hands must be washed immediately and thoroughly if contaminated with blood or other fluids and after removal of gloves or other personal protective equipment
    2. Wash hands for at least 10 seconds before each new client contact and after gloves are removed
  C. Controlling sharp objects
    1. Contaminated needles and other sharp objects must not be bent, recapped, or removed by hand
    2. Immediately after use, contaminated reusable sharp objects must be placed in appropriate containers until properly reprocessed
    3. These containers must be puncture resistant, labeled or color-coded, and leakproof on the sides and bottom
III. Controlling body substances
  A. Specimens of blood or other potentially infectious materials must be placed in a container that prevents leakage during collection, handling, processing, storage, transport, or shipping
  B. Regulated waste must be placed in a container that is closable and constructed to contain all contents and prevent leakage during handling, storage, or transport
    1. Regulated waste includes liquid or semiliquid blood, body wastes, body fluids, or other potentially infectious materials; items caked with dried blood or infectious materials; and contaminated sharp objects
    2. The container shall be color-coded for ease of identification and closed before removal to prevent spillage or protrusion of contents
    3. If the outside of a container is contaminated, it must be placed in a second container and closed before removal
IV. Vaccines
  A. The hepatitis B vaccine and vaccination series should be available to all employees who have occupational exposure
  B. This service must be made available at no cost to the employee
V. Client isolation
  A. Assign an immunocompromised client to a private room or to a room with similarly immunocompromised clients
  B. Identify rooms of clients with airborne infections so that caregivers' susceptibility can be assessed
  C. Avoid roommates if moist body fluids are likely to be sprayed or dispersed about the room
VI. Cleaning
  A. Clean all rooms in which an infected client lives
  B. Clean blood and other body fluid spills with soap and water, a household detergent, or a solution of household bleach and water in a 1:10 dilution

Adapted from U.S. Department of Labor, OSHA: *Universal Precautions.* 1991.

   c. Encourage the client to practice regular oral hygiene, including tartar and plaque control, to reduce oral pathogens
   2. Maintain adequate nutrition and fluid intake
      a. Suggest a high fluid intake to promote frequent urination, which helps flush the client's system of microorganisms
      b. Encourage the client to follow a well-balanced diet, which promotes homeostasis and general resistance to infection
D. Establish an infection-control program
   1. A formal infection-control program is administered by an infection-control department composed of specially educated professionals
   2. Infection-control responsibilities include:
      a. Ensuring staff education
      b. Establishing infection-control procedures
      c. Conducting research on infection-control measures
      d. Providing a liaison to community and other health agencies

NURSING SKILLS

Physical assessment

I. **Overview**
   A. Constitutes an important part of the assessment phase of the nursing process
   B. Must be accurate and thorough to produce appropriate nursing diagnoses
   C. Requires effective communication techniques and interviewing skills
   D. Should be holistic and include a comprehensive health history that explores biopsychosocial factors relevant to the client's health status
   E. Consists of four physical examination techniques in which the nurse uses the senses to gather information about the client
      1. *Inspection:* using sight and smell to collect data (for example, observing the client's gait or detecting a fruity breath odor)
      2. *Palpation:* using touch (fingers and hands) to collect data (for example, taking a radial pulse)
      3. *Auscultation:* using hearing (primarily with the aid of a stethoscope) to detect sounds produced by certain body organs (for example, taking an apical pulse)
      4. *Percussion:* striking one object against another to generate a vibration that produces an audible sound wave (for example, percussing the lung fields); the least likely technique to be used by the novice nurse

II. **Health history**
   A. General health
   B. Childhood illnesses

C. Adult illnesses
D. Psychiatric illnesses
E. Operations
F. Injuries
G. Hospitalizations
H. Medications currently taken
    1.   Prescription
    2.   Nonprescription
I. Diet
J. Exercise
K. Alcohol intake
L. Tobacco use (number of cigarettes or cigars smoked per day)
M. Sleep patterns
N. Family history
O. Appliances (for example, dentures, prostheses, glasses)
P. Allergies
Q. Lifestyle (occupation and leisure-time activities)
R. Relationships with family and friends
S. Menstrual history
T. Client's perception of health
U. Family's or friends' perceptions of client's health
V. Residence (for example, urban or rural, one-story house or high-rise apartment, rent or own)

III. Physical examination
A. General overview (apparent state of health, signs of distress, motor activity, weight, facial expression, grooming, mood, state of awareness)
B. Vital signs
    1.   Blood pressure in both arms in lying, sitting, and standing positions
    2.   Pulses (carotid, abdominal aorta, femoral, tibial, pedal; take pulse bilaterally when possible)
C. Skin (color, moisture, temperature, turgor, presence of lesions; compare bilaterally), nails (compare bilaterally on hands and feet), and hair (dry or oily texture)
D. Eyes (visual acuity of central and peripheral vision)
    1.   Use of glasses, contact lenses, prosthesis
    2.   Presence of eye discharge or inflammation
E. Ears (hearing acuity, presence of cerumen, condition of tympanic membrane)
F. Nose (palpate nose and sinuses; note presence of discharge)
G. Mouth and pharynx (lips, mucosa of mouth, gums, teeth, tongue; ability to swallow and taste; movement of uvula)
H. Neck
    1.   Palpate lymph nodes (preauricular, posterior auricular, occipital, tonsillar, submaxillary, submental, superficial cervical, posterior cervical, deep cervical, and supraclavicular)
    2.   Palpate thyroid
    3.   Palpate trachea
I. Back (inspect and palpate spine and muscles; observe for curvatures)
J. Thorax and lungs (observe, percuss, and auscultate; palpate for respiratory excursion; note presence and type of cough)
K. Breasts and axillae (palpate breasts and nodes in axillae; observe for symmetry, discharge)

L. Heart (auscultate; observe for palpitations, thrills, and heaves)
M. Genitalia (assess penis and scrotum in men, external genitalia and vagina in women) and groin (check for hernia)
N. Motor function
1. Range of motion at all joints
2. Ability to contract all muscles (check muscle tone and strength)
3. Coordination of movements
4. Gait
5. Ability to speak and write
6. Reflexes
O. Sensation (pain and vibration in hands and feet, arms and legs; light touch on abdomen, arms, and legs)
P. Level of consciousness (orientation) and mental status (mood, cognitive functions)
Q. Presence of seizures, tremors, or tics
R. Secondary sex characteristics (hair distribution, voice, and so on)
S. Activity level (note pain, dyspnea, fatigue, or weakness)
T. Voiding and bowel patterns
U. Fluid and electrolyte balance, acid-base balance
V. Pain, infection, bleeding, lesions (note presence and location)

Blood transfusion

I. **Introduction**
A. A blood transfusion is the infusion of blood or blood products into the bloodstream
B. The transfusion can be autologous (the client's blood) or homologous (donor blood)
C. One or more blood transfusions may be performed to replenish the client's blood volume or erythrocytes (red blood cells) or to provide platelets or other coagulation factors
D. The procedure carries risks that can be minimized by carefully assessing the donor's health status, following safe blood administration practices, and knowing how to recognize and manage transfusion reactions

II. **Donor history and screening**
A. Donor blood is unacceptable for use if the donor's history includes any of the following:
1. Viral hepatitis or contact with a hepatitis client within the previous 6 months
2. Blood transfusion within the previous 6 months
3. Previous or current I.V. drug use
4. Exposure to the human immunodeficiency virus
5. Recent allergies or hives
B. Donor blood should not be used if screening tests yield positive results for any of the following:
1. Hepatitis
2. Acquired immunodeficiency syndrome (AIDS)
3. Syphilis
4. Cytomegalovirus

III.   Blood typing and cross matching

A. *ABO blood typing* is a test that identifies the client's blood group (A, B, O, or AB) to check compatibility of donor and recipient blood before transfusion.

1.   Type A blood is that of a person whose erythrocytes contain isoagglutin (antigen) A and antibody anti-B (about 40% of the population)

2.   Type B blood is that of a person whose erythrocytes contain isoagglutin (antigen) B and antibody anti-A (about 10% of the population)

3.   Type O blood is that of a person whose erythrocytes contain neither isoagglutin A nor B but do contain antibodies anti-A and anti-B (about 40% to 45% of the population, known as "universal donors")

4.   Type AB blood is that of a person whose erythrocytes contain both isoagglutins A and B but no antibodies (about 5% to 10% of the population, known as "universal recipients")

B. *Rh typing* is a test that determines the presence or absence of the Rh_o (D) antigen on the surface of red blood cells; an Rh-positive result indicates isoagglutins D, C, and E in erythrocytes

C. *Cross matching* is a test in which the donor's erythrocytes are exposed to the recipient's serum and the donor's serum is exposed to the recipient's erythrocytes; the test is performed to evaluate for agglutination

IV.   Hazards and complications of blood transfusion

A. The recipient of a blood transfusion is at risk for contracting a blood-borne disease such as serum hepatitis, syphilis, malaria, or AIDS

B. Transmission of incompatible or contaminated blood produces agglutination and hemolysis of the donor's erythrocytes by isoagglutinating in the recipient's plasma

C. Too-rapid administration can produce circulatory overload; massive transfusions (5 liters in less than 12 hours) can cause acidosis, hypothermia, citrate overload, hyperkalemia, and dilutional coagulation defects

D. Complications of blood transfusion cause about 3,000 deaths annually in the United States, primarily through serum hepatitis or a hemolytic transfusion reaction

E. Transfusion reactions usually develop during, immediately after, or within 96 hours of the transfusion

F. Delayed complications, which may develop 10 to 120 days after the last transfusion, typically result from disease transmission or sensitization to previous transfusions

V.   Procedures for safe administration

A. Wear gloves when handling blood or blood products

B. Properly collect and label blood and blood products

C. Provide detailed information labels for typing and cross matching samples

D. Obtain appropriate authorization to remove blood from the blood bank

E. Ensure proper client identification by having two nurses compare the recipient's name tag with matching information on the blood label

F. Prepare all necessary equipment in advance

1.   Y-type administration set

2.   Large-gauge needle (19 G or larger)

3.   Blood filter

VI.   Symptoms of transfusion reaction

A. Common symptoms of a transfusion reaction include fever (may be as high as 103° F [39.4° C]), chills, itching, flushing, urticaria, nausea, and vomiting

B. Allergic reactions can produce headache, dyspnea, stridor, and wheezing

C. Hemolytic reactions can lead to chest, flank, or back pain; apprehension or a feeling of impending doom; severe hypotension; spontaneous diffuse bleeding; and anuria

D. Hypervolemia can produce cyanosis, cough, and edema

VII. Managing transfusion reactions

A. Stop the transfusion immediately; if you have been using a Y-type set, infuse normal saline solution at a keep-vein-open rate

B. Notify the physician

C. Obtain a urine sample from the client and send it to the laboratory for analysis; continue to measure and assess urine output hourly

D. Draw a fresh sample of the client's blood and send it to the blood bank or laboratory for analysis

E. Return unused blood to the blood bank for incompatibility and contamination testing

F. Reduce the client's temperature by giving a sponge bath, administering acetaminophen, or lowering room temperature, if necessary; take the client's temperature every half hour until it is normal

G. To treat an allergic reaction, administer antihistamines (and possibly epinephrine or steroids), as ordered

H. To treat a hemolytic reaction, infuse an osmotic diuretic (possibly with sodium bicarbonate and hydrocortisone) and administer vasopressors, as ordered

Arrhythmia interpretation

Nurses who work outside specialty care areas are now routinely assigned to monitor clients for cardiac arrhythmias, whether during an emergency or while on a regular nursing unit. With this duty comes the responsibility to know and understand basic cardiac anatomy and physiology as well as the fundamental components of the electrocardiogram (ECG). Indeed, the health care team's ability to initiate prompt treatment may depend on the nurse's ability to recognize potentially life-threatening ECG changes. The following text reviews the heart's normal conduction system, basic components of the ECG, methods to calculate heart rate, ECG lead placement, and characteristics of and treatment measures for five life-threatening arrhythmias.

Cardiac conduction system

Sinoatrial node

Normally, the heart's electrical impulses originate in specialized conduction cells of the sinoatrial (SA) node, located in the right atrium near the junction of the superior vena cava. The SA node usually discharges at a regular rate of 60 to 100 beats/minute. The impulses then spread throughout atrial tissue via specialized interatrial and internodal pathways, causing atrial depolarization (represented on an ECG strip by P-wave formation). With depolarization, the atria contract, and blood flows to the ventricles. (See *The heart's conduction system,* page 88.)

Atrioventricular node

When the impulses arrive at the atrioventricular (AV) node, a brief delay (0.07 to 0.10 second) permits the atria to contract completely, allowing sufficient time for blood to flow to the ventricles. This delay is represented by a straight line on the ECG strip. If the SA node fails to fire and pace the heart, the junctional tissue around the AV node can serve as a backup pacemaker; its normal rate is 40 to 60 beats/minute.

Bundle of His and bundle branches

After the cardiac impulses leave the AV node, conduction continues rapidly down the bundle of His and the left and right bundle branches, terminating in the many branches of the Purkinje system. Before reaching the Purkinje system, the left bundle branch divides into the anterior and posterior fascicles. Conduction through the His-Purkinje system produces ventricular depolarization (represented on an ECG strip by the QRS complex), immediately followed by ventricular contraction. The pulmonary artery and the aorta then propel blood to the lungs and the rest of the body. Should the SA node and AV junction both fail to depolarize the heart, the His-Purkinje system can initiate an impulse, usually at a rate of 20 to 40 beats/minute.

Ventricular repolarization

Immediately after depolarization, cardiac muscle cells return to a normal state (polarization), ready to accept another electrical stimulus. Repolarization of the ventricles is represented on an ECG strip by T-wave formation. Atrial repolarization, which occurs earlier in the cardiac cycle as the ventricles are depolarizing, is usually obscured by the QRS complex and thus not evident on an ECG strip.

Normal ECG complex

The normal ECG complex consists of the P wave, the PR interval, the QRS complex, and the T wave. (See *Components of an ECG waveform,* page 89.) The *P wave* represents atrial depolarization (the electrical impulse spreading throughout the atrial musculature).

The *PR interval* represents atrial depolarization plus the brief delay of the electrical impulse at the AV node. Measured from the beginning of the P wave to the beginning of the QRS complex, the PR interval has a normal duration of 0.12 to 0.20 second.

CONCEPTS AND SKILLS

The heart's conduction system

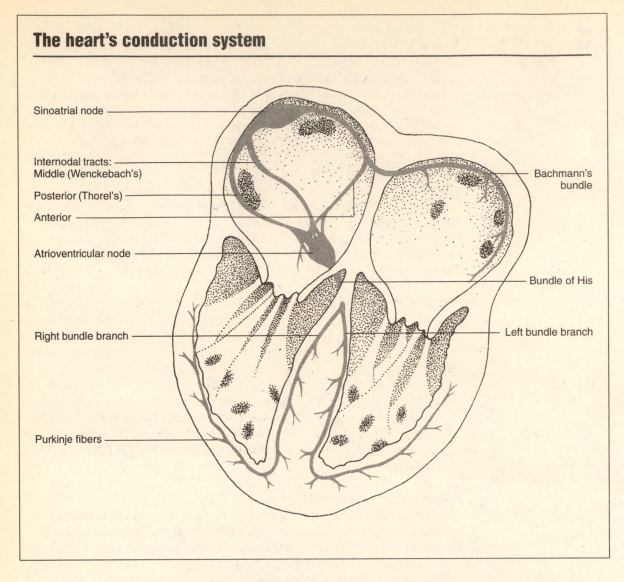

Sinoatrial node

Internodal tracts:
Middle (Wenckebach's)

Posterior (Thorel's)

Anterior

Atrioventricular node

Right bundle branch

Purkinje fibers

Bachmann's bundle

Bundle of His

Left bundle branch

The *QRS complex* represents ventricular depolarization (the electrical impulse spreading throughout the ventricular musculature). Measured from the beginning of the Q wave to the end of the S wave (where the tracing returns to the isoelectric line), the QRS complex has a normal duration of 0.06 to 0.10 second. QRS complexes generally consist of a Q wave (the first negative deflection after a P wave), an R wave (the first positive deflection after a P wave), and an S wave (the first negative deflection after an R wave). Some complexes, however, either begin with a positive deflection (and thus lack a Q wave) or end with one (and thus lack an S wave).

The *T wave* represents ventricular repolarization, or recovery. The point on or near the peak of the T wave is known as the vulnerable period. At this point in the cardiac cycle, even an extremely weak electrical stimulus may produce dangerous rhythm disturbances, such as ventricular tachycardia and ventricular fibrillation.

Components of an ECG waveform

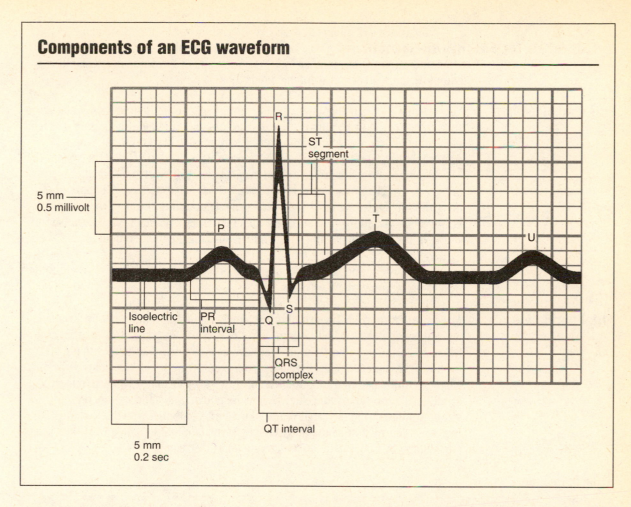

5 mm
0.5 millivolt

R

ST
segment

P

T

U

Isoelectric
line

PR
interval

Q

S

QRS
complex

QT interval

5 mm
0.2 sec

Calculating heart rates

An ECG records the heart's electrical activity on graph paper emitted from the machine at a constant rate. As an aid in heart rate calculation, the graph paper contains small and large boxes that represent time: 0.04 second for each small box and 0.20 second for each large box. Thus, 1,500 small boxes or 300 large boxes represent 1 minute. Additionally, at the top of the paper, vertical lines appear at 3-second intervals.

The nurse can use several methods to calculate the client's heart rate from an ECG strip, as circumstances warrant. The atrial rate (the PP interval) is calculated by measuring the time between two regular consecutive P waves. The ventricular rate (the RR interval) is calculated by measuring the time between two regular consecutive R waves.

If the client's rhythm is regular, the nurse can use one of these methods:
• Count the number of large boxes between two complexes (PP interval or RR interval), and divide 300 by this number (for example, if the nurse counts three large boxes between two R waves, the ventricular rate is 100 beats/minute). This method is faster than the next one discussed but less accurate whenever the interval falls short of a large box, because small boxes are not counted.
• Count the number of small boxes between two complexes (PP interval or RR interval), and divide 1,500 by this number (for example, if the nurse counts 15 small boxes between two R waves, the ventricular rate is 100 beats/minute). This method yields a more accurate answer but takes longer to calculate than the preceding method.

If the client's rhythm is irregular, neither of these methods yields an accurate answer. For irregular rhythms, count the number of QRS complexes in a 6-second strip, and multiply this number by 10 (for example, if the nurse counts 8 QRS complexes in a 6-second strip, the rate is 80 beats/minute).

ECG lead placement

Nurses should become familiar with the monitoring equipment in their work areas so that they can quickly apply ECG leads and obtain a tracing, if necessary. For lead placement, electrodes of most monitoring systems are marked Right Arm, Left Arm, Right Leg, and Left Leg. The client's right leg is used to ground the system.

Many practitioners prefer instead to place the arm electrodes on either side of the chest, directly under each clavicle, and the leg electrodes on the upper abdomen, directly under the ribs. This placement reduces interference from client movements, provides better access to the client in emergencies, and permits monitoring of the three limb leads (I, II, and III) and the augmented limb leads (aV_R, aV_L, and aV_F).

Lead II is commonly used to monitor cardiac rhythms because it provides the best visualization of the P waves.

Atrial fibrillation

Atrial fibrillation is characterized by extremely rapid and totally chaotic atrial activity (approximately 400 beats/minute) that occurs without any effective atrial contraction. Fortunately, the AV node, bombarded by electrical stimuli from the atria, usually blocks most of these impulses from conducting to the ventricles. However, when accompanied by a rapid ventricular rate (greater than 150 beats/minute), atrial fibrillation can produce deleterious hemodynamic effects. A decreased stroke volume (from the rapid ventricular rate), combined with the loss of effective atrial contraction, commonly reduces cardiac output to dangerously low levels, particularly in a client with an underlying heart disease.

Atrial fibrillation

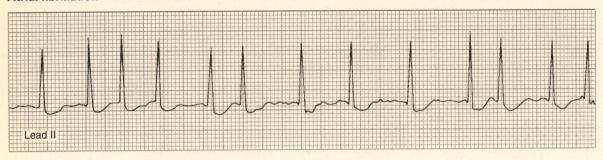

Lead II

ECG characteristics
• No clearly defined or measurable P waves
• Atrial activity characterized by a wavy, irregular, undulating baseline
• An unpredictably irregular ventricular response (RR interval)

Immediate nursing interventions
• Notify the physician.
• Assess the client for signs of decreased cardiac output: falling blood pressure, decreased urine output, and altered level of consciousness.
• Prepare emergency equipment: defibrillator, oxygen, and drugs.

Emergency medical treatments
• Assist with cardioversion or defibrillation if necessary (initially, 50 to 100 joules; may be increased for subsequent attempts).
• Administer drugs, if ordered, such as verapamil (Isoptin), digoxin (Lanoxin), propranolol (Inderal), or quinidine (Quinora).
• Assist in treating the underlying cause.

Premature ventricular contraction

A premature ventricular contraction (PVC) is characterized by early discharge from an irritable focus in the ventricles. Because electrical activity is aberrantly conducted through the ventricles rather than through the heart's normal conduction system, the QRS complex is unusually wide and has a bizarre, distorted configuration. If the client has no underlying heart disease, occasional PVCs have no clinical significance and do not require treatment. Other patterns, however—particularly after an acute myocardial infarction—may progress to more serious arrhythmias, such as ventricular tachycardia and ventricular fibrillation. PVCs are considered life-threatening if they:
• occur more than six times per minute
• have more than one source (multifocal PVCs)
• occur on or near the preceding T wave (R-on-T phenomenon)
• appear at least twice in a row
• have a bigeminal or trigeminal pattern (every second or third beat is a PVC).

ECG characteristics
• Not preceded by a P wave
• Wide, distorted QRS complex (greater than 0.12 second)
• Large T wave in the opposite direction of the QRS complex

Immediate nursing interventions
• Notify the physician.
• Assess the client for signs of decreased cardiac output: falling blood pressure, decreased urine output, and altered level of consciousness.
• Prepare emergency equipment: defibrillator, oxygen, and drugs.

Emergency medical treatments
• Administer drugs, if ordered, such as phenytoin (Dilantin), lidocaine (Xylocaine), procainamide (Pronestyl), or bretylium (Bretylol).
• Assist in treating the underlying cause.

Ventricular tachycardia

Ventricular tachycardia develops when an irritable focus in the ventricles, firing at 150 to 250 beats/minute, takes control of the heart's normal pacing activity. The ventricular beating is unrelated to any atrial mechanism. Sometimes occurring at slower rates of 70 to 130 beats/minute, ventricular tachycardia is also used to describe the client's condition when three or more PVCs occur consecutively. The arrhythmia usually produces significant hemodynamic effects, commonly accompanies an underlying heart disease, and frequently precedes ventricular fibrillation.

CONCEPTS AND SKILLS

Paired PVCs

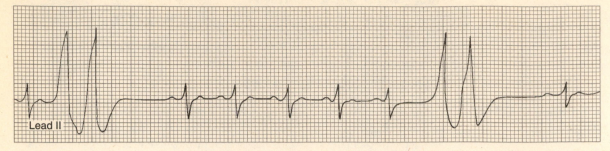

Lead II

Multiform PVCs

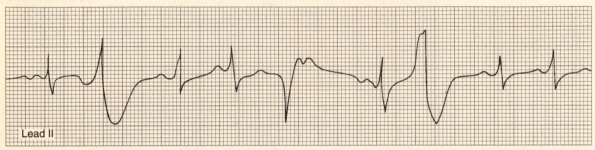

Lead II

Bigeminy

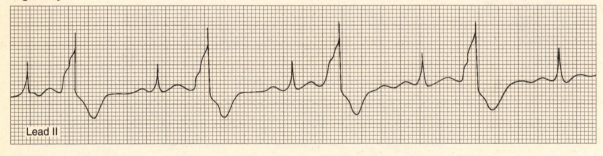

Lead II

R-on-T phenomenon

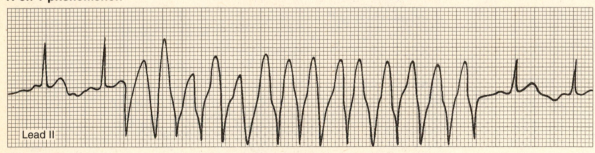

Lead II

Ventricular tachycardia

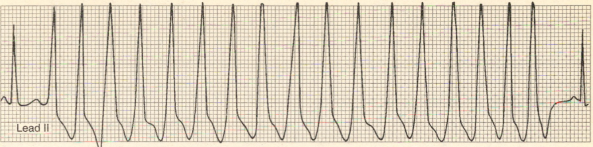

Lead II

ECG characteristics
• Rapid ventricular rate, either regular or slightly irregular
• No relationship to atrial activity
• Wide, distorted QRS complex (greater than 0.12 second)
• Possibly, intermittent P waves unrelated to ventricular activity

Immediate nursing interventions
• Assess the client's level of consciousness; if the client is unconscious, begin cardiopulmonary resuscitation.
• Notify the physician.
• Assess the client for signs of decreased cardiac output: falling blood pressure, decreased urine output, and altered level of consciousness.
• Prepare emergency equipment: defibrillator, oxygen, and drugs.

Emergency medical treatments
Treatment of ventricular tachycardia depends on the degree to which the client is tolerating the rhythm. Unless the client is hemodynamically unstable, drug therapy is preferred over cardioversion. If the rhythm resolves, the team starts a maintenance infusion of the drug that aided resolution. Phenytoin may be administered intravenously to resolve ventricular tachycardia induced by digoxin toxicity.
If the client is awake and alert:
• Administer drugs, if ordered, such as lidocaine, procainamide, or bretylium.
If the client is unconscious or hypotensive or shows signs of angina or congestive heart failure:
• Assist with cardioversion or defibrillation if necessary (initially, 50 joules; may be increased up to 360 joules)
• Administer lidocaine, if ordered.
• Assist in treating the underlying cause.

Ventricular fibrillation

When multiple irritable foci in the ventricles fire off rapidly, the heart cannot respond with any effective contraction, and cardiac output ceases. Death ensues in 3 to 5 minutes unless immediate measures successfully counter this life-threatening arrhythmia.

ECG characteristics
• Totally disorganized, chaotic pattern
• No discernible waves or complexes

Ventricular fibrillation

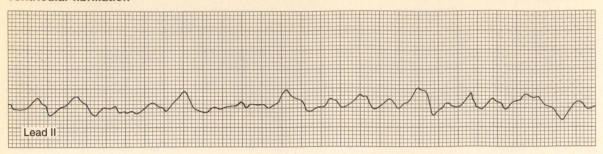

Lead II

Immediate nursing interventions

• Call a code.
• Begin cardiopulmonary resuscitation and continue until help arrives.
• Prepare emergency equipment: defibrillator, oxygen, and drugs.

Emergency medical treatments

• Assist with defibrillation if necessary (initially, 200 joules; may be increased up to 360 joules)
• Administer drugs, if ordered, such as epinephrine, lidocaine, procainamide, and bretylium.
• Draw a sample of the client's blood for arterial blood gas analysis, and administer sodium bicarbonate according to the client's pH level.
• Identify and treat the underlying cause.

Complete heart block (third-degree AV block)

In complete heart block, an underlying disease or drug toxicity prevents the conduction of all atrial impulses to the ventricles. An escape mechanism from the junctional tissue or ventricles takes over and paces the ventricles. Consequently, the atria and the ventricles are controlled by two independent pacemakers firing at two independent rates, with no relationship between atrial and ventricular activity.

Complete heart block

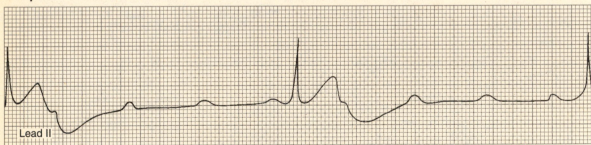

Lead II

ECG characteristics

• Regular atrial rate (PP interval), usually 60 to 100 beats/minute
• Regular ventricular rate, usually 40 to 60 beats/minute (junctional escape rhythm) or 20 to 40 beats/minute (ventricular escape rhythm)
• No relationship of P waves to QRS complexes

Immediate nursing interventions
• Notify the physician.
• Assess the client for signs of decreased cardiac output: falling blood pressure, decreased urine output, and altered level of consciousness.
• Prepare emergency equipment: defibrillator, oxygen, and drugs.

Emergency medical treatments
• Insert a temporary or permanent transvenous pacemaker.
• Administer atropine or isoproterenol (Isuprel), as ordered, if the client is showing signs of decreased cardiac output. These drugs speed up the effective heart rate and improve cardiac output until cardiac pacing is accomplished.

Cardiopulmonary resuscitation

I. Definition and purpose
    A. Cardiopulmonary resuscitation (CPR) is an emergency procedure that consists of artificial respiration and external cardiac massage, instituted after cardiopulmonary arrest
    B. CPR provides tissue oxygenation until normal cardiac function is restored
    C. The basic principles of life support center on the ABCs of CPR: Airway, Breathing, and Circulation

II. Performing CPR
    A. Determine the client's responsiveness by calling, "Are you OK?"
    B. If the client does not respond, call for help
    C. Place the client in the supine position, supporting the head and neck
    D. Open the airway by using the head-tilt, chin-lift maneuver
    E. Look, listen, and feel for signs of breathing
        1. If the client is not breathing, pinch the client's nose and, with your mouth, establish a tight seal over the client's mouth
        2. Ventilate twice; then pause to see whether the client's chest rises
    F. Palpate for the carotid pulse on the near side (keep the client's head tilted with your hand on the forehead)
    G. If the client has no pulse, begin cycles of ventilations with sternal compressions
        1. Check landmarks before placing the heel of the hand on the client's sternum
        2. Perform vertical compressions without bouncing
        3. Try to establish a rate of 80 to 100 beats/minute by counting:
            a. 4 cycles of 15 compressions to 2 ventilations (one rescuer)
            b. 4 cycles of 5 compressions to 1 ventilation (two rescuers)
        4. Make compressions and relaxations of equal duration
        5. Assess each ventilation for proper chest expansion
    H. Periodically assess the client for return of pulse and spontaneous breathing; do not interrupt resuscitation efforts for longer than 5 seconds
    I. Continue CPR until another rescuer relieves you, the client responds, you become too exhausted to continue, or you receive instructions to terminate CPR

Levels of illness prevention

LEVEL	PURPOSE	EXAMPLES OF ANTICIPATORY GUIDANCE
Primary	To prevent trauma or disease	• Child education • Infant immunization • Health screening programs • Accident prevention programs • Parent education classes
Secondary	To delay or stop the progress of an established disease or injury	• Diabetic teaching • Discharge planning • Return demonstration by the client
Tertiary	To maintain an incurably ill client at a maximal activity level	• Referral to self-help groups • Preparation of family for grieving patterns

Anticipatory guidance

I. Introduction
   A. Anticipatory guidance refers to the initiation of interventions before an event occurs to prevent potential problems
   B. If an event can be anticipated, guidance (teaching) increases the likelihood that the event will have a favorable outcome (for example, preparing parents for their child's impending developmental tasks or discussing the ramifications of upcoming surgery with a client)
   C. Anticipatory guidance is inherent in all levels of prevention related to health care (see *Levels of illness prevention*)
   D. With increased emphasis on helping the client achieve and maintain high-level wellness and on involving the client in planning and managing self-care, the nurse's role as teacher has assumed greater importance
   E. Effective teaching strategies incorporate fundamental learning principles

II. Learning principles that aid client teaching
   A. Feedback strengthens learning
   B. Satisfaction from learning increases learning potential
   C. Individualized learning styles necessitate individualized teaching
   D. Active participation by the learner enhances learning
   E. Motivation increases learning
   F. Mutual goal setting produces more meaningful learning
   G. Relevant learning experiences enhance learner motivation
   H. Mild anxiety of the learner can actually benefit learning
   I. Categorization of content facilitates the learning process
   J. The learner's experience and knowledge can enhance future learning

III. Primary client-teaching responsibilities
   A. Orient the client to the hospital environment
   B. Explain all nursing procedures that will be performed as part of the client's care

C. Explain all diagnostic tests, treatments, and medical procedures that the client will undergo, including a discussion of what the client can expect before, during, and after the test, treatment, or procedure
D. Provide written and oral explanations and instructions
E. Determine the client's understanding and perception of health care management, and provide feedback as needed to clarify any concerns or correct any misconceptions the client may have

Discharge planning

I. **Purpose and goals**

A. The overall purpose of discharge planning is to ensure continuity of client care
B. Through effective discharge planning, the nurse accomplishes numerous goals
  1. Helps the client find solutions to health problems on an efficient, timely, economic, and continuous basis
  2. Ensures uninterrupted therapy, which may start in one institution (such as a hospital) but continue in other settings (such as a clinic, the client's home, the physician's office, or a nursing home)
  3. Coordinates quality care provided by multidisciplinary health care professionals
  4. Involves the client and family or friends in discharge planning
  5. Transfers the client safely from:
      a. one hospital unit to another (for example, from acute care to progressive care)
      b. the hospital to the client's home or from the home to the hospital or another facility
      c. one community health care institution to another
  6. Transfers client records and other essential information from one care level to another
  7. Provides individualized planning that reflects the client's special health needs and identifies available and appropriate facilities and services

II. **Principles of discharge planning**

A. Discharge planning should begin on admission, when the client enters the health care system
B. For discharge planning to be effective, the nurse uses a five-step problem-solving approach
  1. Assesses discharge planning needs based on the client's problems
  2. Designs a goal-directed plan
  3. Tests the plan
  4. Evaluates test results
  5. Redesigns the plan as indicated
C. The client and family must assist in the planning process and must receive information about available resources and services
D. A coordinated team approach ensures reliable information and uninterrupted care
  1. Initiates interagency communication (through referrals or written agreements)

2. Establishes contact between the client and the resources and services best suited to the client's needs

E. Integrated discharge planning can resolve complex health problems and produce optimal client recovery

III. Clients with special needs

A. Although every client requires some type of discharge planning, some clients have critical needs that warrant more complex planning

1. Pediatric clients
   a. Children with chronic health problems (such as scoliosis, seizures, asthma, hemophilia, and neurologic conditions)
   b. Children with social problems (such as parental rejection or battered child syndrome)
   c. Premature neonates, those who weigh over 10 lb (4.5 kg), those with an Apgar score of 7 or lower at 5 minutes, and those who have major congenital deformities or disabling birth injuries
   d. Infants or children with severe weight loss (10%), feeding problems, or failure to thrive
   e. Children who have serious illnesses or who undergo unusual surgical procedures

2. Mothers and pregnant clients
   a. Those with a complicated pregnancy, labor, delivery, or postpartum period
   b. Adolescents
   c. Those who lack a support system

3. Medical or surgical clients with acute problems or critical needs (for example, open or infected wounds, ostomies, drainage tubes, extensive casts, injections, special diet instructions or exercises, or medications requiring special considerations, such as insulin)

4. Clients having radical or mutilating surgery that results in a drastically altered lifestyle (such as radical neck surgery, bilateral amputation, cardiovascular surgery, or bilateral nephrectomies)

5. Clients with chronic illnesses or multiple diagnoses (such as cancer, heart disease, and diabetes mellitus)

6. Elderly clients

7. Emotionally disturbed clients

8. Impoverished clients and those without families

B. For clients with special needs, the nurse should arrange community or home health services as part of the discharge plan, as indicated

1. Nursing care (such as an extended care facility, a nursing home, skilled care, or home care)

2. Medical supervision and follow-up

3. Physical, occupational, speech, and other therapies or rehabilitation

4. Supervision and administration of medication

5. Periodic laboratory tests

6. Inhalation therapy

7. Homemaker services

8. Transportation (ambulance or other special vehicles, as required)

9. Special equipment and supplies needed for care at home or in another facility

Part IV

Maintaining homeostasis

Maintaining homeostasis

Introduction

Homeostasis—a state of constancy or equilibrium within the body—is essential for the preservation of life. The body maintains homeostasis through a system of internal control mechanisms that regulate vital functions, including blood pressure, temperature, pH, heart rate, respiratory rate, glandular secretion, and fluid and electrolyte balance.

Various factors (such as acute or chronic illness, trauma, and the pressures of everyday life) may adversely affect homeostasis. The degree to which these stressors alter the body's normal balance depends on the individual's adaptability and ability to cope. Typically, the body responds to stress by activating various regulatory mechanisms (primarily within the vascular system, brain, kidneys, liver, and endocrine system) that produce physiologic changes to bring the body back to normal functional levels. Understanding physiologic responses to stress is crucial to providing appropriate nursing care.

Part IV focuses on major physiologic stressors that can disrupt homeostasis as well as on the internal mechanisms by which the body responds to maintain normalcy. "Inflammation" reviews the cardinal signs of inflammation, factors affecting inflammation, and nursing interventions to prevent complications. "Shock" discusses the pathophysiology of the five types of shock (anaphylactic, septic, cardiogenic, neurogenic, and hypovolemic) and reviews important assessment information and interventions for each specific type. "Pain" includes an overview of pain theories, physiologic responses to pain, and pain management. "Acid-Base Imbalances," "Electrolyte Imbalances," and "Fluid Imbalances" use a nursing-process approach to explain the nurse's responsibilities in identifying and treating these often serious conditions. "Immobility" covers the causes of immobility and its effects on the body and reviews nursing interventions to maintain homeostasis and prevent further complications.

Inflammation

I. **Definition**
   A. The body's response to cellular injury
   B. An immediate, defensive, and beneficial response

II. **Cardinal signs**
   A. Redness (rubor) from dilation of arterioles, which increases blood flow to the injured area
   B. Heat (calor) from increased blood supply to and increased metabolism in the injured area
   C. Pain (dolor) from the release of chemicals, pH changes, and pressure on nerve endings caused by swelling and trauma
   D. Edema from accumulation of fluids in the interstitial tissues of the injured area
   E. Loss of function (functio laesa) from the accumulation of changes affecting normal functioning of the injured tissues
   F. Other changes from the inflammatory response
      1. Migration and extravasation of leukocytes into the injured area
      2. Phagocytosis (engulfing and destruction of irritants, primarily by polymorphonuclear neutrophils, monocytes, and lymphocytes)

3. Walling off by leukocytes to keep the inflammation localized (by cleaning up cellular debris, leukocytes also help resolve inflammation)
4. Exudate formation, produced by the accumulation of interstitial fluids (exudates dilute noxious chemicals in the inflamed area and bring antibodies to tissue defense)
   a. Clear (serous) exudates
   b. Purulent (pus-containing) exudates
   c. Bloody (sanguineous) exudates
5. Cell size changes (metaplasia)
   a. Increased cell size (hypertrophy or hyperplasia)
   b. Decreased cell size (atrophy or hypoplasia)
6. Migration of the inflammation (metastasis) into contiguous tissues (signaled by red streaks radiating along blood vessels)

III.   Systemic signs
A. Fever (from release of pyrogens in the body)
B. Leukocytosis (increased production of white blood cells)
C. Malaise, anorexia, and disability (varying among individuals)
D. Increased sedimentation rate (from changes in blood proteins and effects on red blood cells)

IV.   Factors affecting inflammation
A. Blood supply (inadequate blood supply may prolong inflammation and impair healing)
B. Increased numbers of leukocytes (leukocytes localize inflammation and produce phagocytosis)
C. The client's nutritional status (cellular regeneration requires abundant nutrients, including vitamins A, C, and D; protein; and iron and other minerals)
D. Foreign material in the inflamed area (debris or necrotic cells, dirt, and other foreign substances may prevent healing and lead to infection)
E. Age (children and young adults generally exhibit faster healing and recovery than elderly persons do)

V.   Complications
A. Contracture (shortening or tightening of tissues, causing deformity; contracture involving a joint usually draws the joint into flexion, although it occasionally causes extension)
B. Stricture (scar tissue that encircles a tubular structure—for example, the esophagus—producing a narrowing)
C. Adhesions (bands of granulation, or scar, tissue that bind tissues and organs, producing loss of function and other complications)
D. Hernias (outward bulging of scars)
E. Keloids (excessive growth of scar tissue)
F. Granulomas (accumulation of scar tissue within scar tissue; for example, a neuroma or keloid)

VI.   Resolution of inflammation
A. Resolution (complete remission of signs and symptoms, with no residual evidence of inflammation)
B. Repair (replacement of lost cells with new ones of the same kind)
C. Scar formation (organization of connective tissue cells to form scar tissue)

VII. Nursing implementations for a client with inflammation
   A. Monitor vital signs for indications of developing inflammation: fever; spiking temperatures; increased pulse rate; and early signs of soreness, redness, edema, and rash
   B. Assess a wound for color changes, edema, increased redness or tenderness, and increased drainage, and report any of these findings to the physician (initial serosanguineous drainage should decrease in 24 to 48 hours; purulent drainage signals infection)
   C. Assess drainage from other orifices, and report such signs as yellow sputum, cloudy urine, and diarrhea
   D. Be alert for client complaints of malaise, fatigue, anorexia, and increasing pain as well as for blood chemistry changes (high white blood cell count and sedimentation rate)—all signs of inflammation or infection
   E. Report client complaints of dysuria or burning or frequent urination to the physician
   F. Assess the client's respiratory rate and breath sounds, monitor for pain on respiration, and report any changes to the physician
   G. Record all data and findings on the client's chart

Shock

Shock is a syndrome characterized by excessive reduction of circulating blood volume, resulting in inadequate cell perfusion. Because the cells do not receive adequate nutrition and oxygen, cell death can occur. *Anaphylactic shock* refers to massive vasodilation from release of histamine and an antigen-antibody reaction. Possible causes include insect stings, blood transfusions, and drug allergies. *Septic shock* refers to massive vasodilation from toxic substances released by bacteria. The primary cause is infection by gram-negative organisms or, as in the case of toxic shock syndrome, by gram-positive organisms. In *cardiogenic shock,* left ventricular failure produces circulatory inadequacy. Possible causes include myocardial infarction and cardiac arrest. *Neurogenic shock*—interruption of the sympathetic nervous system—can be caused by spinal cord injuries, damage to the medulla oblongata, or spinal anesthesia. *Hypovolemic shock* refers to excessive loss of body fluid. Possible causes include hemorrhage, burns, adrenal crisis, diarrhea, vomiting, and ketoacidosis.

The three primary physiologic alterations leading to shock are *pump failure* (cardiogenic shock); *volume depletion* from dehydration, hemorrhage, or inadequate fluid replacement (hypovolemic shock); and *vasogenic changes in vasomotor response* (anaphylactic, neurogenic, or septic shock).

This entry first examines aspects of nursing assessment, diagnosis, planning, implementation, and evaluation that are common to all shock types; it then explores assessment and implementation steps specific to each type. For information on pharmacologic therapy, see *Drugs used in shock,* page 104.

Assessment

1. Assess the client for restlessness, anxiety, apprehension, and altered mentation, all caused by decreased cerebral perfusion, with resultant cerebral irritation.
2. Observe the client for color changes—pallor or cyanosis—caused by decreased oxygenation.

MAINTAINING HOMEOSTASIS

Drugs used in shock

Treatment of shock varies according to the factors that precipitate the disorder. Hypovolemic shock must be treated with plasma expanders or blood replacement. Septic shock is treated with antibiotics and volume replacement. Cardiogenic shock is treated with one or more of the following drugs:

• dobutamine (Dobutrex)—increases cardiac output. Its effects are caused by selective $beta_1$-receptor activation, which results in increased output with only minimal increases in heart rate. Because it stimulates $beta_1$ receptors on the vascular beds, dobutamine also causes vasodilation, which decreases left ventricular end diastolic pressure and further improves the pumping efficiency of the heart. It is one of the most useful drugs in treating cardiogenic shock.

• dopamine (Intropin)—dilates coronary, intracerebral, mesenteric, and renal arteries and increases urine output. Dopamine's effects are dose-dependent. At low doses, it activates only dopamine receptors. At higher doses, it activates $beta_1$-receptors, stimulating the heart. At still higher doses, alpha receptors are activated, causing vasoconstriction. Dopamine is especially useful when low cardiac output is complicated by hypotension and low renal output.

• norepinephrine (Levophed)—increases blood pressure and cardiac output, but usually decreases heart rate because of a reflex increase in vagal tone. Norepinephrine stimulates mostly alpha receptors but also will activate $beta_1$ receptors; it has no $beta_2$-receptor activity. Norepinephrine is especially useful when dobutamine or dopamine cannot maintain blood pressure. Because it increases myocardial work and oxygen consumption, it may cause arrhythmias.

• isoproterenol (Isuprel)—causes bronchodilation but also increases heart rate and cardiac output. It has limited use in treating shock because myocardial stimulation may lead to arrhythmias or cardiac decompensation. It is used *only* if the peripheral vascular bed is vasoconstricted or if the client has severe bradycardia.

• vasodilators (such as nitroglycerin [Nitrostat] or sodium nitroprusside [Nipride])—cause peripheral vasodilation, which decreases the force against which the heart has to pump. The net effect is decreased myocardial work and oxygen consumption.

3. Assess the client for inadequate blood pressure—a systolic reading below 80 mm Hg (if the client's blood pressure was normal before the onset of shock)—caused by decreased circulating blood volume or decreased cardiac output.

4. Assess the client for tachycardia. Compensatory central nervous system (CNS) stimulation accompanies a decrease in stroke volume. Cardiac output (CO) can be determined by multiplying the client's stroke volume (SV) by the heart rate (HR): $CO = SV \times HR$.

5. Monitor the client for an elevated respiratory rate—the body's compensatory response to the increased oxygen exchange and carbon dioxide excretion from metabolic acidosis.

6. Monitor the client for inadequate urine output (below 25 ml/hour) caused by decreased renal perfusion.

7. Assess the client for a decreased pH level. Shock causes anaerobic metabolism with resultant lactic acidosis.

8. Assess the client for diaphoresis from inadequate peripheral perfusion.

9. Assess the client for complaints of thirst, which may signal fluid and electrolyte imbalances.

10. Assess the client for clotting alterations, which may indicate decreased perfusion to the liver.

Nursing diagnoses

• Decreased cardiac output related to left ventricular failure, volume depletion, or vasodilation
• Altered tissue perfusion related to decreased myocardial contractility, hypovolemia, or vasogenic changes
• Fluid volume deficit related to excessive fluid loss

• Risk for injury related to sensorimotor deficits or hypotension
• Impaired gas exchange related to altered ventilation-perfusion ratio

Planning and goals

• The client will have adequate cellular perfusion.
• The client will retain renal function.
• The client will suffer no complications.
• The client's and family's anxiety will decrease.

Implementation

1. Position the client to maintain a patent airway and facilitate breathing. Turn the client's head to the side. Remember that a decreased level of consciousness puts the client at risk for aspiration.

2. Maintain complete bed rest for the client to decrease cellular oxygen needs.

3. Plan nursing care that provides the client with rest periods whenever possible.

4. Maintain the client in a flat position or, if possible, use a modified Trendelenburg's position, with the lower end of the bed elevated about 45 degrees and the client's head also slightly elevated. This promotes increased respiratory exchange and increased venous return.

5. Start I.V. fluid therapy, as ordered, adjusting the flow rate according to the client's response to treatment and keeping blood pressure within the range ordered by the physician. This helps maintain adequate perfusion.

6. Administer prescribed volume expanders (such as whole blood, plasma, dextran, or albumin) to increase blood pressure and restore circulating blood volume.

7. Turn the client every 2 hours after being stabilized and maintain proper body alignment to prevent complications from immobility. Use a convoluted foam mattress or air mattress to prevent pressure ulcers.

8. Maintain strict asepsis; the client is susceptible to infection.

9. Monitor the client's urine output hourly to assess renal perfusion and function. Check blood urea nitrogen and creatinine levels.

10. Assess the client every 2 hours for fluid and electrolyte imbalances, such as hyperkalemia from metabolic acidosis.

11. Administer oxygen, as ordered, to increase the amount of oxygen in the blood. Prepare for intubation, if needed.

12. Check vital signs every 15 minutes until the client is stable, then hourly to monitor cellular perfusion.

13. Administer medications intravenously. Poor tissue perfusion results in accumulation and inadequate absorption of medications given subcutaneously or intramuscularly.

14. Administer medications that are appropriate for the type of shock the client has.

15. Assess the client's skin color and temperature, and monitor skin perfusion.

16. Assess bowel sounds and signs of abdominal pain every 8 hours to monitor GI perfusion.

17. Perform hourly neurologic checks to assess CNS perfusion.

18. Attach a cardiac monitor to the client for continuous monitoring. Fluid and electrolyte imbalances can cause arrhythmias.

19. Monitor arterial blood gas measurements and pH levels to detect acidosis and inadequate oxygenation. Shock decreases partial pressure of oxygen (PO_2) and pH. Monitor pulse oximetry for oxygen saturation.

20. Monitor central venous pressure hourly to determine the client's cardiac function and central blood volume. If the client is in an intensive care unit, record other hemodynamic measurements, such as pulmonary capillary wedge pressure (PCWP), as appropriate.

MAINTAINING HOMEOSTASIS

21. Observe the client for common complications—pulmonary edema, congestive heart failure, renal failure, metabolic acidosis, disseminated intravascular coagulation, and toxic effects of medications.

22. Place light bedclothes on the client to prevent chilling or overheating.

23. Provide emotional support to the client and family, especially when the prognosis is uncertain.

Evaluation

• The client's normal blood pressure has been restored.
• The client's fluid and electrolyte levels fall within normal limits.
• The client does not experience pulmonary edema or metabolic acidosis.
• The client's and family's anxieties have decreased satisfactorily.

Anaphylactic shock

Assessment

1. Assess the client for respiratory difficulty, such as dyspnea and wheezing. An allergic reaction causes massive histamine release, resulting in bronchospasm, angioedema, and allergic manifestations.

2. Observe for edema around the site of an insect sting or injection. The site indicates the allergen's source.

3. Observe for general flushing (the skin feels hot to the touch), and check the client's skin for urticaria (hives). These signal an allergic reaction.

4. Observe the client for a voice change and a tight feeling in the throat, which may indicate laryngeal edema.

Implementation

1. Administer epinephrine (1:1,000), 0.1 to 0.3 ml subcutaneously, depending on the client's size. Watch for tachycardia as an adverse reaction. Epinephrine dilates the bronchi and constricts the arterioles and capillaries, thereby reversing the histamine effect. This drug acts quickly but has a short duration.

2. If appropriate, apply a tourniquet to the limb above (proximal to) the site of the insect bite or drug injection to prevent continued absorption.

3. Administer an antihistamine, such as brompheniramine maleate (Dimetane), diphenhydramine hydrochloride (Benadryl), tripelennamine hydrochloride (Pyribenzamine), or chlorpheniramine maleate (Chlor-Trimeton, Teldrin). These drugs replace histamine at the receptor site, preventing histamine action, relieving the client's itching and nasal congestion, and preventing further bronchospasm. (Note, however, that antihistamines cannot reverse the effects of histamine once the effects have occurred.) Also, observe the client for drowsiness, dizziness, and poor coordination. Caution the client to avoid operating hazardous equipment or ingesting alcohol or other depressants while taking these drugs.

4. Administer corticosteroids to decrease inflammation and improve microcirculation.

5. Administer aminophylline (Aminophyllin) for bronchospasm.

6. Instruct the client to wear a medical alert bracelet.

7. Teach the client to carry an epinephrine kit for insect allergies.

Septic shock

Assessment

1. Assess the client for possible causes of septic shock: peritonitis; urinary tract infection; a urinary tract procedure, such as cystoscopy or transurethral resection; general debilitation such as cancer; toxic shock syndrome and food poisoning; and organisms that cause sepsis, including *Pseudomonas, Klebsiella, Proteus,* and *Escherichia coli* (in gram-negative sepsis) and *Staphylococcus* and *Streptococcus* (in gram-positive sepsis).

2. Monitor the client for fever (temperature usually over 104° F [40° C]) and chills. Signs of an overwhelming infection may appear with a sudden onset of shaking chills and high fever, which typically precede a sudden drop in blood pressure and other signs of shock.

3. Observe the client's skin color: gray indicates gram-negative shock, and red indicates gram-positive shock. The client may display increased restlessness, disorientation, and confusion because of anoxia.

4. Assess the client's mental status. Inadequate cerebral tissue perfusion commonly causes anoxia.

Implementation

1. Report any signs of infection. The major goal is to prevent septic shock by preventing overwhelming infection, especially in a client at risk. Because septic shock rapidly progresses to an irreversible state, the client needs prompt, aggressive treatment.

2. Administer oxygen immediately to combat anoxia.

3. Initiate I.V. therapy if it has not already been started. Peripheral blood pooling leads to hypovolemia and can precipitate cardiac arrhythmias.

4. Obtain blood, urine, sputum, and wound cultures—before antibiotic administration, if possible.

5. Administer a broad-spectrum antibiotic initially, then one specific to the organism when it has been identified.

6. Administer a corticosteroid, which decreases inflammation and improves microcirculation.

Cardiogenic shock

Assessment

1. Observe the client for signs and symptoms of myocardial infarction, including a rapid pulse rate and decreased blood pressure. Pump failure commonly follows an infarction.

2. Observe the client for signs and symptoms of cardiac failure, such as neck vein distention, nausea and vomiting, oliguria, cyanosis, dyspnea, and extreme weakness.

Implementation

1. Administer drugs (such as dopamine [Intropin] or dobutamine [Dobutrex]), as ordered, to improve myocardial contractility and increase cardiac output.

2. Administer nitroprusside (Nipride), as ordered, to cause vasodilation, thus decreasing afterload and increasing cardiac output.

3. Be prepared to assist the physician if the client requires an intra-aortic balloon pump (sometimes used in intensive care).

MAINTAINING HOMEOSTASIS

MAINTAINING HOMEOSTASIS

Neurogenic shock

Assessment

1. Assess the client for sudden hypotension, which occurs with an interruption of the sympathetic nervous system and its control of the blood vessels.
2. Observe the client for syncope and altered mental status.
3. Assess the client for hypothermia, which can result from rapid loss of heat caused by peripheral vasodilation or overstimulation of the vagus nerve.
4. Monitor the client for bradycardia resulting from vagal stimulation.

Implementation

1. Administer vasopressors, as ordered. Note that these drugs cause peripheral vasoconstriction, which may lead to complications because of decreased circulation to the kidneys. Drug infiltration can cause subcutaneous necrosis.
2. If the client is receiving vasopressors, monitor blood pressure every 5 minutes and check for cardiac arrhythmias. Observe vital signs every 15 minutes until the client becomes stable.
3. Administer steroids, as ordered.

Hypovolemic shock

Assessment

1. Assess the client for common signs of shock, such as decreased blood pressure, tachycardia, cyanosis, restlessness, anxiety, apprehension, tachypnea, and diaphoresis.
2. Monitor the client for early signs of fluid volume depletion, such as decreased urine output, decreased central venous pressure, restlessness, and tachycardia.

Implementation

1. Replace the client's lost fluids and blood with I.V. fluids, volume expanders, and transfusions of blood or blood products, as ordered.
2. Monitor the client's hemodynamic status, recording blood pressure, central venous pressure, and PCWP, as appropriate.
3. Use antishock trousers, if ordered, in an emergency.

Pain

I.   **Theoretical overview**
  A. Is universally feared (the strongest human fear after the fear of death)
  B. Serves as a bodily protective mechanism (superficial fibers are rich in pain receptors; viscera are not)
  C. Comprises perception and interpretation—a highly complex mechanism
    1.   Specificity theory (traditional theory of pain perception and interpretation)
      a. Stimulus
      b. Receptor
      c. Spinothalamic tract
      d. Thalamus (perception of pain)
      e. Cerebral cortex (interpretation of pain)
        (1) Receptors also respond to cold and pressure
        (2) Pain pathways can be transected and pain still occurs
    2.   Gate control theory (based on the idea that only one major stimulus can be transmitted at a time)
      a. Stimulus
      b. Gate (in substantia gelatinosa)

    c. Gate opens to neural pathway, or conflicting large fiber (general sensory) input closes gate; small fiber input causes pain

    d. Gate closes, responding to impulses from brain stem or central control

II. Reactions to pain perception and interpretation

A. Autonomic
1. Stress response
2. Increased skeletal muscle activity
3. Reflexes (withdrawal from source)
4. Reflex muscular rigidity over affected areas; guarding (protective reflex)
5. Muscle spasms after a fracture

B. Voluntary
1. Grimacing
2. Clenching fists and teeth
3. Pacing floor
4. Twisting and turning
5. Decreasing activity
6. Altering body position

C. Psychological
1. Anxiety, fear, and apprehension (anxiety increases the intensity of pain, which further increases anxiety)
2. Anger and verbalization
3. Decreased sense of control

D. Severe physical or psychological conditions
1. Shock
2. Panic
3. Prolonged pain resulting from fear, depression, insomnia, anorexia, or tension

III. Types of pain

A. Superficial
1. Has abrupt (sharp, prickly) or gradual (burning) onset
2. Is easily localized to one spot

B. Deep
1. Has dull, aching quality that persists; is less easily localized
2. Visceral—caused by spastic contraction of smooth muscle (blood vessels)
3. Referred—pain of a visceral lesion gives the impression of arising in a distant area; for example, shoulder pain experienced in gallbladder disease
4. Central pain—has no peripheral cause but may be caused by injury to the nerve trunk; perception of pain persists after the stimulus is gone; for example, toe pain after leg amputation (phantom limb pain)

IV. Pain management

A. Pharmacologic intervention
1. Nonnarcotic analgesia (inhibits prostaglandin synthesis)
2. Narcotic analgesia (acts centrally to change pain perception and interpretation)

B. Nonpharmacologic intervention
1. Transcutaneous electrical nerve stimulation (TENS)—electronic stimulation of the large fibers to close the gate to painful stimuli (based on the gate control theory)
2. Acupuncture—Chinese method of inserting fine needles at certain sites on the body; how acupuncture works physiologically is uncertain
3. Relaxation techniques—biofeedback, visualization, meditation, and hypnosis can all be useful interventions in pain management

Acid-base imbalances

Acid-base balance refers to the body's hydrogen ion concentration—a measure of the relationship between carbonic acid and bicarbonate (normally a ratio of 1 part carbonic acid to 20 parts bicarbonate). Normal blood has a pH of 7.35 to 7.45. Buffers in the blood, along with the lungs and the kidneys, help maintain acid-base balance.

Buffers are substances in blood that have both acidic and basic properties. The base in the buffer, in the presence of strong acid, neutralizes the acid; or, if the level of base in the blood rises, the buffer acid neutralizes the base. Binding the ions, whether acid or base, prevents the ions from disturbing acid-base balance.

The lungs regulate the amount of carbon dioxide excreted or retained in the body. Cell metabolism yields carbon dioxide as a waste product. Combined with water, carbon dioxide becomes carbonic acid. If the blood becomes too acidic, the person breathes more rapidly and deeply to increase carbon dioxide excretion. Increases in blood alkali make the person's breathing slower and more shallow to retain carbon dioxide.

The kidneys help maintain acid-base balance in several ways. As needed, they excrete or absorb bicarbonate (base), hydrogen ions (acid), and electrolytes, and the distal tubule cells form ammonia (base). For example, if the blood contains too many hydrogen ions, the kidneys retain bicarbonate and sodium, excrete more hydrogen ions, and form ammonia to preserve acid-base balance.

When these mechanisms maintain acid-base balance, pH is slightly alkaline, at 7.35 to 7.45. Other normal values include partial pressure of oxygen in arterial blood (PaO_2), 90±10 mm Hg; partial pressure of carbon dioxide in arterial blood ($PaCO_2$), 35 to 45 mm Hg; HCO_3^- (serum bicarbonate), 22 to 26 mEq/liter; and oxygen saturation, 95% to 98%.

Respiratory acidosis: Carbonic acid excess (▲Pco_2 ▼pH)

Respiratory acidosis occurs when carbon dioxide production in the body tissues exceeds its removal by the lungs, with a resultant increase in the blood's carbon dioxide level. In the blood, carbon dioxide combines with water to form carbonic acid.

Causes
• Health problems that interfere with gas exchange in the lungs; for example, chronic obstructive pulmonary disease, airway obstruction, and open chest wounds

• Health hazards that depress the respiratory center in the medulla; for example, drug overdose or use of narcotics and barbiturates
• Mechanical ventilator that malfunctions or is set to remove too little carbon dioxide

Assessment

1. Assess the client for slow and shallow respirations, which result from central nervous system (CNS) depression.
2. Assess the client for visual disturbances, headache, confusion, drowsiness, and coma, all of which occur because of high levels of carbon dioxide in the CNS.

Diagnostic evaluation

• *PaCO2* level above 45 mm Hg (normal: 35 to 45 mm Hg): This indicates that the lungs are retaining too much carbon dioxide.
• *pH below 7.35* (normal: 7.35 to 7.45): This indicates that the compensatory mechanisms—buffers, lungs, and kidneys—are ineffective.

Nursing diagnoses

• Ineffective breathing pattern related to altered respiratory rate and depth
• Impaired gas exchange related to increased secretions

Planning and goals

• The client will not experience preventable complications.
• The client's blood pH will remain within normal limits.
• As the client's condition improves, the client's and family's anxiety will decrease.

Implementation

1. Place the client on incentive spirometry, and institute deep-breathing exercises every hour. This will increase ventilation, thereby decreasing carbon dioxide retention. Deep breathing prevents hypostatic pneumonia.
2. Observe for a depressed level of consciousness. For an unconscious client, maintain a patent airway and proper ventilation. Intubation and mechanical ventilation may be necessary.
3. Suction as needed to keep the airway clear.
4. Ensure adequate hydration, and use postural drainage and chest physiotherapy to remove secretions.
5. Provide emotional support to the client and family, especially if the prognosis is uncertain.

Evaluation

• The client does not have atelectasis or other respiratory complications.
• The client's blood pH ranges between 7.35 and 7.45, and the PaCO2 level is between 35 and 45 mm Hg.
• The client and family have decreased anxiety.

Respiratory alkalosis: Carbonic acid deficit ($\blacktriangledown$ Pco$_2$ $\blacktriangle$ pH)

Respiratory alkalosis occurs when excessive excretion of carbon dioxide results in decreased levels in the blood.

Causes
• Anxiety resulting in hyperventilation, causing increased carbon dioxide excretion
• Mechanical ventilator that malfunctions or is set improperly, causing increased carbon dioxide excretion

Assessment

1. Determine whether the client has increased rate and depth of breathing (hyperventilation).

2. Check the client for tremulousness, numbness, tingling of digits, or convulsions, all caused by neuromuscular irritability.

Diagnostic evaluation

• *PaCO$_2$ level less than 35 mm Hg* (normal: 35 to 45 mm Hg): This indicates that the lungs are excreting too much carbon dioxide.
• *pH above 7.45* (normal: 7.35 to 7.45): This indicates an ineffective response by the compensatory mechanisms—buffers, lungs, and kidneys.

Nursing diagnoses

• Ineffective breathing pattern related to hyperventilation
• Anxiety related to psychosocial distress

Planning and goals

• The client's blood pH will return to normal.
• The client will not have preventable complications.
• The client and family will have decreased anxiety.

Implementation

1. Help the client breathe into a paper bag to help increase carbon dioxide retention.
2. Administer sedatives to cause respiratory center depression, which will slow respiration.
3. Suggest psychotherapy to decrease severe anxiety.
4. Encourage the client to rest.
5. Check arterial blood gas measurements and report problems to the physician. This prevents potentially dangerous changes in PaO$_2$ and PaCO$_2$ levels.
6. Provide emotional support to the client and family to alleviate anxiety.

Evaluation

• The client's blood pH ranges between 7.35 and 7.45, and the PaCO$_2$ level is between 35 and 45 mm Hg.
• The client has normal breath sounds.
• The client and family have decreased anxiety.

Metabolic alkalosis: Base bicarbonate excess (▲ HCO$_3^-$ ▲ pH)

Abnormal loss of acid ions in the body or excessive retention or ingestion of sodium bicarbonate or other alkali produces metabolic alkalosis.

Causes
• Excess intake of sodium bicarbonate or other alkali (base)
• Loss of hydrochloric acid through gastric suctioning or prolonged or profuse vomiting
• Excess loss of potassium from diarrhea or diuretics

Assessment

1. Assess symptoms related to the cause of alkalosis—irritability, disorientation, tetany, and seizures. Excessive alkali levels cause CNS overstimulation.
2. Check the client for shallow respirations with periods of apnea. If these conditions develop, the lungs are probably retaining carbon dioxide to compensate for increased alkali levels.
3. Monitor the client for an irregular pulse rate, arrhythmias, and muscle twitching, all caused by electrolyte imbalance (low serum potassium and calcium).

Diagnostic evaluation

• *Blood pH over 7.45:* This indicates an ineffective response by compensatory mechanisms—buffers, lungs, and kidneys.
• *Bicarbonate level exceeding 29 mEq/liter:* This confirms alkalosis.

• *Urine pH exceeding 7.0:* This means that the kidneys are excreting bicarbonate and retaining hydrogen ions, resulting in decreased formation of ammonia.

Nursing diagnoses

• Activity intolerance related to impaired metabolism
• Risk for injury related to electrolyte imbalance

Planning and goals

• The client's blood pH will return to normal limits.
• The client will learn how to prevent alkalosis.
• The client and family will have decreased anxiety.

Implementation

1. Permit activity as tolerated. If the client has an electrolyte imbalance, shows disorientation, and experiences convulsions, put the client on bed rest.
2. Treat the cause of alkalosis.
3. Provide emotional support to the client and family.
4. Provide appropriate fluid and electrolyte replacement (the client will need this if vomiting or ion loss from gastric suctioning occurs) and potassium and chloride replacement, as needed.
5. Review laboratory reports to verify that the client's fluid and electrolyte levels remain within normal limits.
6. If excess alkali ingestion caused the imbalance, identify its source. Ask the physician to prescribe a different medication if the client's regular medication caused the alkalosis. To prevent future alkalosis, advise the client to avoid over-the-counter antacid medications.

Evaluation

• The client's blood pH ranges between 7.35 and 7.45 and serum bicarbonate between 21 and 29 mEq/liter.
• The client knows how to prevent alkalosis.
• The client and family have decreased anxiety.

Metabolic acidosis: Base bicarbonate deficit (⬇HCO_3^- ⬇pH)

Metabolic acidosis is an abnormal loss of bicarbonate or excess retention or production of acid ions.

Causes
• Renal failure—retention of phosphate and sulfate ions (acid)
• Severe diarrhea—loss of bicarbonate and sodium ions (base)
• Diabetes mellitus—breakdown of fats, with resulting ketones (acid)
• Prolonged fasting—breakdown of fats
• Excessive exercise, with resultant buildup of lactic acid
• Ingestion of large doses of acidifying salts (for example, ammonium chloride)

Assessment

1. Evaluate the client for apathy, disorientation, and coma, which result from CNS depression.
2. Assess for Kussmaul's respirations. Rapid, deep breathing eliminates carbon dioxide via the lungs.
3. Assess the client for an elevated serum potassium level. Potassium shifts from cells to the plasma, producing an electrolyte imbalance that can cause arrhythmias.
4. If the client has diabetes mellitus or severe diarrhea (loss of bicarbonate and sodium), observe for dehydration. Severe polyuria in diabetes mellitus causes dehydration, which in turn causes excess excretion of water in diarrhea.

Diagnostic evaluation

• *pH below 7.35* (normal: 7.35 to 7.45): This indicates an inadequate response by compensatory mechanisms—buffers, lungs, and kidneys.
• *Bicarbonate level below 21 mEq/liter* (normal: 21 to 29 mEq/liter): This may indicate that bicarbonates are neutralizing the excess acids or that there is an excess loss of bicarbonate.
• *Urine pH below 6.0:* This indicates that the kidneys are excreting hydrogen ions and retaining alkali.

Nursing diagnoses

• Activity intolerance related to impaired metabolic state
• Fluid volume deficit related to increased fluid loss
• Risk for injury related to electrolyte imbalance

Planning and goals

• The client will not have preventable complications.
• The client's blood pH will return to normal limits.

Implementation

1. Maintain the client on complete bed rest to reduce cell metabolism.
2. Treat the cause of acidosis.
3. Administer sodium bicarbonate to correct bicarbonate deficit.
4. Monitor fluid and electrolyte levels frequently; a client with metabolic acidosis always has an imbalance. Check for signs of dehydration and hypovolemic shock.
5. Monitor the client for arrhythmias. Elevated serum potassium levels increase the risk of cardiac rhythm changes.
6. Provide emotional support to the client and family.
7. If diabetic ketoacidosis is the cause, closely monitor blood glucose levels.
8. If the client is in renal failure, start dialysis, the treatment of choice to correct the electrolyte and acid-base imbalance caused by renal failure.
9. Observe the client's level of consciousness. Implement care interventions if the client loses consciousness.

Evaluation

• The client's fluid and electrolyte levels return to normal limits.
• The client's blood pH falls between 7.35 and 7.45, and the serum bicarbonate level is between 21 and 29 mEq/liter.

Electrolyte imbalances

Electrolyte balance is the body's maintenance of normal electrolyte levels. The three electrolytes that have the most frequent imbalances are sodium (135 to 145 mEq/liter), potassium (3.5 to 5 mEq/liter), and calcium (4.5 to 5.8 mEq/liter). The primary extracellular electrolyte, sodium is responsible for intracellular and extracellular movement of water, and a close relationship exists between water balance and sodium concentration. The kidneys regulate the amount of sodium excreted. Potassium, the primary intracellular electrolyte, affects neuromuscular functioning and must be ingested daily. Serum pH directly affects the body's serum potassium concentration. The most plentiful of the electrolytes, calcium plays a major role in bone and tooth formation, affects blood coagulation, and influences cell membrane permeability (specifically, cardiac and neuromuscular functioning). An electrolyte imbalance—an abnormally high or low level of sodium, potassium, or calcium—can result in fluid volume deficit, altered nutrition, and other complications for the client.

Hyponatremia (low serum sodium level)

Assessment	**1.** Assess the client for factors that may be contributing to a low sodium concentration. These may include a prolonged low-sodium diet, fluid replacement with water only (either I.V. or by mouth), tube irrigations with water, use of diuretics, impaired functioning of the adrenal cortex, insufficient aldosterone secretion, and vomiting. **2.** Note manifestations of hyponatremia (weakness, dizziness, fatigue, decreased blood pressure, and abdominal cramps), which occur when the sodium level falls below 135 mEq/liter; they result from the hypotonicity (hypo-osmolarity) of the extracellular fluid. Water moves into the cells, causing them to swell. If the condition is not corrected, the decrease in extracellular fluid can cause symptoms of volume depletion, leading to cardiovascular collapse, seizures, coma, and death.
Nursing diagnosis	Fluid volume deficit related to regulatory failure
Planning and goal	The client's serum sodium level will return to normal limits.
Implementation	**1.** For irrigations, use normal saline solution to replace depleted sodium and to prevent water intoxication. **2.** Cautiously use tap-water enemas. **3.** Provide the client with saline ice chips. **4.** Replace lost body fluids with drinks containing sodium, such as juice and broth. **5.** Teach a client on diuretics about the risk of sodium depletion. Many diuretics act by impairing sodium reabsorption in the renal tubule. **6.** Correct sodium deficiency by using I.V. saline solution as needed. **7.** Restrict such fluids as water to increase the sodium concentration.
Evaluation	The client has a serum sodium level of 138 mEq/liter.

Hypernatremia (high serum sodium level)

Assessment	**1.** Assess the client for factors that may be contributing to a high serum sodium concentration—some combination of decreased intake or increased output of water or increased intake or decreased output of sodium. These factors may include diarrhea, near drowning in salt water, increased insensible loss from rapid respirations, fever, and excessive perspiration. **2.** Assess for muscle weakness; seizures; dry, sticky mucous membranes; and thirst—all caused by hypertonicity of the extracellular fluid, producing water loss from cells and from the brain.
Nursing diagnosis	Fluid volume deficit related to abnormal fluid loss or decreased fluid intake
Planning and goal	The client's serum sodium level will return to normal limits.
Implementation	**1.** Increase the client's water intake to decrease the sodium concentration in the extracellular fluid. **2.** As appropriate, give water with or between tube feedings. **3.** Instruct an elderly client to drink fluids routinely (elderly clients have a decreased perception of thirst).
Evaluation	The client's serum sodium level is 143 mEq/liter.

MAINTAINING HOMEOSTASIS

Hypokalemia (low serum potassium level)

Assessment

1. Assess the client for factors that may be contributing to a low potassium level. These include consuming nothing by mouth for more than 1 day, starvation, lack of potassium replacement in I.V. fluids, use of diuretics (thiazide diuretics and furosemide [Lasix], especially, cause potassium wasting), nasogastric drainage, diarrhea, steroids that increase potassium excretion, and alkalosis, which causes serum potassium stores to enter the cell.
2. Assess the client for muscle weakness, fatigue, abdominal distention, ileus, cardiac arrhythmias, and a flat T wave, all of which may be caused by a disturbance in conduction to the visceral and skeletal muscles.

Nursing diagnoses

• Fluid volume deficit related to abnormal fluid loss
• Altered nutrition (less than body requirements) related to decreased potassium intake

Planning and goal

The client's serum potassium level will return to normal limits.

Implementation

1. Teach the client (especially one taking diuretics) to consume high-potassium foods, including raw greens (spinach), dried fruits (apricots, raisins, peaches), bananas, oranges, and baked potatoes.
2. As indicated, give the client potassium supplements. Dilute liquids by adding ice. Note that potassium supplements taste bad and cause GI irritation. Instruct the client to take supplements with or after meals and a full glass of water or fruit juice.
3. Administer potassium I.V. by slow infusion to replace loss or prevent depletion. Do not exceed 40 mEq/liter nor administer by I.V. bolus. Monitor the client's electrocardiogram. An I.V. bolus or rapid administration can cause cardiac irritability and induce cardiac arrest. Check the client for phlebitis because potassium irritates veins.
4. Monitor for digoxin toxicity, to which a client with a low serum potassium level is especially vulnerable.

Evaluation

The client maintains a serum potassium level of 4 mEq/liter.

Hyperkalemia (high serum potassium level)

Assessment

1. Assess the client for factors that may be contributing to a high serum potassium level. These include severe trauma (such as burns and crushing injuries), impaired renal function, and diabetic acidosis.
2. Assess the client for weakness, paralysis, GI disturbances, arrhythmias, and cardiac arrest, all of which can be caused by an increased depressant effect on the myocardium and skeletal muscles.

Nursing diagnosis

Fluid volume deficit related to abnormal fluid loss

Planning and goal

The client's serum potassium level will return to normal.

Implementation

1. Restrict potassium for a client with impaired renal function, and regularly monitor the client's serum potassium level and renal function.
2. Carefully observe all I.V. infusions that contain potassium. Note the client's response and the infusion rate.
3. Force fluids to flush out the potassium by increasing the client's urine output.

4. Administer cation exchange resins, such as sodium polystyrene sulfate (Kayexalate) with sorbitol, which produce an exchange of sodium ions for potassium ions in the GI mucosa.
5. Administer potassium-excreting diuretics.
6. Perform dialysis as needed. In renal failure, dialysis offers the most effective means to lower the client's potassium level.

Evaluation

The client's serum potassium level is 4.5 mEq/liter.

Hypocalcemia (low serum calcium level)

Assessment

1. Assess the client for factors that may be contributing to a low serum calcium level, including abuse of phosphate-containing antacids, decreased intake of milk and vitamin D, and removal of the parathyroid glands.
2. Assess the client for neuromuscular irritability, Chvostek's sign (twitching of the facial nerve in response to a tap on the nerve), Trousseau's sign (spasm of the forearm on obstruction of its blood supply), tetany (the worst form of tetany is laryngospasm), and muscle twitching. Increased cell membrane permeability causes neuromuscular irritability.

Nursing diagnosis

Altered nutrition (less than body requirements) related to inadequate calcium intake

Planning and goal

The client will maintain a normal serum calcium level.

Implementation

1. Teach the client to use phosphate-containing antacids cautiously and to increase intake of milk, cheese, and vitamin D.
2. Have calcium gluconate on hand to replace decreased calcium levels in an emergency, such as after thyroid surgery when the parathyroid glands may have been removed inadvertently.

Evaluation

The client maintains a serum calcium level of 5 mEq/liter.

Hypercalcemia (high serum calcium level)

Assessment

1. Assess the client for factors that may be contributing to a high serum calcium level, including increased calcium absorption and increased mobilization of calcium from bones (as in hyperparathyroidism, multiple myeloma, and long-term immobility).
2. Assess the client for nausea and vomiting, dehydration, muscle weakness, fatigue, cardiac arrest, and renal calculi.

Nursing diagnosis

Impaired physical mobility related to limited use of extremities

Planning and goal

The client will maintain a normal serum calcium level.

Implementation

1. Limit dietary calcium and avoid vitamin D supplements to decrease the amount of calcium absorbed in the GI tract.
2. Force fluids and acidify urine to prevent the precipitation of calcium calculus that occurs in alkaline urine.
3. Monitor for digoxin toxicity, to which a client with hypercalcemia is especially vulnerable.

MAINTAINING HOMEOSTASIS

Evaluation	The client maintains a serum calcium level of 5.5 mEq/liter.

Fluid imbalances

Sodium balance vitally affects fluid balance. Equivalent amounts of sodium and water that are lost or gained will not change serum osmolarity (tonicity), but the client may show signs of fluid volume deficit or overload.

Fluid volume deficit (dehydration)

Assessment	**1.** Assess the client for dry skin. **2.** Assess the client for decreased skin turgor (after being pinched, the skin remains tented or slowly returns to normal). **3.** Record the client's fluid intake and output. Normally, the body maintains a balance of about 2,300 ml of intake as fluids and food and 2,300 ml of output as sensible or insensible fluid loss. **4.** Weigh the client daily. Each 2-pound weight loss reflects a 1-liter fluid loss. **5.** Assess the client for increased thirst caused by low blood volume; decreased blood pressure; oliguria caused by decreased renal perfusion; tachycardia, a compensatory mechanism to maintain cardiac output in the presence of decreased stroke volume (cardiac output equals heart rate multiplied by stroke volume, or $CO = HR \times SV$); elevated blood urea nitrogen levels (poor perfusion impairs the kidneys' ability to excrete body wastes); and elevated specific gravity, which indicates concentrated urine. **6.** Assess the client for collapsed neck and hand veins, which indicate decreased blood volume.
Nursing diagnosis	Fluid volume deficit related to inadequate fluid intake or abnormal fluid loss
Planning and goal	The client will achieve and maintain adequate hydration.
Implementation	Depends on the cause; may vary from shock treatment (see "Shock," pages 103 to 108) to replacing fluids by oral supplementation and I.V. therapy (see "Acid-base imbalances," pages 110 to 114, and "Electrolyte imbalances," pages 114 to 118)
Evaluation	The client voids at least 40 ml/hour.

Fluid volume overload

Assessment	**1.** Observe the client for edema in the sacrum, scrotum, and feet (edema occurs in dependent parts). **2.** Observe for elevated blood pressure caused by increased cardiac output from fluid volume overload. **3.** Monitor the client for decreased specific gravity caused by hemodilution. **4.** Observe for diluted urine caused by a decreased ratio of solutes to fluid. **5.** Weigh the client daily. Significant weight gain reflects fluid volume overload. **6.** Assess the client for engorged neck and hand veins, which indicate fluid volume overload.

Nursing diagnosis	Fluid volume excess related to increased fluid retention
Planning and goal	The client's circulating blood volume will be within normal limits.
Implementation	**1.** Restrict fluids. **2.** Administer diuretics, as ordered. **3.** Treat the client, if necessary, for congestive heart failure or pulmonary edema.
Evaluation	• The client maintains a stable body weight. • The client displays no overt signs of edema or dehydration.

Immobility

Immobility is a temporary or permanent decrease in the client's ability to move all or part of the body easily or comfortably. Types of immobility include a loss of motor function, a loss of sensory function, and a combined loss of motor and sensory function.

Loss of motor function can produce weakness or paralysis of the muscles, as in quadriplegia (paralysis of all extremities), paraplegia (paralysis of the legs), and hemiplegia (paralysis of one side of the body).

Loss of sensory function can result in blindness, hemianopsia (blindness in half of the field of vision in one or both eyes), agnosia (inability to comprehend or recognize an object), deafness, anesthesia (inability to feel pain or touch), and aphasia (inability to speak intended words or to understand words).

The client can also lose proprioception (awareness of one's position, weight, posture, or equilibrium).

Causes of immobility include:
• trauma (cutting or transection of nerve pathways or muscle fibers to or from affected tissues)
• anoxia (loss of oxygen to cells, resulting in cell death; may accompany hemorrhage or blood loss, excessive swelling, or acid-base imbalances)
• infectious agents (microorganisms exerting toxic effects on cells, either from the organisms themselves or from the toxins they produce)
• degenerative conditions (such as myasthenia gravis and amyotropic lateral sclerosis) that gradually cause tissues to lose function, certain medications (such as anesthetics) and poisons
• treatment for a medical condition (for example, myocardial infarction, surgery, or cast application)
• severe anxiety.

Nursing care focuses on the major goals of maintaining function in unaffected tissues and regaining maximal function in affected tissues, with the client fulfilling usual or new roles within the family and society.

Immobility can affect all of the major body systems. Respiratory and cardiovascular changes affect the rate, depth, and strength of respiratory effort, predisposing the client to anoxia, atelectasis, and pneumonia. To prevent these effects, the client must regularly perform deep-breathing and coughing exercises, frequently change position and, unless contraindicated, increase fluid intake to 3,000 ml daily. The nurse should check vital signs frequently.

Resulting from pressure and stasis, the integumentary effects of immobility include atrophy, tissue breakdown, and pressure ulcers. To prevent these effects, promote proper hygiene, including baths and use of lotions. Use padding, mattresses, protective barriers, and rails to prevent further skin lesions or trauma. Adequately maintain the client's nutritional and fluid intake; frequently change the client's position.

Decreased energy expenditure predisposes the client to anorexia, altered intake, and altered nutrient use and metabolism, resulting in diarrhea, hemorrhoids, and malnutrition. To prevent constipation, increase the client's intake of fluids, especially fruit juices, and of foods that increase dietary bulk (unless contraindicated). Encourage the client to perform range-of-motion and abdominal sitting exercises. Administer a fecal softener or laxative, if ordered. If the client does not have a bowel movement within 3 days, administer an enema. Weigh the client. The client may need to increase nutrient intake via tube feeding or total parenteral nutrition.

Decreased fluid intake and urinary stasis predispose the client to urinary tract infections and formation of renal calculi. To prevent these effects, reduce diet calcium levels and encourage the client to walk or otherwise put stress on the bones routinely. If possible, increase the client's fluid intake to 3,000 ml daily.

Loss of innervation and sensation predisposes the client to muscle spasticity or flaccidity, with such neurologic consequences as altered pain perception, autonomic dysreflexia, confusion, and disorientation. Position the client to maintain joint and body functions. Frequently turn the client from side to side by logrolling if the spinal cord has been damaged. Initiate range-of-motion exercises to affected areas. As needed, perform neurologic checks and obtain physical or occupational therapy consultation.

Endocrine metabolic effects of immobility include predisposition to weight loss; acid-base, fluid, and electrolyte imbalances; stress ulcers; anemia; osteoporosis; pathologic fractures; prolonged healing; amenorrhea; impotence; and loss of libido. Regularly observe the client for these conditions, which may have causes other than immobility.

Immobility can have psychological effects—such as anxiety, fear, and depression—and can even cause death. The client may not be able to obtain employment. Immobility, especially if it is chronic, can adversely affect the ability to develop and maintain social relationships. The client needs emotional support and reassurance from both the family and health professionals. Psychiatric consultation may help during prolonged anxiety and depression. Include family members in the client's care, as feasible, and teach them client care before discharge. Arrange vocational counseling and education as the client requires and requests. Finally, issue continuity of care referrals on the client's transfer or discharge home.

Part V

Review of clinical nursing

Perioperative nursing

Mental health nursing

Maternal-infant nursing

Child nursing

Adult nursing

Perioperative nursing

PERIOPERATIVE
NURSING

Introduction

Perioperative nursing—nursing care provided for a surgical client—comprises three phases: the preoperative period (before surgery), the intraoperative period (during surgery), and the postoperative period (after surgery). Because clients experience varying degrees of anxiety and knowledge deficit related to surgery, careful planning by the nurse can help ensure a positive outcome. Recently, standards of perioperative nursing practice based on the nursing process have been developed to provide guidance to those who work in this important nursing specialty. This section, therefore, uses the nursing process to review the three phases of perioperative nursing.

The first entry, "Preoperative period," examines the role of the nurse in client teaching and in relieving the client's and the family's anxieties. "Intraoperative period" focuses on nursing responsibilities for maintaining safety, monitoring physiologic responses to surgery, and keeping the client comfortable; the entry also reviews general, regional, and local anesthesia. Finally, "Postoperative period" covers routine postoperative nursing care for all surgical clients; potential postoperative problems and complications, with appropriate nursing diagnoses and interventions listed for each potential problem; and recommended postoperative positions, ambulation requirements, and nursing considerations for various surgical procedures.

PERIOPERATIVE NURSING

Preoperative period

Most clients have the following concerns or problems before surgery: incomplete or incorrect information about the surgical procedure, its purpose, and its risks; anxiety (possibly based on past surgery) about the procedure, possible complications, anesthesia, altered body image, and loss of control; lack of trust in health care personnel; and fear of the diagnosis, pain, and death.

Glossary

Anesthesia—loss of pain sensation; may be general, regional, or local
Antidiuretic hormone (ADH)—hormone, released from the pituitary gland, that affects fluid and electrolyte balance
Atelectasis—collapse of the lung alveoli
Central venous pressure gauge—manometer attached to a catheter in a major vein to monitor blood volume and venous return to the heart
Dehiscence—partial or complete separation of wound edges
Evisceration—protrusion of abdominal contents through a surgical incision

Hyperpyrexia—malignant hyperthermia, a complication of anesthesia that usually occurs immediately after surgery
Hypoxemia—deficient blood oxygen level, usually resulting from a ventilation-perfusion imbalance
Incentive spirometry—promotion of deep breathing and full expansion of the alveoli by means of a mechanical device that measures the amount of air the client inhales and exhales
Paralytic ileus—temporary paralysis of the intestines, causing abdominal distention and signs of bowel obstruction

Assessment

NURSING BEHAVIORS	NURSING RATIONALES
1. Assess the client for restlessness, increased verbalization, quiet or withdrawn behavior, feelings of denial, and elevated pulse and respiratory rates.	**1.** All of these are signs of increased anxiety. Virtually every client about to undergo surgery experiences anxiety in some form, from mild to severe.
2. Expect the client to ask questions about the procedure, to cry, and to show anger.	**2.** Questions are normal: knowledge will help speed the client's recovery. Depending on the surgical procedure, the client may experience various stages of loss, including depression and anger.

Nursing diagnoses
- Anxiety related to the impending surgery
- Knowledge deficit related to unfamiliarity with the surgical procedure
- Fear related to the diagnosis

Planning and goals   The client will:
- express fears freely
- be calm and relaxed.

Implementation

NURSING BEHAVIORS	NURSING RATIONALES
1. Increase time spent privately with the client, and encourage the client to express fears.	**1.** Privacy allows the client to express feelings openly. A nurse's presence indicates a concern for the client's well-being, which reduces the client's anxiety.
2. Encourage the client to participate in decision making.	**2.** This increases the client's sense of control and helps maintain self-esteem.
3. Touch the client, if appropriate, while communicating with him.	**3.** Touch expresses caring and has a calming effect.
4. Provide the client with needed information about surgery.	**4.** Education not only promotes trust but also ensures that the client's rights are being upheld.
5. Provide preoperative teaching, as needed.	**5.** Preoperative teaching decreases the client's anxiety, which helps create well-being and comfort. Usually, a client who knows what to expect has fewer complications.
6. Administer sedatives or antianxiety agents, as ordered, the night before surgery, and observe the client for drug effects.	**6.** Sedatives or antianxiety agents decrease anxiety and allow the client restful sleep. Close observation helps detect potential adverse reactions to medication.
7. Administer preoperative medications, such as narcotics (morphine, meperidine) and anticholinergics (atropine, glycopyrrolate), as ordered.	**7.** Narcotics sometimes are given to aid anesthetic induction. Anticholinergics decrease bronchial secretions.

Evaluation   The client approaches surgery with only mild anxiety and freely expresses concerns.

Intraoperative period

In the operating room, the client usually is sedated and under the care of anesthesia personnel. Depending on the surgical procedure, regional or general anesthetic is administered. Expect to assist anesthesia personnel or to monitor the client when local and certain regional anesthesia techniques are used. (See *Types of anesthesia,* page 127.)

Postoperative period

The postoperative period begins when the client is discharged from the operating room to the postanesthesia recovery (PAR) area. During this period, the client must be monitored carefully for vital signs, bleeding, and recovery from anesthesia; life-threatening complications (such as altered respiratory function and decreased cardiac output) can occur during the first few days.

Implementation

NURSING BEHAVIORS	NURSING RATIONALES
1. Maintain basic recovery room priorities, as detailed in steps 2 through 9.	**1.** Priorities are geared toward maintaining vital life functions—patent airway, tissue perfusion, and neurologic integrity—and preventing complications.
2. Check the client's airway regularly, and position the client to prevent aspiration.	**2.** The side-lying position (unless contraindicated) best prevents aspiration.
3. Check the client's circulation; measure vital signs every 15 minutes until the client is stable.	**3.** Many clients have labile vital signs after surgery.
4. Check the client's neurologic function. Note orientation to person, place, and time; check reflexes, sensations, and motor functions.	**4.** The client cannot be discharged from the PAR area until neurologic functions have returned to normal.
5. Check the client's dressing and bedclothes, including underneath the client, for evidence of hemorrhage.	**5.** Gravity may carry drainage under the client. Careful inspection of dressings and bedclothes can detect hemorrhage and ensure prompt treatment.
6. Connect all tubes and catheters.	**6.** This ensures proper tube functioning.
7. Promote client comfort and relieve pain as needed. Do not overlook pain unrelated to the surgical procedure.	**7.** Besides surgery, the client's discomfort may be caused by body position; a full bladder; flatus; hypoxemia; and tight dressings, casts, or bandages.
8. Administer narcotics with great care, and do not administer them if the client's respiratory rate is less than 12 breaths/minute.	**8.** Narcotics administered during the postoperative period can decrease the client's respiratory rate and inhibit recovery from the anesthetic.
9. Ensure the client's safety by keeping the side rails up at all times.	**9.** The client has not fully recovered from anesthesia and is therefore at risk for falling out of bed.

PERIOPERATIVE NURSING

Potential problems for postoperative clients

Altered respiratory function

(related to anesthesia, airway obstruction, pain, chronic obstructive pulmonary disease, or atelectasis)

Assessment

NURSING BEHAVIORS	NURSING RATIONALES
1. Observe the client for dyspnea.	1. Dyspnea indicates impaired ventilation.
2. Observe the client for tachycardia.	2. Tachycardia may indicate hypoxia.
3. Observe the client for decreased breath sounds.	3. Breath sounds decrease in atelectasis because of alveolar collapse.
4. Observe the client for crackles, rhonchi, and stertorous respirations.	4. These indicate airway secretions and possibly an airway obstruction.
5. Assess the client's skin for pallor.	5. Pallor indicates poor oxygenation and a reduced hemoglobin level.
6. Observe the client for anxiety and restlessness.	6. Anxiety and restlessness are early signs of hypoxia caused by cerebral irritability.
7. Monitor the client's PO_2 level to detect any decrease.	7. Impaired ventilation or perfusion causes hypoxemia.
8. Monitor the client's PCO_2 level to detect any increase.	8. Anesthesia or incisional pain can cause hypoventilation, resulting in retention of CO_2.
9. Take and record the client's temperature regularly; be alert for a temperature greater than 100.4° F (38° C).	9. The most common cause of elevated temperature during the first 24 hours after surgery is atelectasis.

Nursing diagnoses
- Ineffective airway clearance related to shallow breathing and incisional pain
- Impaired gas exchange related to postoperative atelectasis

Planning and goal   The client will be free from postoperative respiratory complications.

Implementation

NURSING BEHAVIORS	NURSING RATIONALES
1. Review preoperative teaching of deep-breathing exercises and how and when to change positions.	1. This review of earlier teaching promotes the client's participation in recovery to avoid postoperative complications.
2. Tell the client to turn and perform deep-breathing exercises every hour. Be sure to splint the incision during these exercises by holding a hand over the dressing and applying slight pressure to the incision site.	2. Turning and breathing deeply prevent atelectasis and ventilate the distal alveoli. External splinting decreases pain and allows for increased chest expansion.

Types of anesthesia

I. Regional anesthesia
  A. Effects on the client
    1. Loss of motor and sensory perception to a particular area of the body
    2. Intact consciousness
  B. Common types
    1. *Spinal*—injection of a local anesthetic into the second, third, or fourth lumbar space or the first sacral space
    2. *Epidural*—injection of a local anesthetic into the epidural space
  C. Uses—surgical procedures involving the legs, the lower abdomen, or the perineum
  D. Potential complications
    1. Sympathetic preganglionic block of fibers in the anterior root of the spinal cord, causing vasodilation and reduced venous blood return to the heart
    2. Spinal headache
    3. Respiratory depression (if thoracic, intercostal, or accessory muscles are inadvertently anesthetized)
    4. Overanesthetization of the spinal cord (resulting in the client's inability to breathe; oxygen and ventilatory support are required)
    5. *Other complications*—low blood pressure, depressed myocardium, anaphylactic reaction, seizures, ringing in the ears, facial numbness or twitching, nausea and vomiting
  E. Nursing implementations
    1. Assess the client for hypotension; have a vasopressor, such as ephedrine sulfate (Ephedrine Sulfate Injection) or phenylephrine hydrochloride (Neo-Synephrine), available.
    2. Record the client's respiratory rate and depth.
    3. Assess for return of sensation and motor function below the level of anesthesia; ask the client to move the anesthetized part and to report any perception of touch.
    4. Keep the client flat in bed for about 8 hours after regional anesthesia to prevent spinal fluid leakage, which is thought to cause spinal headache.
    5. Tell the client not to strain when moving in bed or having a bowel movement; straining increases intracranial pressure, which can exacerbate loss of CSF.
    6. If spinal headache occurs, administer an analgesic, keep the client flat, and report the headache to the physician.
    7. Provide adequate hydration to help replace spinal fluid and prevent venous stasis.
    8. Have resuscitation equipment available at all times.
    9. Know the toxic dose of each local anesthetic used during a procedure.

II. General anesthesia
  A. Effects on the client
    1. Produces unconsciousness
    2. Blocks motor and sensory pathways to major nerve and muscle groups
  B. Administration methods
    1. Inhalation gas
    2. I.V. injection
  C. Stages of physiologic changes
    1. Stage I (relaxation)—from initial administration of an anesthetic to loss of consciousness. *Client response:* dizziness, drowsiness, exaggerated hearing, decreased pain sensation
    2. Stage II (excitement)—from loss of consciousness to onset of regular breathing. *Client response:* irregular breathing, increased muscle tone and involuntary motor activity, thrashing and struggling, susceptibility to auditory and tactile stimulation
    3. Stage III (surgical anesthesia)—from onset of regular breathing to cessation of breathing. *Client response:* regular thoracoabdominal breathing, relaxed jaw, loss of pain and auditory sensation, loss of swallowing reflex
    4. Stage IV (danger)—from cessation of breathing to circulatory failure and death. *Client response:* fixed and dilated pupils, rapid and thready pulse, respiratory muscle paralysis
  D. Recovery—gradual, in reverse order of physiologic changes
  E. Nursing implementations
    1. Close operating room doors. Check for proper positioning of the safety belt. Have suction equipment available and working. Minimize room noise.
    2. Provide emotional support.
    3. Avoid stimulating the client. Be available to provide protection or restraint.
    4. Be available to assist anesthesia personnel with intubation. Confirm with them the appropriate times for positioning and scrubbing the client. To prevent impaired circulation, be sure that the client's feet are not crossed.
    5. Be ready to assist in treating cardiac or respiratory arrest. Have emergency drugs and defibrillation equipment available. Document the drug administration.

PERIOPERATIVE NURSING

3. Ensure that the client walks 3 times daily as tolerated.

3. Periodic walking facilitates full chest expansion.

4. Relieve the client's pain by administering narcotics (as ordered), splinting the incision site, and repositioning the client.

4. The client will be unable to perform deep-breathing exercises or cough if pain is too severe.

Evaluation

• The client is free from pulmonary complications.
• The client's arterial blood gas levels and pulmonary function remain within normal limits.

Decreased cardiac output

(related to hemorrhage, vasodilation, or prolonged or insufficient clotting)

Assessment

NURSING BEHAVIORS	NURSING RATIONALES
1. Monitor the client for decreased blood pressure.	**1.** An arterial blood pressure reading of less than 80 mm Hg indicates shock and inadequate tissue perfusion.
2. Monitor the client's urine output, and note any decrease.	**2.** Diminished urine output indicates hypovolemia or poor renal perfusion.
3. Observe the client for a weak, thready, rapid pulse.	**3.** As stroke volume decreases, heart rate increases to maintain the same cardiac output.
4. Monitor the client for decreased central venous pressure (CVP), noting any changes (normal CVP: 6 to 13 cm H_2O).	**4.** A decreased CVP reading indicates hypovolemia, particularly if urine output is also decreased.
5. Observe the client's skin for pallor.	**5.** Pallor indicates decreased peripheral circulation.
6. Observe the client for restlessness.	**6.** Restlessness is an early sign of hypoxia from cerebral irritability.
7. Monitor the client for profuse perspiration and increased drainage from dressings.	**7.** These signs may indicate fluid loss.

Nursing diagnoses

• Decreased cardiac output related to postoperative hypovolemia
• Fluid volume deficit related to hemorrhage or vasodilation
• Altered tissue perfusion related to decreased cardiac output

Planning and goals

• The client's blood pressure will stabilize 1 to 2 hours after surgery.
• The client's pulse rate will remain at 60 to 100 beats/minute.
• The client's urine output will be 30 to 50 ml/hour.

Implementation

NURSING BEHAVIORS	NURSING RATIONALES
1. Check vital signs every 15 minutes until the client is stable, then every half hour for 2 hours, then every 4 hours for 24 hours.	**1.** Shock may occur as a result of anesthesia, blood loss, or medication. As vital signs become more stable, changes occur less frequently.
2. Measure the client's urine output.	**2.** Decreased urine output may indicate hypovolemia or poor renal perfusion. *Caution:* Decreased urine output may also stem from urine retention caused by stress.
3. Check the client's dressing and bedclothes, including underneath the client, for evidence of hemorrhage.	**3.** Hemorrhage or fluid loss may lead to shock. Gravity may carry drainage under the client.

Evaluation   Vital signs are stable, and urine output is adequate.

Altered mental status

(related to anesthesia or hypoxia)

Assessment

NURSING BEHAVIORS	NURSING RATIONALES
1. Assess the client's level of consciousness.	**1.** A client who cannot be aroused has not fully recovered from the anesthesia or may have nervous system damage.
2. Observe the client for decreased reflexes (including the gag, cough, swallow, and deep tendon reflexes).	**2.** Reflexes indicate the client's state of alertness.
3. Observe the client for decreased pupillary response.	**3.** Normally, pupils are the same size and constrict equally to light.
4. Observe the client for neuromuscular irritability.	**4.** After surgery and anesthesia, the client will have an increased response to stimuli.
5. Observe the client for decreased neuromuscular response to stimuli.	**5.** This indicates that the client may not have recovered fully from anesthesia; thus, safety precautions should be taken.

Nursing diagnoses
- Altered cerebral tissue perfusion related to postoperative hypovolemia
- Sensory or perceptual alteration related to postanesthesia effects

Planning and goals
- The client will be mentally alert and oriented after surgery.
- The client will regain all reflex activity.

PERIOPERATIVE NURSING

Implementation

NURSING BEHAVIORS	NURSING RATIONALES
1. Assess the client's orientation and neuromuscular reflex response.	**1.** This assessment helps the nurse determine whether the client has fully recovered from anesthesia.
2. Withhold narcotics or administer in small doses, as ordered.	**2.** Narcotics may further depress the central nervous system (CNS). Until fully recovered from anesthesia, the client does not usually require a full narcotic dose. Narcotics can depress respirations, decrease blood pressure, and alter mentation.

Evaluation

• The client is oriented to time, place, and person.
• The client's reflexes return.

Discomfort and pain

(related to the surgical incision, the client's position, flatus, or a distended bladder)

Assessment

NURSING BEHAVIOR	NURSING RATIONALE
Observe the client for discomfort and its source, such as a catheter, dressing, or cast.	Postoperative discomfort may have many causes that the nurse should rule out before assuming that the incision is the primary source of pain.

Nursing diagnosis   Pain related to incision and tissue trauma

Planning and goal   The client's postoperative pain will be minimal.

Implementation

NURSING BEHAVIORS	NURSING RATIONALES
1. Reposition the client as neccessary to relieve pain, at least every 2 hours.	**1.** The client's position may be a source of discomfort. Repositioning the client and explaining its purpose usually helps.
2. If appropriate, relieve tension on the urinary catheter, loosen bedclothes, and reposition the nasogastric (NG) tube.	**2.** Relieving these sources of discomfort helps achieve the nurse's primary goal: to minimize the client's postoperative pain.
3. Administer narcotics or other analgesics, as ordered. Make sure the client understands how to use patient-controlled analgesia (PCA), if ordered.	**3.** Narcotics act on the CNS to reduce pain perception. Many patients who use PCA fear giving themselves too much medication and need reinforcement about the correct use of PCA.

Evaluation   The client's pain is relieved.

Altered GI function

(related to anesthesia, surgery, obstruction, paralytic ileus, total cessation of bowel function, bowel manipulation, infection, or bacterial overgrowth)

Assessment

NURSING BEHAVIORS	NURSING RATIONALES
1. Observe the client for anorexia.	**1.** Decreased peristalsis from stress increases the potential for poor nutrition.
2. Observe the client for nausea and vomiting.	**2.** Oral fluids given too soon after surgery may lead to nausea and vomiting because of decreased peristalsis.
3. Observe the client for abdominal distention and gas pains.	**3.** These are common postoperative problems as peristalsis returns.
4. Assess the client for absence of bowel sounds.	**4.** Absence of bowel sounds indicates lack of peristalsis and may signal paralytic ileus.
5. Assess the client for diarrhea and incontinence.	**5.** These symptoms may result from increased peristalsis or bacterial overgrowth.

Nursing diagnoses

- Diarrhea related to bacterial overgrowth
- Bowel incontinence related to the client's postoperative status
- Fluid volume deficit related to nausea and vomiting
- Altered nutrition (less than body requirements) related to decreased oral intake

Planning and goals

- The client's GI function will resume a normal pattern.
- The client's fluid and electrolyte balance will be restored.
- The client will be free of discomfort from abdominal distention.

Implementation

NURSING BEHAVIORS	NURSING RATIONALES
1. Withhold food and fluids until bowel sounds return (possibly 2 to 3 days after abdominal surgery).	**1.** This prevents complications of decreased peristalsis resulting from the effects of anesthesia, narcotics, and the stress response, particularly after abdominal surgery.
2. Maintain I.V. access.	**2.** This allows for fluids to be administered until the client's oral intake is adequate.
3. Gradually change the client's diet from clear to regular.	**3.** This provides nutrition consistent with the return of normal bowel functions.
4. Ensure that the client drinks 2 to 3 liters of fluid daily.	**4.** This provides adequate hydration for bowel movement.
5. Ensure that the client walks as tolerated.	**5.** Ambulation prevents constipation and other immobility problems.

PERIOPERATIVE NURSING

6. Insert a rectal tube for 20 minutes every 4 hours.

6. This allows flatus to pass and relieves discomfort.

7. Monitor the client's serum potassium and sodium levels for evidence of depletion; administer potassium I.V. until dietary sources are available.

7. Loss of body fluids during surgery or from NG tube drainage contributes to sodium and potassium depletion.

8. Note signs and symptoms of paralytic ileus: absence of bowel sounds, abdominal distention and discomfort, and nausea and vomiting.

8. Clients with altered GI function are at risk for developing paralytic ileus. Measures designed to provide rest for the GI tract include food and fluid restrictions, NG tube drainage, and I.V. therapy.

Evaluation

- The client's bowel sounds return.
- The client's urine output is 30 ml/hour.
- The client passes stool.
- The client's electrolyte levels are within normal limits.

Decreased urine output

(related to decreased blood volume, anesthesia, stress, increased antidiuretic hormone (ADH) levels, poor position for voiding, or urine retention)

Assessment
NURSING BEHAVIORS

NURSING RATIONALES

1. Monitor the client's urine output.

1. If the client is well hydrated, urine output should resume 6 to 8 hours after surgery.

2. Palpate the bladder above the symphysis pubis to check for distention.

2. A bladder that is not palpable is not distended.

Nursing diagnosis   Altered urinary elimination related to inability to urinate postoperatively

Planning and goal   The client's urine output will resume within 8 hours after surgery.

Implementation
NURSING BEHAVIORS

NURSING RATIONALES

1. Provide 8 to 12 8-oz glasses (2,000 to 3,000 ml) of fluid daily.

1. Adequate hydration prevents urinary stasis. Initially, urine output may be less than 1,500 ml because of body fluid losses and increased ADH levels; however, it should stabilize within 48 hours.

2. Institute measures to induce voiding if urine retention occurs.

2. Running water stimulates voiding, as does pouring warm water over the perineum, which relaxes the sphincter.

3. Insert an indwelling urinary or straight catheter, as ordered.

3. If urine retention occurs, catheterization is necessary.

Evaluation
- The client's urine output is adequate.
- The client voids without difficulty.

Impaired skin integrity

(related to the surgical incision)

Assessment

NURSING BEHAVIORS	NURSING RATIONALES
1. Note signs of wound healing.	**1.** Wound healing occurs in four phases: • Phase I, the inflammatory phase, lasts 1 to 2 days. • Phase II, the collagen deposit stage, begins on the 2nd day; after 7 days, more scar tissue has formed, making the incision stronger; after 14 days, the wound should be strong. • Phase III lasts 2 to 6 weeks; the client should do no heavy lifting during this period. • Phase IV lasts several months; contractures may occur during this period.
2. Note signs of hemorrhage, such as frank or occult bleeding, decreased blood pressure, increased pulse rate, and pallor.	**2.** The greatest risk of hemorrhage occurs during the first 48 hours after surgery.
3. Note signs of infection.	**3.** Fever and incisional redness and swelling after the 3rd postoperative day indicate infection.
4. Assess the client for signs of insufficient abdominal wound healing, including dehiscence (separation of surgical wound layers, producing pink serous drainage; the client feels a pull at the wound site) and evisceration (outright protruding of abdominal contents).	**4.** A client with poor nutrition, cancer, or wound infection is prone to ineffective abdominal wound healing. Dehiscence and evisceration indicate a complete separation of the wound edges, a medical emergency.

Nursing diagnoses
- Impaired skin integrity related to the surgical incision
- Risk for infection related to the surgical incision

Planning and goal   The client's incision will heal without complications.

Implementation

NURSING BEHAVIORS	NURSING RATIONALES
1. If dehiscence or evisceration occurs, notify the physician immediately and cover evisceration with sterile saline solution. Stay with the client, and tell the client not to move or cough. Administer antibiotics if ordered.	**1.** Evisceration is a medical emergency. Covering the evisceration prevents drying and necrosis of abdominal contents. Antibiotics prevent infection.

2. Check the client's dressings and bedclothes, including underneath the client, for excessive drainage and blood, and report any evidence of hemorrhage or shock to the physician.

2. The client may be hemorrhaging and require immediate attention. In some cases, shock may be the only indication of internal hemorrhaging. (See "Shock," pages 103 to 108.)

Evaluation

• The client's wound heals without infection.
• No evidence of hemorrhage appears.

Impaired peripheral circulation

(related to thrombosis or phlebitis)

Assessment

1. Observe the client for Homans' sign.

1. A positive Homans' sign—pain on dorsiflexion of the foot that is referred to the deep posterior calf—indicates phlebothrombosis (clotting without inflammation).

2. Assess the client for pain, warmth, and tenderness in calf muscles.

2. This indicates thrombophlebitis.

Nursing diagnoses

• Altered peripheral tissue perfusion related to immobility
• Risk for injury related to pulmonary embolus

Planning and goal

The client will have adequate peripheral circulation.

Implementation

NURSING BEHAVIORS

NURSING RATIONALES

1. Take the following preventive antithrombus measures:

1. These measures promote peripheral circulation.

• Provide elastic stockings and antiembolitic compression boots.

• Elastic stockings and antiembolitic compression boots compress the superficial veins, increase blood flow through the deep veins, and prevent venous pooling.

• Do not put pressure on the popliteal space.

• Pressure causes blood stasis.

• Do not massage the client's legs.

• This may dislodge a clot.

• Ensure that the client exercises and ambulates soon after surgery.

• Light exercise and periodic walks prevent venous stasis.

2. Treat thrombophlebitis with bed rest, heat, elastic bandages, and anticoagulants.

2. Bed rest promotes healing and prevents clot dislodgment. Heat and elastic bandages increase circulation to the area. Anticoagulants prevent blood clotting.

Evaluation   The client shows no signs of circulatory stasis.

Discharge instructions

Early discharge, which has become common, typically increases client teaching needs. Make sure to provide information about wound care, activity restrictions, dietary management, medication administration, symptoms to report, and follow-up care.

A client recovering from same-day surgery in an outpatient surgical unit must be in stable condition before discharge. This client must not drive home; make sure a responsible adult takes the client home.

PERIOPERATIVE NURSING

Mental health nursing

Introduction

When experiencing the stressors of life, a person tends to respond in a characteristic manner. The person's overall flexibility or rigidity in using this characteristic behavior determines whether the behavior is healthful, unhealthful, or somewhere in between. A healthy person uses numerous and diverse behaviors to manage daily stressors; a person with compromised mental health does not. Instead, the unhealthy person responds to stress by exhibiting a narrow range of behaviors in a manner symptomatic of psychopathology. Using the principles of the nursing process and therapeutic communication as outlined in Part III, this section focuses on clients who demonstrate various types of psychopathology or behaviorial problems: anxiety disorder, substance abuse, depression, suicidal behavior, bipolar disorder (manic phase), schizophrenia, delusions, Alzheimer's disease, domestic violence, obsessive-compulsive behavior, phobias, conversion reactions, anorexia nervosa, and personality disorders. After reviewing this section, you will be better prepared to apply mental health concepts and principles in any clinical setting.

Therapeutic communication

The nurse who provides care for a client with a mental illness uses therapeutic communication to convey acceptance, preserve the client's self-esteem, and gain a greater understanding of how the client perceives the situation. Therapeutic responses encourage the client to continue talking ("Tell me about...," "What happened after...," "I'm not sure what you are saying," or "And then...?"). In contrast, evaluative statements ("You must have felt sad" or "I'll bet you miss your children") close off communication and convey lack of understanding. (For a more detailed review of therapeutic communication, see pages 49 to 52 in Part III.)

The nurse-client relationship

Any therapeutic relationship, including the nurse-client relationship, passes through three phases: the beginning (orientation) phase, the middle (working) phase, and the ending (termination) phase. During the orientation phase, the nurse establishes certain parameters for the relationship, such as the time and duration of nurse-client visits, the responsibilities that each must bear, and the types of issues that they will address. During the working phase, the client actively works on issues germane to managing daily affairs. Although this phase may be emotionally painful, the client must be willing to examine issues with the nurse. During the termination phase, the client and the nurse summarize their work together, and the client plans for the future. If the client and the nurse have become emotionally attached, the termination phase may be painful for both of them. Ideally, termination begins during the first meeting with the nurse, when the parameters of the relationship are negotiated.

How anxiety affects behavior

Anxiety is unexplained discomfort, apprehension, or uneasiness. The energy generated by anxiety can be used constructively or destructively.

Anxiety can be precipitated by unmet expectations that are important to one's self-worth; an actual or perceived threat to one's values, status, prestige, biological integrity, or body image; psychological or physiologic stress; or an adverse reaction to chemical substances (for example, a bad trip after taking LSD).

MENTAL HEALTH NURSING

Glossary

Affective inappropriateness—inappropriate emotional response to a situation; for example, laughing when sad or crying when happy

Agranulocytosis—an abnormal condition of the blood characterized by a severe reduction in the number of granulocytes, resulting in fever, sore throat, and bleeding ulcers of the rectum, mouth, and vagina; may arise as an adverse reaction to neuroleptic drugs or other medications

Ambivalence—simultaneous existence of two opposing feelings, needs, or wishes

Anhedonia—inability to experience pleasure from acts that normally give pleasure

Anticipatory planning—preparing for potential situations and outcomes

Associative looseness—illogical connection of thoughts, so that verbalization is nonsensical or confusing to the listener

Autistic withdrawal—retreat from the external environment through hallucinations, delusions, verbal abuse, refusal to speak, catatonia, or excitation

Confabulation—"stories" told by an individual to fill in memory gaps or to answer questions; the individual considers the "stories" factual

Delusion—false belief to which an individual adheres despite contradictory evidence

Denial—unconscious ego defense mechanism whereby an individual refrains from acknowledging stressful aspects about the self or the environment to ease anxiety

Ego—part of the personality that keeps an individual oriented to reality, enables the individual to solve problems, and mediates between the id and the superego

Free-floating anxiety—anxiety that seems to occur without cause and that produces acute psychic discomfort

Id—part of the personality that houses an individual's needs, drives, and wishes and that has no regard for reality

Identification—unconscious ego defense mechanism whereby an individual takes on characteristics of one or more people

Introjection—unconscious ego defense mechanism whereby an individual incorporates positive or negative aspects of another person or object into the individual's ego (this is the mechanism by which anger is turned inward)

Isolation—unconscious ego defense mechanism that enables an individual to remain unaware of the emotions associated with a thought

Loose ego boundary—failure to distinguish adequately between one's thoughts, wishes, and needs and those of others

Neuroleptic malignant syndrome—potentially fatal reaction to neuroleptic (antipsychotic) drugs, characterized by fluctuating vital signs, altered consciousness, fever, muscle rigidity, diaphoresis, drooling, and an increased white blood count

Primary gain—control of anxiety through manifestation of symptoms

Projection—unconscious defense mechanism of the ego whereby an individual attributes unacceptable ideas, feelings, and impulses to the external environment or to someone else

Psychomotor retardation—slowing of movements to such an extent that the individual appears to perform all physical activity in slow motion

Psychosis—condition characterized by major disturbances in ego functioning

Rationalization—unconscious defense mechanism whereby an individual justifies thoughts, wishes, needs, drives, or actions that would otherwise be unacceptable to the self or others

Reaction formation—unconscious defense mechanism whereby an individual develops behaviors and attitudes that directly oppose the individual's underlying feelings and attitudes

Reframing—altering one's view of a situation

Regression—unconscious defense mechanism whereby an individual returns to an earlier, less mature level of functioning

Repression—unconscious defense mechanism whereby an individual keeps unacceptable ideas, impulses, or feelings from conscious awareness

Secondary gain—any benefit that an individual experiences as a result of having a symptom or illness

Situation repetition—characteristic bothersome or problematic behaviors that are repeated during the course of therapy

State anxiety—anxiety experienced under specific conditions

Superego—part of the personality that is commonly called the conscience and that has no regard for reality

Tardive dyskinesia—side effect of long-term phenothiazine therapy; symptoms include gait disturbances and involuntary, bizarre movements of the face, tongue, and neck

Trait anxiety—anxiety experienced most of the time regardless of the circumstances

Undoing—unconscious ego defense mechanism whereby an individual acts to reverse the effects of a previous act

Withdrawal—adverse physical and psychological reactions to abstinence from a substance to which the individual has become addicted

Responses to anxiety

EMOTIONAL RESPONSES	COGNITIVE RESPONSES	PHYSICAL RESPONSES
• Worry • Irritability • Apprehension • Vague discomfort • Expectation of danger • Tendency to cry easily • Lack of self-confidence	• Rumination • Forgetfulness • Poor concentration • Blocking of thoughts • Inattentiveness • Distractibility • Preoccupations	• Restlessness • Tremulousness • Increased pulse and respiratory rates • Elevated blood pressure • Muscle tightness • Nausea • Dizziness • Fatigue • Urinary urgency or frequency or both • Constipation or diarrhea

Anxiety has emotional, cognitive, and physical manifestations, which the nurse must consider when planning care. (See *Responses to anxiety*.) Regardless of the underlying psychopathology, the nurse must assess the client's anxiety level because this guides the choice of nursing interventions. For example, a client with a moderate anxiety level is able to problem solve with assistance and commonly benefits from relaxation techniques. In contrast, a client with severe or panic-level anxiety cannot problem solve and needs much guidance, support, and structure from the nurse. (See *Anxiety levels and nursing implications,* page 140.)

A client with mild anxiety can function well and needs no assistance from the nurse. A client with moderate anxiety will require some assistance because of selective inattention and an inability to provide the self-structure needed to remain focused. A client with severe anxiety will require much assistance from the nurse because of an inability to solve problems and a preoccupation with internal experience. A client at the panic level of anxiety is at risk for harming himself or others because of distortions of reality.

Research and technology

As health care professionals strive to understand what causes mental illness, research and technology continue to play significant roles. Psychobiological research has become increasingly important to the study of mental health. For example, researchers have associated structural and biochemical changes in the brain with schizophrenia and have linked heredity with schizophrenia and mood disorders. Technological procedures, such as positron emission tomography (PET scan), have enabled researchers to visualize the effects of medication or acute symptoms (such as hallucinations) on brain activity. Despite these advances, a simple explanation for mental illness has not been revealed; causation appears to be multidimensional, with psychological, biological, social, and cultural factors affecting human behavior (see *Review of major mental illnesses,* pages 141 and 142).

Working with groups

Nurses are expected to have group skills so that they can work therapeutically with clients in a group setting. Nurses can facilitate such therapeutic groups as educational groups, skills in living groups, parenting groups, support groups, and socialization groups. (*Note:* Having group skills does *not* mean the nurse is permitted to conduct group psychotherapy. Conducting group psychotherapy requires a master's degree and at least 2 years' supervision in psychotherapy.)

MENTAL HEALTH NURSING

Anxiety levels and nursing implications

The following chart presents manifestations of and nursing implications for the four primary levels of anxiety.

ANXIETY LEVEL	MANIFESTATIONS	NURSING IMPLICATIONS
Mild	• Alertness • Maximal problem-solving ability • Enhanced learning	• Client can be fully responsible for self.
Moderate	• Selective inattention • Impaired problem solving • Complaints of feeling "uptight," "on edge," or nervous	• Help client talk through situation and label feelings. • Use relaxation techniques.
Severe	• Narrowed attention • Inability to grasp meanings • Inability to problem solve • Clingy or demanding behavior • Many physiologic signs, including increased blood pressure, dry mouth, restlessness, and muscular tightness	• Client needs structure and direction. • Do not force client to make decisions. • Provide one-on-one supervision. • Give p.r.n. medication for escalating anxiety, as ordered. • Provide a nonstimulating environment. • Use touch carefully. Do not physically touch the client without first obtaining permission or explaining what you are doing; a severely anxious client may misinterpret touch as an attack. • Maintain a calm, soothing tone of voice. • Act as a focal point, taking over the interaction and actively directing the client's attention to the nurse. This usually has a calming effect on the client. • Dress conservatively to maintain a soothing environment; bright coloring can overstimulate severely anxious and manic clients.
Panic	• Inability to solve problems • Client feels detached from body or may feel "unreal" • Breathing problems • Loss of contact with reality • Inability to recognize familiar objects or persons • Erratic behavior	See nursing implications for severe anxiety.

Working with clients in small groups has many benefits, for both the nurse and client. Because the nurse works with several clients simultaneously, the technique is cost effective. Also, it allows the nurse to observe interaction patterns, and permits situation repetition. Being in a group allows clients to receive feedback from peers, to practice new interactional and coping skills, and to see that others have had similar experiences. It also helps them meet unfulfilled needs for belonging and acceptance, and gives them a chance to network.

To work with groups, the nurse must understand group dynamics and therapeutic communication. The nurse also must establish group standards or rules—for example, who has access to what group members say (confidentiality); who is responsible for determining content and keeping the group focused (leadership and responsibility); and will smoking, eating, drinking, interrupting, or swearing be permitted (norms).

Review of major mental illnesses

A client with any of the following illnesses manifests problems with anxiety. Accurate assessment of the client's anxiety level will enable the nurse to implement appropriate and effective interventions.

DSM-IV DIAGNOSIS	COMMON BEHAVIORAL MANIFESTATIONS	DEFENSE MECHANISMS	SELECTED BIOPHYSICAL FACTORS	COMMON MEDICATION
Schizophrenia	Ambivalence, associative looseness, affective disturbance, autistic withdrawal, social inappropriateness, emotional detachment, anhedonia, lack of motivation, mistrust	• Failure of repression • Projection • Regression	• Genetics • Structural changes in the brain • Disturbance in dopamine transmission	• Antipsychotics (neuroleptics, major tranquilizers)
Delusional disorder (paranoid)	Suspiciousness, hypervigilance, aloofness, hostility, aggressiveness	• Projection	• Genetics	• Antipsychotics (neuroleptics, major tranquilizers)
Generalized anxiety disorder	Feeling of dread; tension; tendency to worry too much; motor tension; physical symptoms, such as palpitations, dry mouth, feelings of suffocation, abdominal distress; inability to sleep; chronic anxiety	• None	• Genetics • Defect in neurochemical regulation	• Antianxiety agents (anxiolytics, minor tranquilizers) • Tricyclic antidepressants
Simple phobia and social phobia	Intense anxiety if in contact with phobic object or situation; behaviors designed to avoid object or situation; life possibly very constricted	• Displacement • Avoidance • Projection • Regression	• Deficit in neurochemical regulation	• Antianxiety agents • Monoamine oxidase inhibitors
Obsessive-compulsive neurosis	Social constriction due to time-consuming rituals; feelings of inner tension; sleep disturbance; worrying; anxiety; veiled anger; emotional constriction	• Repression • Isolation • Reaction formation • Undoing	• Deficit in neurochemical regulation	• Tricyclic antidepressants (such as clomipramine [Anafranil]) • Serotonin reuptake inhibitor (such as paroxetine hydrochloride [Paxil]) or fluoxetine hydrochloride [Prozac])
Eating disorders (anorexia nervosa and bulimia nervosa)	Perfectionist; desire to please; preoccupied with food and with physical appearance; body image distortion; controlling; exercising despite fatigue; uncontrolled binging (bulimia); purging (bulimia)	• Regression • Denial • Avoidance • Undoing	• Biophysical factors under study	• Tricyclic antidepressant (such as amitriptyline [Elavil]) • Serotonin reuptake inhibitor (such as fluoxetine hydrochloride [Prozac])
Panic disorder	Sudden, unpredicted, intense fear that something terrible is about to happen; palpitations; trembling; hot flashes or chills; fear of losing control or losing one's mind; afraid of being alone; constriction of social activities	• None (defenses fail)	• Mitral value prolapse may be present • Increased norepinephrine • Genetics • Lactic acid sensitivity	• Tricyclic antidepressants • Antianxiety agents (benzodiazepines)

(continued)

Review of major mental illnesses *(continued)*

DSM-IV DIAGNOSIS	COMMON BEHAVIORAL MANIFESTATIONS	DEFENSE MECHANISMS	SELECTED BIOPHYSICAL FACTORS	COMMON MEDICATION
Major depression	Loss of appetite; sleep disturbance; extreme fatigue/loss of energy; low self-worth; social isolation; psychomotor retardation; constipation; hopelessness; powerlessness	• Introjection • Regression • Identification • Turning in of affect	• Genetics • Decreased serotonin and norepinephrine • Disturbance in circadian rhythm	• Antidepressants
Bipolar disorder, manic	Expansiveness; grandiosity; impaired judgment; flight of ideas; emotional lability; hyperactivity; inability to sleep; social inappropriateness; irritability and/or anger when limits are imposed; sexual acting out	• Denial	• Genetics • Increased serotonin and norepinephrine • Disturbance in circadian rhythm	• Antimanic (lithium) • Anticonvulsants such as carbamazepine (Tegretol) and valproic acid (Depakene)
Borderline personality disorder	Rage; intense relationships; feelings of emptiness; exploitative/manipulative; demanding; extreme self-centeredness; impulsivity; feelings of entitlement; labile mood; sexual acting out; self-destructive behaviors	• Splitting • Idealization • Devaluation • Projective identification	• None known	• None, unless needed for anxiety or underlying depression

Phases of a group

As is true in a one-to-one relationship, groups go through three phases: orientation, working, and termination. Common behaviors exhibited by group members during the orientation phase include politeness, strained silences, and self-protective actions; they also question the purpose of the group as well as the qualifications of the leader. Conflicts are addressed directly and openly during the working phase; commitment to the work of the group is high and members care about one another, show support for each other, and exhibit risk-taking. During the termination phase, members express their feelings about the group ending, review the group experience, and plan for the future.

Leading a group

The group leader, or facilitator, has multiple functions:
• to keep the group focused
• to facilitate the group process (how members respond to each other and the topic being discussed), when appropriate
• to screen group members, when appropriate
• to evaluate outcomes.
Types of group leadership styles include authoritarian (directive), democratic (consensus), facilitative (growth promoting, processing), and laissez-faire (lacking in direction and purpose). (See *Leadership styles*.)

To facilitate a therapeutically oriented group, the nurse can use various strategies. For example, to start a new session, briefly review the last session, and then ask how things have gone since then. When appropriate, respond to themes. For instance, say, "At least three people have talked about staying balanced. Perhaps it would be useful to examine what staying balanced means to each of us."

Leadership styles

Leadership style affects group outcome; the style used depends upon the outcome desired. Here are four leadership styles, their strengths and limitations, and occasions for the use of each style.

STYLE	STRENGTHS	LIMITATIONS	WHEN TO USE
Democratic (consensus)	• All participate in decision making • Group consensus reached	• Personal growth limited • Group process not attended to unless it interferes with decision making	• Committee meetings • Team conferences
Authoritarian (directive)	• Maintains organization during times of crisis • The immediate task is accomplished quickly	• Growth of members limited • Group process not attended to	• During crisis; for example, a code blue or disruptive behavior needing immediate control
Facilitative (growth-promoting)	• Personal growth maximized • Cohesiveness and sense of personal commitment high	• Not good when immediate action is required to maintain safety	• Growth groups • Therapy groups
Laissez-faire (lacking in direction and purpose)	• No restraints on members	• No structure to follow • Commitment to group low • No cohesiveness among members	• Social gatherings where structure or completing a task is not important

Other phrases the nurse can use to help a group move along include:

"I sense a lot of feeling in the group today. What's up?"

"I wonder if all the small talk is keeping us from dealing with what we need to deal with today."

"Life is often unfair. Would someone like to tell us how they have managed to deal with this?"

"Who would like to begin today?"

"What's happened since our last meeting (or class or session)?"

Dealing with problems within a group

When a group is cohesive, members have the potential to experience maximal growth because they are committed to themselves as well as to fellow participants. This commitment allows members to risk dealing with sensitive issues within the group. Threats to group cohesion include:
• transient group members
• poorly selected group members
• cliques
• competition
• transference and countertransference
• unacknowledged conflict
• lack of privacy
• irregular meetings.
These threats can be diffused through various interventions.

Before the first group meeting, the nurse should screen the participants to determine their appropriateness; individuals who are blatantly psychotic, acutely manic, or experiencing dementia are not suitable candidates for an interpersonal issues group intended to enhance self-insight and personal growth. If consistent attendance is important, this requirement should be made known during the first group meeting and members who cannot commit to regular attendance should be excluded. Acknowledge the presence of any cliques and assist clique members and others in analyzing this phenomenon. If competition or unacknowledged conflict exists among group members, acknowledge it, state observations, and seek feedback about what is happening. Transference, where unresolved issues of group members are projected onto other members or the group leader, is identified and members assist in responding to the incident. Countertransference, where unresolved issues of the nurse interfere with the ability to work objectively with the group, requires immediate peer supervision and use of a coleader for firsthand feedback. Meet at least once a week to communicate the importance of the group work to be done. Provide privacy by arranging for sessions to be held in an enclosed area that is not visually accessible to others and in which comments cannot be overheard by nonparticipants.

Many individuals find that participating in therapeutic groups designed to examine their own behavior is threatening. To protect themselves, these individuals may respond by exhibiting problem behaviors (see *Problem behaviors in a group*) or signs of resistance. Common signs of resistance include:
• missing sessions
• rescuing others
• projecting blame
• showing up late
• engaging in small talk
• changing the subject
• forming cliques
• verbally attacking other members or the leader.
The nurse employs various interventions to address these resistance behaviors.

The nurse should acknowledge a member's absence or chronic lateness, seek clarification about the meaning of the behavior, and assist the member to formulate theories and solutions about being consistently late. When one member "rescues" another, point out the behavior and ask the rescuer what prompted it; also ask the one "rescued" to provide feedback about the rescuer's behavior. If members project blame, ask them to identify the parts of the situation for which they are responsible and to focus on the actions under their control. Observe patterns of engaging in small talk or changing the subject; comment on the observations made and ask if the group members have any ideas about what is happening or what the group is trying to avoid. If cliques form, state specific indicative behaviors among group members and ask both clique and nonclique members to analyze what is happening in the group. A verbal attack by one group member on the group leader or another member requires immediate intervention—have the attacker nonabrasively state the issue and ask those attacked to provide feedback; help the attacker analyze the intent of the behavior and assist all group members in identifying boundary issues.

Problem behaviors in a group

Common problems encountered within groups are listed below along with possible causes. It is important for the nurse to remember that these behaviors are intended to protect the person who is engaging in them.

PROBLEM BEHAVIOR	POSSIBLE CAUSE
Conflict	• Attempt to focus attention elsewhere • Lack of knowledge as to how to resolve issues in a healthy manner • Highly charged issue • Transferences and countertransferences
Group gets sidetracked	• Unclear focus • Group members with limited intellectual capacity or inability to consider a wide range of ideas • Lack of group structure • Avoidance of painful issues • Leader does not effectively assist group members in analyzing what is happening within the group
Member approaches group leader outside group to discuss group business	• Inability to confront issues directly • Attempt to manipulate leader to gain power • Lack of understanding about how groups work • Lack of clarity about group rules • Testing behavior • Fear of reprisal within group • Attempt to seek attention to fill inner void
Member uses strong or offensive language	• Attempt to control others • Testing behavior • Self-protection • Poor communication skills
Member exhibits minimal or no active participation	• Anxiety • Previously "squelched" • Uncertain of group rules • Fear that expressed ideas may lead to more work
Loquacious (dominating) member	• May become anxious with silence • May feel overly responsible for outcome • Attempt to feel important • Avoidance of painful issues • Attempt to control outcome through bulldozing

MENTAL HEALTH NURSING

Crisis intervention

An event that disrupts a person's usual manner of coping with stress can precipitate a crisis. Such an event may be situational (such as divorce), maturational (occurring when a person enters a new developmental phase of life or career), or adventitious (caused by uncontrolled events, such as flood, war, or assault). An event that triggers a crisis in one person may not do so in another.

According to Aguilera, three balancing factors offset a crisis: realistic perception of the event, adequate emotional support, and adequate coping mechanisms. Absence of any of these factors predisposes a person to crisis.

A crisis develops in four phases. During *phase one,* a specific situational, maturational, or adventitious event occurs. During *phase two,* the person feels threatened and tries to deal with the event by using the usual coping methods. *Phase three* occurs if the usual coping methods fail. This phase is marked by disorganization, which leaves the person feeling overwhelmed and at loose ends. Phase three persists until the person finds new ways to cope, or until the old ways work. During *phase four,* the crisis resolves and the person returns to a pre-crisis level of functioning—or to a higher or lower level of functioning. Crisis intervention aims to restore at least a pre-crisis level of functioning and to prevent untoward emotional sequelae.

The following clinical situation focuses on a client who requires crisis intervention.

Clinical situation

You are on duty in the emergency department (ED) at 7 p.m. this evening when Judy Rose, age 24, a deeply religious woman, is brought in by the police. During triage, she sits stiffly, clutching her coat tightly around her and keeping her head down. "I'm so ashamed," she says in a barely audible voice. "It's all my fault." She does not raise her head to answer questions. She repeatedly says, "I don't know what to do." You find out that Ms. Rose lives alone, that her parents live in a nearby city, and that she has a married sister who lives within 5 miles of the hospital. She has few friends.

During the medical examination (performed using the hospital's rape protocol), Ms. Rose tries to maintain her composure, but she cannot help crying at times. The examination reveals small lacerations of the external genitalia and vagina as well as scratches on her face, throat, breasts, arms, and legs.

Following completion of the rape protocol examination, Ms. Rose tells you she is afraid to leave the hospital and return to her apartment because the rapist has her purse containing identification and house keys. After much persuasion on your part, Ms. Rose agrees to contact her sister.

While waiting for her sister to arrive, Ms. Rose sits in her cubicle crying softly. She says she can't understand how God could let this happen to her, that she was a virgin, and now she is "nothing more than a dirty rag that no one would ever want."

"I guess it doesn't make any difference what happens now," she says. "No one will ever want me."

Assessment

NURSING BEHAVIORS	**NURSING RATIONALES**
1. Initially, assess Ms. Rose's physical condition.	**1.** When a client presents with a physical condition and a psychological one, the physical condition (lower-level need) must be assessed before psychological intervention can take place.
2. Assess Ms. Rose's level of anxiety.	**2.** Nursing interventions are based on the client's presenting level of anxiety. Nursing interventions will change as the client's anxiety level fluctuates.
3. Assess for balancing factors: • realistic perception of the event • adequate social supports • adequate coping skills.	**3.** Absence of any of the balancing factors will prolong the crisis.

4. Refer Ms. Rose to a rape counselor, who can provide ongoing support.

4. Nurses in the ED do not provide support once the client leaves the hospital. Follow-up counseling will help the client put the rape into perspective and move along with her life.

Nursing diagnoses

- Rape-trauma syndrome related to failure of coping skills
- Self-esteem disturbance related to the client's perception that she is no longer an acceptable marriage partner
- Spiritual distress related to a violation of the client's deeply held moral code

Planning and goals

- Ms. Rose's immediate physical and safety needs will be met.
- Ms. Rose will seek follow-up counseling where she will:
—gain cognitive mastery over the rape and begin to express her feelings (such as fear, anger, and self-blame).
—regain a sense of safety.
—verbalize reestablishment of self-esteem.
—recognize that God was not responsible for the rape.

Implementation

NURSING BEHAVIORS	NURSING RATIONALES
1. Do not leave Ms. Rose alone.	**1.** The nurse's calming influence can prevent the client from becoming more overwhelmed by the rape experience. The client needs to feel safe at this point.
2. Ask Ms. Rose where she is experiencing pain.	**2.** This question helps the client focus on something specific; it also communicates the nurse's caring and concern.
3. Assist Ms. Rose with completing the hospital's rape protocol.	**3.** Because of her traumatic experience, the client will need assistance with completing the hospital's rape protocol, which includes documenting her condition and validating that she indeed was raped. Her anxiety level will fluctuate, making it difficult for her to concentrate on the tasks at hand.
4. Offer Ms. Rose a cleansing douche, mouthwash, and other supplies after all evidence has been gathered; help her clean up if she cannot care for herself.	**4.** The client may feel the need to "wash away" the traumatic experience. Symbolically, this cleaning can help the client put the experience behind her. The nurse's assistance conveys caring and concern.
5. When her anxiety level is at or below the moderate level, ask Ms. Rose to tell you about the rape, letting her set the pace. Phrase your questions and comments with care and sensitivity.	**5.** This approach promotes the client's eventual cognitive mastery over the rape experience, decreasing her tendency to withdraw and to feel guilt and shame. Thoughtlessly worded comments and questions ("Were you really raped?") convey doubt and project blame. In contrast, a carefully worded statement ("I'd like to hear about what happened") conveys the nurse's desire to understand the client's experience.
6. Help Ms. Rose to identify her most immediate concern.	**6.** With this concrete focus to her thoughts, the client can begin to regain control of her life.

7. Ask Ms. Rose to name someone who can stay with her for the next 24 to 48 hours.

7. During this interval, the client's anxiety level will fluctuate, and she may experience flashbacks to the rape. Having a trusted friend or family member around can ease her anxiety and help her cope with periodic waves of anxiety and fear.

8. Give Ms. Rose the names and telephone numbers of appropriate community resources. If possible, introduce Ms. Rose to a rape counselor *before* she leaves the ED.

8. Explaining about community resources lets the client know that she will not be abandoned. Giving her the information in writing increases the probability that she will contact someone for rape counseling. Establishing contact with the rape counselor before leaving the ED will decrease the client's sense of aloneness and better assure that she will seek follow-up rape counseling.

Clinical situation
(continued)

Ms. Rose accepts rape counseling. In the weeks after the rape, the counselor explores the event with her and works with her to strengthen her coping skills.

Implementation (rape counseling)
NURSING BEHAVIORS

NURSING RATIONALES

1. Encourage Ms. Rose to recall how she has dealt with past traumatic events.

1. Recalling past success in dealing with trauma shows the client that she will be able to cope with this unwanted experience just as she has coped with others.

2. Help Ms. Rose talk about the rape and vent her feelings.

2. Thorough venting of emotions helps mobilize the client's energies and decreases her sense of helplessness, powerlessness, and self-doubt. Talking about the rape helps the client put the traumatic experience into perspective, permitting self-growth and healing. Unexpressed feelings may lead to depression and other symptoms in the future.

3. Help Ms. Rose examine any differences in her lifestyle that have resulted from the rape.

3. This self-examination helps the client determine whether she is giving this experience more power in her life than she would like, and helps her gain a realistic perception of the rape.

4. Encourage Ms. Rose to recall enjoyable relationships with men.

4. Recalling enjoyable relationships helps prevent the client from viewing all men as potential rapists.

5. Have Ms. Rose examine how she views herself.

5. The client's concept that she is "dirty" must be vigorously challenged. She cannot regain self-esteem if she thinks negatively about herself.

6. Talk with Ms. Rose about her spiritual beliefs. If appropriate, consider seeking pastoral assistance for her.

6. The client's spiritual condition should not be ignored. For the deeply religious client, restoration of her faith in God may enhance healing.

7. Discuss Ms. Rose's thoughts and feelings about prosecuting her attacker.

7. This discussion conveys that the client has the option to take direct action against her attacker. Under no circumstances, however, should the nurse coerce the client into prosecuting.

8. Teach Ms. Rose defensive living techniques (such as the safest place to park the car, especially at night) that will increase her sense of power and control.

8. The client may unwittingly make herself vulnerable to rape because of naivete. Increasing her sense of power and control will enhance her feeling that she is free to come and go as she pleases.

Evaluation

• Ms. Rose states she no longer fears being raped again and pursues her life as she did before the rape.
• Ms. Rose verbalizes reestablishment of self-esteem and states that, although she would not have chosen a rape experience, it is now a part of her history and a part of who she is.
• Ms. Rose anticipates a bright future.

Anxiety disorders

The client with an anxiety disorder experiences overwhelming anxiety, which interferes with the quality of life. To relieve the anxiety, the client develops a variety of symptoms, which may or may not control the anxiety. Types of anxiety disorders include panic disorder, generalized anxiety disorder (GAD), obsessive-compulsive disorder (OCD), phobia, and post-traumatic stress disorder (PTSD).

Panic disorder

Persons who experience panic disorder suffer unpredictable, paralyzing attacks of panic. Many cannot identify trigger events and live in constant fear of having an attack. To avoid public embarrassment, they may refuse to leave home, and may then concurrently develop agoraphobia (fear of public and open places). According to research, there is a correlation between lactic-acid buildup and panic attacks; aerobic exercise can precipitate panic attacks in some persons.

Generalized anxiety disorder

Persons with GAD experience moderate to severe levels of anxiety during most waking hours. They worry excessively about many things and cannot feel calm or relaxed in situations that most persons do not perceive as particularly stressful. Because their anxiety is so pervasive, it affects most areas of their lives.

Obsessive-compulsive disorder

Persons with OCD experience unwanted, bothersome thoughts (obsessions), which cause severe anxiety. To relieve the anxiety, they perform repetitive acts (compulsions), which should not be interrupted once begun. They spend a great deal of emotional energy containing their underlying anxiety and maintaining control of themselves and life situations. They frequently use the defense mechanisms of denial, isolation, reaction formation, and undoing.

Fear of losing control and fear of losing the esteem of others are central issues for persons with obsessions and compulsions. Perfectionistic, overly conscientious, and filled with self-doubt, they have trouble being spontaneously emotional because of their intense underlying need to stay "in control" and not make waves. They have intense needs for love, affection, and belonging.

If persistent anxiety interferes with therapy, benzodiazepines may be prescribed to relieve anxiety and help the client participate in other therapies. Although psychotherapy has not been particularly useful in treating OCD, behavioral techniques have proven effective.

Phobia

A phobia is an irrational fear of something that in reality can cause little, if any, harm. Phobias serve the purpose of externalizing anxiety. Once the anxiety has been projected onto the unconsciously chosen object, anxious feelings can be displaced onto the object, which can then (ideally) be avoided. Forced contact with the phobic object or situation may precipitate panic. Persons experiencing phobias have underlying needs for love, affection, and belonging.

Phobias become problems if they expand or if the object cannot be successfully avoided. When this happens, the person's ability to meet daily commitments is impaired. Behavioral techniques, such as desensitization and distraction, have provided relief for clients with phobias.

Somatoform disorder

A somatoform disorder is the literal transference of inner conflict onto a body part, often resulting in crippling. Individuals with somatoform disorders channel anxiety through a body system. Channeling anxiety in this manner usually succeeds because the person is unaware of uncomfortable amounts of anxiety.

Symptoms of a somatoform disorder are not under voluntary control and suggest a physical disorder with a psychogenic origin. Physical symptoms are not consistent with the presence or degree of underlying pathophysiology. At an affective level, persons with somatoform disorders do not experience emotional distress over life events, but are keenly aware of uncomfortable somatic sensations, for which they seek treatment.

Examples of somatoform disorders include hypochondriasis, conversion reaction, and somatization disorder (Briquet's syndrome). Most people who experience conversion reactions accept their condition with a complacency known as *la belle indifference*.

In caring for a client with a somatoform disorder, the nurse must not force the client to renounce symptoms, no matter which symptoms the client exhibits. Doing so will only heighten the anxiety and prolong the condition. For example, a client who experiences a conversion reaction must not be forced to accept the reality implied by diagnostic results.

Post-traumatic stress disorder

PTSD may develop in individuals who have witnessed or experienced life-threatening trauma. It may follow a traumatic event, such as a serious threat or harm to one's physical well-being (as from rape); sudden loss of home or community (as from an earthquake); or witnessing an event that results in serious injury or death of another person. The characteristic symptoms of PTSD include persistent reexperiencing of the traumatic event (such as in flashbacks and nightmares); avoidance of feelings and other stimuli associated with the trauma; a sense of emotional numbness and detachment; and symptoms of increased arousal, such as sleep disturbances, difficulty concentrating, irritability, hypervigilance, and startle response (an exaggerated response to stimuli). Acute PTSD resolves spontaneously; chronic or delayed PTSD requires intervention.

The nurse plays an essential role in assessing the client with PTSD and in making appropriate referrals. Regardless of the cause, a crucial component of intervention is encouraging the client to express and share emotions associated with the trauma.

Comparing the anxiety disorders

Anxiety disorders are described briefly in the chart below. A combination of drug therapy and behavioral or cognitive approaches is used to treat these disorders.

DISORDER	DESCRIPTION	TREATMENT
Generalized anxiety disorder	Excessive worry about many life circumstances; anxiety persists during most waking hours	• Relaxation exercises • Cognitive reframing • Benzodiazepines
Obsessive-compulsive disorder	Overwhelming need to carry out a stereotypical act to relieve anxiety precipitated by an obsessive thought	• Behavioral techniques, such as response prevention and thought stopping • Tricyclic antidepressants
Panic disorder	Unpredictable attacks of intense anxiety lasting a few minutes to several hours	• Benzodiazepines • Antidepressants • Relaxation exercises
Post-traumatic stress disorder	Reexperiencing the original traumatic event; may be acute, delayed, or chronic	• Benzodiazepines • Antidepressants • Cognitive therapy • Group therapy • Hypnosis
Simple phobia	Avoidance of something that in reality is harmless	• Benzodiazepines • Desensitization • Distraction
Social phobia	Avoidance of social situations that in reality are not life-threatening	• Social skills training • Benzodiazepines

The three clinical situations that follow focus on a client experiencing OCD, a client with delayed PTSD, and a client with a phobia and a somatoform disorder. (For details on classifications of anxiety disorders, see *Comparing the anxiety disorders.*)

Clinical situation #1: Obsessive-compulsive disorder

Sarah Minor, age 40, is seeing you on an outpatient basis at a community mental health center. Although her colleagues consider her a top-notch travel agent, she seldom feels she has done her job well enough.

For the past 6 weeks, the resulting anxiety has greatly interfered with her ability to eat and sleep. She sleeps only 3 hours at a time and cannot eat more than a few bites of "health food" at each meal. She also spends a great deal of time thinking and talking about what she should have done or should be doing. An exceptionally neat person, she spends about $1\frac{1}{2}$ hours each morning dressing and applying makeup. She calls her husband at work throughout the day to make sure he is all right, and she calls the children when they get home from school to check on them. She says she becomes tense when things do not go well or when she has to make spur-of-the-moment changes.

Mrs. Minor tells you she is a super-organized person who easily becomes upset if the house is messy or if her three high-school–age children fail to follow the daily schedule she establishes for them. She came to the mental health clinic because she felt exhausted and believed her life was getting out of control.

Assessment

NURSING BEHAVIORS	NURSING RATIONALES
1. Assess Mrs. Minor's anxiety level and underlying needs.	1. Identifying the client's anxiety level and underlying needs allows the nurse to plan appropriate care.
2. Assess which types of events in Mrs. Minor's environment precipitate her obsessive-compulsive behavior.	2. Identifying the factors that precipitate a client's obsessive-compulsive behavior enables the nurse to engage in anticipatory planning with the client to manage her anxiety.
3. Assess Mrs. Minor's eating and sleeping patterns.	3. The client's level of disturbance in eating and sleeping indicates the amount of anxiety she is experiencing.
4. Assess Mrs. Minor's expectations of her meetings with you, and help her set appropriate goals.	4. Setting goals enables the nurse and the client to monitor the client's progress and provides clues about the appropriateness of the client's expectations of herself and others.
5. Assess Mrs. Minor's expectations of her family: Does she see family members as autonomous individuals? How does she feel when family members do not behave as she expects?	5. Inappropriate expectations of others can reflect an individual's problems with autonomy and feelings of self-worth. The obsessive-compulsive client typically feels a great need to control everyone around her and derives her sense of worth from being perfect. For example, she may not be satisfied with the way others do their jobs.
6. As therapy proceeds, assess changes that occur in Mrs. Minor's coping skills.	6. Assessing changes in the client provides clues to the effectiveness of the treatment plan.

Nursing diagnoses
- Anxiety related to fear of losing control of the environment
- Sleep pattern disturbance related to the client's underlying anxiety

Planning and goals
- Mrs. Minor will develop new coping skills.
- Mrs. Minor will identify factors that precipitate her obsessive-compulsive behavior and plan accordingly.
- Mrs. Minor will relinquish her need to control others.
- Mrs. Minor will sleep for at least 6 hours at a time and feel rested on arising.

Implementation

NURSING BEHAVIORS	NURSING RATIONALES
1. Instruct Mrs. Minor to keep a daily journal of her thoughts, feelings, and actions to identify those that immediately precede the onset of her obsessive-compulsive behavior.	1. Obsessive-compulsive behavior reflects severe anxiety. Therefore, the time to process such behavior with the client is after the anxiety level falls to moderate or below. (Also remember that compulsions should not be forbidden or interrupted because doing so escalates the client's anxiety.) A journal helps the obsessive-compulsive client identify anxiety-precipitating factors and can provide a sense of being in control.

2. Help Mrs. Minor engage in anticipatory planning.

2. Anticipatory planning helps the obsessive-compulsive client feel in control of potentially anxiety-producing situations. By interrupting the pattern of automatically exhibiting obsessive-compulsive behavior, the client can learn new coping skills.

3. With Mrs. Minor, plan ways for her to improve sleeping and eating patterns.

3. Sleep deprivation and inadequate food intake interfere with one's ability to manage anxiety.

4. Help Mrs. Minor identify her expectations of herself and others.

4. Obsessive-compulsive people typically set themselves up for failure because their unrealistically high expectations mean they cannot accept anything less than perfection in themselves or others.

5. Help Mrs. Minor identify what she would like to accomplish through therapy, and instruct her to write down specific, limited goals.

5. Identifying therapeutic goals helps the obsessive-compulsive client examine her expectations in terms of personal achievement. Eventually, she should be able to relinquish responsibility for what rightfully belongs to others. For example, she should not hold herself responsible if her teenage children ignore their homework or decide to wear unironed clothing.

6. Plan meetings with Mrs. Minor, her husband, and their children. In these sessions, help all family members accomplish the following:
• Identify what they are willing to do and are capable of doing.
• Agree on standards for family responsibilities.
• Identify each family member's individual responsibilities.
• Practice age-appropriate autonomous behaviors.

6. Meetings like these help the client become more objective about her expectations of herself and others. Increased objectivity leads to a stronger and healthier self-concept, which should enable her to relinquish inappropriate controlling behaviors. For each family member, learning to function responsibly yet autonomously contributes to personal growth as well as to healthy family functioning.

7. Ask Mrs. Minor to write down three alternative daily schedules.

7. This is a relatively nonthreatening way to introduce the obsessive-compulsive client to the concept of flexibility. Once she is comfortable with thinking in terms of alternative plans, she will be able to try them.

8. Encourage Mrs. Minor to work with creative media—for example, woodworking, sanding, sculpting, painting, and modeling with clay.

8. Participation in such activities increases the client's self-confidence by releasing creative energies.

9. Teach Mrs. Minor techniques for response prevention and thought stopping, and encourage her to engage in relaxation exercises several times a day.

9. Engaging in relaxation exercises and response prevention techniques will help dissipate the client's anxiety and interrupt her automatic obsessive-compulsive behavior.

Evaluation

• Mrs. Minor regains a healthy sleeping pattern and eats adequate portions of nutritious food.
• Mrs. Minor no longer calls her husband and children needlessly while she is at work.

MENTAL HEALTH NURSING

• Mrs. Minor expresses her thoughts openly, without undue concern for others' approval.
• Mrs. Minor relinquishes responsibility for her husband's and children's behaviors.

Clinical situation #2: Post-traumatic stress disorder

Lee Jaslow, age 35, returned from active duty in the Gulf War 6 months ago. He is sitting in his yard with his wife when a passing car backfires loudly. He throws himself over his wife and tells her he'll protect her from the SCUD missile attack.

Over the next few weeks, Mr. Jaslow has trouble sleeping, awakening from horrific nightmares. He is irritable with his family and coworkers, and frequently looks over his shoulder to scan the sky for SCUD missiles. When he tells his wife they must build a shelter for protection, she convinces him to seek treatment at a local mental health center. Reluctantly, he agrees, although he fears being labeled "weird" or "crazy."

Assessment

NURSING BEHAVIORS	NURSING RATIONALES
1. Assess Mr. Jaslow's anxiety level and evaluate the pervasiveness of his anxiety.	**1.** The client's anxiety level dictates the type of nursing intervention. Pervasive anxiety may indicate the need for a p.r.n. medication order.
2. Assess the nature and duration of Mr. Jaslow's symptoms.	**2.** This will help determine if the client's post-traumatic stress response is delayed, chronic, or acute.
3. Assess precipitating factors for flashbacks.	**3.** If precipitating factors can be identified, they can be anticipated. This assessment also helps determine if the client's anxiety is well-contained. If the anxiety occurs only during flashbacks and not at other times, it is well-contained. If anxiety occurs randomly, it is not well-contained or limited to a specific cue.
4. Assess Mr. Jaslow's coping skills.	**4.** This assessment provides information about the adequacy of the client's current and past coping skills. He may need to learn new coping skills.

Nursing diagnosis

Post-trauma response related to unassimilated wartime experiences

Planning and goals

• Mr. Jaslow will gain cognitive mastery over his wartime experiences.
• Mr. Jaslow will verbalize feeling safe at work and at home.

Implementation

NURSING BEHAVIORS	NURSING RATIONALES
1. Teach Mr. Jaslow about PTSD.	**1.** The client needs to know he is not "weird" or "crazy." Gaining knowledge about PTSD will help him feel in control and allow him to make plans for recovery.

2. Use active listening to help Mr. Jaslow talk about his wartime experiences in detail.

2. Until the client relives his experiences in an accepting atmosphere, he will be unable to gain cognitive mastery over them. He probably feels guilty about surviving the war when others did not. Through active listening, the nurse can help him gain objectivity over his experiences.

3. Help Mr. Jaslow establish a healthy daily routine.

3. The client needs structure in his daily routine to help him feel safe. Adequate rest and exercise will help him manage his anxiety.

4. Refer Mr. Jaslow to an appropriate PTSD support group.

4. An appropriate support group is a safe place in which the client can confront his trauma. It also provides a social support system of others with whom he can identify and who can validate his experiences.

5. Administer medications, as ordered and needed.

5. Several types of medications have been useful in treating PTSD. Antidepressants may relieve depression, improve sleep, and reduce intrusive thoughts, jumpiness, and explosive anger. Benzodiazepines help reduce anxiety and improve sleep. Lithium controls mood swings and angry outbursts. Beta blockers (such as propranolol) relieve agitation and anxiety.

Evaluation	• Mr. Jaslow sleeps at least 6 consecutive hours per night. • Mr. Jaslow's concentration is restored. • Mr. Jaslow is no longer hypervigilant. • Mr. Jaslow states that he feels safe. • Mr. Jaslow no longer experiences flashbacks precipitated by previous triggers.

Clinical situation #3: Phobia with somatoform disorder (conversion reaction)

Hugo Hinks, age 12, weighs 200 lb (90.7 kg) and is 4′ 10″ (147 cm) tall. His mother brought him to the emergency department (ED) because his legs suddenly became paralyzed as he was getting ready to leave for school. When the ED nurse asked Hugo what happened, he stated calmly that he couldn't move his legs. As Hugo was preparing for examination by the ED physician, the nurse noticed that Hugo's mother undressed him and did not let him do anything for himself. Then she spontaneously said, "Hugo never manages to dress without my being around to help him."

Because the physician could find no physiologic cause for the paralysis, Hugo was transferred from the ED to an inpatient adolescent treatment center for further evaluation. As he is being admitted to the treatment center, Mrs. Hinks tells the admitting nurse that Hugo has been in counseling for the past 2 months because he is afraid to go to school. Furthermore, she continues, Hugo's frequent absences from school caused him to fail the 6th grade last year, and she is afraid this is going to happen again.

When the nurse asks Hugo why he doesn't like school, Hugo says that the other kids tease him about his name and his weight. He was a "normal" kid, he says, "just like everybody else," until he was 10 years old. Hugo impresses the nurse as being sad and lonely.

MENTAL HEALTH NURSING

As the admission procedure continues, Mrs. Hinks reveals to the nurse that Mr. Hinks died 2 years ago, and she has felt painfully lonely and lost without him. After talking about this for several minutes, Mrs. Hinks concludes by saying, "My baby Hugo is my whole life now."

Assessment

NURSING BEHAVIORS	NURSING RATIONALES
1. Assess Hugo's anxiety level. (It will probably be minimal because his conversion reaction successfully keeps anxiety out of his awareness.)	**1.** Nursing interventions are based on the client's level of anxiety.
2. Assess the underlying needs of Hugo and his mother.	**2.** Identifying their underlying needs allows the nurse to plan appropriate nursing care.
3. Assess Hugo's eating patterns: What types of food does he usually eat? When does he eat? What does food mean to him?	**3.** The overweight adolescent client may have a habit of stuffing himself with food (with his mother's approval) to fulfill unconscious, unmet needs.
4. Assess the nature and extent of Hugo's relationships with peers: Does he have a best friend? Has he joined any clubs? Does he ever stay overnight at a friend's house or ask others to stay overnight with him? How does he respond to peers on the unit?	**4.** Peer relationships are important to the adolescent. When classmates call him names, he experiences an assault to his self-concept, and their ostracism prevents him from engaging in age-appropriate social activities. Indeed, the client may not know how to engage in such activities. When he can identify the sources of stress, he will be able to plan ways to deal with unresolved conflicts. When he has learned more effective coping techniques, he will not need his present defenses, which are hindering his development.
5. Assess the extent of Hugo's paralysis and the purpose it serves.	**5.** The client's primary gain is relief from anxiety; a secondary gain will be not having to grow up and leave his mother. One parent has "abandoned" him through death, so he may fear losing his mother as well. He will need to learn different coping skills to develop into a healthy, self-confident adolescent.
6. Assess the effects of Mrs. Hinks on Hugo's behavior.	**6.** A child's symptoms commonly result from underlying tension in the home. Mrs. Hinks's unmet needs may be causing her to hinder Hugo's development by actively reinforcing his school phobia. As a result, she literally forces him to stay close to her.

Nursing diagnoses
- Altered family processes related to role changes resulting from the father's death
- Impaired social interaction related to immaturity of the mother and son
- Altered growth and development related to exploitation of the child by the mother

Planning and goals
- Hugo will demonstrate age-appropriate behaviors.
- Hugo will develop new coping skills.
- Hugo will overcome his school phobia and return to school.
- Mrs. Hinks will receive counseling to resolve situational and maturational issues.

MENTAL HEALTH NURSING

Implementation

NURSING BEHAVIORS	NURSING RATIONALES
1. Develop a healthy adult-child relationship with Hugo.	**1.** The nurse can foster appropriate adult-child interaction patterns by forming a healthy relationship with the adolescent client. A client who feels comfortable in the relationship will be able to explore thoughts and feelings honestly—in the case of this client, thoughts and feelings about his father's death, his body size, his lack of friends, and the gains he receives from allowing his mother to baby him.
2. Instruct Hugo to keep a detailed journal for 2 days to record his thoughts and feelings.	**2.** A journal provides a way for the client to become more aware of his inner experiences. Showing it to the nurse is one way for him to share his burdens and receive nonjudgmental feedback.
3. Assist Hugo to participate in activities he can complete successfully.	**3.** Successful participation in activities helps the client build self-confidence.
4. Include Hugo in activities with peers.	**4.** In group settings, the client can practice relating to peers and discover that he is not the only boy in the world with problems. This will decrease his feelings of being different and weird. Developmentally, Hugo needs to identify with his peer group.
5. Deal with Hugo's paralysis in a matter-of-fact manner; do not insist that he walk.	**5.** The paralysis exists to control the client's anxiety. Prematurely demanding that he walk or become independent will only prolong his paralysis.
6. Focus on Hugo's abilities, and give him positive reinforcement for his accomplishments.	**6.** The nurse's encouragement builds the client's self-confidence.
7. Help Hugo use problem-solving skills to design effective methods for dealing with stress.	**7.** Learning to use problem-solving skills expands the client's repertoire of coping skills. Hugo can begin making conscious choices about how he will respond to life's stressors.
8. Help Hugo implement a plan to become more independent by making friends with a peer, by getting involved in a sport, and by getting out of the house on his own. For example, have Hugo ask a peer to go to the movies with him.	**8.** These strategies will help the client achieve greater autonomy. Age-appropriate activities will build his social network and support system.
9. Collaborate with the treatment team to establish a desensitization program for treatment of Hugo's school phobia. Involve Hugo, Mrs. Hinks, his teacher, counselor, and relatives in this plan.	**9.** The longer the school-phobic client remains out of school, the more difficult it will be for him to return. Because the extent of the client's arrested development is directly related to the length of time he remains out of school, a desensitization program should be implemented as quickly as possible.

MENTAL HEALTH NURSING

10. Help Mrs. Hinks find a counselor to explore the ways she is using Hugo to meet her needs.

10. With counseling, the client's mother should be able to let her son grow away from her.

Evaluation

• Hugo asserts himself with his mother and other adults, even though they may initially object to his new behaviors.
• Hugo establishes spontaneous relationships with peers on the unit.
• Hugo contacts a peer to visit him at the hospital.
• Hugo chooses a well-balanced diet and begins to lose weight.
• Hugo can talk about his anxiety and is no longer school phobic or paralyzed.
• Mrs. Hinks develops relationships with peers, engages in activities outside the home, and expresses a desire for Hugo to engage in his own activities.
• Mrs. Hinks plans to continue her therapy.

Depression and attempted suicide

Depression is an acutely painful psychic experience. It sometimes occurs, paradoxically, when life seems to be going well. At the extreme ends are clients who are actively suicidal and those who are mildly depressed. Every clinically depressed person struggles with dependency, anger, ambivalence, and painfully low self-esteem; is often immobilized by lack of energy and anhedonia; and has difficulty externalizing anger (energy). Such a person experiences life as dull and boring. Intense sadness, hopelessness, guilt, and indecisiveness overwhelm the person, who commonly exhibits such somatic symptoms as anorexia, insomnia, constipation, headache, backache, and psychomotor retardation. (See *Forms of depression and nursing implications*.)

Effective emergency intervention should be based on an assessment of the client's lethality. For this, the nurse uses a lethality scale, which considers such factors as the client's age, employment status, availability of support systems, and intended manner of committing suicide. Adolescents and young adults (age 15 to 24) and elderly white males over age 80 are the two groups at highest risk for suicide. (For indicators of suicidal behavior, see *Identifying the suicidal client*, page 160, and *Classifying suicidal behavior*, page 161.)

The following clinical situation focuses on the client who has attempted suicide.

Clinical situation

Grace Danes, age 30, was transferred to your inpatient psychiatric treatment facility last night. One week ago, she tried to asphyxiate herself with carbon monoxide. After spending the week in intensive care, she was transferred to your facility because she threatened to "do the job right next time."

You learn from the head nurse that Mrs. Danes is newly divorced, has two preschool-age children, is herself a nurse, and has never been hospitalized for mental illness. However, she has received periodic counseling over the past several years for depression. She is receiving 150 mg of amitriptyline (Elavil) daily, 100 mg at bedtime and 50 mg at 9 a.m.

When you meet Mrs. Danes, she is lying on her bed and staring at the ceiling. Her hair is matted, she is wearing no makeup, and her clothing is soiled and wrinkled. She doesn't look at you or speak when you introduce yourself.

Forms of depression and nursing implications

Use this chart to review commonly observed forms of depression and related nursing implications.

FORM	CHARACTERISTICS	NURSING IMPLICATIONS
Seasonal affective disorder	• Onset between mid-October and mid-November • Remission occurs between mid-February and mid-April • Signs and symptoms of dysthymia	• Advise the client to use bright lights and go outdoors as much as possible. • If possible, advise client to purchase full-spectrum lights designed specifically to treat this disorder. • Suggest that the client vacation in the winter, rather than the summer, and in a place with longer daylight hours.
Dysthymia	• Depressed mood • Poor appetite • Low energy level or fatigue • Feelings of hopelessness • Poor concentration • Sleep pattern disturbances • Low self-esteem • Difficulty making decisions	• Help the client identify activities that promote well-being. • Help the client establish a healthy daily routine. • Assist the client in setting realistic goals.
Severe depression	• Severe manifestations of dysthymia • Limited ability to respond to stimuli • Severe psychomotor retardation or agitation • Limited ability to perform life-sustaining activities • Severe anhedonia • Feelings of worthlessness • Excessive guilt • Morbid thoughts, preoccupation with death	• Provide a structured daily routine. • Do not give the client choices. • Make the client engage in activities. • Use compliments sparingly. Ill-timed compliments indicate insensitivity to the client's inner pain and may precipitate regression or a suicide attempt. • Assist the client with self-care activities until energy returns. • Make decisions for the client until energy returns.
Psychotic depression	• Characteristics of severe depression • Hallucinations, delusions, or both	• Intervene as for a severely depressed client. • Orient an hallucinatory or delusional client to reality, as needed. • Provide a consistent environment.

MENTAL HEALTH NURSING

Assessment

NURSING BEHAVIORS

1. Assess Mrs. Danes's potential for another suicide attempt: What methods did she use in previous attempts? Does she acknowledge that she still has suicidal intentions? If she is still suicidal, how specific is her plan for a future attempt? What support systems are available to her?

NURSING RATIONALES

1. Taken together, the answers to these questions indicate the seriousness of the client's suicide attempt and the degree of risk that another attempt will be made. Depending on the outcome of the nurse's assessment, the client may be placed on suicide precautions. (If the client is unresponsive to queries, the nurse must rely on secondary data and observational skills.)

Identifying the suicidal client

In hospitalized clients, the nurse should stay alert for the following signs, which suggest suicidal tendencies:
• Unexpected calmness
• Insistence on obtaining or using grounds privileges
• Change in behavior patterns.

Also, the nurse may feel uneasy about a client, sensing that the client is suicidal. If this or any of the above signs is present, be prepared to use the following interventions:
• If the client's behavior has changed, ask the client what these changes mean.
• Place the client on suicide precautions.
• Ask the client, "Are you suicidal?"
• Consult with nurse-colleagues, other health care team members, and the client's physician.
• Document your observations and actions.
• Don't promise to keep secrets. Sometimes, a client will ask a nurse to keep something confidential in advance; if the information needs to be shared, the promise can cause problems.

2. Determine Mrs. Danes's ability to meet self-care needs: grooming, hygiene, nutrition, and elimination.

2. A severely depressed client does not have the energy to perform simple daily activities. If basic self-care needs are not being met, the client's sense of unworthiness is confirmed.

3. Assess Mrs. Danes's underlying feelings, noting signs of hopelessness. Observe the degree of congruency between her feelings and her actions and words: Does she ignore you or tell you to go away?

3. A despairing client is at high risk for suicide. Depression will not lift until despair abates. Ignoring the client or leaving her room will further intensify feelings of worthlessness.

4. Assess how Mrs. Danes interacts with peers, staff, and visitors, noting any persistent patterns: Does she initiate interaction, or does she wait for others to approach her? How does she cope with disappointments and frustrations?

4. Theoretically, the nurse should observe in the client the same behavioral patterns that created problems before hospitalization (repeating these patterns in the hospital is called situation repetition). Having observed the behavioral patterns, the nurse is better prepared to help the client change them.

5. Assess Mrs. Danes's ability to set realistic goals in the hospital and after discharge.

5. Setting unrealistic or unattainable goals leads to failure, which lowers self-esteem and intensifies despair. These conditions predispose the client to attempt suicide.

6. Assess Mrs. Danes's expectations of herself, her children, her former husband, and her friends.

6. A client who is prone to depression typically relies on others to make the client happy. When others do not meet unrealistic expectations, the client feels unloved, unwanted, inadequate, and angry.

7. Determine which resources, including family, friends, employer, religious organization, and postdischarge follow-up (such as an outpatient group), are available to Mrs. Danes after discharge.

7. Lack of social support systems predisposes the depressed client to suicide. A client with diverse support systems is less likely to require further hospitalization.

Classifying suicidal behavior

A brief method of classifying the suicide risk for a given client is shown here. No matter how low the risk assessed, all threats of suicide must be taken seriously.

LOW RISK	MODERATE RISK	HIGH RISK
• Verbal threat • No specific plan • Gesture with no threat to life	• Verbal threat • Specific plan • Lethal plan • Attempt made where rescue is possible	• Verbal threat • Specific plan • Lethal plan • Attempt made where rescue is highly unlikely

Nursing diagnoses

- Risk for violence (self-directed) related to underlying despair
- Dressing or grooming self-care deficit related to lack of energy
- Impaired social interaction related to lack of energy
- Sleep pattern disturbance related to underlying anxiety

Planning and goals

- Mrs. Danes will remain safe from suicidal impulses while hospitalized.
- Mrs. Danes will meet self-care needs.
- Mrs. Danes will not lose weight while hospitalized.
- Mrs. Danes will sleep 6 to 8 hours at night by the time of discharge.
- Mrs. Danes will develop a positive attitude about herself, other people, and the future by the time of discharge.
- Mrs. Danes will initiate interactions with peers, staff, and family by the time of discharge.
- Mrs. Danes will set daily, weekly, and postdischarge goals that are specific and attainable.

Implementation

NURSING BEHAVIORS

NURSING RATIONALES

1. Ask Mrs. Danes whether she is suicidal now.

1. Directly asking the client whether she is suicidal conveys the nurse's caring attitude and lack of fear concerning the client's underlying self-destructive impulses. This approach often deters subsequent attempts because the client recognizes that someone understands her pain.

2. Place Mrs. Danes on suicide precautions when warranted.

2. This measure alerts the nursing staff to pay close attention to the client and to monitor her activity carefully. It also conveys to the client that staff members really care.

3. Monitor Mrs. Danes's energy level and sleep patterns.

3. The client's energy level and sleep patterns provide clues to the depth of her depression. As her energy level rises, her potential for suicide increases.

4. Monitor Mrs. Danes's verbal and nonverbal behaviors for congruency.

4. A depressed client may act as if she feels better when she does not.

5. Until Mrs. Danes has more energy, provide help with all self-care needs, and do not ask her to make decisions or to take any initiative.

5. Early on during hospitalization, a depressed client may be unable to make any decision, and insisting that she do so will only frustrate the nurse and seriously damage the client's already low self-esteem. The nurse cannot make the client dependent; instead, responding to the client's dependency needs will have the opposite effect over time.

6. When Mrs. Danes has more energy, encourage her to perform self-care activities.

6. Self-care has a positive effect on the client's self-esteem, helps her to externalize energy, and provides meaningful activity. (Keep in mind, however, that the client who looks and acts better may not feel better and thus may remain at risk for suicide.)

7. When Mrs. Danes shows signs of improvement, be cautious about prematurely complimenting her; instead, say something like, "I see you have done this; what does it mean?" or "How are you feeling?"

7. Prematurely complimenting a depressed person may trigger a suicide attempt or the return of symptoms. The client may interpret the compliments as lack of understanding that the client is still experiencing inner pain. Thus, the client may take action to communicate this clearly to her caregivers.

8. Continually validate with Mrs. Danes the meaning of her behavior. For example, you might say, "I see you've applied makeup and have on a new outfit. What does this mean?" or "I sense you are down today. Tell me what's happening."

8. This approach conveys the nurse's interest and desire to understand the client's inner experience. It also provides good role modeling for making overt that which is covert.

9. Provide prompt care for any physical symptoms, such as constipation, anorexia, insomnia, and muscle aches.

9. Besides conveying the nurse's care and concern, this approach demonstrates a willingness to meet the client's dependency needs and recognizes the legitimacy of the client's symptoms.

10. Ask Mrs. Danes how she feels.

10. Talking about feelings lessens their impact on the client.

11. Insist that Mrs. Danes attend all unit activities and therapy sessions; give her no choice, even if she refuses.

11. Given a choice about attending unit activities and therapy sessions, a depressed client usually declines. However, insisting that the client attend helps to externalize her energies and decrease her social isolation. In contrast, allowing the client to vegetate subtly communicates to the client that staff members do not care about her or have given up on her.

12. Help Mrs. Danes identify people she can turn to for help when she begins to feel overwhelmed again.

12. Developing and using a support system help the client stave off hopelessness, thus decreasing the likelihood of suicide attempts.

13. Administer an antidepressant to Mrs. Danes as ordered, and monitor its effects. (*Note:* Typically, a larger dose is given at bedtime, a smaller dose in the morning.)

13. Pharmacologic intervention is commonly used to relieve depression. A loaded dose of antidepressant at bedtime promotes sleep, and the mood-elevating effect carries over to the next day. If the client needs another dose, it is usually smaller and given early in the day.

14. Assist Mrs. Danes in contacting friends or family.

14. Besides decreasing the client's social isolation, this measure teaches the client to take the initiative to get her needs met.

15. If Mrs. Danes asks you to leave or tries to push you away, tell her that you plan to stay for a specified number of minutes; do not leave at her request.

15. Remaining with the client for an allotted time conveys a willingness to meet her dependency needs and affirms the nurse's value of her as a person.

16. Assign accomplishable tasks to Mrs. Danes when her energy level rises—for example, preparing coffee for herself or helping to prepare the evening snack.

16. Accomplishing tasks strengthens the client's pride and self-esteem. (Remember, be careful about prematurely complimenting the client. She will experience satisfaction as her depression lifts.)

17. Have Mrs. Danes list her daily and weekly goals and the resources needed to meet them.

17. Listing one's goals can lead to greater success in achieving them: The client feels a strengthened commitment to the goals and can visualize her progress toward them. Identifying needed resources improves planning for goal attainment.

18. Discuss and evaluate the results of Mrs. Danes's trial home visits.

18. Setting and meeting goals while hospitalized can be easier than setting and meeting goals on the outside. Evaluating trial home visits lets the client more accurately assess how to meet her needs once discharged.

19. Ask Mrs. Danes to outline what she wants from herself and others.

19. Understanding her wants will help the client develop realistic expectations of herself and others.

20. Have Mrs. Danes list her strengths and her plans for using them to get her needs met.

20. Listing her strengths will improve the client's self-concept, boost her sense of autonomy, and provide tangible evidence that she must assume responsibility for her life.

21. Help Mrs. Danes work on problem areas one at a time—for example, finding qualified child care, coping with divorce, obtaining employment, and managing loneliness.

21. Working on problem areas one at a time makes them manageable and provides a sense of accomplishment as each problem is resolved. Specifying problem areas helps the client focus on them; however, several sessions may pass before the client can define her problem areas clearly. Thereafter, she can begin to formulate specific strategies for dealing with them.

22. Engage in structured anticipatory planning with Mrs. Danes as needed. For example, you might ask, "If your child gets sick and you are supposed to go to work, what can you do?" or "If the nursing supervisor says she doesn't like something about your nursing care, what can you do [or say]?"

22. Anticipatory planning prepares the client to remain in control when things go awry after she leaves the hospital. She will not be easily overwhelmed by helplessness and inadequacy if she has taken the time to plan her responses to problems.

MENTAL HEALTH NURSING

23. Role-play with Mrs. Danes so she learns how to negotiate with various resources to get specific needs met. Ask her questions like these:
• How can you negotiate child care on your terms?
• How can you negotiate flexible working conditions?
• How can you work with the children's paternal grandparents?

24. Help Mrs. Danes formulate a specific plan for outpatient follow-up.

23. Directly asking for need fulfillment is a new skill for the depressed client, who typically imagines that others automatically know her needs. Learning to negotiate takes practice, but the client is rewarded with greatly increased self-control and a sense that she has options. Assertiveness training may enhance her negotiating ability.

24. The client will need support and reinforcement while she is learning new coping behaviors. If she devises the follow-up plan herself, she will be more likely to adhere to it.

Evaluation

• Mrs. Danes does not attempt suicide while receiving treatment.
• Mrs. Danes assumes full responsibility for self-care, consuming an adequate diet and keeping personal belongings in order.
• Mrs. Danes sleeps 6 to 8 hours every night.
• Mrs. Danes interacts spontaneously with staff, peers, and visitors.
• Mrs. Danes identifies realistic weekly goals related to home, work, child care, social life, and meeting personal needs.
• Mrs. Danes develops specific and realistic expectations for herself and for significant others.
• Mrs. Danes develops a support system for getting her needs met.

Bipolar disorder, manic

In a client with bipolar disorder, mood swings can range from great elation and activity (manic phase) to extreme hopelessness, sadness, and lassitude (depressive phase). This entry focuses on the client during the manic phase. (See *Characteristics of bipolar disorder* for a brief comparison of the manic and depressed phases.)

During the manic phase, the client commonly exhibits excessive motor activity and may become highly irritable if caregivers place limits on behavior. The client also demonstrates disturbed thought processes that lead to socially inappropriate behavior. Because the client lacks self-pacing and problem-solving abilities, care and treatment focus on slowing the client's movements and activities. Otherwise, a manic client can die of self-induced exhaustion or injury. Potential for suicide increases when the client's mood is changing from mania to depression or from depression to mania, and suicide precautions may be needed.

Clinical situation

Peter Cox, age 46, is a stockbroker and avid stamp collector. Married and the father of five teenage children, he has been treated by a psychiatrist for the past 20 years for episodes of mood swings. He was taking lithium but stopped 1 month ago after losing thousands of dollars in the stock market. Today he is being admitted to the psychiatric unit.

Characteristics of bipolar disorder

MANIC PHASE

- Irritability
- Hyperactivity
- Impulsiveness
- Gregariousness
- Impaired nutrition
- Sleep disturbance
- Emotional lability
- Disruptive behaviors
- Thought disturbances
- Social inappropriateness
- Overinflated sense of self
- Refusal to take medication

DEPRESSED PHASE

- Guilt
- Anxiety
- Anorexia
- Dependency
- Constipation
- Hopelessness
- Helplessness
- Self-derogation
- Low self-esteem
- Boredom or fatigue
- Sleep disturbances
- Somatic complaints
- Social withdrawal
- Internalized anger

His wife reports that for the past 3 weeks, Mr. Cox has been calling all his clients five to six times a day and telling them about fantastic stock tips. She also says he has slept no more than 3 hours each night, staying awake to rearrange his stamp collection. Convinced that he owns many million-dollar stamps, he has been waking the entire family several times nightly to boast about his collection. Mr. Cox will begin receiving 600 mg of lithium three times daily on admission to the hospital.

Assessment

NURSING BEHAVIORS

1. Assess Mr. Cox's anxiety level by evaluating his speech and thought patterns, degree of orientation, affect and mood, and ability to meet personal needs.

2. Assess Mr. Cox's anxiety level.

3. Assess Mr. Cox's rest and activity patterns.

4. Throughout his hospitalization, assess Mr. Cox's mood swings (for example, from elation to anger).

5. Assess Mr. Cox for patterns of manic and depressive episodes.

NURSING RATIONALES

1. This provides evidence about the client's level of elation.

2. Identifying the client's anxiety level allows the nurse to plan appropriate care (see *Anxiety levels and nursing implications,* page 140).

3. During a manic episode, physical complications of exhaustion can cause death unless the client's activity is properly managed. The client may sleep and eat sparingly, unable to stay still long enough to do either.

4. Mood lability is common during a manic episode. During an acute manic episode, the client is typically impulsive and at risk for harming himself or others.

5. If patterns can be detected accurately, the nurse and other health care professionals can initiate appropriate treatment interventions.

MENTAL HEALTH NURSING

6. Assess Mr. Cox for positive and adverse effects of lithium (see *Selected drugs commonly used in mental health nursing,* pages 201 to 211). Monitor the serum drug level daily until it reaches 0.6 to 1.2 mEq/liter.

6. The client may require up to 3 weeks of lithium therapy before positive results are evident. While on the drug, the client can become toxic at any time because lithium's narrow therapeutic window is highly individualistic.

7. Assess Mr. Cox's understanding of his discharge plans.

7. The client who does not understand his discharge plans or who thinks them unimportant will probably not comply with them.

Nursing diagnoses
- Risk for injury related to impaired judgment
- Altered nutrition (less than body requirements) related to hyperactivity
- Altered thought processes related to compromised ego functioning
- Sleep pattern disturbance related to high energy level and distractability

Planning and goals
- Mr. Cox will not harm himself while hospitalized.
- Mr. Cox will not weigh less than _____ lb (_____ kg) by discharge.
- Mr. Cox will regain control of his thought processes.
- Mr. Cox's normal sleep pattern will return.
- Mr. Cox will demonstrate a stable mood.

Implementation

NURSING BEHAVIORS

NURSING RATIONALES

1. Arrange for one nurse per shift to care for Mr. Cox.

1. This arrangement promotes consistency of care and, by controlling the client's exposure to interpersonal stimuli, helps to decrease his anxiety.

2. Decrease stimuli in Mr. Cox's environment: Do not encourage him to participate in competitive games, and keep him out of busy areas, such as the dayroom and nursing stations.

2. Because of impaired thought processes, the manic client has a tendency to become overloaded by environmental stimuli. With fewer stimuli, he may get more rest and enjoy more sedentary activities.

3. Channel Mr. Cox's energy in one direction, and pace his activities: Walk slowly with him, and suggest quiet activities, such as making collages and folding laundry.

3. Slow-paced activities decrease the client's energy expenditure, prevent overstimulation, and sometimes have a soothing effect.

4. If quiet activity does not decrease Mr. Cox's energy expenditure, involve him in activities that exercise the large muscles, such as ripping rags, throwing a ball, or walking. Be sure to monitor him for signs of exhaustion.

4. Active exercise is sometimes required to dissipate the tremendous amount of energy within the client.

5. Give Mr. Cox nutritious foods that he can eat on the run.

5. To prevent nutritional depletion, allow the client to eat on the run.

6. Establish a bedtime ritual for Mr. Cox, and give him sleep medication, as ordered and needed.

6. Sometimes an established bedtime ritual is soothing for the manic client.

7. If a mood swing to depression seems imminent, implement suicide precautions for Mr. Cox.

7. The client is at increased risk for suicide during mood swings.

8. Discuss with Mr. Cox the events surrounding his manic or depressive episodes, such as major holidays, vacations, increased expectations at work, the birth of a child, visits from relatives, and a change in medications.

8. Identifying a consistent pattern of precipitating events enables the nurse to use anticipatory planning to reduce manic episodes.

9. Administer lithium as ordered, and evaluate its effects. If unpleasant side effects develop, teach Mr. Cox how to manage them, and notify the physician.

9. Lithium restores the body's chemical balance and thereby helps control manic episodes. If lithium proves ineffective, the physician may order carbamazepine (Tegretol) or valproic acid (Depakene).

10. Help Mr. Cox plan for compliance with his treatment plan after discharge.

10. If the client is involved in discharge planning, he will be more likely to comply with treatment.

11. Involve Mr. Cox's family in discharge planning, and encourage their participation in follow-up care.

11. Careful lifestyle management can help control this chronic illness. However, family members are likely to be ignorant about home management of a loved one with this disorder, so they appreciate receiving information. Furthermore, family members who participate in discharge planning are more likely to follow through with the plan than those who do not participate.

Evaluation

- Mr. Cox engages in goal-directed activity and no longer exhibits disturbed thinking.
- Mr. Cox eats his meals quietly with the other clients.
- Mr. Cox sleeps through the night.
- Mr. Cox's weight falls within the range established for him.
- Mr. Cox did not harm himself or others during his hospitalization.
- Mr. Cox is adequately maintained on lithium, expresses a desire to follow the medication regimen, understands why he must take the drug, knows its side effects and how to manage them, and has a plan for getting serum drug levels analyzed once a month.

Schizophrenia

People with major distortions in ego functioning experience serious disturbances in all areas of their lives, having impaired reality testing and a compromised ability to relate with others. Common signs of impairment in reality testing include bizarre behaviors, inability to assume responsibility for oneself, and misinterpretation of environmental stimuli. Major disturbances in ego functioning can result from functional causes such as acute psychosis or from underlying organic causes related to drug ingestion, high fever, an accumulation of toxins in the body, or dementia.

Schizophrenia is a brain disease characterized by neurotransmitter imbalances and structural changes within the brain. Distorted thought processes make living with this disease a challenge. Signs and symptoms of schizophrenia include hallucinations, delusions, loose associations, catatonic behavior, flat or inappropriate affect, compromised ability to manage daily affairs, social inappropriateness, aberrant speech patterns, and anhedonia.

MENTAL HEALTH NURSING

Consider the clinical situation of Mrs. Sara Smith (see below), medically diagnosed as having schizophrenia on the basis of what have become known as the four A's of schizophrenia: affective inappropriateness, ambivalence, associative looseness, and autistic withdrawal.

Clinical situation

Sara Smith, age 38, was admitted to the hospital 1 week ago. Her mother, age 70, brought Sara to the hospital after she attempted to burn down the mother's house. The mother provided the following information about her daughter: Mrs. Smith had few friends in high school, has never been employed, and had been married for 6 months when her first episode of emotional illness occurred. Mrs. Smith's husband divorced her after 2 years of marriage, at which time she moved in with her mother.

During the past 16 years, Mrs. Smith has been hospitalized 10 times for recurring episodes of schizophrenia. Between hospitalizations, she attends day treatment and is maintained on fluphenazine (Prolixin), 50 mg I.M. every 2 weeks.

Six weeks ago, Mrs. Smith stopped attending day treatment and refused to go to the clinic for her fluphenazine injections. One week ago, voices told Mrs. Smith that she deserved to die by fire because she was evil and nobody liked her.

In the hospital, Mrs. Smith has difficulty performing activities of daily living, spends most of her time alone, declines to participate in unit activities, and exhibits bizarre speech patterns. She has been observed wearing mismatched clothing and applying makeup inappropriately. Her conversation does not always flow logically, and her affect is flat. Since admission, she has been receiving 10 mg of haloperidol (Haldol) three times daily instead of fluphenazine.

You will serve as Mrs. Smith's primary nurse until she is discharged.

Assessment

NURSING BEHAVIORS

1. Observe Mrs. Smith's responses as you introduce yourself and establish the parameters of your relationship: Does she establish eye contact with you? How does she hold her body? What is her affect? Does she initiate physical contact with you?

2. Assess Mrs. Smith's underlying need.

3. Determine Mrs. Smith's ability to meet self-care needs: Is she well groomed? Does she have body odor? Is her immediate area tidy? Who does her laundry? Does she have personal hygiene articles (comb, brush, toothbrush, and so forth)?

4. Identify Mrs. Smith's safety needs: Can she manage smoking without supervision? What happens when she leaves the unit by herself? How aware is she of what is happening in her external environment?

NURSING RATIONALES

1. Initially, the nurse's presence may make the client uncomfortable, and the client may respond either by refusing to acknowledge the nurse or by cursing and demanding that the nurse leave. Careful observation enables the nurse to determine the client's anxiety level and need for space.

2. Identifying the client's underlying need allows the nurse to plan appropriate nursing care.

3. The client's self-care habits provide clues about her anxiety level and ability to function. Poor hygiene may result from perceptual distortions and disturbed thought processes. An untidy environment often symbolizes internal disorganization.

4. The more disorganized the client's thought processes, the less she will be able to function without supervision. If she still hears voices that tell her she must die by fire, she is at risk for harming herself or others.

Helping the client cope with hallucinations

This chart details the progression of behaviors and sensations that a schizophrenic client may experience just before and during a hallucination and describes nursing interventions that may help the client cope with these occurrences.

After a hallucination, the client may be exhausted. Be sure to allow time for the client to rest or sleep.

BEHAVIORS AND SENSATIONS	NURSING INTERVENTIONS
The client feels anxious or lonely and attempts to cope by daydreaming or seeking out a trusted person.	• Lack of structure and feelings of loneliness may precipitate hallucinations. Therefore, provide the client with a highly structured daily routine and engage the client in a structured activity to dissipate anxiety and feelings of loneliness. •*Do not* allow the client hours of free time.
The client experiences increasing anxiety, which leads to a state of alertness. The client becomes preoccupied with internal sensations (such as voices and images) and starts to respond to them. Aware that the sensations are internal, the client attempts to control them.	• Help the client compare internal sensations with external reality. • Engage the client in a structured activity. • Teach the client to hum, whistle, or talk out loud to "crowd out" internal sensations. • Ask the client to identify concrete things in the external environment.
As internal sensations become increasingly dominant, the client has trouble controlling them, and eventually yields to them.	• Talk to the client about external reality. • Ask the client to compare the hallucination with external reality. • Use self as a focal point to get the client's attention and the client to focus on what you are doing and saying. • Instruct the client to firmly tell the hallucination to go away. • Engage the client in a large-muscle activity.
The client becomes immersed in internal sensations and feels powerless over them. Depending on the nature of the hallucination, the client may become very frightened.	• Have the client focus on external reality. • Do whatever is necessary to get the client's attention. • Maintain a firm but kindly tone of voice.

MENTAL HEALTH NURSING

5. As you continue to work with Mrs. Smith, assess her for hallucinations or delusions: What is the nature of the hallucination or delusion? When does it occur? How often? Can you identify a consistent precipitating event?

5. Initially, the nurse can obtain information about the hallucination by allowing the client to describe it. After grasping the nature of the hallucination, however, the nurse should provide the client with a concrete focus. (See *Helping the client cope with hallucinations.*)

6. Monitor Mrs. Smith's patterns of interaction: Does she interact with roommates? If so, how? With whom does she spend her time, and what do they do? Does she have visitors? If so, who? How does she respond to them? What happens when her mother comes to see her?

6. Monitoring the client's interactions provides information about her social skills, her ability to meet interpersonal needs, and the extent of her social withdrawal.

7. Keeping in mind that Mrs. Smith has a history of noncompliance with her medication regimen, assess her response to her medication: What side effects, if any, are bothering her? How well does the medication control her symptoms? Does she show signs of tardive dyskinesia? How does she perceive her medication regimen?

7. Many clients stop taking their medications after discharge. Understanding why this happens enables health care professionals and the client to plan how to resolve the issue in an effort to ensure compliance and reduce recidivism.

8. Assess the nature and extent of Mrs. Smith's support systems and social networks, keeping in mind that her mother is elderly and may not live much longer.

8. With only one family member in the support system, the client will probably become acutely ill if that person dies or otherwise withdraws support. Research shows that broad social support systems help clients remain healthier for longer periods.

9. As Mrs. Smith prepares for her return to the community, assess her ability to terminate the nurse-client relationship.

9. Unless termination is carefully planned, the client may interpret it as rejection by the nurse. If this happens, she will have difficulty forming other relationships.

10. At the time of discharge, assess Mrs. Smith's goals: Are they specific or vague? Are they attainable? Do they include other people?

10. If the client does not know what she will be doing after discharge, the likelihood of future hospitalizations increases greatly. If her goals do not include activities with others, she will probably experience painful loneliness and withdraw, becoming a recluse.

Nursing diagnoses
- Risk for violence (self-directed or directed at others) related to acting on command hallucination
- Impaired social interaction related to lack of interpersonal skills
- Sensory or perceptual alterations (auditory) related to altered ego functioning
- Bathing or hygiene self-care deficit related to disturbed thought processes
- Dressing or grooming self-care deficit related to disturbed thought processes

Planning and goals
- Mrs. Smith will not experience physical harm while in the hospital.
- Mrs. Smith will no longer hear voices or will learn to control them.
- Mrs. Smith will understand the purpose and importance of her medication and will not experience undesirable side effects.
- Mrs. Smith will establish a relationship with her primary nurse, refer to other clients by name, and make eye contact when talking with others.
- Mrs. Smith will identify at least three resources she can use to maintain her mental health after discharge.
- Mrs. Smith will perform self-care without assistance.

Implementation
NURSING BEHAVIORS

NURSING RATIONALES

1. Structure a no-demand relationship with Mrs. Smith; that is, move slowly, speak softly, do not ask questions, and use touch sparingly.

1. Using a no-demand approach acknowledges the client's need for privacy and will eventually allow trust to develop. The schizophrenic client has great difficulty forming relationships because of lack of trust, and the need for interpersonal safety is so great that the client may require weeks or months to establish a relationship with the nurse. (However, becoming overly attached to the nurse is not uncommon once rapport has been established.)

2. Provide a highly structured and predictable daily routine for Mrs. Smith: Do not vary the daily routine. Assign consistent caregivers. Assist with self-care activities as needed. Give her a written schedule of activities.

2. A structured and predictable daily routine decreases client anxiety and promotes the development of trust. A predictable routine also simplifies the amount of information the client must process.

3. Do not allow Mrs. Smith access to matches.

3. As long as a client hears voices telling her to die by fire, she is at risk for setting herself on fire or starting a fire on the unit. A client who smokes should be carefully supervised.

4. Keep the unit doors locked, and accompany Mrs. Smith when she leaves the unit.

4. At this time, the client's reality-testing and problem-solving capabilities are impaired, so her safety would be jeopardized if she left the unit by herself.

5. When Mrs. Smith is actively hallucinating, determine the nature of the hallucination; then use one or both of the following techniques:

5. The techniques listed below can help to interrupt the hallucination and reorient the client to reality:

• Involve the client in a structured activity, such as walking, bedmaking, playing table tennis, or doing laundry.

• Besides channeling the client's anxiety, structured activity interrupts the hallucination by providing the client with a new focus.

• Acknowledge the client's underlying feeling, and provide reality orientation. For example, you might say, "I don't hear any voices. But I sense that you are frightened."

• This approach can provide a new focus for the client. If it fails, the nurse may try involving the client in structured activity or permitting the client to rest. Many clients are tired after experiencing a hallucination because of the tremendous energy drain.

6. When Mrs. Smith's anxiety has lessened and she has formed a working relationship with you, gently direct her toward improving social skills and planning for discharge, as follows:

6. By the completion of the orientation phase of the nurse-client relationship, enough trust will have been established for the nurse to help the client function at a higher level.

• Provide structured activities, such as baking projects, grooming, group quilting, and eating meals together, that also involve roommates, other clients, or visitors.

• Engaging in activities with others counters the client's tendency to withdraw and remain lonely. In addition, group activities promote development of social skills and a sense of camaraderie. As her social skills develop, the client will also show improvement in self-care capabilities.

• Ask Mrs. Smith about her experiences with medications: What does being on medication mean to her? How does the medication affect her? What prompts her to stop taking her medication?

• As long as the client remains noncompliant with her medication regimen, she is at risk for continuing the cycle of hospitalization, discharge, and rehospitalization. Understanding the client's perspective enhances the nurse's ability to help the client formulate a plan that promotes compliance.

• Underscore the importance of compliance to Mrs. Smith. Give her written information about her medication, and help her devise a plan that promotes compliance.

• If the client helps to make decisions about her treatment plan, she will be more likely to comply.

• Work with Mrs. Smith's case manager to plan an outreach program for Mrs. Smith.

• The client's ability to remain in the community may improve if someone is available whenever she needs assistance.

MENTAL HEALTH NURSING

• Involve Mrs. Smith in anticipatory planning by asking these questions: How will she manage when her mother is no longer around? Does she see herself ever working outside the home? What would she like most from life?

• Begin to terminate your relationship with Mrs. Smith before her discharge date. As the discharge date approaches, review the relationship you have shared and what you have accomplished together. Encourage Mrs. Smith to express her feelings (and discuss your feelings) about the termination. Ask if she would like to accomplish anything else with you before she is discharged. Observe her for signs of difficulty with termination.

• Review the purposes of follow-up care with Mrs. Smith, and encourage her to plan for continuing postdischarge care and for managing her daily affairs. Help her find acceptable answers to these questions: How will she get to and from day treatment? Whom can she rely on in time of need? How will she relieve boredom and loneliness? How will she manage her money? What kind of structured routines can she incorporate into each day?

7. Before she leaves the hospital, help Mrs. Smith make contacts in the community. For example, encourage her to participate in church activities or to perform volunteer work at a local library.

• Anticipatory planning allows the client to think about situations that might occur after discharge. If they do occur, the client is better prepared to take constructive action.

• Clients sometimes become overly attached to therapists once basic trust has been established. If termination is painful or perceived as rejection, the client may revert to previous behavioral patterns. Thus, the nurse should help the client interpret termination and plan for it. In particular, the client needs to plan for transferring newly learned interpersonal skills to situations outside the hospital.

• Although devising specific postdischarge plans demands considerable forethought, such planning can greatly reduce the incidence of future distress that could progress to overwhelming crisis. (In many settings, the case manager participates in discharge planning long before the client is released.)

7. Establishing community contacts builds the client's social networking skills, enhances her social support, and demonstrates that she can intervene actively on her own behalf.

Evaluation

• Mrs. Smith no longer hallucinates, or she takes action to control hallucinations.
• Mrs. Smith independently manages her daily care.
• Mrs. Smith's thoughts are rational.
• Mrs. Smith interacts appropriately with staff, selected peers, and visitors.
• Mrs. Smith can state the primary actions of her medications, expresses a willingness to comply with the medication regimen after discharge, and has a plan for managing adverse reactions.
• Mrs. Smith successfully completes termination with the nurse with no return of symptoms.
• Mrs. Smith has arranged to attend a structured day treatment program 5 days a week, has joined a community support group composed of former clients, and has the names and phone numbers of five people she can contact if she needs help after discharge.
• Mrs. Smith knows the name and phone number of her case manager.

Delusions

A delusion is a false belief to which a person adheres despite contradictory evidence. The most common types include *delusions of grandeur* (belief that one is highly important, famous, or powerful), *delusions of persecution* (belief that one is being persecuted or harmed by others or the environment), and *delusions of reference* (belief that one is connected to events unrelated to the individual; for example, the belief that one is responsible for all the evil in the world because the individual once "did something bad").

A delusional person's beliefs are steadfast; pointing out contradictory evidence reinforces rather than dissipates the delusional thinking. For the nurse, the most effective approach involves listening to the content of the delusion for clues to the client's underlying needs and conflicts. The nurse can then respond to the need rather than to the delusion. The nurse should also keep in mind that an actively delusional client, particularly one who is paranoid, commonly experiences severe to panic-level anxiety.

Persons with full-blown paranoid delusions exhibit extreme suspiciousness about those around them, believing others are out to "get" them. Thus, they spend an inordinate amount of time protecting themselves from perceived dangers that do not actually exist.

Clinical situation

The local police brought Charles Cain to the hospital 3 days ago; he was examined in the emergency department (ED) and then admitted to your psychiatric unit. In the ED, Mr. Cain's daughter relayed the following information to the attending physician: Mr. Cain, age 45, has been periodically suspicious of family, neighbors, and coworkers for the past 6 months. About 3 weeks ago, he became convinced that they hated him and were out to get him. No amount of talking would change his mind. To protect himself, Mr. Cain moved out of his home, quit his job, and disappeared; he did not tell anyone where he was. Three days ago, he returned home to do away with his wife and began breaking dishes and throwing canned goods around the kitchen. He repeatedly screamed at his wife, "I won't let you kill me! I'll kill you first!" At this point, Mr. Cain's 23-year-old daughter summoned the police.

Since his admission to your unit, Mr. Cain has kept to himself. He refuses medication—claiming that it is poison—and frequently assumes a karate stance when approached. His appearance is disheveled, and he has severe body odor. He does not sleep well at night because "I have to be sure no one will do me in while I'm asleep." His facial muscles are drawn, his brows are knit, and he peers sideways in a classically suspicious manner.

Mr. Cain, who has no previous history of psychiatric hospitalization, is to receive 10 mg of loxapine succinate (Loxitane) four times a day until his symptoms abate. You are assigned to care for Mr. Cain for the remainder of his hospitalization.

Assessment

NURSING BEHAVIORS

1. Initially, assess Mr. Cain's response to you, noting his body language, verbalizations, and tone of voice.

NURSING RATIONALES

1. This assessment provides clues about the client's anxiety level and his level of trust in the nurse.

2. Note whether Mr. Cain is suspicious of you, and be especially aware of staring, pressured speech, tight facial muscles, clenched fists, and darting eyes.

2. These are signs of impending violence; the client is literally defending himself. The nurse must respect the client's need for space.

3. Determine how safe Mr. Cain feels in the hospital by observing the following behaviors: Where does he stand or sit? With whom does he interact? When does he let his guard down?

3. The client who does not feel safe will constantly devote his energies to defending himself and thus will probably avoid interaction with everyone.

4. Assess Mr. Cain's overall self-care ability, including his ability to meet personal needs: grooming, hygiene, laundry, bedmaking, nutrition, elimination, and rest.

4. Characteristically, the client is too busy protecting himself to take care of personal needs. This assessment provides information about the pervasiveness of the client's anxiety.

5. Once you have established a relationship with Mr. Cain and have begun working with him, assess what he was like before he became ill. How long has he been delusional? How steadfast is the delusion?

5. This information provides the nurse with standards for measuring the client's progress and clues to formulating realistic treatment goals and outcome behaviors.

6. Finally, assess Mr. Cain's expectations of his wife, other family members, friends, and coworkers.

6. Unclear, unrealistic, or unverbalized expectations can lead to misinterpretation of others' behavior when others do not behave as the client desires or expects.

Nursing diagnoses
- Bathing or hygiene self-care deficit related to spending energy on self-protection
- Dressing or grooming self-care deficit related to spending energy on self-protection
- Risk for violence (other directed) related to delusions of persecution
- Sleep pattern disturbance related to underlying fear and inability to relax

Planning and goals
- Mr. Cain will not harm himself or others while hospitalized.
- Mr. Cain will comply with his medication regimen.
- Mr. Cain will regain his normal level of functioning.
- Mr. Cain will regain his reality-testing ability.
- Mr. Cain will adequately perform self-care.
- Mr. Cain will sleep 6 to 8 hours at night.

Implementation

NURSING BEHAVIORS

NURSING RATIONALES

1. Establish a nonthreatening, therapeutic relationship with Mr. Cain, using the following guidelines:
- State verbal requests clearly.
- Do not demand verbal responses from him.
- State the purpose of each contact with him.
- Keep contacts short, frequent, and goal-directed.
- Give him choices when possible.
- Approach him slowly, maintaining adequate space between you.
- Clarify who you are each time you approach him.
- Do not corner him.
- Watch him for signs of impending violence.

1. A suspicious client may strike out if he perceives a threat to himself. Enhancing his feeling of safety requires a structured and absolutely predictable environment. The client will not have the energy to invest in healthy behavior (for example, interaction with others) if he feels the constant need to be on guard. The nurse should be direct, goal-oriented, and businesslike with him; this will help to allay some of his anxiety. Remember, lower-level needs supersede higher-level needs—until the client's need for safety is met, he cannot get well.

• Do not gang up on him with other staff.
• Do not assume anything about what he knows. Explain all schedules and procedures to him.
• Keep other clients from wandering too near him.
• Assign one staff person per shift to him.
• To use his pooled energy, involve him in large-muscle activity.

2. Adapt unit routines to Mr. Cain's needs, as follows:
• Allow him to shower before or after scheduled showering hours.
• Allow him to have a unit tray or to go to the dining area before or after dining hours, or allow him to be first in line to choose his spot.
• Negotiate a sleeping plan with him so he can relax and sleep.
• Inform him about unit routines in a matter-of-fact way.

2. Giving the client as much power in the environment as possible will help him feel less threatened—less like someone is out to get him. This is not the time to adhere rigidly to rules designed for the convenience of the system. As his efforts at self-preservation consume less of his energy, more energy will become available for engaging in unit routines. The nurse cannot let his self-care needs go unmet; this would further convince him that no one cares what happens to him.

3. Work with Mr. Cain to determine when he will be most cooperative in taking his medication:
• Ask whether he prefers tablets or liquid.
• Determine whether he responds better if he is allowed to dispense his own medication from the bottle or jar.
• Ask whether he wants to be the first or last client to receive medication.
• Ask what he would like to know about the medication that would enable him to take it.

3. The nurse's goal is to increase the client's feeling of safety. He may be willing to take the medication if he feels he has some control. Only as a last resort should he be forced to take the medication; holding him down and giving him an injection will greatly increase his anxiety.

4. As Mr. Cain's anxiety decreases, talk with him about any changes that may have occurred during the past year: Did his wife take a job outside the home? Was he relieved of certain responsibilities at work? Did the last child leave home for college? Are his parents in poor health? Is he feeling dissatisfied with how his life is going?

4. If the client can identify factors that precipitated his illness, he may be able to prevent future delusional episodes through anticipatory planning. (*Note:* A brain lesion can also cause sudden, aberrant behavior. This possibility should be discussed in a staff conference.)

5. Teach Mr. Cain about his medication if he will be taking it on an outpatient basis.

5. The client will probably require psychotropic medication for 6 months to 1 year; understanding the medication's intended action and knowing how to manage side effects can significantly increase compliance with treatment.

Evaluation

• Mr. Cain does not harm himself or others during his hospitalization.
• Mr. Cain expresses willingness to comply with his medication regimen.
• Mr. Cain expresses readiness to return to work, his family, and other activities.
• Mr. Cain is no longer delusional.
• Mr. Cain showers daily, interacts with peers, and manages self-care needs.
• Mr. Cain goes to sleep readily and arises feeling well rested.

MENTAL HEALTH NURSING

Alzheimer's disease

Organic mental disorders (OMDs), which affect millions of people, may be acute and reversible or chronic and irreversible. Alzheimer's disease, a chronic OMD that affects up to 10% of those over age 65, is progressive and eventually fatal. Onset is commonly insidious. As the brain deteriorates, personality changes occur, along with marked declines in memory, self-care capability, and ability to perform routine tasks. In the last phase of the disease, the client is incontinent; becomes progressively immobile, bedridden, and nonverbal; and does not recognize loved ones. The client with a chronic OMD typically lives with family members until caring for the client and protecting the client from harm become unmanageable. The family must then make the painful decision either to transfer their loved one to a long-term care facility or to bring help into their home.

Recently, tacrine hydrochloride (Cognex) has been used to improve the memory of clients with mild to moderate Alzheimer's disease. Although some measure of success has been attained in prolonging functional ability, this drug does not permanently arrest disease progression.

The following clinical situation focuses on the client with onset of Alzheimer's disease.

Clinical situation

Mildred Wall, age 65, lives at home with her husband; their four children are grown. A florist, Mrs. Wall owns her own business. During the past year, her husband relates, she has become forgetful and absent-minded and has had occasional outbursts of anger, which are atypical for her.

One month ago, Mrs. Wall started withdrawing from social activities and began refusing to go to the florist shop. She said she was tired and didn't need to waste her time in meaningless activities. Her husband has noticed that she frequently misidentifies people, does not remember simple things unless prompted, makes up stories about events, and rarely uses people's names. Sometimes at night Mrs. Wall becomes agitated and wanders around the house. If Mr. Wall asks what she is doing, Mrs. Wall tells him it is none of his business.

Because of his concern about her, Mr. Wall insisted that his wife have a complete physical examination; yesterday, the physician informed the couple that Mrs. Wall has Alzheimer's disease. Mr. Wall has decided that his wife will remain at home until he can no longer care for her—but he confided to the office nurse that he feels inadequate to care for his wife because he knows so little about her illness. A referral to a visiting nurse association has been made.

Assessment

NURSING BEHAVIORS

1. Initially, assess Mrs. Wall's physical status and safety needs: coordination, continence, ability to chew and swallow, physical strength, vision, gait, and tendency to wander.

2. Assess Mrs. Wall's mental status: recent and long-term memory; orientation to time, place, and person; ability to perform familiar tasks; patterns of forgetfulness; and response to the disease.

NURSING RATIONALES

1. The nurse can use baseline data to measure the disease's progression. Nursing interventions will be tailored to the client's ability to function.

2. This information also provides a baseline for measuring progression of the disease. Nursing interventions will be based on the client's degree of memory impairment.

3. Assess the impact of Mrs. Wall's illness on her husband: Does he feel overburdened? Is he grieving? Can he maintain his social interests? Does he feel angry or guilty?

4. Over time, assess the progression of Mrs. Wall's disease: Does she turn on the stove and wander away? Does she wander from the house and get lost? Does she drive unsafely? Can she meet hygiene needs? Is she eating nutritious foods? Is she in full control of bladder and bowel elimination? Can she perform household tasks?

3. A sense of duty may be forcing the client's husband to assume more responsibility than he can handle. In such situations, the primary caregiver rapidly becomes overburdened, and social support systems shrink because the caregiver spends more and more time with the spouse. The caregiver also may feel embarrassed and ashamed about the spouse's condition.

4. As the client becomes increasingly disoriented, the spouse will need greater assistance in managing home care (see *Global deterioration scale for cognitive decline and Alzheimer's disease,* pages 178 and 179).

Nursing diagnoses

- Risk for injury related to impaired cognition
- Anticipatory grieving related to loss of ability to function
- Altered family processes related to role changes necessitated by the client's condition

Planning and goals

- Mrs. Wall will remain free from serious injury.
- Mrs. Wall will maintain the ability to engage in familiar activities and to meet personal hygiene and grooming needs as long as possible.
- Both Mr. and Mrs. Wall will engage in healthy grieving about Mrs. Wall's illness.
- Mr. Wall will anticipate role changes as his wife's condition deteriorates.
- Mr. Wall will seek out information about Alzheimer's disease.

Implementation

NURSING BEHAVIORS

NURSING RATIONALES

1. Initiate health assessments by the visiting nurse every 3 weeks.

1. A 3-week interval between home visits is long enough to allow observable changes to develop yet short enough to prevent the client and her husband from feeling abandoned. During these visits, the visiting nurse should encourage Mr. and Mrs. Wall to discuss how the disease is affecting them. At times, the client may express acute sadness about her debilitating illness. Attentive listening by the nurse can provide a source of comfort. If Mrs. Wall exhibits denial, the visiting nurse should not insist that the client grieve her loss.

2. Have Mr. Wall establish a daily routine for Mrs. Wall.

2. A daily routine helps preserve the client's memory function so she stays reality oriented and functional.

3. Label and color-code any objects that Mrs. Wall has difficulty identifying.

3. Knowing an object's name helps the client use it appropriately and avoid confusion.

4. Ensure that someone is available to help Mrs. Wall with grocery lists, cleaning, and other home tasks.

4. Mrs. Wall's participation in home tasks promotes healthy functioning and enhances the client's self-esteem.

MENTAL HEALTH NURSING

Global deterioration scale for cognitive decline and Alzheimer's disease

LEVEL	CLINICAL PHASE	CHARACTERISTICS	FUNCTIONAL ABILITY	NURSING CONSIDERATIONS
1	Normal	• No subjective complaints of memory loss • No objective evidence of memory deficit on clinical interview	• No impairment	• None
2	Forgetfulness (normal for age)	• Subjective complaints of slight memory loss (for example, forgetting the location of reading glasses or the name of a former associate) • No objective evidence of memory deficit on clinical interview • No objective deficits in employment or social situations	• No impairment (but appropriate subjective concern about memory loss)	• None
3	Early confusional (borderline Alzheimer's disease)	• Clear-cut deficits that become apparent to others (tendency to get lost, decline in job performance, forgetfulness of recent events, difficulty in finding the right word in conversation) • Objective evidence of deficits in memory and concentration (obtained only during an intensive interview conducted by a trained geriatric psychiatrist) • Attempts by the client to deny and hide cognitive impairment • Mild to moderate anxiety about symptoms	• Inability to perform in demanding employment and social interactions (evident to intimates and associates)	• Help the client devise ways to manage job performance (for example, writing notes to oneself, planning each day, keeping one's environment free of clutter, and attending to one task at a time).
4	Late confusional (mild Alzheimer's disease)	• On clinical interview, demonstration of several cognitive deficits (decreased knowledge of current and recent events, slightly impaired memory of personal history, concentration deficit elicited on serial subtractions) • Commonly, no deficit in orientation to time and person, recognition of familiar faces, or ability to travel to familiar locations • Use of denial as the dominant defense mechanism • Tendency to be overwhelmed when confronted with a complex task • Flattening of affect and withdrawal from challenging situations	• Decreased ability to handle finances and marketing	• Help the client grieve the loss of function. • Do not insist that the client "face reality." No useful purpose would be served. • Advise the family that the client can probably perform simple household tasks with prompts, and help them plan accordingly. • Help the client anticipate and plan for various situations.
5	Early dementia (moderate Alzheimer's disease)	• Inability to recall major aspects of one's life (familiar addresses and telephone numbers, the names of certain relatives, the name of the high school or college from which the client graduated) • Disorientation to time (date, day of the week, or season) or to place • Difficulty in counting back from 40 by 4s or from 20 by 2s • Retention of basic facts about self and family members	• No assistance required with toileting or eating but may require coaxing to bathe • Occasional difficulty in choosing the proper clothing to wear	• Have a family member assist the client with clothing selection. • Help the client follow established routines for self-care. • Keep demands on the client simple. • Closely observe the client during meals for signs of choking.

Global deterioration scale for cognitive decline and Alzheimer's disease

(continued)

LEVEL	CLINICAL PHASE	CHARACTERISTICS	FUNCTIONAL ABILITY	NURSING CONSIDERATIONS
6	Middle dementia (moderately severe Alzheimer's disease)	• Occasional inability to recall the spouse's name • Retention of ability to distinguish between strangers and family and friends and to recall own name • Virtual ignorance of all recent events and experiences • Retention of certain aspects of past life (though sketchy) • General unawareness of surroundings, the year, and the season • Possible difficulty in counting backward from 10 or in counting forward • Occasional ability to travel to familiar locations (but the client usually requires a travel escort)	• Personal or hygienic dysfunction, or both (progression: difficulty in dressing properly; need for assistance with bathing, possibly developing into a fear of bathing; inability to handle mechanics of toileting, leading to urinary and bowel incontinence)	• Help the caregiver develop a daily routine that meets the caregiver's needs as well as the client's. • Refer the caregiver to a support group and a home health care agency if the caregiver has not already contacted these resources for respite. • At the appropriate time, help the caregiver talk through the decision to have the client placed in an extended care facility. • If the client is institutionalized, refer to visiting family members and friends by proper name ("Mrs. Wall, your husband George is here to see you"), and avoid inappropriate humor ("Look at this handsome young fella who has come to see you").
7	Late dementia	• Apparent inability of the brain to tell the body what to do • Loss of verbal skills (the client merely grunts) • Loss of basic psychomotor skills such as the ability to walk • Urinary and bowel incontinence	• Speech and motor dysfunction (progression: limited vocabulary, unintelligible phrases and grunting, loss of all motor abilities, stupor, coma)	• Attend to the bedridden client's skin integrity and range of motion. • Anticipate and meet the client's needs.

Reprinted with permission of The Free Press, a Division of Simon & Schuster, from *Alzheimer's Disease: The Standard Reference*, by Barry Reisberg, M.D. ©1983 by Barry Reisberg, M.D.

5. Write down Mrs. Wall's routines and procedures, put a large clock in a prominent spot, and hang signs showing the day and date.

5. These orientation aids will help the client stay reality-oriented and functional.

6. Give Mr. Wall the name and telephone number of an Alzheimer's support group.

6. A support group can help Mr. Wall mourn his loss and decrease his burden and sense of loneliness. The group will also provide him with valuable information about Alzheimer's disease and suggestions for managing his wife's care.

7. Teach Mr. Wall the predictable progression of Alzheimer's disease.

7. To make sound decisions about disease management, the client's caregiver needs information about the illness.

8. Help Mr. Wall identify areas where he needs assistance in managing his wife at home, such as respite care, meal preparation, and toileting.

8. Identifying his needs will reduce Mr. Wall's anxiety and enhance his ability to remain in control of this situation.

9. Write down at least three options for each problem identified.

9. Having at least three options for solving each problem gives the client's spouse a sense of being in control rather than feeling trapped or limited.

10. Give Mr. Wall information about community resources available to help him, such as weekend respite care, day care for persons with Alzheimer's disease, and home health aide services.

10. Community resources can help the client's spouse manage care so that the client need not enter an extended-care facility until the late stage of her illness.

Evaluation

• Mrs. Wall demonstrates ability to meet her physical, safety, and hygiene needs with minimal assistance.
• Mrs. Wall continues to participate in daily household tasks.
• Mr. Wall joins a weekly Alzheimer's disease support group.
• Mr. Wall does not feel over burdened by his wife's illness, and he uses community resources for help when needed.
• Mr. Wall maintains his social network.
• Mr. Wall engages in anticipatory problem solving to meet Mrs. Wall's increasing dependency needs.

Substance abuse

Some people discover that certain chemical substances appear to relieve their anxiety, boredom, depression, or feelings of inadequacy. Over time, continual intake of a chosen substance becomes abusive, tolerance develops, and the person must ingest increasingly larger quantities to obtain the desired effects. Continued substance abuse leads to physiologic and psychological changes. Some family members, friends, and coworkers may notice these changes and "protect" the abuser, either by excusing misbehavior at home or by taking on extra work to make up for the abuser's decreased productivity on the job. Others may be slow to recognize that alcohol abuse is adversely affecting the abuser as well as family, friends, and associates. (See *Stages of alcohol addiction* for a summary of behaviors commonly observed as a person develops dependency on alcohol.)

Health professionals typically see a substance abuser for the first time when the client seeks treatment for a related health problem, such as gastric ulcers, malnutrition, or hepatitis. The abuser may be admitted to a general hospital directly or through the emergency department—for example, following an accident or overdose. Lack of cause-and-effect insight makes treating such a client a challenge for nurses (see *Treating alcohol abuse,* page 182). Because most substance abusers do not view themselves as having a problem, they do not initiate treatment for their abusive behavior. Furthermore, they overuse the defense mechanisms of denial, rationalization, and projection, and they make considerable use of negative manipulation.

The following clinical situation focuses on a client whose alcoholism has come to light after an automobile accident that resulted in a charge of driving while intoxicated.

Stages of alcohol addiction

STAGE	BEHAVIOR
Preaddiction	
Experimental use	The client drinks alcohol for the first or second time and begins to learn about its effects.
Responsible use	The client drinks alcohol in moderation; use does not harm the client or others.
Occasional misuse	Intake occasionally puts the client over the legal blood alcohol limit.
Addiction	
Early phase (regular misuse)	• Intake usually puts the client over the legal blood alcohol limit. • Drinking relieves such symptoms as anxiety. • Drinking helps the client cope. • The client is preoccupied with drinking. • Intake is rapid. • The client has hangovers. • The client minimizes intake when discussing it with others. • The client sneaks drinks. • Blackouts begin. • Personality changes occur.
Middle phase (dependency)	• The client sets out to drink. • Problems of alcohol abuse begin. • The client begins to lie about drinking. • The client begins to feel guilty about drinking. • The client loses friends and interests. • Blackouts increase. • The client makes excuses for drinking. • The client's alcohol tolerance increases. • The client begins to lose control and can no longer predict what will happen once drinking starts.
Late phase (extreme or complete dependency)	• The client cannot be without alcohol. • Physiologic symptoms develop if the client stops drinking. • The client drinks until the supply is gone, then searches for more. • Alcohol becomes more important to the client than anything else. • The client drinks to feel "normal." • The client changes drinking places to hide the problem's severity from others. • Moral deterioration occurs. • Tolerance for alcohol decreases. • Thinking is impaired. • The client drinks in the morning. • The client may change jobs or move to another city to "start over again," only to resume the drinking pattern (geographic cure).

MENTAL HEALTH NURSING

Clinical situation   Allan Maze, a 38-year-old business executive, is under observation at a local hospital for 3 days following an automobile accident that left him with head injuries and suspected internal injuries. Within 10 hours of admission, the nurse notes that Mr. Maze is experiencing vivid hallucinations. In reviewing his chart, the nurse notes that Mr. Maze's blood alcohol content was 0.25 on admission.

Treating alcohol abuse

TREATMENT RECOMMENDATIONS	ASSESSMENT FACTORS	RATIONALES
Monitor alcohol intake	• Consumes fewer than 6 drinks/week • Blood alcohol content (BAC) 0.14 or less • Benign scores on Western Personality Inventory (WPI) subscales • Benign family history	• Increased awareness of intake may prevent future problems.
Limit alcohol intake	• BAC between 0.15 and 0.17 • Benign WPI subscale scores • History of exceeding the legal blood alcohol limit more than four times/year • History of consuming more than 10 drinks/week	• Client is at risk for developing alcohol dependency; limiting intake now helps prevent increased future intake.
Abstain from alcohol; use support and counseling services: Alcoholics Anonymous, inpatient treatment, family counseling	• BAC greater than 0.18 • Significant WPI subscale scores • History of daily alcohol consumption • History of consuming more than 15 drinks/week • Family history of alcohol abuse • Extreme defensiveness about use of alcohol • Multiple drug use • Presence of blackouts, personality changes, other problems related to use of alcohol • Inability to control alcohol intake • Previous conviction for driving while intoxicated or previous treatment for alcohol abuse • Presence of family problems related to client's alcohol abuse	• Data indicative of addiction, which is best controlled by abstinence. • Abstinence is best maintained with the help of a support group. • Inpatient treatment may be indicated for the client assessed as at high risk for dying or for doing harm to self or others. • Alcohol abuse potentiates problems within the family (alcoholism is a family disease).

Assessment

NURSING BEHAVIOR

Assess Mr. Maze for alcohol withdrawal (see *Recognizing alcohol withdrawal syndrome* and *Selected substances of abuse*, pages 184 and 185).

NURSING RATIONALE

The client requires protective nursing measures during withdrawal. Physical restraints should be used only as a last resort; ideally, one-on-one care should be provided for the client if symptoms progress beyond mild tremors, diaphoresis, nausea, nervousness, tachycardia, and increased blood pressure.

Clinical situation
(continued)

After Mr. Maze recovers from the effects of withdrawal, he tells the nurse that he began consuming alcoholic beverages at age 14 and has averaged about a fifth (25.6 oz) of bourbon daily for the past 2 years. The medical staff discovers that Mr. Maze, who is 5′ 11″ (180 cm) tall and weighs 150 lb (68 kg), has a gastric ulcer and slight cirrhosis of the liver. His blood pressure has been stable at 160/110 mm Hg.

MENTAL HEALTH NURSING

Recognizing alcohol withdrawal syndrome

Use this chart to review alcohol withdrawal syndrome, keeping in mind that the client should have one-on-one care as symptoms worsen. For nursing management, use restraints only as a last resort; restraining the client will heighten anxiety and increase agitation.

SIGNS AND SYMPTOMS	ONSET AND DURATION	NURSING MANAGEMENT
Mild tremors, diaphoresis, nausea, nervousness, tachycardia, increased blood pressure	Signs and symptoms may occur within 4 to 6 hours after the last drink.	• Carefully monitor the client's behavior. • Seek the physician's order for medication to relieve withdrawal symptoms. • Talk to the client about symptoms, and remain with the client once withdrawal begins. • Monitor the client's vital signs.
Increased tremors, hyperactivity, insomnia, anorexia, disorientation, delusions, transient visual hallucinations, tachycardia	Signs and symptoms commonly occur 8 to 10 hours after the last drink.	• Administer medications, as ordered, to relieve withdrawal symptoms. • Remain with the client and orient to reality. • Keep the room free from distractions and unnecessary noise. • Monitor the client's vital signs as able.
Same as those listed above plus persistent hallucinations, nausea, and vomiting; withdrawal seizures may also occur 7 to 48 hours after last drink.	Signs and symptoms occur 12 to 48 hours after the last drink	• Remain with the client. • Monitor the client's vital signs as able. • Institute seizure precautions. • Administer anticonvulsant medications as ordered. • Offer fluids and light foods, as tolerated, during periods of lucidity. • Maintain a peaceful environment.
Delirium tremens (withdrawal delirium, which lasts 2 to 3 days), disorientation, fluctuating consciousness, hallucinations, agitation, and low-grade fever	Signs and symptoms most commonly occur 48 to 72 hours after the last drink, but may not arise until 7 days after.	• Remain with the client. • Monitor the client's vital signs as able. • Maintain a peaceful environment. • Offer fluids and light foods, as tolerated, during periods of lucidity. • Administer medications, as ordered.

MENTAL HEALTH NURSING

Assessment

NURSING BEHAVIORS

After his withdrawal from alcohol, assess Mr. Maze's physical condition, giving priority to his gastric ulcer, nutritional status, blood pressure, weight, and signs of liver damage.

NURSING RATIONALES

The client's lower-level needs must be met before the nurse can address higher-level needs. Therefore, the client's physiologic problems, if any, must be carefully assessed and monitored as a first priority.

Clinical situation
(*continued*)

Once his physical condition is stabilized, Mr. Maze is transferred to an inpatient treatment program because of an intervention by his wife, boss, and children. Mrs. Maze relates that her husband's drinking has caused much worry in the family and that the children, embarrassed, refuse to invite other youngsters to their home. She also says that she frequently covers for him so he will not lose his job.

Selected substances of abuse

The chart below lists various substances of abuse, signs of withdrawal, and corresponding nursing interventions. During the acute withdrawal stage (detoxification), the nurse may administer medications intended to prevent or minimize the severe consequences of withdrawal, such as seizure or delirium.

SUBSTANCE	WITHDRAWAL SIGNS	NURSING IMPLICATIONS
Alcohol (beer, wine, liquor)	• Mild tremors • Diaphoresis • Nervousness • Increased blood pressure • Increased heart rate	• Monitor client's vital signs. • Obtain order for benzodiazepines to relieve withdrawal signs. • Remain with client and monitor behavior. • Promote sleep and rest.
	• Moderate to severe tremors • Appetite loss • Disorientation • Hallucinations • Delusions	• Monitor client's vital signs. • Administer benzodiazepines, as ordered. • Maintain a quiet environment. • Remain with client.
	• Persistent hallucinations • Grand mal seizures	• Monitor client's vital signs. • Remain with client. • Administer anticonvulsants, as ordered. • Take seizure precautions. • Minimize environmental stimulation. • Offer foods and fluid when client is lucid.
	• Delirium tremens • Sleeplessness • Tachycardia • Hallucinations	• Monitor client's vital signs. • Remain with client. • Minimize environmental stimulation. • Offer foods and fluids, as tolerated.
Opiates (such as morphine and heroin)	• Lacrimation • Runny nose • Yawning • Diaphoresis • Tachycardia • Fever • Insomnia • Muscle aches • Drug craving • Nausea or vomiting • Dilated pupils • Chills	• Monitor client's vital signs. • Remain with client. • Offer foods and fluids, as tolerated. • Provide a soothing environment. • If ordered, wean client by offering small doses of opiate. • If ordered, administer methadone.
Central nervous system stimulants Amphetamines	• Depression • Fatigue • Agitation • Suicidal thoughts • Paranoia • Disorientation • Insomnia or hypersomnia	• Monitor client's vital signs. • Monitor client for suicidal ideation. • Promote sleep and rest. • Administer antidepressants, if ordered. • Remain with disoriented or frightened client; orient client to reality.
Cocaine, crack cocaine	• Depression • Fatigue • Agitation • Suicidal thoughts • Paranoia • Insomnia or hypersomnia	• Monitor client's vital signs. • Monitor client for suicidal ideation. • Promote sleep and rest. • Administer antidepressants, if ordered. • Remain with disoriented or frightened client; orient client to reality.

Selected substances of abuse *(continued)*

SUBSTANCE	WITHDRAWAL SIGNS	NURSING IMPLICATIONS
Hallucinogens Lysergic acid diethylamide (LSD)	• Flashbacks at a later time	• Administer diazepam, as ordered, if client has severe anxiety during flashbacks.
Phencyclidine (PCP)	• Depression • Lethargy • Craving	• Monitor client's vital signs. • Monitor client for suicidal ideation. • Promote sleep and rest. • Administer antidepressants, if ordered. • Remain with disoriented or frightened client; orient client to reality.
Marijuana (cannabis)	• Insomnia • Irritability • Anorexia • Agitation • Restlessness • Tremors • Depression	• If client is depressed, attend to physiologic and safety needs. • Know that physicians rarely order medication to ease withdrawal.

Assessment

NURSING BEHAVIORS

NURSING RATIONALES

1. Provide opportunities for Mr. Maze to discuss being in a residential treatment program.

1. The client will probably be angry and resistive to treatment; unless he can vent these feelings, they may interfere with his participation in the program. Beware of the client who is eager to receive treatment under forced circumstances: he is most likely conning himself and the staff.

2. Ask Mr. Maze which areas of his life are causing him the most serious problems.

2. The nurse's and the client's perceptions of his problems may differ, but the nurse must work with the client's perceptions, seeking information about them as needed. Typically, the client cites other people or his job as most problematic for him and makes heavy (and convincing) use of denial and rationalization. The nurse must be careful not to be deceived. (See *How alcohol abuse affects quality of life*, page 186.)

3. Assess Mr. Maze's capacity to handle stress at home, at work, and in social situations: What does he do when he feels pushed? How often does he ask for assistance? Does he take on too many projects? Is he gregarious or retiring?

3. This assessment provides information about the consistency of the client's behavior in various situations.

4. Assess Mr. Maze's willingness to adopt a lifestyle free from substance abuse.

4. When the client's history indicates that he is at high risk for death from alcohol, unwillingness to consider an abstinent lifestyle indicates the intensity of his denial.

How alcohol abuse affects quality of life

Alcohol abuse has widespread effects, causing changes in virtually every aspect of a person's life. This chart delineates the changes that may occur.

ASPECT OF LIFE	EFFECTS OF ALCOHOL ABUSE
Economic	• Deteriorating financial status as abuser spends increasing amounts of money on alcohol
Emotional	• Embarrassment • Guilt • Defensiveness about alcohol consumption • Use of defense mechanisms, such as denial, rationalization, and minimization
Family	• Codependency and loss of self-identity in family members • Broken promises by abuser • Conflict and strife within family over abuser's drinking problem
Legal	• Traffic violations • Bar fights or other altercations resulting in arrest
Leisure	• Abandonment of formerly satisfying activities as alcohol use occupies increasing amounts of time
Mental	• Impaired judgment while inebriated • Blackouts or episodes of amnesia
Occupational	• Decreasing quality of work • Decreasing productivity • Absenteeism (*Note:* Occupation usually is the last area to be affected.)
Physical	• Deteriorating health, as manifested by such problems as hypertension, gastritis, head and neck cancers, or hangovers
Sexual	• Impotence • Careless sexual behavior during blackouts or while inebriated
Social	• Loss of friends because of unacceptable behavior • Constriction of social circle as drinking companions replace friends or as abuser spends more time drinking alone at home
Spiritual	• Engaging in activities contrary to abuser's previous value system (such as lying, stealing, cheating, or acting in an offensive manner)

Nursing diagnoses
• Risk for injury related to alcohol-induced impaired judgment during withdrawal
• Ineffective denial related to perceived threat to sense of competence
• Ineffective family coping (compromised) related to codependency of family members

Planning and goals
• Mr. Maze will experience an uncomplicated recovery from alcohol withdrawal.
• Mr. Maze will lose no more weight while in the hospital, reduce blood pressure to the normal range for his age, and show no signs of GI bleeding before discharge from the residential treatment center.
• Mr. Maze will recognize that alcohol is creating problems in his life.
• Mr. Maze will develop specific plans for abstinence from alcohol and for managing stress.
• Mr. Maze and his family will join appropriate support groups.

Implementation

NURSING BEHAVIORS	NURSING RATIONALES
1. Provide care for Mr. Maze during withdrawal, as follows:	**1.** During withdrawal, Mr. Maze must have his physical needs met to prevent injury and complications.
• Give medications for restlessness and insomnia, as needed and ordered.	• Sleep disturbances will further stress Mr. Maze. Medications for restlessness and insomnia may help to decrease the intensity of withdrawal. A benzodiazepine such as diazepam (Valium) is typically prescribed to decrease the effects of withdrawal.
• Give Mr. Maze at least 10 8-oz glasses (2,500 ml) of fluids daily unless otherwise ordered. Offer favorite juices every other hour, and limit intake of caffeinated drinks.	• Monitoring fluid intake helps maintain the client's physiologic well-being.
• Record Mr. Maze's fluid intake and output.	• The fluid intake and output record provides data about the client's physiologic status.
• Encourage Mr. Maze to ambulate as much as possible.	• Early ambulation helps maintain the client's self-esteem and prevent complications from immobilization.
• Assess Mr. Maze's vital signs every 4 hours.	• Vital signs indicate the client's physiologic status. For example, an elevated pulse rate may indicate gastric bleeding or withdrawal.
• Provide physical protection as needed to ensure Mr. Maze's safety; use restraints only as a last resort.	• For the client who is out of touch with reality during withdrawal, restraints are frightening and will increase agitation.
• Note any behavioral changes, such as agitation or hyperactivity, and provide care as needed. If Mr. Maze is confused or agitated, stay with him and orient him to reality as needed. Provide a soothing, nonstimulating environment, particularly if he is hallucinating.	• During delirium tremens, the client's behavior is erratic and must be monitored continually to ensure his safety.
• Provide a special-duty nurse, if possible, until delirium tremens has passed.	• Having someone with him during delirium tremens makes the client's experience less frightening. If he is hallucinating or having delusions, he will need a great deal of environmental structuring and reality orientation.
• Implement seizure precautions.	• This is a safety measure to protect the client from harm. For a person experiencing withdrawal, seizures are not unusual.
2. Provide care for Mr. Maze during his recovery from withdrawal and early residential treatment, as follows:	**2.** After withdrawal, the client may not feel well for a while. His condition should be carefully monitored to prevent complications.
• Monitor Mr. Maze's blood pressure and pulse rate daily.	• A pulse rate above 100 beats/minute may indicate an adverse condition such as internal bleeding.

MENTAL HEALTH NURSING

• Provide small, frequent, nutritious meals high in vitamins and carbohydrates and with normal protein and fat composition. Give vitamin B supplements as ordered.

• The underweight client, unable to tolerate large amounts of food at a single meal, will be more apt to eat if given small portions. When possible, provide meals that he enjoys (encourage the family to bring in his favorite foods). Vitamin B supplements may be ordered to correct a deficiency in vitamin B.

• Weigh Mr. Maze weekly, keeping in mind that he is about 20 lb (9.1 kg) underweight.

• Weekly weighing is part of monitoring the client's progress.

• Test Mr. Maze's stools for occult blood weekly.

• A weekly guaiac test provides information about the client's progress, especially if he has a history of gastric ulcer.

3. Encourage Mr. Maze to talk about all facets of his condition and treatment, as follows:

3. Talking helps the client vent his feelings and frees him to participate in treatment.

• Ask Mr. Maze to describe the events leading up to his admission to the alcohol treatment program. To keep the discussion going, use such phrases as: "Tell me more," "And then?" "I can tell you still have a lot of feeling about this," "What did _____ say (do)?" and "What did you do when _____ said (did) that?"

• In talking about his situation, the client should eventually be able to adopt a more objective view of himself. The nurse should be cautious about using confrontational techniques, which may increase the client's defensiveness.

• In an accepting, nonjudgmental manner, discuss Mr. Maze's use of alcohol with him.

• A nonjudgmental approach conveys to the client the nurse's ability and willingness to understand his situation without making him feel guilty.

• When Mr. Maze uses denial, rationalization, or projection, consider redirecting him by saying, "I'm not clear about what this has to do with you."

• Redirecting the client's statements may eventually reduce his use of these defense mechanisms. As mentioned earlier, however, the nurse must avoid premature or ill-timed confrontation, which increases defensiveness.

• Help Mr. Maze examine how he responds to stressors at home, at work, and in social situations.

• Self-examination helps the client recognize the pervasiveness of his stress. At that point, he may be able to identify other ways to cope with it.

4. Refer Mr. Maze to Alcoholics Anonymous (AA) or a similar support system while he is still a client in the treatment program.

4. The client will need continuing postdischarge care to maintain abstinence. Initiating community support before discharge helps ensure his continuing participation afterward.

5. Assist Mr. Maze to practice new coping skills, such as relaxation techniques, reframing, and anticipatory planning.

5. Learning new coping skills requires practice. For the alcoholic client, practicing these skills while still in the treatment program will reduce his tendency to revert to self-destructive coping methods.

6. Review with Mr. Maze his plan for staying sober. (A realistic plan must include Mr. Maze's acknowledgment that he has a problem, his admission that he cannot stay sober by himself, and his active participation with others who are maintaining abstinence.) Help him identify specific methods for adopting an abstinent lifestyle.

6. Planning for an abstinent lifestyle is crucial: If the plan is not specific, the client will revert to old coping patterns. A client who has put his plan into action before discharge will fare better than one who waits until after discharge.

7. If Mr. Maze is scheduled for disulfiram (Antabuse) therapy, teach him the interactional effects of disulfiram and alcohol: severe nausea and vomiting, flushed face, rapid pulse and respirations, and reduced blood pressure.

7. Teaching the client about disulfiram is necessary to ensure his compliance and to reduce the risk of severe adverse reaction from consuming alcohol while taking disulfiram. Because of his slight cirrhosis of the liver, Mr. Maze may not be a candidate for disulfiram or naltrexone.

8. Help Mr. Maze's family become active in an appropriate support group, such as Al-Anon, Alateen, or ACOA (Adult Children of Alcoholics).

8. Many nonaddicted family members have been codependents and enablers. All family members must adopt new coping skills to achieve healthy family functioning.

Evaluation

• Mr. Maze's blood pressure is normal.
• Mr. Maze gains at least 5 lb (2.3 kg) and shows no signs of GI bleeding.
• Mr. Maze freely acknowledges the problems created by alcohol ingestion and makes restitution with his employer and family.
• Mr. Maze participates in six stress-management group sessions and identifies specific strategies for managing stress.
• Mr. Maze develops a workable, realistic, and specific plan for maintaining abstinence.
• Mr. Maze joins AA while in the hospital and plans to continue attending AA meetings (with a peer) after discharge.
• Members of Mr. Maze's family attend appropriate support groups at least once weekly.

Anorexia nervosa

Anorexia nervosa and bulimia nervosa, two major forms of eating disorder, result in death for 5% to 15% of the persons they affect. The incidence of eating disorders is particularly high among adolescent girls from highly competitive, upwardly mobile families.

The warning signs of anorexia nervosa include loss of 25% or more of the person's body weight without apparent cause, severe curtailment of food intake, intense fear of gaining weight, amenorrhea, exercising to excess despite fatigue, denial of hunger, and peculiar patterns of handling food. Onset generally occurs between ages 12 and 18.

MENTAL HEALTH NURSING

The warning signs of bulimia nervosa include weight control by vomiting or other means of purging, extreme eating patterns ranging from binging to fasting, consumption of high-calorie foods during binges, secretiveness about food intake, maintenance of body weight within 10 to 15 lb of normal despite apparent consumption of large amounts of food, and depression following a binge (the person can be at risk for suicide at this time). Onset generally occurs between ages 18 and 30.

Persons with these two eating disorders share many characteristics, including:
• excessive concern about food and weight control
• use of extreme measures to control weight (starvation, purging)
• perfectionistic self-expectations
• concern about how one is viewed by others
• eagerness to please and make a good impression
• underdeveloped sense of personal identity
• discomfort in social situations
• unresolved issues of autonomy
• underlying needs for love, affection, and belonging.

The anorexic client and the bulimic client also display distinct behavioral differences. For example, when the client is finally hospitalized for treatment of anorexia nervosa, malnutrition is apparent (see *Anorexia nervosa and bulimia nervosa: Client behaviors* for more information). It is not unusual for a client with anorexia nervosa to weigh as little as 70 or 80 lb (31.8 or 36.3 kg). In most cases, the client must weigh at least 90 lb (40.8 kg) before psychotherapy can be initiated successfully.

The goal of treatment for the anorexic client is reversal of weight loss; for the bulimic client, interruption of the binging-purging pattern. Overall, treatment is aimed at helping the individual understand the underlying issues that caused the eating disorder.

The following clinical situation focuses on nursing care for the client with anorexia nervosa.

Clinical situation

Sandi Brent, age 17, has been admitted to your unit in the hospital for treatment of severe weight loss. Sandi is 5′ 6″ (168 cm) tall and weighs 85 lb (38.6 kg). She has been in counseling at a community mental health center for the past 2 months but was admitted to the hospital when her weight dropped below 90 lb (40.8 kg).

Sandi, who lives with her parents and three younger siblings, is an honor student and president of the student council. She works hard to please her teachers and her parents.

According to her history, 6 months ago Sandi decided to lose 25 lb (11.3 kg) so others would find her more attractive and she would look slimmer in her graduation pictures. When she attained her goal of 110 lb (50 kg), she decided to continue dieting in the firm belief that her ability to lose weight and remain thin would demonstrate her self-discipline and ability to succeed.

On your unit, Sandi becomes extremely upset when anyone tries to get her to eat, saying that the sight of food nauseates her. When she does eat, she complains of feeling bloated and needs to go to the bathroom immediately. Sandi says she does not understand why everyone is so concerned about her weight. She just feels fat and does not want to be any heavier. Sandi rarely socializes with the other teenagers on the unit, preferring to spend time in solitary activity. When she does socialize, she appears uncomfortable and sometimes makes tactless remarks.

MENTAL HEALTH NURSING

Anorexia nervosa and bulimia nervosa: Client behaviors

ANOREXIA NERVOSA

- Denies that the eating pattern is abnormal
- Loses significant amounts of body weight
- Is introverted
- Copes with stress by starving
- Denies feeling fatigued
- Exercises compulsively
- Tightly controls food intake
- Is unlikely to abuse alcohol
- Feels powerful after abstaining from food

BULIMIA NERVOSA

- Recognizes that the eating pattern is abnormal
- Keeps weight within a normal range
- Appears extroverted
- Copes with stress by binging
- Admits feeling fatigued
- May or may not exercise strenuously
- Is unable to control food intake
- May abuse alcohol
- May be suicidal after binging

Assessment

NURSING BEHAVIORS

1. Assess Sandi's physical condition, noting her weight, body temperature, vital signs, electrolyte levels, fluid intake and output, and skin condition.

2. After Sandi's weight reaches at least 90 lb, assess her thoughts and feelings about food and ideal body weight: What is the origin of her thoughts and feelings? How realistic are they?

3. Assess Sandi's underlying needs.

4. Assess Sandi's previous eating patterns and the events surrounding her decision to begin dieting: What primary gain does she derive from dieting? What are the secondary gains?

5. Assess Sandi's self-expectations and her perception of what others expect of her, including parents, siblings, teachers, friends, and boys.

6. Assess the interaction patterns in Sandi's family, along with her parents' expectations for her.

NURSING RATIONALES

1. Sandi's physiologic state needs careful monitoring because cardiac arrest from potassium deficiency is not uncommon. She will not have the ability to participate in psychotherapy until her weight stabilizes at a minimum of 90 lb.

2. The nurse should listen for indications of the client's self-expectations and perceptions of what others expect of her.

3. Identifying Sandi's underlying needs allows the nurse to plan appropriate care and intervene accordingly.

4. This assessment may lead the client to reveal problems with autonomy and identity. Commonly, a primary gain for the anorexic adolescent girl is control of underlying anxiety created by conflicts stemming from arousal of autonomy issues. Secondary gains include the attention she now gets because of the weight loss and relief from age-appropriate responsibilities. Overall, remaining excessively thin shields the client from having to face issues surrounding her emergence into womanhood.

5. Anorexic clients typically have unusually high self-expectations and distorted views of what others expect of them.

6. Many families of anorexic clients stress appearances and "doing the right thing." If Sandi is striving to be the perfect daughter, her ability to master the developmental tasks of adolescence will be hindered.

Nursing diagnoses	• Ineffective denial related to uncertainty about the future
	• Altered nutrition (less than body requirements) related to fear of becoming fat
	• Body image disturbance related to distorted perception of body size

Planning and goals	• Sandi will increase her weight to at least 105 lb (47.6 kg).
	• Sandi's physiologic processes will be within normal limits.
	• Sandi's anxiety about having a heavier body will decrease to tolerable limits.
	• Sandi will formulate a healthy self-concept.
	• Sandi will engage in age-appropriate behavior with peers.

Implementation

NURSING BEHAVIORS	NURSING RATIONALES
1. Offer highly nutritious foods every 3 hours. After Sandi eats a meal or snack, observe her closely for at least 90 minutes.	**1.** Sandi cannot ingest large quantities of food at one time. Initially, she is anxious about eating and fearful of becoming obese; unobserved, she may resort to vomiting in order to keep her weight down.
2. Help Sandi participate in sedentary diversional activities for at least 4 hours daily, and encourage her to stay in bed at least 7 hours every night; restrict strenuous exercise.	**2.** Until Sandi reaches a weight of at least 90 lb, conserving her energy is vital to prevent further weight loss and body stress.
3. Ask Sandi what she achieves by maintaining such a low body weight.	**3.** For the anorexic client, food is closely linked to the underlying maturational issue of control. The thinner she becomes and the less she eats, the more powerful she feels. Thus, the client consumes small quantities of low-calorie, low-carbohydrate foods and will become extremely anxious if forced to eat foods she perceives as fattening. No matter how painfully thin the anorexic client becomes, she sees a fat person in the mirror, so she is afraid to eat and "get fatter."
4. Assign Sandi to a therapy group composed of clients with similar problems.	**4.** In group therapy, the client will feel less isolated and lonely when she discovers that others experience similar struggles. As she develops a healthier perspective, she will stabilize at a weight negotiated between the therapist and her. She will also begin to separate what she wants from what she thinks others want for her.
5. Ask Sandi what would happen if she maintained her weight at 110 lb (20 lb [9 kg] below her ideal weight of 130 lb [59 kg]).	**5.** This question challenges the client to think about her decision to maintain an extremely low body weight.
6. Ask Sandi to describe the events surrounding her dieting behavior.	**6.** This question encourages Sandi to evaluate the validity of her thoughts about thinness. Eventually, she will discover other ways to control her life besides self-induced starvation.

MENTAL HEALTH NURSING

7. Institute the treatment program designed for Sandi by the treatment team, and follow the plan precisely. Be aware that Sandi may try to pit staff members against each other or to play on staff members' sympathies to bring about changes in the plan.

7. Until her weight reaches 90 lb, the client is placed on restricted activity to conserve her energy. After reaching 90 lb, she is typically started on a combination of behavior modification and psychotherapy. Because of the nature of this illness, the treatment plan must be followed exactly. Initially, the client may try to thwart the plan's success. However, as she gains insight into her underlying needs, she should become more cooperative.

8. Instruct Sandi to write down her weekly goals.

8. This exercise helps Sandi develop a firmer sense of self as an autonomous being. She needs to learn how to differentiate what she wants for herself from what she thinks others want for her.

9. Teach Sandi assertiveness skills.

9. The ability to express her wants freely will enhance the client's self-identity and empower her to manage her affairs actively and responsibly.

10. Arrange for family sessions that will examine family dynamics related to issues of power, control, and decision making. (*Note:* Family therapy is typically conducted either by nurses prepared at the master's level or by other appropriately licensed health care providers.)

10. Anorexia nervosa in one or more family members is often symptomatic of underlying conflict in the family unit. Working with each family member allows the therapist to help them clarify individual issues, relieving the client's burden of "carrying" the problems of other members. Sessions should take place at least once a week, with all members present. If they refuse to attend and the client returns to the same environment that precipitated her eating disorder, her chances for sustained recovery will be jeopardized. If the family unit develops awareness, family tensions will decrease, and each member will become more comfortable functioning autonomously. Overall, the need to present a united front will be greatly reduced.

MENTAL HEALTH NURSING

Evaluation

- Sandi's vital signs, electrolyte levels, and fluid intake and output are within normal limits.
- Sandi states that she is pleased with her appearance when her weight reaches 105 lb.
- Sandi verbalizes an understanding that what she wants for herself is separate from what she thinks others want for her.
- Sandi reestablishes an old friendship and says she enjoys the renewed relationship.

Borderline personality disorder

Clients with personality disorders control anxiety by adopting behavior patterns that interfere with their ability to adapt to daily stressors and establish healthy relationships. The personality disorders fall into three major groups. (See *The personality disorders*.)

Most clients with personality disorders are treated as outpatients. However, those with borderline personality disorder (BPD) may be hospitalized after a self-destructive act such as a suicide attempt. Typically, clients with BPD attempt suicide when feeling abandoned; their goal is to get others to take care of them.

The following clinical situation focuses on a client with BPD.

Clinical situation

Danielle Wyatt, age 32, is admitted to the psychiatric hospital after attempting suicide. During the 3 days since her admission to your unit, she has caused dissension among the staff and has displayed temper outbursts when limits are set on her behavior. She often lingers near the nurse's station.

Yesterday, Ms. Wyatt inflicted wounds on her lower arms with a paper clip when her husband failed to appear during visiting hours. She says she can relate to only two people on the unit: you and a new social worker. During report today, you learn that she has been telling other patients they are receiving substandard care because one of the staff nurses is a recovering alcoholic.

Assessment

NURSING BEHAVIORS	NURSING RATIONALES
1. Assess Ms. Wyatt's underlying needs.	**1.** The client most likely has an underlying fear of abandonment, resulting in an intense need for interpersonal safety as well as needs for recognition, self-esteem, and achievement.
2. Evaluate Ms. Wyatt's pattern of self-destructive behavior.	**2.** This provides information about the client's impulse control and the potential for future self-destructive acts.
3. Assess Ms. Wyatt's ability to process what she experiences.	**3.** Lack of problem-solving skills and inability to process experiences leaves the client powerless over her self-destructive behavior. Also, she is likely to distort reality.

Nursing diagnoses

- Risk for self-mutilation related to a history of self-inflicted injury
- Impaired social interaction related to inability to process interpersonal experiences

Planning and goals

- Ms. Wyatt will refrain from self-destructive behavior while hospitalized.
- Ms. Wyatt will learn how to process experiences before and after taking action.

The personality disorders

The personality disorders fall into three groups, or clusters, shown in this chart. Clients with cluster A personality disorders are characteristically aloof and restrained in relationships; others may describe them as odd or strange. Clients with cluster B disorders typically are dramatic, unrestrained, and unpredictable. Those with cluster C disorders are overly apprehensive about the present and future, and worry about failing.

PERSONALITY DISORDER	CLIENT DESCRIPTION
CLUSTER A	
Schizotypal personality disorder	• Is sometimes labeled a "healthy" schizophrenic • May be viewed as odd or eccentric • Has poorly developed social skills • Has strained and uncomfortable relationships • Is easily overwhelmed by too much social or interpersonal stimuli
Paranoid personality disorder	• Uses projection • Is extremely suspicious of others' motives • Is very guarded in relationships • Is very private • Expects to be exploited or harmed by others • Questions others' loyalty • Reads hidden meaning into harmless remarks or events • Does not forgive slights, insults, or injuries
Schizoid personality disorder	• Is emotionally cold and detached • Is withdrawn and controlled • Cannot form warm, spontaneous relationships • Usually lives alone or in parents' home • Has little need for friendships or intimacy • Has a solitary lifestyle • Seems indifferent to praise or criticism
CLUSTER B	
Narcissistic personality disorder	• Cannot empathize with others because of intense need for love and admiration • Demands much time and attention from others • Feels entitled • Is arrogant and haughty • Expects to be recognized as superior without commensurate achievements
Histrionic personality disorder	• Controls anxiety through dramatic presentation of self • Uses attention-seeking behaviors and flattery to get others to meet needs • Is overly concerned with physical attractiveness • Cannot tolerate delayed gratification • Has a seductive appearance or behavior • Becomes anxious when limits are placed on attention-seeking behaviors
Borderline personality disorder	• Has a poorly developed sense of self • Struggles with overwhelming feelings of anger and anxiety • Views situations in extremes (all good or all bad) • Has intense fear of abandonment • Feels empty and devoid of substance • Needs others around to maintain a sense of self (you + me = self)

(continued)

MENTAL HEALTH NURSING

The personality disorders (continued)

PERSONALITY DISORDER	CLIENT DESCRIPTION
Antisocial personality disorder	• Is aggressive and impulsive • Acts out conflicts within social contexts • Has no regard for rules and norms • Lacks remorse • Takes no responsibility for outcomes of own behavior • Blames others when things go wrong • Believes others are unreliable • Must have immediate gratification • Disregards the truth • Has a poor work history • Cannot sustain a monogamous relationship

CLUSTER C

Passive-aggressive personality disorder	• Is not aware of underlying anger • Procrastinates • Is habitually late and keeps others waiting • Does not uphold own end in a situation requiring follow-through • Is full of excuses • Controls others through inaction • Becomes anxious if not in control
Dependent personality disorder	• Is unable to be assertive • Remains in abusive situations • Falls apart if significant other leaves or dies • Does not trust own judgment • Feels incapable of managing on own • Needs excessive reassurance and advice • Lacks self-confidence • Will go to extremes to get nurturance from others
Obsessive-compulsive personality disorder	• Controls anxiety through extreme orderliness, cleanliness, and punctuality • Needs to be in control • Is excessively devoted to work and productivity • Is overly conscientious • Is unable to discard worn or useless objects • Is reluctant to delegate tasks to others • Hoards supplies for future catastrophes
Avoidant personality disorder	• Remains aloof in relationships • Wants friendships but can form them only if assured of not getting hurt or shamed • Does not like surprises • Is preoccupied with fear of being criticized or rejected in social situations • Feels inferior to others

Implementation

NURSING BEHAVIORS	NURSING RATIONALES
1. Develop a behavioral contract with Ms. Wyatt.	**1.** Clients with BPD benefit from written contracts that reduce the ambiguity in the relationship and define the parameters of acceptable behavior. Having such a contract also reduces splitting.
2. Engage Ms. Wyatt in role playing.	**2.** This technique provides opportunities for the client to try out different roles and practice viewing situations from different perspectives. Over time, she may develop empathic skills.

MENTAL HEALTH NURSING

3. Teach Ms. Wyatt how to engage in anticipatory planning.

3. This teaching helps the client develop new coping skills and feel empowered.

4. Meet daily with staff to ensure that Ms. Wyatt's plan of care is current and understood by all.

4. Consistency helps the client feel safe. All staff must follow the agreed-upon plan. The client will stop testing limits when she realizes that the plan of care is followed consistently.

5. Have Ms. Wyatt process her behavior with a staff person regularly.

5. This lays the foundation for development of problem-solving skills and will help the client develop empathy.

Evaluation

- Ms. Wyatt delays acting out when feeling alone or anxious.
- Ms. Wyatt exhibits the ability to see how her behavior affects others.
- Ms. Wyatt exhibits the ability to identify and plan for situations that precipitate acting out.
- Ms. Wyatt does not exhibit behavior that is harmful to herself or others while hospitalized.

Domestic abuse

Physical, emotional, and sexual abuse is common in families and constitutes an urgent mental health issue. Recipients of abuse are primarily women (battered wives), children, the elderly, the infirm, and the physically or mentally handicapped. Unfortunately, despite its shattering effects, family abuse is usually difficult to prove or even to stop. Lack of tangible evidence makes emotional and sexual abuse more difficult to prove than physical abuse. Family sexual abuse may continue for years because of the shame and guilt associated with revealing it.

Abused children commonly become abusive parents, in turn raising the next generation of abusers. In abusive families, seemingly mild stressors can precipitate abusive episodes.

Persons unfamiliar with abuse may be overwhelmed when they must assist recipients of abuse. Thus, nurses must be aware of their own feelings about abuse so that they can assist both the abuser and the abused.

The following clinical situation focuses on nursing care for an abused child and her family.

Clinical situation

Louise, age 2, is admitted to your pediatric unit at 4:30 p.m. from the emergency department (ED). She has bruises on her back and a spiral fracture of her left upper arm, which has been put in a cast. The ED report indicates that Louise's father, who has been unemployed for 6 months, became upset with her when she wet her pants while playing. According to him, he placed Louise firmly on her potty chair and told her not to move. When she got off the potty chair in "direct defiance" of his authority, he grabbed her arm and put her back on the chair to show her that he was the boss. When she screamed, he spanked her. Louise's screaming was so persistent, and her arm looked so reddened and swollen, that her mother—8 months pregnant with twins—convinced Louise's father that they should bring her to the ED.

In the pediatric unit, both parents express their concern about Louise to the nursing staff. They say that the father did not intend to hurt her—that he was only trying to teach her to be obedient. However, when the nurse-manager indicates a desire to talk more about Louise's broken arm, the parents become angry and quickly leave the hospital, saying they will be back later. Louise cries and calls after her departing parents, "Come back! Me be good. Me be good girl."

Assessment

NURSING BEHAVIORS	NURSING RATIONALES
1. Perform a physical assessment of Louise: Is she well nourished? Does she have unexplained marks or bruises on her body? Are her height and weight appropriate for her age?	**1.** A physical assessment provides baseline data about the abused child's condition; subsequent progress is measured against baseline findings.
2. Assess Louise's response to her broken arm.	**2.** An abused child may react passively to pain from a broken arm.
3. Assess Louise's response to being hospitalized and separated from her parents.	**3.** The child's response provides information about her developmental level and current care needs. Louise probably has never been away from her parents overnight. From her perspective, she has been abandoned.
4. When her parents return later in the evening, assess Louise's usual routine. Have the parents describe Louise's bedtime and toileting habits, and ask them to identify her favorite foods, toys, and play activities.	**4.** The abused child's adjustment to hospitalization will be enhanced if her normal routine is followed as closely as possible. Furthermore, this information facilitates individualized nursing care.
5. Assess Louise's response to her parents: Does she flinch when either parent reaches out to touch her? Does she avoid eye contact with either parent?	**5.** This assessment provides further information about the existence of abuse. A nurse who suspects child abuse is expected to follow the reporting protocol mandated by agency and state laws.
6. Assess the parents' willingness to help the staff care for Louise.	**6.** If the parents are willing to help with care of the abused child, they and the nursing staff have an opportunity to form a working relationship. In addition, increased familiarity will help everyone feel more at ease during the child's hospitalization.
7. Assess the underlying needs of each family member, keeping in mind that their needs will probably differ.	**7.** Identifying each family member's underlying needs will allow the nurse to plan appropriate care. Louise will no doubt need to feel safe in this new environment.
8. Assess Louise's parents for predisposing factors of child abuse.	**8.** Child abuse is highly correlated with abuse of drugs (including alcohol) and with unemployment, debt, lack of knowledge about child behavior, lack of social supports, inadequate housing, limited coping abilities, and marital strife. Referral to a social service agency may bring help to the abused child's family.

| **Nursing diagnoses** | • Altered parenting related to father's lack of knowledge about normal growth and development, and family stressors (father out of work and mother pregnant with twins)
• Risk for injury related to the father's lack of coping skills |

| **Planning and goals** | • Louise will recover uneventfully from her physical injury.
• Louise will sleep, eat, and play at a level appropriate for her age.
• Louise's parents will attend hospital-sponsored parenting classes.
• Louise's parents will contact appropriate community resources. |

Implementation

NURSING BEHAVIORS

1. Monitor Louise's physical progress. Check the cast for tightness every hour for the next 24 hours (see *Cast care,* page 357, for more information).

2. Give Louise age-appropriate toys for acting out her feelings.

3. As much as possible, follow Louise's usual daily routines.

4. Enhance Louise's sense of security in the hospital as follows:
• Remain with her until she falls asleep.
• Provide comfort measures before putting her to bed (holding, rocking, stroking, hugging, reading a story).
• If possible, let the child take a favorite toy or blanket to bed.
• Talk with her about when her mother will return (for example, "Mommy will come back after you eat breakfast").
• Be alert to Louise's concern for her mother's whereabouts.

5. Encourage her parents to help with Louise's care. Because a toilet training episode precipitated the abusive incident, be sure the parents understand that young children commonly revert to bed-wetting and thumb-sucking when hospitalized.

6. Teach the parents about cast care.

NURSING RATIONALES

1. Any physical injury must be attended to first. Lower-level needs must be met before higher-level needs.

2. In the young child with a limited vocabulary (around 200 words), play provides a way to express underlying feelings. At any age, unexpressed thoughts and emotions connected with being abused can predispose a child to dysfunctional behavior later in life.

3. Familiar routines promote the abused child's trust and decrease her anxiety about hospitalization.

4. These measures help provide security for the abused child in a strange environment. At such a vulnerable age, she is acutely aware of being separated from her parents, especially her mother, and may even think they have abandoned her. She may fear strangers. She also may start to fall asleep and then suddenly awaken when the nurse leaves the room.

5. Working with the parents gives the nurse opportunities to evaluate parent-child interactions and to provide positive reinforcement for their care as appropriate.

6. Proper cast care will help prevent further injury to the arm after the child is discharged.

MENTAL HEALTH NURSING

7. Give the parents appropriate information about management of infants and preschool-age children, and discuss "What if?" situations.

7. Anticipatory planning prepares the parents for the likely recurrence of situations that have triggered angry outbursts—and possibly abuse of their child—in the past. Ideally, instead of automatically reverting to abusive behaviors when such situations occur, the parents can develop and use new coping skills. Contrary to popular belief, the abusive parent usually loves the child. Removing the child from the parental home is not always the best way to manage child abuse.

8. With Louise's parents, discuss the various stressors in their lives and how they would like to handle these stressors.

8. This form of anticipatory planning can lay the groundwork for developing new problem-solving and coping skills. Expanded coping skills should decrease the parents' tendency to displace their frustrations onto the child.

9. Give the parents the names, addresses, and telephone numbers of appropriate community agencies.

9. People are more likely to use information when it is readily available. Furthermore, use of appropriate resources can greatly enhance parents' coping skills by increasing their social networking; social support positively affects a person's ability to manage stressors.

Evaluation

- Louise's broken arm heals without complications.
- Louise interacts spontaneously with the nurses and participates in age-appropriate play activities.
- Louise's parents begin attending meetings of Parents Anonymous, a support group for parents who abuse their children.
- Louise's father agrees to work with the social services department to obtain financial assistance and job placement.
- Louise's parents begin parenting classes by (date).

Selected drugs commonly used in mental health nursing

This chart presents information about drugs commonly prescribed for psychiatric disorders, including the drug action, dosage, and common side effects. Nursing considerations focus on patient comfort and teaching; side effects appear in italicized type in this column.

DRUG AND USUAL ADULT DOSAGE	ACTION	NURSING CONSIDERATIONS AND POSSIBLE SIDE EFFECTS
Antianxiety drugs (used to treat anxiety disorders)		
Benzodiazepines Alprazolam (Xanax): 0.25 to 0.5 mg P.O. b.i.d. or t.i.d. Chlordiazepoxide (Librium): 5 to 25 mg P.O. t.i.d. or q.i.d. Clonazepam (Klonopin): 0.05 to 0.2 mg/kg/day P.O. Diazepam (Valium): 2 to 10 mg P.O. b.i.d. to q.i.d. Lorazepam (Ativan): 2 to 6 mg P.O. daily in divided doses	Produce a calming effect by enhancing the action of the inhibitory neurotransmitter gamma-aminobutyric acid (GABA)	• To reduce *daytime sedation,* ask the physician for an order for a smaller dosage and allow the client to nap during the day until the body adjusts to the medication. • Offer sugar-free drinks and candy to relieve *dry mouth.* • To avoid *orthostatic hypotension,* have the client rise slowly. • Because of *lethargy* and *drowsiness,* advise the client to avoid driving or operating heavy machinery.
Antihistamine Hydroxyzine (Atarax, Vistaril): 50 to 400 mg P.O. daily in divided doses	A histamine₁-receptor blocking agent, acts as a nonspecific central nervous system (CNS) depressant	• To reduce *daytime sedation,* ask the physician for an order for a smaller dosage and allow the client to nap during the day until the body adjusts to the medication. • Offer sugar-free drinks and candy to relieve *dry mouth.* • To avoid *orthostatic hypotension,* have the client rise slowly. • Because of *lethargy* and *drowsiness,* advise the client to avoid driving or operating heavy machinery. • May be particularly useful in clients with anxiety or insomnia caused by *itching* or *pruritus.*
Antidepressants (used to treat depression)		
Tricyclics Amitriptyline (Elavil): 75 to 150 mg/day P.O.	Blocks reuptake of norepinephrine and serotonin into CNS neurons	• Before starting therapy, document the client's baseline pulse rate, blood pressure, and electrocardiogram (ECG). Monitor these periodically to detect *hypotension* or *arrhythmias.* • This drug is associated with a high incidence of *drowsiness,* especially when therapy begins. Some clinicians prefer to administer the entire daily dose at bedtime to minimize daytime drowsiness. • To reduce *orthostatic hypotension,* instruct the client to rise slowly when shifting to an upright position. Measure and document the client's supine and standing blood pressure; withhold the drug and inform the nurse-manager if systolic pressure drops more than 30 mm Hg. • Offer sugar-free drinks and candy to relieve *dry mouth.* • To detect *urine retention,* monitor urine output. Inform the nurse-manager if output is low.

(continued)

Selected drugs commonly used in mental health nursing *(continued)*

DRUG AND USUAL ADULT DOSAGE	ACTION	NURSING CONSIDERATIONS AND POSSIBLE SIDE EFFECTS
Antidepressants *(continued)*		
Amoxapine (Asendin): 50 mg P.O. t.i.d.	Blocks reuptake of norepinephrine and serotonin into CNS neurons; also may block postsynaptic dopamine receptors	• Before starting therapy, document the client's baseline pulse rate, blood pressure, and ECG. Monitor these periodically to detect *hypotension* or *arrhythmias.* • This drug is associated with a high incidence of *drowsiness,* especially when therapy begins. Some clinicians prefer to administer the entire daily dose at bedtime to minimize daytime drowsiness. • To reduce *orthostatic hypotension,* instruct the client to rise slowly when shifting to an upright position. Measure and document the client's supine and standing blood pressure; withhold the drug and inform the nurse-manager if systolic pressure drops more than 30 mm Hg. • Offer sugar-free drinks and candy to relieve *dry mouth.* • To detect *urine retention,* monitor urine output. Inform the nurse-manager if output is low.
Desipramine (Norpramin): 100 to 200 mg/day	Blocks reuptake of norepinephrine and serotonin into CNS neurons	• Before starting therapy, document the client's baseline pulse rate, blood pressure, and ECG. Monitor these periodically to detect *hypotension* or *arrhythmias.* • This drug may cause *drowsiness,* especially when therapy begins. Some clinicians prefer to administer the entire daily dose at bedtime to minimize daytime drowsiness. • To reduce *orthostatic hypotension,* instruct the client to rise slowly when shifting to an upright position. Measure and document the client's supine and standing blood pressure; withhold the drug and inform the nurse-manager if systolic pressure drops more than 30 mm Hg. • Offer sugar-free drinks and candy to relieve *dry mouth.* • To detect *urine retention,* monitor urine output. Inform the nurse-manager if output is low.
Doxepin (Sinequan): 75 to 150 mg/day	Blocks reuptake of norepinephrine and serotonin into CNS neurons; also may have anxiolytic effects	• Before starting therapy, document the client's baseline pulse rate, blood pressure, and ECG. Monitor these periodically to detect *hypotension* or *arrhythmias.* • Associated with a high incidence of *drowsiness,* especially at the start of therapy. Some clinicians prefer to administer the entire daily dose at bedtime to minimize daytime drowsiness. • This drug is a good choice for anxious clients. • To reduce *orthostatic hypotension,* instruct the client to rise slowly when shifting to an upright position. Measure and document the client's supine and standing blood pressure; withhold the drug and inform the nurse-manager if systolic pressure drops more than 30 mm Hg. • Dilute the oral concentrate with juice; do not mix drug with soda because they are incompatible. • Offer sugar-free drinks and candy to relieve *dry mouth.* • To detect *urine retention,* monitor urine output. Inform the nurse-manager if output is low.

Selected drugs commonly used in mental health nursing *(continued)*

DRUG AND USUAL ADULT DOSAGE	ACTION	NURSING CONSIDERATIONS AND POSSIBLE SIDE EFFECTS
Antidepressants *(continued)*		
Imipramine (Tofranil): 50 to 150 mg/day P.O. as maintenance dose	Blocks reuptake of norepinephrine and serotonin into CNS neurons	• Before starting therapy, document the client's baseline pulse rate, blood pressure, and ECG. Monitor these periodically to detect *hypotension* or *arrhythmias*. • Some clinicians prefer to administer the entire daily dose at bedtime to minimize daytime *drowsiness*. • To reduce *orthostatic hypotension,* instruct the client to rise slowly when shifting to an upright position. Measure and document the client's supine and standing blood pressure; withhold the drug and inform the nurse-manager if systolic pressure drops more than 30 mm Hg. • Offer sugar-free drinks and candy to relieve *dry mouth.* • To detect *urine retention,* monitor urine output. Inform the nurse-manager if output is low.
Trimipramine (Surmontil): 75 to 200 mg/day	Blocks reuptake of norepinephrine and serotonin into CNS neurons	• Before starting therapy, document the client's baseline pulse rate, blood pressure, and ECG. Monitor these periodically to detect *hypotension* or *arrhythmias*. • To reduce *orthostatic hypotension,* instruct the client to rise slowly when shifting to an upright position. Measure and document the client's supine and standing blood pressure; withhold the drug and inform the nurse-manager if systolic pressure drops more than 30 mm Hg. • Instruct the client to avoid over-the-counter sympathomimetics. • Advise the client to take drug with food or milk if it causes *GI upset.* • Offer sugar-free drinks and candy to relieve *dry mouth.* • To detect *urine retention,* monitor urine output. Inform the nurse-manager if output is low.
Monoamine oxidase (MAO) inhibitors		
Isocarboxazid (Marplan): 10 to 30 mg/day	Increases levels of CNS catecholamines by blocking their metabolism by MAO	• To reduce *orthostatic hypotension,* instruct the client to rise slowly when shifting to an upright position. Measure and document the client's supine and standing blood pressure; withhold the drug and inform the nurse-manager if systolic pressure drops more than 30 mm Hg. • Warn the client to avoid foods high in tyramine or tryptophan (such as Chianti wine, aged hard cheese, beer, hard liquor aged in wooden casks, avocados, chicken livers, bananas, chocolate, soy sauce, and meat tenderizers), large amounts of caffeine, and nonprescription drugs to prevent *hypertensive crisis.* • Offer sugar-free drinks and candy to relieve *dry mouth.* • To detect *urine retention,* monitor urine output. Inform the nurse-manager if output is low. • Advise the client to avoid driving or operating heavy machinery because this drug may cause *drowsiness.*

(continued)

MENTAL HEALTH NURSING

Selected drugs commonly used in mental health nursing *(continued)*

DRUG AND USUAL ADULT DOSAGE	ACTION	NURSING CONSIDERATIONS AND POSSIBLE SIDE EFFECTS
Antidepressants *(continued)*		
Phenelzine (Nardil): 15 to 60 mg/day	Increases levels of CNS catecholamines by blocking their metabolism by MAO	• To reduce *orthostatic hypotension,* instruct the client to rise slowly when shifting to an upright position. Measure and document the client's supine and standing blood pressure; withhold the drug and inform the nurse-manager if systolic pressure drops more than 30 mm Hg. • Warn the client to avoid foods high in tyramine or tryptophan (such as Chianti wine, aged hard cheese, beer, hard liquor aged in wooden casks, avocados, chicken livers, bananas, chocolate, soy sauce, and meat tenderizers), large amounts of caffeine, and non-prescription drugs to prevent *hypertensive crisis.* • Offer sugar-free drinks and candy to relieve *dry mouth.* • To detect *urine retention,* monitor urine output. Inform the nurse-manager if output is low. • Advise the client to avoid driving or operating heavy machinery because this drug causes *drowsiness* more often than other MAO inhibitors.
Tranylcypromine (Parnate): 30 to 60 mg/day P.O.	Increases levels of CNS catecholamines by blocking their metabolism by MAO	• To reduce *orthostatic hypotension,* instruct the client to rise slowly when shifting to an upright position. Measure and document the client's supine and standing blood pressure; withhold the drug and inform the nurse-manager if systolic pressure drops more than 30 mm Hg. • Warn the client to avoid foods high in tyramine or tryptophan (Chianti wine, aged hard cheese, beer, whiskey and other hard liquor aged in wooden casks, avocados, chicken livers, bananas, chocolate, soy sauce, meat tenderizers, salami, bologna, preserved meats), large amounts of caffeine, and self-medication with nonprescription drugs (especially cold, hay fever, and diet preparations) to prevent *hypertensive crisis.* • Offer sugar-free drinks and candy to relieve *dry mouth.* • To detect *urine retention,* monitor urine output. Inform the nurse-manager if output is low. • Advise the client to avoid driving or operating heavy machinery because this drug may cause *drowsiness.*
Miscellaneous antidepressants		
Bupropion (Wellbutrin): 100 to 150 mg P.O. t.i.d.	Exact mechanism of antidepressant effect unknown; used as a second-choice drug in patients who do not respond well to tricyclic antidepressants	• This drug should not be administered to clients with eating disorders because of the high risk of induced seizures. • Withhold medication and contact physician if CNS effects, such as *agitation* or *insomnia,* occur. • Offer sugar-free drinks and candy to relieve *dry mouth.* • This drug is not recommended for breast-feeding mothers or pregnant women. Educate female clients about birth control while taking this medication. • Monitor for *orthostatic hypotension.* • Monitor for *weight gain.* Rapid weight gain should be reported to the physician immediately, and measurement of intake and output instituted.

Selected drugs commonly used in mental health nursing (continued)

DRUG AND USUAL ADULT DOSAGE	ACTION	NURSING CONSIDERATIONS AND POSSIBLE SIDE EFFECTS
Antidepressants (continued)		
Fluoxetine (Prozac): Initially, 20 mg/day in the morning, then increase as tolerated	Blocks reuptake of serotonin	• To reduce *orthostatic hypotension,* instruct the client to rise slowly when shifting to an upright position. Measure and document the client's supine and standing blood pressure; withhold the drug and inform the physician if systolic pressure drops more than 30 mm Hg. • Avoid administering late in the day or at bedtime because this may cause *insomnia.* If the client is taking more than 20 mg/day, give divided doses at breakfast and lunch. • Offer sugar-free drinks and candy to relieve *dry mouth.* • To detect *urine retention,* monitor urine output. Inform the nurse-manager if output is low.
Paroxetine hydrochloride (Paxil): 20 to 50 mg P.O. q.d.	Inhibits reuptake of serotonin	• This drug should not be used in combination with an MAO inhibitor; fatal reactions have been reported. Allow 14 days between stopping paroxetine therapy and initiating MAO inhibitor therapy as well as between stopping MAO inhibitor therapy and starting paroxetine therapy. • Advise clients to refrain from ingesting alcohol while taking paroxetine. • Offer sugar-free drinks and candy to relieve *dry mouth.* • Inform clients that some side effects, such as nausea and dizziness, may abate after 4 to 6 weeks. • Tell clients not to take over-the-counter (OTC) medications without consulting the physician or pharmacist.
Sertraline (Zoloft): 50 mg P.O. daily	Inhibits reuptake of serotonin	• This drug should not be used in combination with an MAO inhibitor; fatal reactions have been reported. Allow 14 days between stopping sertraline therapy and initiating MAO inhibitor therapy as well as between stopping sertraline therapy and starting sertraline therapy. • Observe for signs of *hyponatremia,* especially in older patients or patients also taking diuretics. • Advise clients to refrain from ingesting alcohol while taking sertraline. • Tell clients not to take OTC medications without consulting physician or pharmacist.
Trazodone (Desyrel): 150 to 400 mg/day P.O.	Blocks reuptake of norepinephrine and serotonin into CNS neurons	• To reduce *orthostatic hypotension,* instruct the client to rise slowly when shifting to an upright position. Measure and document the client's supine and standing blood pressure; withhold the drug and inform the nurse-manager if systolic pressure drops more than 30 mm Hg. • Offer sugar-free drinks and candy to relieve *dry mouth.* • To detect *urine retention,* monitor urine output. Inform the nurse-manager if output is low. • Advise the client to avoid driving or operating heavy machinery because this drug may cause *drowsiness.*

(continued)

MENTAL HEALTH NURSING

Selected drugs commonly used in mental health nursing *(continued)*

DRUG AND USUAL ADULT DOSAGE	ACTION	NURSING CONSIDERATIONS AND POSSIBLE SIDE EFFECTS
Antidepressants *(continued)*		
Venlafaxine hydrochloride (Effexor): 75 mg P.O. daily	Inhibits reuptake of serotonin	• This drug should not be used in combination with an MAO inhibitor; fatal reactions have been reported. Allow 14 days between stopping venlafaxine therapy and initiating MAO inhibitor therapy as well as between stopping MAO inhibitor therapy and starting venlafaxine therapy. • This drug should be given in divided doses and taken with food to avoid nausea. • Venlafaxine should not be abruptly discontinued. • Advise clients to refrain from ingesting alcohol while taking venlafaxine. • This drug may cause sexual dysfunction. • Offer sugar-free drinks and candy to relieve *dry mouth.* • This drug may increase blood pressure. Monitor the client's blood pressure for the first 6 weeks.
Mood stabilizers (used to treat bipolar manic disorder)		
Carbamazepine (Tegretol): Initially, 200 mg P.O. b.i.d., then 200 to 600 mg P.O. in divided doses	Exact mechanism unknown	• This drug may be used in clients who do not respond to or tolerate lithium. • This drug should not be administered to breast-feeding clients. • Monitor cardiac functioning because heart block may occur. • If the drug is discontinued, the client must be weaned. • Monitor blood urea nitrogen values and be alert for indications of renal failure. • Instruct patient about CNS effects, such as *drowsiness, dizziness,* and *unsteadiness.* • Monitor electrolytes if *vomiting* or *diarrhea* occurs for more than one day. • Watch for signs of *blood dyscrasias,* such as aplastic anemia or agranulocytosis. • Be aware that an increased risk of neurotoxicity exists when carbamazepine is used with lithium.
Lithium carbonate (Eskalith, Lithane, Lithobid, Lithonate, Lithotabs): 1,800 to 2,400 mg during acute mania; 300 to 1,200 mg/day in divided doses for maintenance	Reduces hyperactivity by altering cationic exchange at the sodium-potassium pump	• Emphasize the need for routine blood studies, especially at the start of therapy, to monitor for therapeutic levels and prevent toxicity. Therapeutic levels are usually 0.6 to 1.2 mEq/liter. • Monitor for excessive *weight gain.* • Offer sugar-free drinks and candy to relieve *dry mouth.* • To relieve *hand tremors,* have the client perform an activity that controls tremors, such as sewing or writing. • Monitor *diarrhea* for severity. Have the client wash rectal area as often as needed. Report this side effect to the nurse-manager. • Monitor laboratory results. Report a white blood cell (WBC) count over 11,000/microliter to the nurse-manager. • If signs of toxicity occur, notify the nurse-manager or supervisor and withhold the medication. Signs and symptoms of toxicity include persistent nausea and vomiting, severe diarrhea, ataxia, blurred vision, tinnitus, excessive output of dilute urine, increasing tremors, muscle irritability, mental confusion, nystagmus, and seizures (in order of severity). • Advise the client to avoid driving or operating heavy machinery because this drug may cause *drowsiness.* • Document findings. To help prevent toxicity, ensure adequate daily fluid intake.

Selected drugs commonly used in mental health nursing *(continued)*

DRUG AND USUAL ADULT DOSAGE	ACTION	NURSING CONSIDERATIONS AND POSSIBLE SIDE EFFECTS
Mood stabilizers *(continued)*		
Valproic acid (Depakene): 15 to 60 mg/kg/day P.O. in divided doses	Exact mechanism not fully understood	• This drug may be used in clients who do not respond to or tolerate lithium. • Instruct client about potential *drowsiness.* Allow client to nap if drowsy. • Be alert for signs of *blood dyscrasias,* such as anemia or agranulocytosis. • Perform an alcohol assessment. Warn client that alcohol may potentiate CNS effects; instruct client to avoid alcohol.
Antipsychotic agents (used to treat schizophrenia and other psychotic disorders)		
Chlorpromazine (Thorazine): 200 to 800 mg/day P.O.	Relieves symptoms of psychosis by blocking postsynaptic dopamine receptors in the CNS	• Because this drug is associated with a high incidence of *sedation,* advise the client not to drive or operate heavy machinery. • To reduce *orthostatic hypotension,* instruct the client to rise slowly when shifting to an upright position. Measure and document the client's supine and standing blood pressure; withhold the drug and inform the nurse-manager if systolic pressure drops more than 30 mm Hg. • Offer sugar-free drinks and candy to relieve *dry mouth.* • To detect *urine retention,* monitor urine output. Inform the nurse-manager if output is low. • To minimize *weight gain,* monitor food intake, offer low-calorie snacks, and encourage as much physical activity as possible. • To prevent *photosensitivity,* do not allow the client to sunbathe. Instruct the client to apply a sunscreen before going outdoors and to wear long-sleeved garments. • Reassure the client that *blurred vision* decreases after 1 or 2 weeks. Do not ask the client to perform activities requiring the eyes to accommodate (such as reading or handwork) until this side effect diminishes. • Monitor bowel movements. If *constipation* occurs, document it and ask the nurse-manager about a laxative order. Offer high-fiber foods. • *Akathisia* may occur within the first few weeks of therapy. Signs and symptoms, which usually disappear spontaneously, include restlessness and agitation; inability to sleep or sit down; and fright, anger, terror, or rage. Compare the client's behavior with his pre-therapy behavior to distinguish true akathisia from psychopathology. • *Parkinsonism* may occur during the first few weeks of therapy, usually abating 2 to 3 months after stabilization of the drug regimen. Depending on the severity of symptoms (cogwheel muscular rigidity, stooped posture and shuffling gait, tremor affecting fine motor coordination, masklike expression, and hypersalivation and drooling), the clinician may reduce the dosage, switch to another drug, or prescribe an antiparkinsonian drug. • *Dyskinesia* and *dystonia* may occur suddenly within the first few weeks of therapy but usually abate within 2 weeks. Signs and symptoms include coordinated, involuntary rhythmic movements; uncoordinated, spastic movements of the neck, face, eyes, and muscles; and twisting of the neck. If necessary to manage the client's reaction, administer an anticholinergic agent, as ordered. • *Tardive dyskinesia* may occur if the client takes the drug for prolonged periods, especially if the client is elderly or has brain damage. Signs and symptoms, which may be permanent, include coordinated rhythmic mouth and tongue movements and involuntary sucking, chewing, licking, grimacing, and blinking. Observe the client for early signs (blinking and fine vermiform tongue movements), and conduct screening tests every 3 months.

(continued)

Selected drugs commonly used in mental health nursing *(continued)*

DRUG AND USUAL ADULT DOSAGE	ACTION	NURSING CONSIDERATIONS AND POSSIBLE SIDE EFFECTS
Antipsychotic agents *(continued)*		
Chlorpromazine *(continued)*		• *Neuroleptic malignant syndrome* may occur after short-term use of antipsychotic (neuroleptic) drugs. Signs and symptoms of this potentially fatal reaction include fluctuating vital signs, altered consciousness, increased WBC count, fever, muscular rigidity, diaphoresis, and drooling. As ordered, administer bromocriptine to counter these symptoms. • *Agranulocytosis* may occur after short-term use of antipsychotic drugs. Signs and symptoms of this potentially fatal reaction include sore throat, fever, decreased WBC count, and oral ulcers. Place the client in reverse isolation and administer antibiotics, as ordered.
Chlorprothixene (Taractan): 75 to 200 mg/day	Relieves symptoms of psychosis by blocking postsynaptic dopamine receptors in the CNS	• See *Chlorpromazine* for nursing considerations and common side effects.
Clozapine (Clozaril): Initially, 25 mg P.O. daily or b.i.d., increased in 25- or 50-mg increments up to a daily dosage of 300 to 450 mg	Binds to dopamine receptors	• This drug is used in clients who have not responded to other neuroleptic agents. • Watch for signs of *agranulocytosis;* draw blood weekly and carefully monitor WBC count. • *Seizures* may occur. Warn patients not to operate heavy machinery or a motor vehicle while taking this drug. • Tell clients not to take OTC medications without consulting physician. • Lactating clients should not breast-feed their children while taking this drug.
Fluphenazine decanoate (Prolixin Decanoate): 12.5 to 100 mg I.M. q 1 to 4 weeks Fluphenazine enanthate (Prolixin Enanthate): 12.5 to 100 mg q 1 to 2 weeks Fluphenazine hydrochloride (Prolixin): 2 to 30 mg/day I.M. or 2.5 to 10 mg P.O. q 6 to 8 hours	Relieves symptoms of psychosis by blocking postsynaptic dopamine receptors in the CNS	• See *Chlorpromazine* for nursing considerations and common side effects.
Haloperidol (Haldol): 0.5 to 5 mg b.i.d. or t.i.d.	Relieves symptoms of psychosis by blocking postsynaptic dopamine receptors in the CNS	See *Chlorpromazine* for nursing considerations and common side effects.
Loxapine succinate (Loxitane): 60 to 100 mg/day P.O.	Relieves symptoms of psychosis by blocking postsynaptic dopamine receptors in the CNS	See *Chlorpromazine* for nursing considerations and common side effects.

Selected drugs commonly used in mental health nursing *(continued)*

DRUG AND USUAL ADULT DOSAGE	ACTION	NURSING CONSIDERATIONS AND POSSIBLE SIDE EFFECTS
Antipsychotic agents *(continued)*		
Perphenazine (Trilafon): 4 to 64 mg/day P.O. in divided doses	Relieves symptoms of psychosis by blocking postsynaptic dopamine receptors in the CNS	• See *Chlorpromazine* for nursing considerations and common side effects.
Risperidone (Risperdal): 1 to 6 mg b.i.d.	Interferes with binding of dopamine to D_2 interlimbic region of the brain, serotonin (5-HT_2) receptors, and alpha adrenergic receptors in the occipital cortex.	• This drug has proven effective in certain clients who have not responded well to traditional antipsychotic therapy. • Sedation and drowsiness are the most common side effects. Instruct clients not to drive or operate machinery until the drug's effects have been established. • Less common effects include dry mouth, constipation, urine retention, tachycardia, elevated liver function tests (AST, ALT), headache, transient blurred vision, and insomnia. • Advise clients to rise slowly from a supine or sitting position to prevent orthostatic hypotension, which is characterized by dizziness or light-headedness. • Urge clients to consult their physicians before breast-feeding.
Thioridazine (Mellaril): 200 to 800 mg/day P.O. in divided doses b.i.d. to q.i.d.	Relieves symptoms of psychosis by blocking postsynaptic dopamine receptors in the CNS	• See *Chlorpromazine* for nursing considerations and common side effects.
Trifluoperazine (Stelazine): 4 to 40 mg/day in divided doses	Relieves symptoms of psychosis by blocking postsynaptic dopamine receptors in the CNS	• See *Chlorpromazine* for nursing considerations and common side effects.
Antiparkinsonian agents (used to treat extrapyramidal side effects)		
Anticholinergics Benztropine mesylate (Cogentin): 1 to 4 mg/day P.O. or I.M.	Counters extrapyramidal reactions to antipsychotic drugs by blocking central cholinergic receptors and restoring the balance of acetylcholine and dopamine in the basal ganglia	• Offer sugar-free drinks and candy to relieve *dry mouth*. • Monitor bowel movements. If *constipation* occurs, document it and ask the nurse-manager about a laxative order. Offer high-fiber foods. • May impair short-term memory.
Biperiden (Akineton): 2 to 6 mg/day P.O., I.V., or I.M.	Counters extrapyramidal reactions to antipsychotic drugs by blocking central cholinergic receptors and restoring the balance of acetylcholine and dopamine in the basal ganglia	• Offer sugar-free drinks and candy to relieve *dry mouth*. • Monitor bowel movements. If *constipation* occurs, document it and ask the nurse-manager about a laxative order. Offer high-fiber foods. • May impair short-term memory.

(continued)

MENTAL HEALTH NURSING

Selected drugs commonly used in mental health nursing *(continued)*

DRUG AND USUAL ADULT DOSAGE	ACTION	NURSING CONSIDERATIONS AND POSSIBLE SIDE EFFECTS
Antiparkinsonian agents *(continued)*		
Antihistamines Diphenhydramine (Benadryl): 75 to 200 mg/day in 3 to 4 divided doses P.O.	A histamine$_1$-receptor blocking agent; also blocks central cholinergic receptors	• May cause *sedation*. Client should avoid hazardous activity until CNS effects are known. • Offer sugar-free drinks and candy to relieve *dry mouth*.
Trihexyphenidyl (Artane): 6 to 10 mg/day P.O.	Counters extrapyramidal reactions to antipsychotic drugs by blocking central cholinergic receptors and restoring the balance of acetylcholine and dopamine in the basal ganglia	• Offer sugar-free drinks and candy to relieve *dry mouth*. • Monitor bowel movements. If *constipation* occurs, document it and ask the nurse-manager about a laxative order. Offer high-fiber foods. • May impair short-term memory
Dopaminergic agents (used to reverse neuroleptic malignant syndrome)		
Bromocriptine (Parlodel): 1/2 to 2 1/2 mg "snap-tabs" P.O. b.i.d.	Stimulates postsynaptic dopamine receptors	• Cardiovascular side effects limit use. Watch for *hypotension,* especially at the start of therapy.
Drugs used in early recovery from alcohol or opioid abuse		
Disulfiram (Antabuse): 125 to 500 mg/day	Inhibits the body's ability to metabolize alcohol	• Be alert for signs and symptoms of a disulfiram reaction, such as flushing, pulsating headache, nausea, violent vomiting, sweating, confusion, weakness, slurred speech, tachycardia, chest pain, hypotension to shock level, arrhythmia, marked respiratory depression, convulsion, and sudden death. • Because disulfiram therapy can cause liver toxicity, liver function tests should be done monthly for the first 6 months of therapy and every 6 months thereafter. • Caution clients to avoid alcohol while taking this drug and for 2 weeks after discontinuing it. • Check with the physician about concurrent use of other drugs. • Administer doses at bedtime, if necessary, to prevent daytime sedation. • Advise clients that side effects (GI disturbances, headache, tremor) will subside within 2 weeks of using the drug.
Naltrexone hydrochloride (ReVia, Trexan): 25 to 50 mg/day	Blocks the effects of opioids by competitive binding at opioid receptor sites	• Be alert for signs and symptoms of opioid overdose syndrome, such as coma, flaccid paralysis, miosis, and respiratory depression. • Caution clients to avoid alcohol and opiates while on this drug. Overdose is likely because naltrexone causes an inability to experience the effect of either substance. • Caution clients not to use OTC drugs, which may contain small amounts of opioids. • Urge clients to wear an ID bracelet or necklace indicating naltrexone use.

MENTAL H
NU

Selected drugs commonly used in mental health nursing *(continued)*

DRUG AND USUAL ADULT DOSAGE	ACTION	NURSING CONSIDERATIONS AND POSSIBLE SIDE EFFECTS
Anticonvulsants (used to treat convulsive disorders)		
Barbiturates Phenobarbital (Barbita): 100 to 300 mg/day Primidone (Mysoline): maintenance dose is 250 mg P.O. t.i.d. or q.i.d.	Exact mechanism unknown; may facilitate the actions of the inhibitory neurotransmitter	• Used for prophylaxis of various seizure types, principally tonic-clonic seizures and partial seizures. • Primidone is partially metabolized to phenobarbital, which adds to its anticonvulsant effects. • Therapeutic effects require close monitoring of blood levels, especially early in therapy. Therapeutic levels of phenobarbital are 15 to 40 mcg/ml; primidone, 6 to 12 mcg/ml. • Selection is based on the type of seizure and may require multiple drug regimens. • Some degree of *CNS depression* is common to all anticonvulsants and frequently decreases or disappears with continued use. By starting low and gradually increasing the dose, this side effect may be minimized. • Clients should be cautioned to avoid hazardous activities that require mental alertness or physical coordination until the drug's effects are known. • Clinicians should be alert to the signs that precede the onset of *drug-induced cutaneous lesions* and reactions, including *high fever, severe headache, stomatitis, rhinitis, urethritis,* and *conjunctivitis.* • Blood counts, hepatic function, and renal function should be tested prior to and periodically throughout therapy. Drug levels should also be monitored routinely. • *Bone marrow depression* progressing to fatal aplastic anemia has occurred with nearly all anticonvulsants. Clients should report any unusual bruising, bleeding, or signs of infection (sore throat, fever). • A causal relationship between many anticonvulsants and birth defects in epileptic women has not been clearly established despite the 2 to 3 times greater incidence of birth defects when these agents are taken in the early stages of pregnancy. • Epileptic pregnant women taking barbiturates or primidone should receive prophylactic vitamin K one month prior to and during delivery to reduce the chance of drug-induced hemorrhagic disease of the newborn. Neonates should also receive vitamin K immediately after birth.

MENTAL HEALTH NURSING

Maternal–newborn nursing

Introduction

This section presents essential information about nursing care of the childbearing family, applying the nursing process to care delivered during the antepartal, intrapartal, postpartal, and neonatal periods. To promote the concept of family-centered maternity care, each clinical situation integrates physiologic, psychological, and sociocultural adaptations that accompany childbearing and explores the effects of these changes on the pregnant client and her family.

The review begins with a clinical situation involving oral contraception, a commonly used method of family planning. The text then presents information on nursing care during the three trimesters of the antepartal period, focusing first on a normal pregnancy and then on some of the complications that can occur during this period. The section concludes by examining normal and high-risk conditions associated with the intrapartal, postpartal, and neonatal periods.

Glossary

Acrocyanosis—bluish discoloration of a newborn's extremities

Atony—lack of muscle tone

Cephalopelvic disproportion (CPD)—incompatibility of the fetal head with the diameters of the maternal pelvis

Certified nurse-midwife—member of the obstetric team who manages perinatal and gynecologic clients who lack complications

Chloasma—irregular facial pigmentation, usually on the cheeks, forehead, and nose, that occurs during pregnancy

Colostrum—watery secretion from the breast after delivery; it contains some immune properties and is higher in protein than breast milk

Dystocia—abnormally difficult labor

Effacement—thinning and shortening (obliteration) of the cervix during labor, reported in percentages from 0% to 100%

Electronic fetal monitoring (EFM)—use of a direct or indirect device to assess the fetal status and uterine activity

Expected date of delivery (EDD)—due date established by calculations, ultrasound, or amniocentesis (replaces "expected date of confinement")

Fetal station—relationship of the fetal presenting part to the maternal ischial spines; measured in centimeters

Gravida—pregnant woman; also, the number of pregnancies, including the current one

Kernicterus—abnormal toxic accumulation of bilirubin in the brain tissues resulting from hyperbilirubinemia; may cause brain damage and neonatal death

Lanugo—fine downy hair that appears on the fetal body at about 20 weeks' gestation

Lecithin/sphingomyelin ratio (L/S ratio)—ratio of lecithin to sphingomyelin in amniotic fluid; useful in predicting fetal lung maturity

Lochia—postpartal vaginal discharge containing debris from the uterus, such as blood, decidual tissue, mucus, and epithelial cells

Oxytocin—posterior pituitary hormone that stimulates uterine contractions and also initiates the letdown reflex of lactation

Pathological jaundice—yellowness of the skin and hyperbilirubinemia in the newborn within the first 24 hours after birth

Perinatal period—the time from conception through postpartum; also, the time extending from completion of the 20th to 28th week of gestation and ending 28 days after birth

Quickening—fetal movement as perceived by the pregnant woman, first noticed between the 16th and 20th weeks of gestation

Souffle—soft, blowing sound auscultated as fetal blood flows through the umbilical arteries (funic souffle) or as maternal blood enters the uterine arteries (uterine souffle)

Vernix—cheesy substance that covers and protects the fetal body

MATERNAL-NEWBORN NURSING

FAMILY PLANNING

The client desiring to use contraception

Family planning involves exercising choices to prevent or achieve pregnancy and to control the timing and number of pregnancies. Contraceptive methods are widely used in family planning as a result of changing attitudes, improved technology, economic considerations, and mass media coverage of family planning issues. The client should receive information about contraceptive methods and procedures (their effectiveness, cost, contraindications, and adverse reactions) as well as information about community resources available to the family. Factors involved in selection of a contraceptive method include its effectiveness, the client's age and lifestyle, and partner support.

The following clinical situation focuses on the care of a client desiring to use contraception.

Clinical situation

Sheri Carter, age 24, appeared at the Health Department Family Planning Clinic requesting a prescription for oral contraceptives. She and her husband have two young daughters, ages 2 and 4, and at present do not want to have any more children. (For more information on contraceptives and how they disrupt the normal menstrual cycle, see *The menstrual cycle,* and *Contraceptive technology,* pages 216 and 217.)

Assessment

NURSING BEHAVIORS

1. Review Mrs. Carter's general health history for cancer of the reproductive organs, thrombophlebitis, hypertension, liver dysfunction, renal disease, diabetes mellitus, sickle cell disease, epilepsy, migraine disorder, breast-feeding, suspected pregnancy, and cigarette smoking. Determine whether her family history includes hypertension, heart disease, diabetes mellitus, neurologic diseases, or cancer.

NURSING RATIONALES

1. Information obtained from the client's health history may identify the client as being at risk for complications. *Absolute* contraindications for oral contraceptives include malignancy of the reproductive system, hypertension, pregnancy, and liver dysfunction. The remaining conditions listed are relative contraindications; that is, oral contraceptives may be used cautiously. Clients over age 35 are at increased risk for a fatal heart attack if they smoke more than 15 cigarettes a day and take oral contraceptives. For a breast-feeding client, the physician may prescribe progesterone only or low-dose combination oral contraceptives. Milk supply may decrease. Low-dose oral contraceptives may be prescribed for a diabetic client with no vascular complications. The Food and Drug Administration revised its stand on oral contraceptives, stating that for healthy, nonsmoking women over age 40, the benefits (such as decreased menstrual cramps and increased cycle regularity) may outweigh the risks.

The menstrual cycle

The hypothalamus stimulates the anterior pituitary to accelerate secretion of the gonadotropic hormones: follicle-stimulating hormone (FSH) and luteinizing hormone (LH).

FSH stimulates the ovum to mature. The graafian follicle secretes estrogen. Elevated estrogen levels inhibit production of FSH. Increased LH levels contribute to ovulation.

Calculation of the fertile period is based on the approximate life of the sperm (72 hours) and the egg (24 hours). The corpus luteum secretes progesterone. Elevated progesterone levels inhibit LH production.

If fertilization does not occur, the corpus luteum regresses, estrogen and progesterone levels drop, and menses occurs approximately 14 days after ovulation. If fertilization does occur, the corpus luteum continues to produce progesterone until the placenta is formed.

MENSTRUAL CYCLE

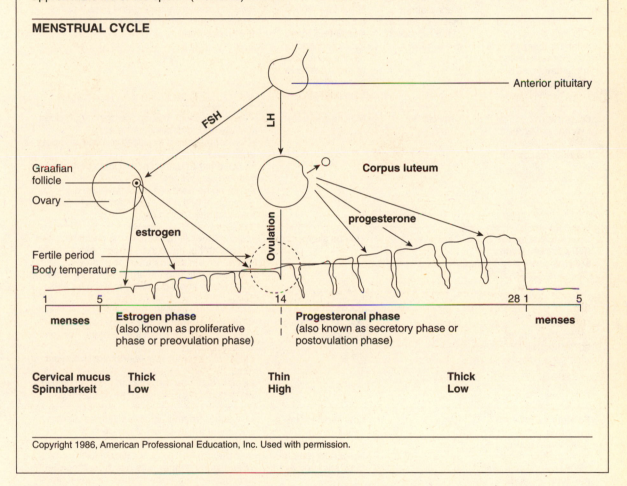

2. Review Mrs. Carter's menstrual history (age at onset of menses, interval between periods, duration and amount of flow, and any problems) and obstetric history (for each pregnancy, date of child's birth, sex, weight, duration of pregnancy, type of delivery, and any complications).

2. Oral contraceptive use affects the reproductive system. A complete menstrual and obstetric history is important in determining the safety of using oral contraceptives.

Contraceptive technology

When discussing contraception with clients, emphasize the following for all contraceptive methods:
• importance of history, physical examination, and diagnostic tests
• protection against sexually transmitted diseases offered by barrier methods
• proper use
• possible adverse reactions
• importance of follow-up examinations.

METHOD AND ACTIONS	CONTRAIN-DICATIONS	POTENTIAL PROBLEMS	CLIENT TEACHING
Intrauterine device (IUD) Not fully understood: IUD may cause an inflammatory process that interferes with implantation; 95% effective	Pelvic infections, uterine abnormalities, cancer of the reproductive organs	Increased menstrual flow, abdominal cramps, expulsion, infection, ectopic pregnancy, uterine perforation (many IUDs have been withdrawn from market)	• Teach the client to check string placement after each menstrual period and before coitus. • Advise her to follow manufacturer's timetable for replacement.
Diaphragm Mechanical barrier; 81% effective within 4 hours of placement	Cervicitis	May be allergenic	• Teach the client to keep the diaphragm clean and dry and to check it for holes. • Tell her to leave it in place for at least 6 hours after coitus. • Advise her to use a spermicidal agent along with the diaphragm. • Caution her that she must have the diaphragm refitted after significant weight gain or loss and after childbirth.
Spermicidal agent (jelly, cream, foam, suppository) Chemical barrier; 82% effective	Cervicitis	May be allergenic	• Instruct the client to insert the agent high into the vagina not more than 1 hour before coitus, and to remain supine after insertion. • Advise her to use the agent with a condom. • Tell her to avoid douching for 6 hours after coitus.
Condom Mechanical barrier; 90% effective	None	May be allergenic; may tear	• Advise the client to make sure her partner leaves a small space in the tip of the condom when applying. • Instruct her on proper condom use to avoid tears. • Emphasize that the condom must be held in place during withdrawal to prevent spillage.
Fertility awareness methods Abstinence during the fertile period, determined by one or more methods (calendar method, basal body temperature graph, and cervical mucus test); 75% effective	None	Low reliability because of difficulty in determining the fertile period; may reduce spontaneity	• Calendar (rhythm) method: Tell the client to document the duration of her periods and to presume that ovulation occurs 14 days before menses. • Basal body temperature graph: Tell the client to document her body temperature over time and to presume that a drop in temperature followed by a sustained increase indicates ovulation. • Cervical mucus test: Teach the client that the spinnbarkeit is high at ovulation. The client must be self-disciplined, keep accurate records, and be prepared to cope with unexpected pregnancy.

Contraceptive technology *(continued)*

METHOD AND ACTIONS	CONTRAIN-DICATIONS	POTENTIAL PROBLEMS	CLIENT TEACHING
Oral contraceptives (such as estrogen and progestin combination) Prevents ovulation; 98% effective	Reproductive system cancers, hypertension, pregnancy, liver dysfunction	Spotting, nausea, vomiting, breast tenderness, hyperglycemia, thrombophlebitis	• Inform the client of health benefits, such as decreased menstrual cramps and increased cycle regularity.
Medroxyprogesterone acetate (Depo-Provera; 150 mg administered I.M. every 3 months) Suppresses release of gonadotropic hormones and prevents ovulation; 99% effective	Pregnancy, liver disease, undiagnosed vaginal bleeding, breast cancer, blood clotting disorders, cardiovascular disease	Changes in menstrual cycle, weight gain, headache, nervousness, fatigue	• Teach the client that this drug prevents pregnancy for 3 months. • Inform her that most women can conceive within 12 months after last dose. • Counsel client about side effects to promote long-term compliance.
Levonorgestrel (Norplant System; subdermal implant consisting of six silastic capsules) Prevents ovulation and stimulates production of thick cervical mucus, which inhibits sperm penetration; 99% effective	Pregnancy, liver disease, undiagnosed vaginal bleeding, breast cancer, blood clotting disorders, cardiovascular disease	Irregular menstruation, spotting, amenorrhea, weight gain, headache	• Inform the client that capsules must be replaced every 5 years. • Counsel the client about potential side effects, such as menstrual irregularities.
Tubal ligation Interruption of fallopian tube passageways; 99.6% effective (40 to 75% reversible)	Client-specific surgical risks	Menstrual disorders; discomfort from CO_2 during laparoscopy; problems of laparotomy, such as infection, hemorrhage, and anesthesia complications	• Advise the client to approach the procedure as irreversible. • Demonstrate aseptic incision care. • Inform her that the procedure can be reversed in 40% to 75% of clients.
Vasectomy Interruption of vas deferens passageways; 99.6% effective (29 to 85% reversible)	Client-specific surgical risks	Autoimmune response; surgical complications	• Advise the client to approach the procedure as irreversible (although reversal may be possible). • Suggest an alternative contraceptive method until a sperm count confirms the procedure's effectiveness. • Teach incision care.

3. Assess the results of Mrs. Carter's diagnostic tests: Papanicolaou (Pap) smear, hemoglobin, hematocrit, and urinalysis.

3. The Pap smear is a cytologic examination that detects cellular abnormalities. Use of oral contraceptives is contraindicated in the presence of malignant cell growth. Data from routine tests, such as hemoglobin and hematocrit measurements and urinalysis, help determine the client's health status.

4. Assess the results of Mrs. Carter's physical examination.

4. A physical assessment, including a pelvic examination, is necessary to determine the client's health status as well as any risks and contraindications associated with oral contraceptive use.

5. Assess Mrs. Carter's learning needs: What does she know about oral contraceptive use? What concerns does she have about using an oral contraceptive? What are her expectations of this contraceptive method?

5. The effectiveness and safety of oral contraceptives depend greatly on the client's knowledge of and compliance with the chosen method. The nurse uses information obtained during the interview to plan appropriate teaching.

Nursing diagnoses

- Risk for injury related to lack of knowledge about contraceptive medication administration
- Altered nutrition (less than body requirements) related to vitamin B_6 and folic acid deficiencies
- Noncompliance related to lack of knowledge about medication administration

Planning and goals

- Mrs. Carter will relate significant aspects of her health history when interviewed.
- Mrs. Carter will describe the routine for taking an oral contraceptive.
- Mrs. Carter will be able to recognize possible adverse reactions to oral contraceptives.
- Mrs. Carter will return for her scheduled follow-up appointments.
- Mrs. Carter will ask questions to indicate her need for information.
- Mrs. Carter will be satisfied with the contraceptive method she chooses.

Implementation

NURSING BEHAVIORS

NURSING RATIONALES

1. Teach Mrs. Carter the routine for taking oral contraceptives. (Sample routine: Starting on the 5th day of the menstrual cycle, or the Sunday after the start of menses, take one pill per day at the same time each day for 21 days, then stop taking the medication. Menses should start within 1 to 4 days. Repeat the routine.) Be sure she understands the following considerations:

- If the medication is accidentally omitted for 1 day, she should continue the prescribed routine and take the missed pill, using a second (backup) form of contraception for the remainder of the cycle if more than one pill is missed.
- If menses does not occur after the medication is stopped, she should resume the routine on the 7th day and repeat the cycle.

1. The client must understand her responsibility for taking the oral contraceptive as scheduled to ensure its effectiveness. Because it contains a combination of estrogen and synthetic progesterone, the oral contraceptive increases the body's levels of these hormones, thereby inhibiting secretion of gonadotropic hormones and preventing ovulation. The hormones also affect the endometrial lining of the uterus so that, if ovulation and fertilization occur, interference with nidation may occur. An additional form of contraception should be used for at least the 1st month of oral contraceptive use.

• If menses does not occur after the second regimen, she should contact the physician.

2. Teach Mrs. Carter the possible adverse reactions to oral contraceptives (fluid retention, weight gain, breast tenderness, headache, breakthrough bleeding, chloasma, acne, yeast infection, nausea, and fatigue), and urge her to report any of these to the physician.

2. Changing the dosage or type of oral contraceptive sometimes relieves adverse reactions. The physician may decide to discontinue the oral contraceptive if the client reports any danger sign indicating a complication, such as thrombophlebitis, hypertension, or severe depression.

3. Instruct Mrs. Carter on the dietary needs of a woman who is taking an oral contraceptive. Tell her to increase her intake of foods high in vitamin B_6 (wheat, corn, liver, meat) and folic acid (liver and green, leafy vegetables).

3. About 20% to 30% of oral contraceptive users have dietary deficiencies of vitamin B_6 (pyridoxine) and folic acid. Moreover, health care professionals are increasingly speculating that oral contraceptive users should increase their intake of vitamins A, B_2, B_{12}, C, and niacin.

4. Urge Mrs. Carter to return for her scheduled follow-up appointments, and explain their importance. (Suggested schedule: in 6 to 12 weeks, then in 6 months, then yearly.)

4. During follow-up visits, health care professionals can validate proper use of oral contraceptives, detect and treat adverse reactions, perform Pap smears if indicated, and answer any health-related questions that the client may ask.

Evaluation

• Mrs. Carter cooperates in providing health history information.
• Mrs. Carter describes the routine for administering the oral contraceptive correctly.
• Mrs. Carter describes adverse reactions to oral contraceptives and states her responsibility to report any that occur.
• Mrs. Carter makes an appointment for her next visit.
• Mrs. Carter states that this method of birth control is acceptable.

ANTEPARTAL PERIOD

The client and family during the antepartal period

The antepartal period extends from conception to the onset of labor. During this time, care of both mother (client) and fetus focuses on health maintenance and prevention of complications. The family's physiologic, psychological, and sociocultural adaptations to the pregnancy are considered when planning and providing care, so the nurse also plays a role as teacher and counselor to the family. The three-part clinical situation that follows focuses on care of the client and family during pregnancy.

Clinical situation

Nursing care during the first trimester of pregnancy and prenatal screening

Peggy Nance, age 28, stopped taking birth control pills 5 months ago with the hope of becoming pregnant. She is seeing the physician today because she has missed two menstrual periods and has experienced some early morning nausea and vomiting. If confirmed, this will be her first pregnancy. She is married; her blood type is A, Rh-negative.

Assessment

NURSING BEHAVIORS	NURSING RATIONALES
1. Assess Mrs. Nance's general health history for diabetes mellitus, cardiac disease, anemia, renal disease, rickets, and sexually transmitted diseases.	**1.** Pregnancy is a normal condition. A general health history that includes any of the listed conditions identifies the client as at high risk for pregnancy-related complications.
2. Assess Mrs. Nance's family health history.	**2.** Genetically transmitted diseases should be identified and considered in the care plan for the pregnant client.
3. Assess Mrs. Nance's menstrual history.	**3.** The client's menstrual history can help health care professionals identify potential problems and determine the client's expected date of delivery (EDD). To determine the EDD, use Nägele's rule: Note the 1st day of the last normal menstrual period, count back 3 months, then add 7 days. For example, assume the 1st day of the woman's last normal menstrual period was October 10. Subtract 3 months (July 10), then add 7 days for a July 17 EDD.
4. Assess Mrs. Nance's obstetric history, including gravida (the number of pregnancies, including the current one; also the term used for a pregnant woman) and para (the number of past pregnancies of at least 20 weeks' gestation; also the term used for a woman who has given birth to a viable fetus or infant).	**4.** Useful information from previous pregnancies includes (for each pregnancy) the type of delivery, the length of gestation, the length of labor, the size of the newborn, and information about any problems that occurred. Many hospitals use the *GTPAL* system to document previous pregnancies. *G* stands for the number of pregnancies; *T*, the number of term infants born; *P*, the number of preterm infants born; *A*, the number of pregnancies ending in spontaneous or elective abortion; and *L*, the number of living children. Multiple gestation does not change *G* (gravida) or *P* (para).
5. Assist with the physical assessment of Mrs. Nance, beginning with measurement of vital signs and fundal height (see *Typical uterine changes during pregnancy*).	**5.** Physical assessment helps determine the client's health status and its potential influence on the pregnancy. The nurse can compare baseline information with normal body changes during pregnancy. Approximate fundal height related to weeks of gestation is as follows: 12 weeks, symphysis pubis; 20 to 24 weeks, umbilicus; 36 weeks, xiphoid; 40 weeks, lightening—between the xiphoid and the umbilicus.
6. Assess Mrs. Nance's abdominal wall for striae gravidarum (the shiny white lines called stretch marks), linea nigra (a dark line extending from the umbilicus to the symphysis pubis), and diastasis recti abdominis (separation of the rectus abdominis muscles).	**6.** Striae gravidarum result from the stretching, rupture, and atrophy of the deep connective tissue. Linea nigra results from hormonal changes. Diastasis recti abdominis may occur when tension strains the muscles late in pregnancy.

Typical uterine changes during pregnancy

Beginning at the 20th week, fundal height equals gestational age, plus or minus 2 cm.

UTERUS	NONPREGNANT	PREGNANT (AT TERM)
Length	6.5 cm	32 cm
Width	4 cm	24 cm
Depth	2.5 cm	22 cm
Weight	50 g	1,000 g

Fundal height related to gestational weeks

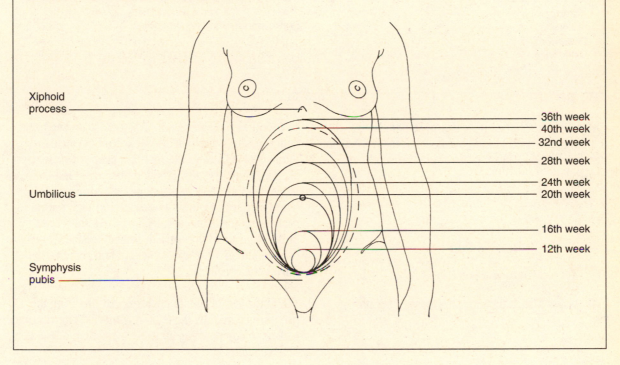

7. Assess Mrs. Nance for enlargement of breast tissue, nipples, and Montgomery tubercles; darkened areolae; and colostrum.

7. Breast enlargement results from hormonal changes that prepare the breasts for lactation. Darkened areolae result from increased melanotropin. Colostrum, the first secretion from the breasts, is the precursor of milk.

8. Assess Mrs. Nance's weight gain (Suggested: 1 to 2 lb during the first trimester and 1 lb per week during the second and third trimesters, for a total of 25 to 30 lb above prepregnancy weight).

8. Weight gain should be consistent and associated with balanced nutrition. No sudden increase in weight should occur.

MATERNAL-NEWBORN NURSING

Influence of hormones on pregnancy

HORMONE	FUNCTION
Placental hormones	
Human chorionic gonadotropin (HCG)	HCG causes the production of estrogen and progesterone during the first trimester.
Estrogen, progesterone	Estrogen and progesterone are necessary to maintain the pregnancy.
Human placental lactogen (HPL)	HPL is necessary for fetal cell growth and preparation for lactation.
Human chorionic somatomammotropin (HCS)	Same as HPL.
Pituitary hormones	
Anterior Prolactin	Prolactin stimulates milk production.
Posterior Oxytocin	Oxytocin stimulates the myometrium and initiates the letdown reflex.

9. Assess Mrs. Nance for cardiovascular changes, including increased blood volume, elevated fibrinogen levels, increased pulse rate, and decreased blood pressure.

9. Blood volume increases 30% to 50% during pregnancy, peaking at about 28 weeks, but because the number of cells does not increase proportionately, pseudoanemia results. Elevated fibrinogen levels are a normal response to pregnancy-related hormonal changes. Cardiac output increases and total peripheral resistance decreases, leading to an increased pulse rate. Blood pressure decreases to slightly below normal at 8 to 12 weeks' gestation and remains so during the pregnancy.

10. Assess Mrs. Nance for shortness of breath.

10. Shortness of breath near term results from the pressure exerted by the enlarging uterus. The rib cage widens to compensate, allowing more than adequate lung capacity.

11. Assess Mrs. Nance for gastrointestinal changes, such as heartburn, flatulence, and constipation.

11. Heartburn, flatulence, and constipation are common during pregnancy because of interference with GI motility. Decreased peristalsis results from high progesterone levels and the pressure of the enlarging uterus.

12. Assess Mrs. Nance for renal changes, including increased urine production, decreased urine specific gravity, occasional glucosuria, urinary frequency, and urinary stasis.

12. Increased renal blood flow increases the glomerular filtration rate. Glucosuria may occur because of the lower renal threshold (lactosuria may occur in late pregnancy). Any glucosuria should be investigated. Pressure from the enlarged uterus causes urinary frequency in the first and third trimesters. The stretched and dilated ureters contribute to urinary stasis.

External female reproductive organs and landmarks

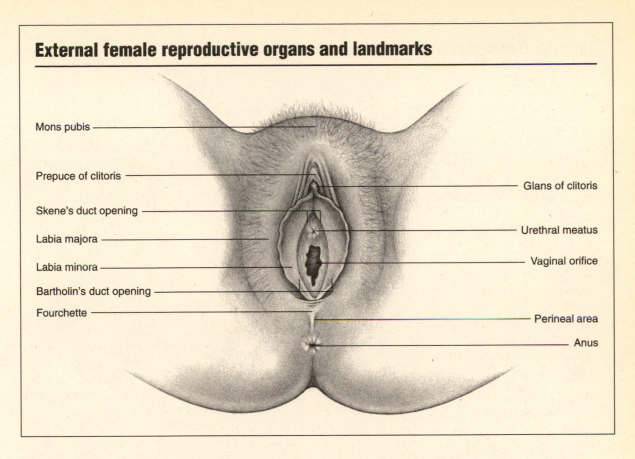

Mons pubis

Prepuce of clitoris

Skene's duct opening

Labia majora

Labia minora

Bartholin's duct opening

Fourchette

Glans of clitoris

Urethral meatus

Vaginal orifice

Perineal area

Anus

13. Assess Mrs. Nance for endocrine changes (see *Influence of hormones on pregnancy*).

13. The placenta and pituitary gland produce hormones that influence pregnancy.

14. Assist with the internal and external pelvic examinations. (See *External female reproductive organs and landmarks* and *Internal female reproductive organs and landmarks,* page 224.)

14. During the pelvic examination, assessment of external organs may reveal discharges, growths, and other abnormalities. Assessment of internal organs provides information related to confirmation of pregnancy, length of gestation, and risk factors. In addition to the routine pelvic examination, the bony pelvis is measured to predict adequacy for labor and delivery. The female pelvis is broader and lighter in construction and has a wider pubic arch (>90 degrees) than the male pelvis.

15. Observe Mrs. Nance for presumptive signs and symptoms of pregnancy: amenorrhea, nausea, vomiting, urinary frequency, breast tenderness, quickening, increased vaginal secretions, Chadwick's sign, changes in skin pigmentation (darkened areolae, linea nigra, chloasma), and fatigue.

15. Amenorrhea, nausea, vomiting, urinary frequency, and breast tenderness are expected body responses to pregnancy; however, they may result from other conditions. Quickening is fetal movement as perceived by the mother. Increased vascularity to the vaginal epithelium causes increased secretions and bluish color of the vagina (Chadwick's sign). Darkening of skin pigmentation results from hormonal interactions. Fatigue accompanied by the need for more sleep may be noted early in pregnancy.

Internal female reproductive organs and landmarks

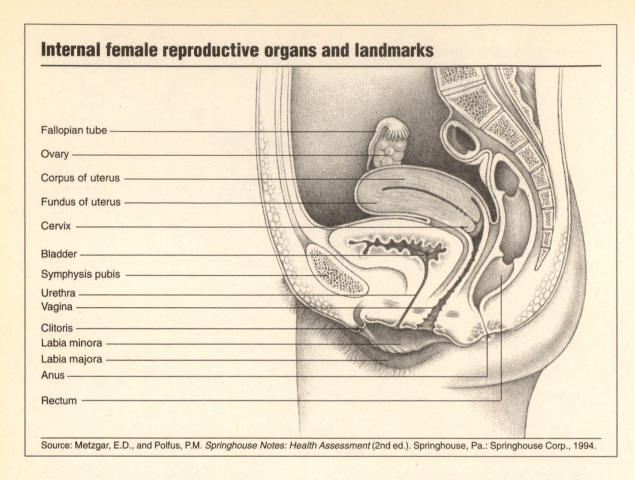

Fallopian tube
Ovary
Corpus of uterus
Fundus of uterus
Cervix
Bladder
Symphysis pubis
Urethra
Vagina
Clitoris
Labia minora
Labia majora
Anus
Rectum

Source: Metzgar, E.D., and Polfus, P.M. *Springhouse Notes: Health Assessment* (2nd ed.). Springhouse, Pa.: Springhouse Corp., 1994.

16. Observe Mrs. Nance for probable signs and symptoms of pregnancy: weight increase, ballottement, Goodell's sign, Hegar's sign, Braxton Hicks contractions, and a positive pregnancy test.

16. These signs and symptoms usually indicate pregnancy but may have other causes. The products of conception (such as the developing zygote, blood, and amniotic fluid) contribute to weight gain. Ballottement describes rebound of the fetus when palpated by the examiner. Goodell's sign is softening of the cervix. Hegar's sign is softening of the lower uterine segment. Braxton Hicks contractions are uncoordinated contractions of the uterus as it enlarges. Pregnancy tests are not 100% accurate and therefore are inconclusive alone.

17. Assess Mrs. Nance for positive signs and symptoms of pregnancy: fetal movement felt by the examiner, the fetal outline seen on X-ray or ultrasonography, and fetal heart tones (FHTs). Follow these steps to detect FHTs:
• Locate the fetus's back.
• Place an electronic monitor or fetoscope over the back.
• Note the heart rate for 1 minute.
• Record the location and rate.
• Differentiate FHTs from other sounds, such as uterine souffle (the swishing sound of blood pulsating

17. Positive signs and symptoms confirm pregnancy. Fetal movement can be palpated by the examiner late in the second trimester. An X-ray is considered teratogenic in early pregnancy. Ultrasonography is currently considered safe throughout pregnancy. FHTs are best heard through the infant's back. After 12 weeks, FHTs may be heard with an electronic monitor; after 16 to 20 weeks, with a fetoscope. Normal range is 120 to 160 beats/minute.

Maternal and newborn laboratory values

TEST	NONPREGNANT WOMEN	PREGNANT WOMEN	POSTPARTAL WOMEN	TERM NEWBORNS
Hemoglobin	12 to 16 g/dl	11 to 15 g/dl	11 to 15 g/dl	15 to 20 g/dl
Hematocrit	37% to 48%	36% to 46% (32% to 35% indicates physiologic anemia)	32% to 46%	43% to 61%
Red blood cells	4 to 5 million/µl	3.8 to 4.4 million/µl	3.8 to 4.4 million/µl	5 to 6 million/µl
White blood cells	5,000 to 10,000/µl	5,000 to 12,000/µl	5,000 to 16,000/µl (possibly up to 25,000/µl)	10,000 to 30,000/µl
Platelets	150,000 to 400,000/mm³	150,000 to 400,000/mm³	150,000 to 400,000/mm³	100,000 to 280,000/mm³
Serum glucose	65 to 105 mg/dl	Below 120 mg/dl	Below 120 mg/dl	First 24 hours; 40 to 100 mg/dl
Glucola screen	Below 140 to 150 mg/dl	Below 140 to 150 mg/dl	(Not performed)	(Not performed)
3-hour glucose tolerance test (3GTT)	1-hour: below 190 mg/dl 2-hour: below 165 mg/dl 3-hour: below 145 mg/dl	1-hour: below 190 mg/dl 2-hour: below 165 mg/dl 3-hour: below 145 mg/dl	(Not performed)	(Not performed)
Hemoglobin A₁C	6% to 8%	6% to 8%	(Not performed)	(Not performed)
Serum bilirubin (total)	(Not performed)	(Not performed)	(Not performed)	Cord blood: Below 2.8 mg/dl At 24 hours: 2 to 6 mg/dl At 3 to 5 days: 4 to 6 mg/dl
Urine protein	Negative	Negative or trace	Negative to +1 False-positive may occur due to lochia	Negative
Urine glucose	Negative	Negative or +1	Negative to +1 False-positive may occur due to lochia	Negative

through the uterine artery and corresponding to the maternal heartbeat) and funic souffle (the swishing sound of blood pulsating through the umbilical cord and corresponding to the fetal heartbeat).

18. Assess the results of Mrs. Nance's diagnostic laboratory tests, as follows:

18. Routine laboratory tests are performed to contribute data to the health assessment of the client and fetus and to establish baseline information.

• hemoglobin, hematocrit, complete blood count

• These tests will be repeated periodically throughout the pregnancy to monitor for abnormalities. (See *Maternal and newborn laboratory values*, page 225.)

• blood type, Rh factor, and indirect Coombs' test

• The blood type and Rh factor are important for predicting possible incompatibilities, which may occur with an Rh-negative client. The Coombs' test detects maternal antibodies that could harm the fetus.

• genetic tests—sickle cell disease, alpha-fetoprotein (AFP)

• Pregnant women with sickle cell disease are considered to be at high risk because of a decrease in their blood's oxygen-carrying potential. Testing also is important because sickle cell disease is genetically transmitted. Elevated AFP may indicate neural tube defects, such as anencephaly, encephalocele, and spina bifida.

• serology

• Serologic tests are performed to screen for syphilis.

• autoimmunodeficiency syndrome (AIDS) and hepatitis screening

• AIDS screening is performed for clients in high-risk groups, such as I.V. drug users. The Centers for Disease Control and Prevention now recommends hepatitis B screening of all prenatal patients.

• routine urinalysis

• Routine urinalysis is done to rule out such problems as glucosuria and urinary stasis. (For related information, see *Common genitourinary infections*, page 228.)

• urinary chorionic gonadotropin (UCG)

• The presence of UCG is the basis of the pregnancy test and will be positive.

• cervical smears for sexually transmitted diseases (gonococcus, beta-streptococcus, chlamydia)

• These infectious agents are detrimental to the pregnancy. Their effects are described in *Nursing care of a pregnant client with an infection,* and *High-risk maternal and newborn problems,* pages 312 to 314.

19. Assess the health status and risk behaviors of Mrs. Nance's husband.

19. Sexual partners with high-risk behaviors can transmit disease to the pregnant client and her fetus.

Nursing care of a pregnant client with an infection

DISORDER	MATERNAL-FETAL PROBLEMS
Toxoplasmosis	Toxoplasmosis is a protozoal infection commonly acquired by eating raw or undercooked meats or by contact with infected animal feces. The mother may be asymptomatic or develop symptoms of a systemic infection. The disorder is associated with abortion, stillbirth, neonatal death, and congenital anomalies in the fetus and neonate.
Syphilis	If the mother is infected early in pregnancy (up to the 18th week), the spirochete will not cross the placental barrier. If the mother is treated during this period, the fetus will not be infected. If the mother is infected after the 18th week, the fetus may be infected. When the mother is treated with penicillin or an accepted substitute, the fetus also will be treated.
Gonorrhea	Gonorrhea present at the time of delivery may cause a serious postpartal maternal infection. It also may cause blindness (if not treated with a prophylactic medication) in the newborn exposed to the organisms during delivery.
Chlamydia	Chlamydia, a sexually transmitted disease, is a bacterial infection that may cause neonatal conjunctivitis and pneumonia. Pregnant women are treated with erythromycin to avoid exposing the fetus in utero to possibly teratogenic therapy. The postpartal mother and neonate receive tetracycline.
Autoimmunodeficiency syndrome (AIDS)	AIDS may be transmitted to the fetus in utero or perinatally. Children born to infected mothers have a 25% to 35% chance of acquiring the AIDS virus. High-risk mothers (such as I.V. drug abusers and those who are HIV positive) should be counseled regarding AIDS prevention and ways to stop AIDS transmission. Partners with high-risk behaviors should be identified as well.
Rubella	Rubella during early and middle pregnancy may severely affect the fetus, resulting in eye and ear defects, mental disorders, growth retardation, and cardiac conditions. Plan postpartal immunizations.
Cytomegalovirus (CMV)	CMV may cause intrauterine fetal death, mental retardation, cerebral palsy, and hearing deficits. CMV is detected by urinalysis and by antibody screening. CMV has no effective treatment.
Herpes simplex virus type 2 (HSV-2)	HSV-2 may cause an overwhelming viral infection in the newborn who is exposed during delivery. Delivery by cesarean section is recommended if the amniotic fluid is negative for herpesvirus antibodies. Herpes cultures should be obtained from the newborn 24 to 48 hours after delivery.
Hepatitis B (HBV)	This viral infection is acquired through sexual contact, I.V. drug use, exposure to infected blood, and artificial insemination of infected semen. Transmission to the fetus or neonate is via vaginal secretions, amniotic fluid, maternal blood, saliva and, possibly, breast milk. Hepatitis B can cause acute and chronic hepatitis, cirrhosis, and hepatocellular carcinoma. As many as 40% to 60% of infants will develop HBV if exposed late in the third trimester to an active, untreated maternal infection.
Human parvovirus B19	This airborne viral infection can produce rash, fever, malaise, myalgia, upper respiratory infection, hydrops fetalis, and stillbirth. There is no vaccine.

MATERNAL-NEWBORN NURSING

Common genitourinary infections

The following table presents three of the most common genitourinary infections, along with associated physical characteristics, chief complaints, treatments, and effects on pregnancy.

INFECTION	DISCHARGE	CHIEF COMPLAINT	TREATMENT	EFFECT ON PREGNANCY
Bacterial vaginosis	White to gray; fishy odor	Itching	Metronidazole	Preterm labor, chorioamnionitis
Candidiasis	Thick, white; yeast odor	Itching	Azole topicals	Common in pregnancy and diabetes
Trichomoniasis	Yellow to green; foul odor	Frothy discharge	Metronidazole	Premature rupture of membrane, preterm labor, postpartal endometritis

20. Perform a psychosocial assessment of Mr. and Mrs. Nance, beginning with the couple's psychological adaptation to the first trimester of pregnancy.

20. Psychosocial assessment data will help the nurse anticipate the couple's needs. The major psychological task of the first trimester is accepting the pregnancy (for example, the expectant mother may state, "I am pregnant," or the expectant father may state, "She is pregnant, and I am the father."). Excitement, ambivalence, and apprehension are normal for both expectant parents. The expectant father may experience *couvade*—symptoms of pregnancy, such as nausea, fatigue, and weight gain.

21. Assess Mrs. Nance's learning needs.

21. The client needs to understand the changes that will take place in her body during pregnancy so she will not become alarmed about normal changes and will be aware of and report any unusual or unexpected changes.

22. Assess Mrs. Nance's support systems. Ask her to identify two or three persons she can depend on to be available and helpful to her during this pregnancy.

22. Planning appropriate care requires the nurse to have knowledge of the persons emotionally close to the client, such as spouse, parents, siblings, and friends.

23. Assess the Nances' economic status.

23. Determining whether the family has a stable source of income to meet medical expenses and other basic needs is important for planning the family's health maintenance care and adequate prenatal care for the client.

24. Assess the stability of the Nances' living conditions.

24. Adequate housing is essential for the client and her expanding family.

25. Assess the family's ethnic and cultural values, beliefs, and practices.

25. Understanding ethnic and cultural factors helps the nurse understand variations in the family's adaptation to pregnancy. For example, pregnancy and birth may be viewed from a number of perspectives—as a natural occurrence, a sickness, a crisis, or a developmental stage—and each may influence the family's adaptation to pregnancy. Knowing the client's ethnic and cultural values, beliefs, and practices is important for planning individualized care with minimal risk of making inappropriate generalizations within or across various ethnic and cultural groups.

Nursing diagnoses
- Altered health maintenance related to possible lack of resources
- Risk for fluid volume deficit related to nausea and vomiting of early pregnancy

Planning and goals
- The results of Mrs. Nance's health history and physical and diagnostic examinations will be within normal limits.
- Mrs. Nance will be able to describe the warning signs of pregnancy complications.
- Mrs. Nance will discuss concerns about her pregnancy related to personal and family psychosocial needs.
- Mrs. Nance will return for routine follow-up visits.

Implementation
NURSING BEHAVIORS

NURSING RATIONALES

1. Teach Mrs. Nance the warning signs of pregnancy-related complications: vaginal bleeding, gush of fluid from the vagina, persistent vomiting, chills and fever, abdominal pain, visual disturbances, severe headache, and swelling of the face and hands.

1. These warning signs indicate complications, such as spontaneous abortion, fluid and electrolyte imbalance, pregnancy-induced hypertension, and infection. Any of these signs should be reported immediately because early detection is important to the success of treatment.

2. Explain that Mrs. Nance should not take any medication unless it is prescribed by the physician.

2. Many medications are teratogenic, especially in the first trimester, when the fetal organs are developing.

3. Teach Mrs. Nance the suggested treatment for nausea and vomiting (morning sickness).

3. Nausea and vomiting can be managed by eating dry crackers before rising; eating small, frequent, high-protein meals; and avoiding spicy and fried foods.

4. Stress the importance of regular health supervision during pregnancy. A suggested routine includes monthly visits through 32 weeks' gestation, bimonthly visits through week 36, and weekly visits from week 37 until delivery.

4. The quality of prenatal care has a great impact on the well-being of the mother and the fetus. Besides enabling the physician to detect and treat problems promptly, prenatal visits provide an opportunity for teaching the client about pregnancy, labor and delivery, and postpartum and newborn care.

MATERNAL-NEWBORN NURSING

5. Give Mrs. Nance an opportunity to ask questions and talk about her expectations.

5. Listening to the client helps to establish a communicative, positive, caring nurse-client relationship. It also provides an opportunity, early in the pregnancy, for the nurse to initiate appropriate referrals to community resources for the client who is isolated or who may need help with material resources (such as food and housing). Discussing ethnic or cultural beliefs and practices may identify some that should be considered in implementing care.

Evaluation

• The results of Mrs. Nance's health history and physical and diagnostic examinations are within normal limits.
• Mrs. Nance describes the warning signs of pregnancy complications and the importance of reporting them.
• Mrs. Nance verbalizes gradual acceptance of the body changes of early pregnancy.
• Mrs. Nance identifies sources of emotional and material support adequate to meet personal and family needs during this pregnancy.
• Mrs. Nance has made an appointment for her next visit.

Clinical situation

(continued)

Nursing care during the second trimester of pregnancy

Peggy Nance is now in the 5th month of her pregnancy, which has progressed without complications. During her routine visit today, she indicates that she has some questions about hygiene and activity.

Assessment

NURSING BEHAVIORS	NURSING RATIONALES
1. Assess for maternal and fetal well-being.	**1.** The routine assessments made during each prenatal visit are necessary for determining maternal-fetal well-being and for early detection of possible complications.
2. Assess Mrs. Nance's vital signs.	**2.** An elevated temperature may indicate infection. Elevated blood pressure may indicate early preeclampsia.
3. Weigh Mrs. Nance, and record her weight.	**3.** Weight gain of 1 lb/week during the second trimester is expected. Sudden weight gain may indicate fluid retention.
4. Listen for FHTs. Note funic souffle and uterine souffle.	**4.** FHTs should be audible with a fetoscope at this time.
5. Measure fundal height.	**5.** At 20 weeks' gestation, the fundus should be palpable near the umbilicus.
6. Assess for quickening.	**6.** The client should be feeling fetal movement daily, starting within the 18th to 20th week of gestation.

7. Review the results of Mrs. Nance's routine laboratory tests, including urinalysis (glucose and albumin levels) and blood tests (hemoglobin and hematocrit levels).

7. A pregnant woman's urine may contain glucose; if so, further investigation is needed. The urine should not contain albumin. A hemoglobin level of 11 g/dl and a hematocrit value of 35% are acceptable for a pregnant woman during the second trimester.

8. Perform a psychosocial assessment of Mr. and Mrs. Nance, beginning with the couple's psychological adaptation to the second trimester of pregnancy.

8. Psychosocial assessment will help the nurse anticipate the Nances' future needs. A growing awareness of the fetus as a separate being is important for beginning the maternal-fetal relationship (for example, the client should now be able to state, "I am going to have a baby," or both parents may state, "We are going to have a baby."). Failure to acknowledge quickening or to begin planning for the baby may represent dysfunctional adaptation or lack of information.

9. Assess Mrs. Nance's learning needs. What questions does she have about her health and the health of the fetus?

9. During the second trimester, the mother is usually receptive to teaching that focuses on personal care and may also have many questions about the fetus.

10. Assess Mrs. Nance's emotional, economic, and social support systems.

10. Stable and supportive relationships and adequate financial and social support are important for the physical and psychological well-being of the expectant mother throughout her pregnancy.

Nursing diagnoses
- Fluid volume excess related to the effects of estrogen
- Risk for injury related to possible complications of pregnancy
- Altered health maintenance related to knowledge deficit regarding changes that occur during second trimester
- Self-esteem disturbance related to the changes of pregnancy

Planning and goals
- Mrs. Nance's pregnancy will continue without complications.
- Mrs. Nance will describe the adaptations she makes in her daily activities during pregnancy.
- Mrs. Nance will discuss how to cope with the common annoyances of pregnancy.
- Mrs. Nance will describe the dietary adjustments necessary during pregnancy.
- Mrs. Nance will ask questions about fetal development.
- Mrs. Nance will keep appointments for routine health supervision during pregnancy.

**MATERNAL-
NEWBORN
NURSING**

Implementation
NURSING BEHAVIORS

NURSING RATIONALES

1. Teach Mrs. Nance about general health measures and common concerns, as described in 2 through 15 below. Remember to teach on the client's level, allow time for questions, and validate the client's understanding.

1. The second trimester is the ideal time for teaching during pregnancy. Usually the client is feeling well and has worked through the tasks of the first trimester. The nurse should assess the client's knowledge level to establish a realistic teaching plan.

2. Explain to Mrs. Nance the safety precautions she should take when exercising.

2. The client should take safety precautions when exercising and should not exercise to the point of fatigue. Walking in fresh air is recommended.

3. Discuss proper bathing techniques.

3. When bathing, the client should cleanse her breasts first, using nothing that will cause nipple dryness. Daily tub baths or showers are acceptable in early pregnancy. However, as the pregnancy progresses, poor balance may interfere with taking tub baths.

4. Explain the importance of dental care.

4. The pregnant client should continue to have regular dental checkups but should avoid X-rays.

5. Tell Mrs. Nance to avoid douching.

5. Douching is contraindicated.

6. Caution Mrs. Nance about immunizations.

6. The client should not receive immunizations with live viruses such as rubella.

7. Advise Mrs. Nance about what to wear during pregnancy.

7. The client should wear a supportive bra and shoes with low heels and should avoid wearing restrictive clothing.

8. Discuss travel restrictions that Mrs. Nance should adhere to during the pregnancy.

8. If traveling a long distance by car, the pregnant client should stop and walk every 2 hours. Also, the client should not travel in an unpressurized airplane and before taking any airplane trip should consult the physician or nurse about additional restrictions.

9. Encourage Mrs. Nance to refrain from tobacco and alcohol.

9. Studies indicate that mothers who smoke tend to have low-birth-weight babies. The effects of alcohol are discussed in *High-risk maternal and newborn problems,* pages 312 to 314.

10. Review with the couple any restrictions on sexual intercourse that apply, discuss alternative methods of showing affection, and encourage open communication between the partners.

10. Restrictions may vary from abstinence to no restrictions at all. The client should abstain from intercourse if she has experienced unexpected complications from the pregnancy. If appropriate, the nurse should recommend changes in position or alternative methods of showing love and affection. Open communication between the couple helps them deal constructively with their sexual needs and concerns.

11. Teach Mrs. Nance how to prevent or minimize constipation and hemorrhoids.

11. The pregnant client should not use laxatives or enemas to alleviate constipation. Adequate fluids, raw fruit and vegetables, and regular exercise usually are sufficient to manage the problem. Hemorrhoids commonly accompany constipation; correcting the constipation should help. In addition, the physician may prescribe medication to manage hemorrhoids.

12. Teach Mrs. Nance how to manage leg aches and cramps.

12. To relieve leg aches and cramps, the client should extend and elevate her legs and dorsiflex her feet. If discomfort persists, the physician may suspect a calcium-phosphorus imbalance, requiring an adjustment in the client's milk intake.

(Text continues on page 236.)

MATERNAL-
NEWBORN
NURSING

Nutrient needs during pregnancy

NUTRIENT	AMOUNT (set by National Research Council)		REASONS FOR INCREASE	FOOD SOURCES
	NONPREGNANT ADULT (AGES 19 TO 24)	PREGNANT ADULT		
Protein	46 g	60 g	• Rapid fetal tissue growth • Amniotic fluid • Placenta growth and development • Maternal tissue growth: uterus, breasts • Increased maternal circulating blood volume, hemoglobin increase, plasma protein increase • Maternal storage reserves for labor, delivery, and lactation	Milk Cheese Eggs Meats Grains Legumes Nuts
Calories	2,100	2,400 (or 300 more than nonpregnant adult)	• Increased energy needs • Protein sparing	Carbohydrates Fats Protein
Minerals				
Calcium	800 mg	1,200 mg	• Fetal skeletal formation • Fetal tooth bud formation (development of enamel-forming cells in gum tissue) • Increased maternal calcium metabolism	Milk Cheese Whole grains Leafy vegetables Egg yolk
Phosphorus	800 mg	1,200 mg	• Fetal skeletal formation • Fetal tooth bud formation • Increased maternal phosphorus metabolism	Milk Cheese Lean meats
Iron	18 mg	18+ mg (and 30- to 60-mg supplement)	• Increased maternal circulating blood volume, increased hemoglobin • Fetal liver iron storage (primarily in third trimester) • High iron cost of pregnancy	Liver Meats Eggs Whole or enriched grains Leafy vegetables Nuts Legumes Dried fruits
Iodine	100 mcg	125 mcg	• Increased basal metabolic rate • Increased thyroxine production	Iodized salt
Magnesium	300 mg	450 mg	• Coenzyme in energy and protein metabolism • Enzyme activator • Tissue growth, cell metabolism • Muscle action	Nuts Soybeans Cocoa Seafood Whole grains Dried beans and peas

(continued)

Nutrient needs during pregnancy. (continued)

NUTRIENT	AMOUNT (set by National Research Council)		REASONS FOR INCREASE	FOOD SOURCES
	NONPREGNANT ADULT (AGES 19 TO 24)	PREGNANT ADULT		
Vitamins				
A	4,000 IU	5,000 IU	• Cell development, tissue growth • Fetal tooth bud formation • Fetal skeletal formation	Butter, cream Fortified margarine Green and yellow vegetables
D	400 IU	400 IU	• Absorption of calcium and phosphorus • Mineralization of bone tissue • Fetal tooth bud formation	Fortified milk Fortified margarine
E	12 IU	15 IU	• Tissue growth • Cell wall integrity • Red blood cell integrity	Vegetable oils Leafy vegetables Cereals Meats Eggs, milk
C (ascorbic acid)	45 mg	60 mg	• Tissue formation and integrity • Cement substance in connective and vascular tissues • Increased iron absorption	Citrus fruits Berries Melons Tomatoes Chili peppers Green peppers Green leafy vegetables Broccoli, potatoes
Folic acid	400 mcg	800 mcg (and 200- to 400-mcg supplement)	• Increased metabolic demand in pregnancy • Prevention of megaloblastic anemia in high-risk clients • Increased heme production for hemoglobin • Production of cell nucleus material	Liver Green leafy vegetables
Niacin	13 mg	15 mg	• Coenzyme in energy metabolism and protein metabolism	Meats Peanuts Beans and peas Enriched grains
Riboflavin	1.2 mg	1.5 mg	• Coenzyme in energy metabolism and protein metabolism	Milk Liver Enriched grains
Thiamine	1 mg	1.3 mg	• Coenzyme in energy metabolism	Pork, beef, liver Whole or enriched grains Legumes
B_6 (pyridoxine)	2 mg	2.5 mg	• Coenzyme in protein metabolism • Increased fetal growth requirement	Wheat, corn Liver, meats
B_{12}	3 mcg	4 mcg	• Coenzyme in protein metabolism, especially vital cell proteins such as nucleic acid • Red blood cell formation	Milk Eggs Meats, liver Cheese

Fetal circulation

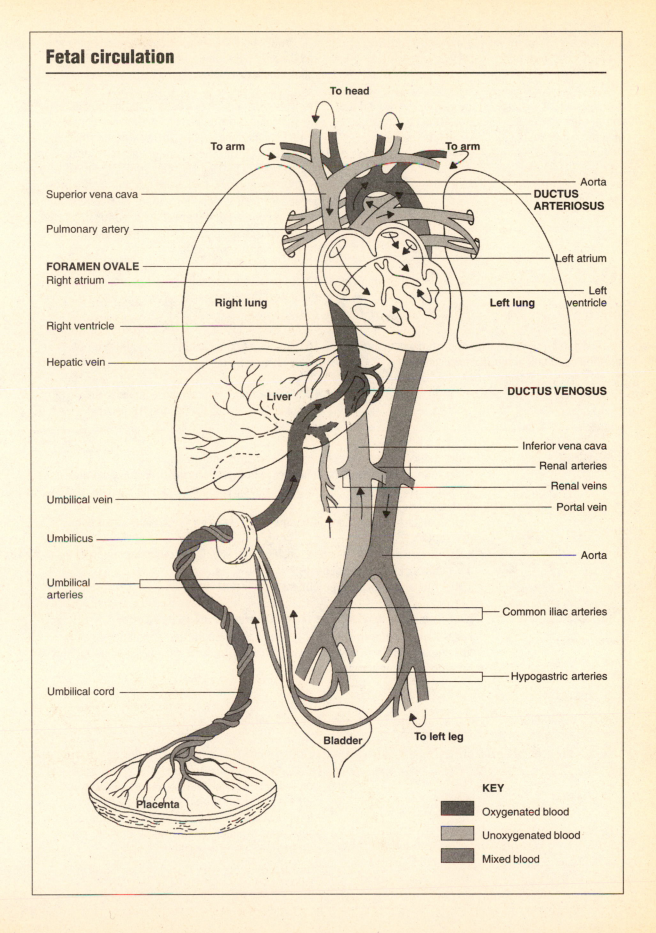

To head

To arm

To arm

Superior vena cava

Pulmonary artery

FORAMEN OVALE

Right atrium

Right ventricle

Hepatic vein

Liver

Right lung

Umbilical vein

Umbilicus

Umbilical
arteries

Umbilical cord

Placenta

Bladder

To left leg

Aorta

**DUCTUS
ARTERIOSUS**

Left atrium

Left
ventricle

Left lung

DUCTUS VENOSUS

Inferior vena cava

Renal arteries

Renal veins

Portal vein

Aorta

Common iliac arteries

Hypogastric arteries

KEY

Oxygenated blood

Unoxygenated blood

Mixed blood

MATERNAL-
NEWBORN
NURSING

13. Teach Mrs. Nance how to manage backache.

13. Proper body mechanics, sufficient rest periods, and the pelvic rocking exercise will help relieve the client's back discomfort.

14. Instruct Mrs. Nance on the elements of sound nutrition during pregnancy, emphasizing the importance of sufficient protein, calories, calcium, and iron.

14. The pregnant client's diet should be nutritionally adequate and individualized to reflect her choice of foods (see *Nutrient needs during pregnancy*, pages 233 and 234). The client should increase her daily intake of protein by 10 g (for cell growth) and calories by 300 (for energy). Increased calcium intake is needed for fetal skeletal formation. Increased iron intake is recommended to meet the need for increased maternal circulation and, in the third trimester, for the fetal liver to store iron.

15. Teach Mrs. Nance the basics of fetal development.

15. To provide answers to Mrs. Nance's questions about fetal development, see *Fetal circulation*, page 235.

16. Provide Mrs. Nance with opportunities to ask questions and talk about her expectations.

16. Listening to the client helps establish a positive nurse-client relationship.

17. Schedule Mrs. Nance's next prenatal visit (4 weeks).

17. This complies with the acceptable schedule of prenatal visits during the second trimester.

Evaluation

• Mrs. Nance's pregnancy continues to progress normally.
• Mrs. Nance describes how to take care of herself during pregnancy, including information on general health practices, changes in diet, and management of common annoyances.
• Mrs. Nance asks questions about the progress of her pregnancy and the fetus's development.
• Mrs. Nance describes her relationships with significant others as supportive and her family resources as adequate.
• Mrs. Nance makes an appointment for her next visit.

Clinical situation

(continued)

Nursing care during the third trimester of pregnancy

Peggy Nance is now in her 8th month of an uncomplicated pregnancy. She states that she is looking forward to having her baby, and she has questions about how to prepare for labor and delivery.

Assessment

NURSING BEHAVIORS

NURSING RATIONALES

1. Assess the general health of Mrs. Nance and the fetus.

1. The routine assessments made during each prenatal visit are necessary for determining maternal-fetal well-being and for early detection of possible complications. The client should gain about 1 lb/week. Blood pressure rises slightly but should not increase above prepregnancy levels by more than 30 mm Hg systolic or 15 mm Hg diastolic.

2. Perform a psychosocial assessment of Mr. and Mrs. Nance: What information do they have about labor and delivery? Do they have questions about preparing for their infant's care? Assess the couple's psychological adaptation to the third trimester of pregnancy.

2. The couple's major developmental task is preparing for childbirth and care of the newborn. Thus, both parents need information that will enable them to cope successfully with labor and delivery, and their activities during this time should reflect psychological adaptation to the third trimester of pregnancy. These activities, such as preparing a nursery and attending childbirth education classes, provide the couple with opportunities to rehearse their anticipated roles. Such statements as "I am going to be a mother" and "I am going to be a father" indicate positive identity adaptation.

Nursing diagnoses

- Ineffective individual coping related to the situational crisis of labor and delivery
- Body image disturbance related to body changes in the client during the third trimester

Planning and goals

- Mr. and Mrs. Nance will describe their preparations for labor and delivery and will attend prenatal classes.
- Mrs. Nance will ask questions that indicate her need for information about caring for her infant.
- Mrs. Nance will describe the warning signs of labor and the appropriate response to them.
- Mrs. Nance's pregnancy will reach term without complications.

Implementation
NURSING BEHAVIORS

NURSING RATIONALES

1. Teach Mr. and Mrs. Nance techniques to prepare for labor and delivery, and suggest they attend prenatal classes—for example, Lamaze, Read, or Bradley.

1. The better prepared the couple is, the less fear they are likely to have. Class objectives include preparing for the physical experience of labor and delivery, gaining knowledge of the experience, learning coping techniques, understanding the value of a support person's involvement, and focusing on birthing as a positive experience. If the couple has children, discuss related concerns and refer them to a sibling education class.

2. Teach the premonitory (warning) signs of labor:

2. When the client notices these warning signs, she should prepare for the onset of labor.

- lightening

- Lightening describes the descent of the fetus; the woman breathes more easily.

- urinary frequency

- Frequency returns when lightening occurs, as the uterus puts pressure on the bladder.

- weight loss

- Some women lose 1 to 2 lb of body weight because of hormonal changes.

- bloody show

- When the mucus plug is discharged, capillary bleeding may occur, making the discharge pink or bloody.

MATERNAL-NEWBORN NURSING

Monitoring uterine contractions

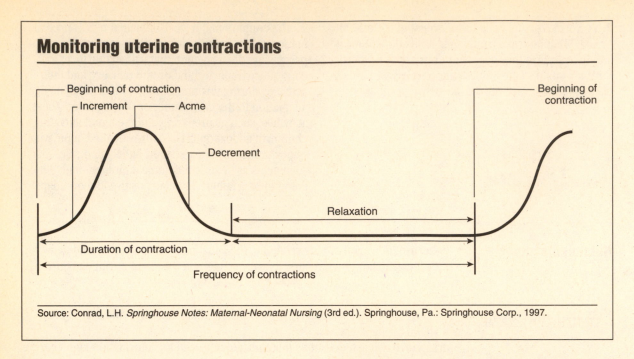

- Beginning of contraction
- Increment
- Acme
- Decrement
- Beginning of contraction
- Relaxation
- Duration of contraction
- Frequency of contractions

Source: Conrad, L.H. *Springhouse Notes: Maternal-Neonatal Nursing* (3rd ed.). Springhouse, Pa.: Springhouse Corp., 1997.

• spurt of energy

• Some women experience increased energy as the basal metabolic rate rises.

• rupture of membranes

• If the membranes rupture prematurely, the client should report it immediately. Fetal heart tones must be checked because they are the most reliable evidence of fetal status.

• Braxton Hicks contractions (see *Monitoring uterine contractions*).

• Braxton Hicks contractions are irregular uterine contractions that do not produce cervical effacement and dilation.

3. Because Mrs. Nance is Rh-negative, make sure she has an indirect Coombs' test at 28 weeks, 34 weeks, and then every 1 to 2 weeks until delivery. After delivery, administer $Rh_o(D)$ immune globulin (Rh_oGAM) I.M., as ordered.

3. The indirect Coombs' test detects Rh-positive antibodies in maternal blood. Rh_oGAM should be given to all unsensitized women at 28 or 34 weeks, and then again within 72 hours of delivery.

4. Schedule Mrs. Nance's routine return visit.

4. Return visits are scheduled every 2 weeks during the 8th month and weekly during the 9th month. The physician may perform an internal pelvic examination to detect cervical changes during the last month.

Evaluation

• Mr. and Mrs. Nance attend prenatal classes and describe them as helpful.
• Mrs. Nance describes the warning signs of labor and the appropriate responses.
• Mrs. Nance's pregnancy progresses to term without complications.

Caring for the client with a threatened or inevitable abortion

TYPE	SYMPTOMS	NURSING CONSIDERATIONS
Threatened abortion	Vaginal bleeding, cramping, cervix remains closed	• Maintain the client on bed rest with a light diet. • Instruct the client to avoid any kind of straining. • Administer a mild sedative as ordered. • Keep a perineal pad count to determine blood loss. • Tell the client to restrict sexual intercourse.
Inevitable abortion	Vaginal bleeding, cramping, cervical dilation, rupture of membranes	*Complete abortion* • Keep a complete perineal pad count and save all tissue samples. • Replace blood or fluid loss as necessary. *Incomplete abortion* • Same as above. • Assist with dilatation and curettage.

Interruption of an early pregnancy

Abortion is the term used to describe termination of a pregnancy when gestation is less than 20 weeks. Possible causes of unintentional abortion include abnormal products of conception, infection, hormonal imbalances, and reproductive tract abnormalities. (See *Caring for the client with a threatened or inevitable abortion,* and *Complications of early pregnancy,* page 240. For information on preterm labor, see *Preterm labor,* page 241.)

Clinical situation

Ruby Reed arrives at the emergency department complaining of severe abdominal cramps. Appearing quite distraught, she relates that she is 3 months pregnant and is afraid she is losing her baby. Mrs. Reed has some vaginal bleeding, and a pelvic examination reveals some cervical dilation.

Assessment

NURSING BEHAVIORS	NURSING RATIONALES
1. Assess Mrs. Reed for signs of inevitable abortion: bleeding, abdominal cramps or pain, cervical dilation, and rupture of membranes.	**1.** An inevitable abortion cannot be halted. The uterus is contracting to empty its contents; the cervix is dilating to expel the uterine contents.
2. Observe Mrs. Reed's vital signs for indications of shock or infection.	**2.** The client may show signs of shock related to blood loss. Infection is also possible.
3. Observe Mrs. Reed's and her partner's emotional status, assessing for fear, guilt, and anxiety.	**3.** Expectant parents may think they have "done something wrong" to cause the abortion and may be extremely frightened about the outcome.

Nursing diagnoses

• Risk for injury related to possible hemorrhage and infection
• Dysfunctional grieving related to loss of the fetus

MATERNAL-NEWBORN NURSING

Complications of early pregnancy

CONDITION	DEFINITION	SIGNS AND SYMPTOMS	TREATMENT	NURSING CONSIDERATIONS
Ectopic pregnancy	Pregnancy outside the uterine cavity (the fallopian tube is the most common site)	• Signs and symptoms of pregnancy • Rupture at 6 to 12 weeks (usually) • Possible vaginal bleeding • Severe pain in lower abdomen • Vaginal tenderness • Shock	• Salpingectomy • Salpingostomy and tubal repair	• Assess the client for bleeding and pain. • Prepare the client for abdominal surgery. • Provide emotional support to the client.
Hydatidiform mole	Abnormal pregnancy that results in a grapelike cluster of vesicles	• Incidence in two age-groups: under 20 and over 40 • Rapid uterine growth • Nausea and vomiting • Elevated levels of chorionic gonadotropin • Uterine bleeding in first and second trimesters • Symptoms of preeclampsia	• Hysterotomy • Hysterectomy • Dilatation and curettage	• Prepare the client for the procedures. • Allow the client to verbalize her feelings. • Stress the importance of follow-up care (a high incidence of choriocarcinoma is associated with hydatidiform mole). • Plan birth control for at least 1 year.
Hyperemesis gravidarum	Persistent vomiting during pregnancy, thought to be caused by high chorionic gonadotropin levels or psychological problem	• Nausea and vomiting • Weight loss • Fatigue • Signs of dehydration • Signs of starvation	• Antiemetics • I.V. fluids (vitamins and electrolytes) • Quiet environment • Sedation • Counseling	• Provide treatment as ordered. • Allow the client to verbalize her feelings.
Incompetent cervix	Failure of the cervix to remain closed, resulting in abortion at 18 to 20 weeks' gestation	• Signs and symptoms of inevitable abortion	• Cerclage of the cervix (using Shirodkar technique or McDonald technique) for future pregnancies	• Assist with the procedure. • Provide emotional support to the client. • Maintain bed rest for 24 hours after cerclage.

Planning and goals

• Mrs. Reed will not develop complications, such as infection or shock.
• Mrs. Reed will express knowledge of her condition and of the procedures being performed.
• Mrs. Reed will not exhibit signs of extreme anxiety and fear.
• Mrs. Reed will have an opportunity to begin grieving.
• Mrs. Reed will identify her support system and available resources.

Implementation

NURSING BEHAVIORS	NURSING RATIONALES
1. Explain all procedures to Mrs. Reed.	**1.** Explanation promotes client trust and helps reduce anxiety.
2. Estimate Mrs. Reed's blood loss, recording the number of perineal pads used, the degree of pad saturation, and a description of pad contents.	**2.** A pad count helps estimate the client's blood loss and risk for hemorrhagic shock. A description of pad contents helps in determining whether an abortion has occurred.

Preterm labor

Preterm labor begins between the 20th and 37th weeks of gestation. The following table provides a quick-reference overview of preterm labor: its incidence, symptoms, risk factors, treatments, and associated nursing care.

Incidence and etiology
- From 8% to 19% of all births
- From 75% to 80% of all neonatal mortality and morbidity
- Pathophysiology related to increased estrogen, fetal stress, increased stretch of uterine muscle, increased prostaglandins, increased maternal oxygen

Symptoms
- Uterine contractions palpable, more than 4 per hour, greater than 30 seconds in duration
- Cervix effaced and dilated
- Increased vaginal drainage

Risk factors
- Medical and pregnancy history factors (such as previous preterm delivery, diethylstilbestrol exposure, cervical shortening)
- Current pregnancy problems (such as multiple gestation, pregnancy-induced hypertension, infection, premature rupture of membranes)
- Socioeconomic factors (such as age extremes, insufficient prenatal care, education)
- Lifestyle habits (such as nutrition or substance abuse)

Treatments
- Tocolytics (magnesium sulfate, ritodrine, terbutaline)
- Glucocorticoids (betamethasone)
- Medical therapy (cervical cerclage, bed rest)

Nursing care
- Discuss risks related to preterm delivery with client and her support system.
- Teach self-care measures.
  - Increase fluid intake to 2 to 3 quarts/day.
  - Empty bladder every 2 hours while awake.
  - Follow activity restrictions (bed rest, lay on left side).
  - Avoid nipple stimulation.
  - Use home monitoring techniques.

---

3. Save any tissue passed vaginally.

3. Any tissue passed will be examined to help determine whether all the products of conception were expelled (complete abortion) or only a portion (incomplete abortion).

4. Assist with blood typing and crossmatching.

4. The client's blood is typed and crossmatched in preparation for replacement of blood or blood products if necessary.

5. Monitor Mrs. Reed's vital signs frequently.

5. Changes in vital signs (elevated temperature and pulse rate, lowered blood pressure) may be early indicators of complications, such as infection and hemorrhage.

6. If the abortion is incomplete, prepare for dilatation and curettage (D&C).

6. If a portion of the products of conception is retained, the uterus will not contract effectively, and the client will be at risk for hemorrhage. Any retained products are removed by D&C.

7. Allow Mrs. Reed time to talk about her experience. Explore expressed feelings of inadequacy, guilt, anger, and fear. Provide appropriate information.

7. The client needs to mourn her loss before she can consider the possibility of a future pregnancy. Initial feelings of shock and disbelief are normal. Grieving may last for 6 to 24 months.

MATERNAL-NEWBORN NURSING

Evaluation

- Mrs. Reed does not develop complications.
- Mrs. Reed verbalizes understanding of what happened with her pregnancy.
- Mrs. Reed begins to use positive coping strategies to deal with her anxiety.
- Mrs. Reed begins to express her feelings about the loss of her pregnancy.

Maternal diabetes mellitus

The normal physiologic changes of pregnancy increase a woman's need for insulin. If the woman is healthy, the body compensates for this need. If the woman is diabetic or develops gestational diabetes mellitus, these normal changes create additional stress. Because of the higher incidence of maternal and fetal complications associated with the pregnancy of a diabetic woman, such a woman should receive close supervision when planning a pregnancy, during pregnancy, and throughout the postpartum period. Signs and symptoms of gestational diabetes disappear when the pregnancy ends. A follow-up oral glucose tolerance test (OGTT) is done 6 weeks after delivery, or after cessation of breast-feeding. The nurse can optimize the client's physiologic and psychological responses to pregnancy and diabetes. (See *How maternal hyperglycemia affects the fetus and the neonate.*) Roughly one-third of clients with gestational diabetes mellitus develop diabetes mellitus within 8 years of delivery.

Clinical situation

Cindy Baker is a 26-year-old primigravida in her 8th month of pregnancy. She has been diabetic since age 15. Her insulin dosages have been adjusted throughout her pregnancy, and she has been conscientious about her prenatal care. Mrs. Baker's physician will perform tests today to decide how to manage the remainder of her pregnancy.

Assessment

NURSING BEHAVIORS

1. Determine maternal well-being by performing routine prenatal assessments of vital signs, weight gain, and fundal height.

2. Assess for signs and symptoms of complications, as follows:

- preeclampsia

- polyhydramnios

- urinary tract infection

NURSING RATIONALES

1. Routine prenatal assessments contribute data that help determine the client's general well-being. In particular, the fundal height provides information related to fetal size and possible polyhydramnios.

2. Pregnant diabetic women are at high risk for complications.

- The vascular disturbances associated with diabetes mellitus predispose the pregnant diabetic woman to preeclampsia.

- Polyhydramnios, an excessive amount of amniotic fluid, is thought to result from fetal metabolism and is usually associated with fetal problems.

- The pregnant diabetic woman is prone to urinary tract infections because glucosuria provides a good medium for bacterial growth.

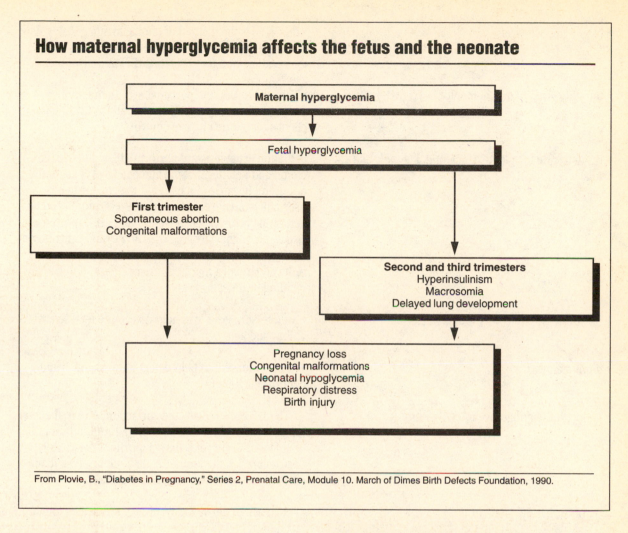

How maternal hyperglycemia affects the fetus and the neonate

Maternal hyperglycemia

Fetal hyperglycemia

First trimester
Spontaneous abortion
Congenital malformations

Second and third trimesters
Hyperinsulinism
Macrosomia
Delayed lung development

Pregnancy loss
Congenital malformations
Neonatal hypoglycemia
Respiratory distress
Birth injury

From Plovie, B., "Diabetes in Pregnancy," Series 2, Prenatal Care, Module 10. March of Dimes Birth Defects Foundation, 1990.

• vaginitis

• ketoacidosis.

3. Determine fetal well-being by listening for fetal heart tones (FHTs) and measuring fetal size, noting macrosomatia (large body size) or intrauterine growth retardation (IUGR).

4. Assess the results of Mrs. Baker's diagnostic tests, as follows:

• The pathology of diabetes mellitus plus the increased vaginal secretions of pregnancy increase the pregnant diabetic woman's susceptibility to yeast infections.

• The nausea and vomiting common in early pregnancy may increase the potential (present in all diabetics) for ketoacidosis.

3. Fetal well-being primarily depends on the degree to which the mother's diabetes is controlled. FHTs and fetal size are routine assessments. Because of glucose metabolism and fat deposits, the infant usually is large, increasing the risk that cephalopelvic disproportion will develop. Poor placental functioning because of severe uncontrolled maternal diabetes may cause IUGR.

4. Diabetes mellitus affects the small blood vessels at the placental site, causing the placenta to degenerate early. Stillbirths occur more often after 36 weeks of gestation. Diagnostic tests help in determining the optimal time for delivery.

- blood glucose levels

- An OGTT is the method of choice for diagnosing diabetes. Testing blood glucose levels four times a day is the ideal method for regulating diet and insulin dosage.

- monthly glycosylated hemoglobin (Hgb A$_2$) test

- This test reveals the percentage of hemoglobin to which glucose is bonded permanently, reflecting the client's long-term glucose control.

- urine testing for glucose, acetone, ketones, and estriols

- Routine urine tests are performed for glucose, acetone, and ketones, but the glucose level is generally not useful because glucose spill may occur in any pregnant woman's urine. Estriol levels, monitored to determine fetal-placental well-being, are expected to rise as pregnancy progresses. The normal estriol level at 40 weeks' gestation is 12 mg/24 hours. Drastically reduced levels (4 mg/24 hours or below) indicate impending fetal death.

- ultrasonography (every 4 to 6 weeks)

- An ultrasonogram can help determine fetal size, viability, and age.

- amniocentesis

- Amniocentesis can help detect abnormalities and confirm lung maturity.

—lecithin-sphingomyelin (L/S) ratio

—The L/S ratio reflects the surfactant level in the fetal lungs. A ratio of 1:1 indicates immature lungs; a ratio of at least 2:1 indicates lung maturity. A 3:1 ratio is desirable when the mother is diabetic because diabetes tends to produce inaccurate elevation.

—phosphatidyl glycerol (PG)

—Absence of phosphatidyl glycerol indicates immature lungs.

—Nile blue test

—The Nile blue test demonstrates the presence of fat cells. Normally, the level rises.

—bilirubin level

—The bilirubin level should fall, indicating fetal hepatic maturity.

—creatinine level

—The creatinine level should rise, indicating fetal renal maturity.

—gross appearance of fluid

—The amniotic fluid is observed for vernix, meconium, blood, and other substances that indicate the condition of the fetus.

- serum alpha-fetoprotein test at 16th week

- The fetus of a woman with diabetes is at greater risk for neural tube defects.

- nonstress test (NST)

- During the NST, a screening test to determine fetal well-being, the FHT is electronically monitored for about 30 minutes in relation to fetal movement. The NST aims to detect at least two instances of fetal movement with corresponding acceleration of the FHT of

15 beats/minute for 15 seconds or longer within any 10- to 20-minute period. If this occurs, the test is recorded as reactive, and the client is scheduled for a repeat test in a week. The desired result is reactive. A nonreactive test is a negative finding, indicating the need for further study.

• stress tests (oxytocin challenge test [OCT] and the contraction stress test)	• The stress tests, usually reserved for monitoring fetal well-being in high-risk pregnancies, involve electronic monitoring of the FHT during a uterine contraction. Oxytocin (Pitocin) is administered to stimulate uterine contractions until three contractions occur within any 10-minute period. The fetal heart rate is observed for decelerations occurring with or after contractions, indicating poor placental oxygen reserve. The desired result is negative. Three contractions with no decelerations constitute a negative OCT. Any sign of deceleration results in a positive OCT and warrants a follow-up examination by the physician.
• daily fetal movement counts, starting at 28th week.	• This promotes daily maternal awareness of fetal movement.
5. Assess Mrs. Baker's learning needs concerning diabetes and prenatal care.	**5.** Obtaining this information enables the nurse to plan appropriate care for the mother and fetus and provides a helpful focus for client teaching.

Nursing diagnoses
- Risk for injury related to the complications associated with diabetes
- Altered nutrition (less than body requirements) related to the effects of placental hormones on glucose metabolism
- Noncompliance related to required frequent monitoring and prenatal visits

Planning and goals
- Mrs. Baker will describe her responsibility for insulin regulation and will be conscientious in administering her insulin.
- Mrs. Baker will describe her diet and the importance of following it strictly.
- Mrs. Baker will verbalize knowledge of the diagnostic tests and the implications of their results.
- Mrs. Baker will maintain personal hygiene with the goal of preventing infection and will seek treatment promptly if an infection develops.
- Mrs. Baker will accept the need for close medical and nursing supervision during her pregnancy.

Implementation
NURSING BEHAVIORS

NURSING RATIONALES

1. Teach Mrs. Baker how diet, exercise, and insulin regulation help control diabetes. Review use of capillary glucose monitoring system.

1. The client must understand diabetes and her role in controlling it. Diet is regulated individually in response to the needs of pregnancy. Planned exercise plays an important part in controlling blood glucose levels. In early pregnancy, insulin needs will probably decrease. During middle and late pregnancy, however, as the placenta forms and functions, it produces estrogen, progesterone, and human placental lacto-

MATERNAL-NEWBORN NURSING

gen—which alter the effectiveness of insulin—and insulinase, an enzyme destructive to insulin. Therefore, insulin needs during this time usually increase. Insulin coverage for the pregnant diabetic woman is typically accomplished by using both regular and longer-acting insulin at various times throughout the day.

2. Teach Mrs. Baker about the indications and procedures for fetal tests.

2. Insulin requirements change during pregnancy. Fetal status and compromise must be identified.

3. Teach Mrs. Baker general health measures related to diabetes mellitus.

3. General health measures related to diabetes mellitus include skin care, exercise, treatment of infection, and prevention of hypoglycemic reaction and metabolic acidosis.

4. Schedule return visits for Mrs. Baker on a weekly basis, as appropriate. Make sure she receives follow-up care with a diabetologist.

4. The pregnant diabetic woman is examined every 2 weeks during early pregnancy and, beginning around the 7th month, weekly or more often, as necessary. For information about the potential for labor, delivery, and postpartal problems (including dystocia, induction of labor, cesarean section, fetal distress, and postpartal bleeding), see "Concepts of labor and delivery," page 253, and *Postpartal complications,* pages 279 and 280.

5. Allow time for Mrs. Baker to express concerns and ask questions.

5. Therapeutic communication promotes a positive pregnancy outcome.

Evaluation

• Mrs. Baker manages her diet and insulin regulation without problems.
• Mrs. Baker asks questions about the diagnostic tests and discusses the results.
• Mrs. Baker verbalizes the importance of careful personal hygiene in preventing infection.
• Mrs. Baker makes an appropriate follow-up appointment.
• Mrs. Baker maintains normal blood glucose levels (euglycemia) during pregnancy.

Pregnancy-induced hypertension

Preeclampsia and eclampsia—forms of pregnancy-induced hypertension (PIH) that can occur after the 20th week of gestation—are characterized by the cardinal signs of hypertension, proteinuria, and edema. Eclampsia occurs with the onset of seizures. Predisposing factors include primigravida status, multiple pregnancy, diabetes mellitus, hydatidiform mole, poor maternal nourishment, and extremes of maternal age. Complications of preeclampsia and eclampsia are related to decreased uteroplacental blood flow and include abruptio placentae, disseminated intravascular coagulation, premature labor, cerebrovascular accident, and fetal death. (See *Nursing care of a pregnant client with a cardiovascular disorder, Nursing care during fetal distress,* page 248, and *High-risk conditions associ-*

Nursing care of a pregnant client with a cardiovascular disorder

CONDITION	IMPLICATIONS
Vena cava syndrome (supine hypotensive syndrome)	Vena cava syndrome occurs when something interferes with blood flow to the right atrium. This may occur if the near-term or full-term pregnant woman lies on her back, with the weight of the uterus compressing the inferior vena cava. The symptoms are dizziness, tingling of the extremities, circumoral pallor, and faintness. The client should lie on her side to relieve pressure on the inferior vena cava and restore circulation.
Chronic hypertension	Although a client with chronic hypertension develops the condition before pregnancy, her blood pressure will rise with each pregnancy and will not return to the prepregnancy level. Because it interferes with oxygen supply, chronic hypertension poses a danger to the mother and the fetus.
Anemia • First trimester: Hemoglobin below 12 g/dl Hematocrit below 37% • Second and third trimesters: Hemoglobin below 11 g/dl Hematocrit below 35%	Maternal problems associated with anemia include abortion, infection, preeclampsia, premature labor, and heart failure. Fetal problems associated with anemia include growth retardation, morbidity, and mortality. Treatment includes an iron-rich diet, vitamin C, and folic acid. Additionally, the physician may prescribe an iron supplement (for example, ferrous sulfate). If so, teach the client to take the supplement between meals with a source of vitamin C, and to include roughage and fluids in her diet because iron may cause constipation. Also caution the client that iron will make her stools black.
Heart disease	The normal physiologic changes of pregnancy are stressful to the client with heart disease. Periods of increased risk include: • around the 28th week of gestation, when the blood volume increase peaks, resulting in additional stress on the heart • during the second trimester, when an elevated basal metabolic rate increases maternal-fetal oxygen requirements • during labor and delivery, at which time epidural or caudal anesthesia is recommended (forceps may be used to prevent pushing) • during the 1st postpartal week as body fluid levels return to normal. Care focuses on adequate rest; prevention of infection; diet management; and controlled, cautious weight loss.

MATERNAL-NEWBORN NURSING

ated with hemorrhage in late pregnancy, page 250, for related information.) The following clinical situation focuses on care of the pregnant woman with preeclampsia.

Clinical situation   Rita Clancy, a 38-year-old primigravida, is in her 8th month of pregnancy. During a routine checkup today, the nurse notes a weight gain of 8 lb since Mrs. Clancy's last visit. Mrs. Clancy remarks that she's had to remove her rings because her fingers are swollen. Her blood pressure is 144/92 mm Hg.

Assessment

NURSING BEHAVIORS

1. Assess Mrs. Clancy for signs of preeclampsia and eclampsia.

NURSING RATIONALES

1. Preeclampsia can be mild or severe. If mild preeclampsia is untreated or does not respond to treatment, severe preeclampsia may follow, accompanied by additional signs and symptoms. If the client has a seizure, she is considered eclamptic.

• Signs of mild preeclampsia include:
—hypertension: a blood pressure of 140/90 mm Hg, a systolic measurement 30 mm Hg above normal, or a diastolic measurement 15 mm Hg above normal (taken at 6-hour intervals)

Nursing care during fetal distress

Fetal distress is caused primarily by decreased oxygen supply to the fetus. The decrease may be maternal or fetal in origin.

MATERNAL-RELATED CAUSES	FETAL-RELATED CAUSES	FETAL DISTRESS SIGNS
• Anemia • Hypertension or hypotension • Preeclampsia • Abruptio placentae • Placenta previa • Medication • Prolonged contraction • Pressure on the placenta	• Prolapsed cord • Knotted cord • Nuchal cord	• Fetal hyperactivity • Meconium-stained amniotic fluid, except in a known breech presentation • Persistent fetal bradycardia (below 100 beats/minute) or tachycardia (above 180 beats/minute) or loss of beat-to-beat variability

FETAL DISTRESS PATTERN GRAPHS

Continuous electronic monitoring can identify fetal heart rate patterns that indicate fetal distress and its possible cause.

Early deceleration (related to head compression)

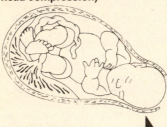

Head compression

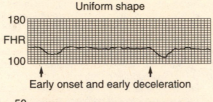

Uniform shape

Early onset and early deceleration

uterine contraction

Nursing interventions
Continue observation. This pattern usually indicates head compression as the fetal head passes through the birth canal.

Late deceleration (related to uteroplacental insufficiency)

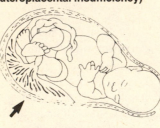

Compression of vessels

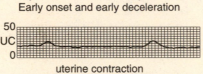

Uniform shape

Late onset and late deceleration

uterine contraction

Nursing interventions
• Stop oxytocin if in progress, and replace I.V. fluid.
• Change the client's position to the preferred left-side-lying position.
• Check blood pressure and pulse rate.
• Administer oxygen.
• Notify the physician.

Variable deceleration (related to umbilical cord compression)
The first deceleration is V-shaped; the second, U-shaped. Transitory acceleration precedes or follows the deceleration. The fetal heart rate may fall below 100 beats/minute.

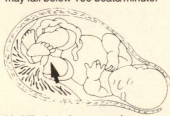

Umbilical cord compression

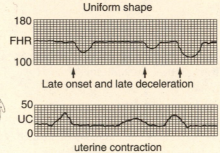

Variable shape

Variable onset and variable deceleration

uterine contraction

Nursing interventions
• Stop oxytocin if in progress, and replace I.V. fluid.
• Change the mother's position.
• Check for a prolapsed cord.
• Check blood pressure and pulse rate.
• Administer oxygen.
• Notify the physician.
• Prepare to assist with drawing a blood sample from the fetal scalp.

—proteinuria: trace to 2+ (< 5 g/24 hours)
—edema: weight gain over 1 lb/week.

• Signs of severe preeclampsia include:
—hypertension: a blood pressure of 160/110 mm Hg, sustained for 6 hours with the client at rest
—proteinuria: 3+ to 4+ (5 g/24 hours)
—pitting edema: generalized (4+)
—oliguria: urine output 400 ml or less/24 hours
—other indications: headache, nausea, vomiting, visual disturbances (blurriness, dimness), hyperreflexia, epigastric pain.

• Signs of eclampsia include those of preeclampsia accompanied by seizures or coma.

2. Determine fetal well-being by assessing fetal heart tones.

2. Continuous fetal monitoring is recommended for early detection of fetal distress.

3. Assess Mrs. Clancy's general well-being, noting any early signs of preeclampsia, such as swelling of the fingers and weight gain from fluid retention. Assess deep tendon reflexes and clonus.

3. Consistent prenatal care is essential to detect the early signs of preeclampsia, which may go unnoticed by the client. Deep tendon reflexes should be of moderate strength (+2 to +3). Clonus should be absent.

4. Assess Mrs. Clancy's dietary intake.

4. Sodium, protein, and fluid intake are pertinent factors in assessing individual needs related to pregnancy-induced hypertension.

5. Assess laboratory results: hematocrit, serum creatinine, blood urea nitrogen, and serum sodium.

5. Hematocrit increases from decreased intravascular volume. All other values will increase as a result of decreased glomerular filtration rate, increased vascular resistance, and decreased plasma and blood volume.

MATERNAL-NEWBORN NURSING

Nursing diagnoses
• Risk for fluid volume deficit related to fluid shift to the interstitial spaces
• Altered nutrition (less than body requirements) related to protein loss in urine
• Risk for maternal or fetal injury related to decreased tissue perfusion
• Ineffective individual coping related to unexpected pregnancy complication

Planning and goals
• Mrs. Clancy will describe the warning signs that indicate she needs immediate attention.
• Mrs. Clancy will describe the required alterations to her diet and activity.
• Mrs. Clancy will continue to receive prenatal care under closer surveillance.
• Mrs. Clancy will exhibit decreased severity of signs and symptoms of preeclampsia.

Implementation
NURSING BEHAVIORS

NURSING RATIONALES

1. Teach Mrs. Clancy self-care as follows:

1. Mrs. Clancy needs instruction for self-care at home.

• bed rest in the left-side-lying position

• Bed rest in a left-side-lying position promotes better circulation.

High-risk conditions associated with hemorrhage in late pregnancy

CONDITION	DEFINITION	SIGNS AND SYMPTOMS	TREATMENT	NURSING CONSIDERATIONS
Placenta previa	Placenta located over or near the cervical opening	• *Painless* bleeding in third trimester • Signs of hemorrhage • Signs of fetal distress • Predisposing factor: multiparity in older women • Intermittent bleeding	• Hospitalization • Bed rest • Diagnosis by sonogram	• Do not perform a pelvic examination. • Explain procedures to the client. • Monitor maternal and fetal condition. • Prepare the client for delivery.
Total	Placenta lies over the cervical opening — mucus plug		• With frank bleeding—delivery always by cesarean section	
Partial	Placenta covers only part of the cervical opening — mucus plug		• Delivery usually by cesarean section	
Marginal	Low implantation near the cervical opening — mucus plug		• Delivery occasionally by cesarean section	
Abruptio placentae	Premature separation of the placenta from the uterine wall	• Concealed (hidden) or apparent hemorrhage • *Painful* bleeding in third trimester • Boardlike abdomen (with shock or fetal distress)	• Replacement of blood loss • I.V. fluids • Vaginal delivery if possible; otherwise, cesarean delivery	• Explain procedures to the client. • Monitor maternal and fetal condition. • Prepare the client for delivery. • Maternal cocaine use is a predisposing factor.
Total	Completely separated			
Partial	Partly separated	• Predisposing factors: preeclampsia, eclampsia, multiparity, and endocrine imbalances • Complication: hypofibrinogenemia		

• quiet environment

• A nonstimulating environment is an essential aspect of treatment for preeclampsia.

• sedation (usually phenobarbital)

• Sedation may be given to enhance relaxation.

• high-protein, moderate-salt diet

• A high-protein, moderate-salt diet is recommended to replace protein loss and to control fluid retention.

• daily weight

• The client should be weighed daily and instructed to report a sudden increase in weight. Sudden weight gain usually results from fluid retention.

• signs indicating progression to severe preeclampsia: generalized edema, decreased urine output, headache, visual disturbances, nausea and vomiting, epigastric pain, and hyperreflexia.

• Signs indicating progression to severe preeclampsia should be reported promptly so that treatment can be started to prevent preeclampsia.

2. Schedule twice-weekly return visits for Mrs. Clancy.

2. Frequent visits are necessary for prompt detection of changes in the client's condition.

Clinical situation
(continued)

Two days after her office visit, Rita Clancy calls to report a 2-lb weight gain. She also has nausea and a persistent headache and is puffy around her eyes. The physician admits her to the hospital for treatment to prevent eclampsia.

Implementation
NURSING BEHAVIORS

1. Provide a darkened, quiet room for Mrs. Clancy, and limit visitors.

2. Take Mrs. Clancy's blood pressure every hour, or more frequently if indicated.

3. Maintain Mrs. Clancy on strict bed rest; position her in the left-side-lying position, with the bed side rails up and padded.

4. Insert an indwelling urinary catheter.

5. Administer medications as ordered. Medications that may be given include magnesium sulfate (I.M. or I.V.), phenobarbital, and vasodilators, such as hydralazine and methyldopa.

NURSING RATIONALES

1. A darkened, quiet room reduces stimuli and enhances relaxation.

2. Frequent blood pressure readings aid in determining the effectiveness of treatment.

3. Restricting activities is an attempt to promote relaxation; lying on the left side promotes circulation; keeping the side rails up is a safety precaution.

4. An indwelling urinary catheter is inserted to determine the client's hourly urine output. The urine is then tested for the protein level. Urine output should equal at least 30 ml/hour.

5. Magnesium sulfate, a central nervous system depressant, decreases neuromuscular irritability. After administering the drug, the nurse routinely checks that the client's deep tendon reflexes are present, that her respiratory rate is at least 14 breaths/minute, and that her urine output is at least 30 ml/hour. The antagonist calcium gluconate should be kept available in case the client becomes too depressed from magnesium sulfate. Phenobarbital, a sedative, promotes relaxation in mild preeclampsia. Hydralazine and methyldopa cause vasodilation, thereby lowering blood pressure.

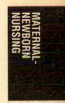
MATERNAL-NEWBORN NURSING

Induction of labor

Induction of labor refers to initiation of labor by artificial methods after the period of viability. It may be indicated when continuing the pregnancy would put the client or fetus at risk. Care of the client whose labor is augmented by infusion of oxytocin (a potent drug that causes myometrial contractions) is similar to care of the client undergoing induction of labor.

Indications	• Fetal postmaturity • Dystocia • Mild preeclampsia • Premature or prolonged rupture of membranes • Maternal diabetes mellitus
Contraindications	• Cephalopelvic disproportion • Hypertonic uterine patterns • Prolonged fetal distress • Uterine inertia • Severe preeclampsia • Prolapsed cord • Complete placenta previa
Nursing care	• As ordered, dilute oxytocin and infuse in secondary I.V. line at initial dosage of 1 to 2 milliunits/minute. Adjust dosage every 30 minutes. Use regulating device to ensure accurate dosage. • Apply electronic fetal monitor (EFM), and obtain 15- to 20-minute tracing and nonstress test before labor induction. • Monitor fetal and uterine responses per continuous EFM. • Observe for side effects of oxytocin: —fetal distress —tetanic contractions (which occur when uterus does not return to resting tone and when contractions are more frequent than every 2 minutes and last more than 60 seconds) —hypertension —water intoxication (indicated by nausea and vomiting, hypotension, tachycardia, and arrhythmias). • Discontinue drug if side effects occur. • Stay with client.
Nursing diagnoses	• Risk for maternal or fetal injury related to side effects of oxytocin • Pain related to uterine contractions

6. If ordered, monitor fetal heart tones continuously. Other tests, such as the nonstress test, oxytocin challenge test, amniocentesis, and fetal movement count, may be ordered.

6. The fetus may indicate distress because of placental insufficiency. Monitoring fetal well-being promotes a positive fetal outcome.

7. Monitor Mrs. Clancy for signs of labor.

7. A woman with preeclampsia is likely to experience premature labor.

8. Monitor Mrs. Clancy for signs of approaching eclampsia: severe headache, hyperreflexia, visual disturbances, epigastric pain, and nausea and vomiting. Immediately report any of these to the physician.

8. Careful monitoring for and prompt reporting of these signs help ensure early treatment to prevent seizures. If the client's condition worsens, the physician may decide to induce labor (see *Induction of labor*) or perform a cesarean section. If a seizure occurs, the client will remain at risk for seizures for 48 hours postpartum.

9. Continue to monitor laboratory results. Obtain liver enzyme tests and a platelet count, as ordered, to rule out HELLP syndrome (hemolysis, elevated liver enzymes, and low platelet count).

9. HELLP syndrome sometimes is associated with severe preeclampsia. Limited blood flow and vasospasms result in life-threatening complications.

10. Prepare for seizure care if needed. Have the following equipment available: artificial airway, padded side rails, suction equipment, oxygen equipment, and emergency tray.

10. Preeclamptic women are at risk for seizures. Anticipatory care includes adequate preparation for seizures. The emergency tray will contain either bolus doses of diazepam (Valium) or magnesium sulfate to control imminent or actual seizures.

11. Spend time with the Clancys, giving them opportunities to ask questions and express their feelings.

11. Considered at high risk, the client will probably have many fears about her own and her fetus's condition.

Evaluation

• Mrs. Clancy's vital signs and laboratory values return to normal (or labor is induced).

INTRAPARTAL PERIOD

Concepts of labor and delivery

Fetal habitus (attitude)

The term *fetal habitus,* or *attitude,* refers to the relation of fetal parts to one another. The relation usually is one of flexion; that is, legs flexed against the trunk, arms flexed across the chest, and so on. Any unflexed part presents a potential problem for labor and delivery.

The fetal head is the most significant body part because it is the least malleable (see *Fetal head diameters,* page 254). Suture lines allow for molding of the fetal head during labor and delivery. They meet to form the anterior and posterior fontanelles; the location of the fontanelles is helpful in assessing fetal position. Suture lines also allow for rapid growth during the infant's 1st year.

Lie, presentation, presenting part

Fetal lie refers to the relationship of the long axis of the fetus to the long axis of the mother.

Fetal presentation refers to the part of the fetus closest to the internal os of the mother's cervix. Various fetal presentations are possible. (See *Fetal positions and variations in presentation,* page 255.)
• In a cephalic presentation, any part of the head can present, including the occiput or vertex, brow, or face.
• In a transverse presentation, the back or shoulders present, and vaginal delivery is not possible.
• In a breech presentation, the buttocks (frank breech), one or both feet (footling breech), or both the buttocks and feet (complete breech) are the presenting part.

MATERNAL-NEWBORN NURSING

Fetal head diameters

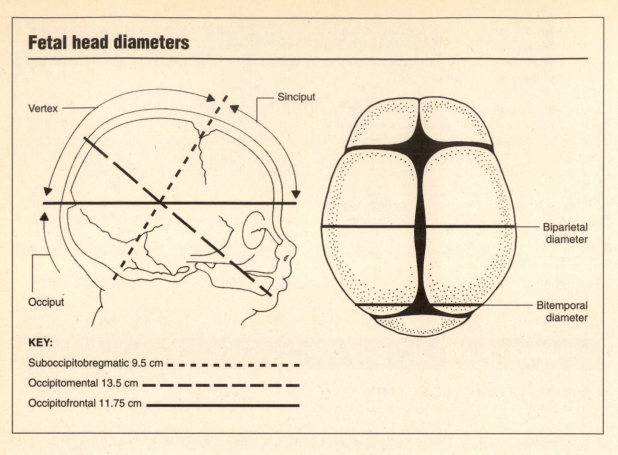

KEY:

Suboccipitobregmatic 9.5 cm — — — — — — — — — — —

Occipitomental 13.5 cm — — — — — — — — —

Occipitofrontal 11.75 cm ————————————

Fetal position and fetal station

Fetal position describes the relationship of the presenting part to the mother's pelvis, which is divided into the following quadrants:

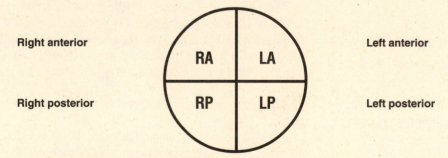

Right anterior   Left anterior

Right posterior   Left posterior

The examiner can determine fetal position through vaginal examination, location of fetal heart tones, Leopold's maneuvers, and ultrasonography or X-ray. During a vaginal examination, the examiner first determines the presenting part (location of the suture lines and fontanelles) and then determines whether the presenting part is directed toward the right or left side of the mother and toward the symphysis pubis (anterior) or the sacral area (posterior). For example, in the left occipital anterior (LOA) position, the presenting part is the occiput, and it is directed toward the left side of the pelvis and toward the symphysis pubis. (The middle initial represents the presenting part.) Occipital anterior is the preferred delivery position because the fetal head can extend under the arch of the symphysis pubis; LOA is the ideal position because, with the fetus lying on the mother's left side, oxygen supply to the client and the fetus is maximized. With occipital posterior, the occiput attempts to extend into the sacral area.

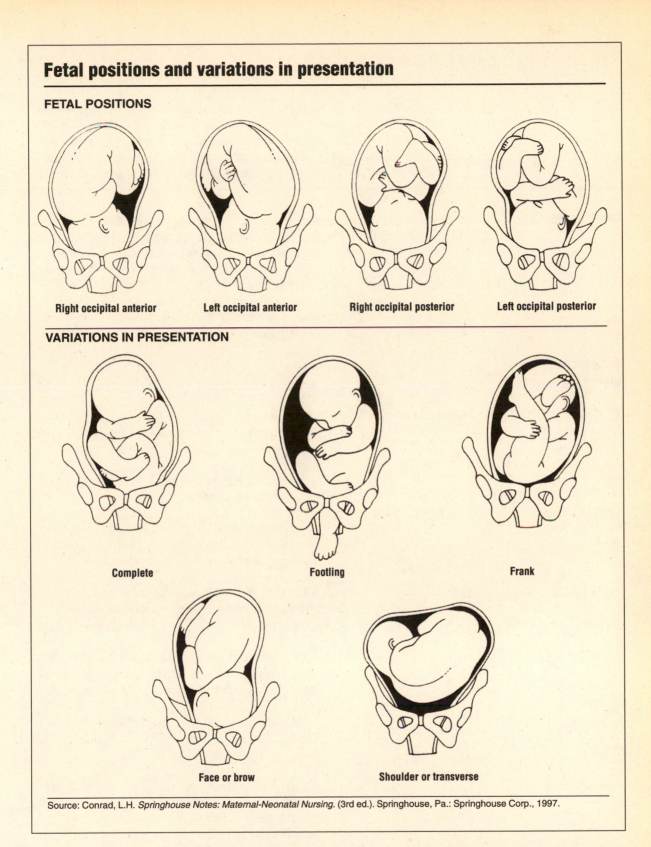

Fetal positions and variations in presentation

FETAL POSITIONS

Right occipital anterior   Left occipital anterior   Right occipital posterior   Left occipital posterior

VARIATIONS IN PRESENTATION

Complete   Footling   Frank

Face or brow   Shoulder or transverse

Source: Conrad, L.H. *Springhouse Notes: Maternal-Neonatal Nursing.* (3rd ed.). Springhouse, Pa.: Springhouse Corp., 1997.

Fetal station, also called *degree of engagement,* is the location of the presenting part in relation to the mother's ischial spines (see *Measuring fetal station,* page 257). Fetal station can be determined by vaginal examination.

The client during the intrapartal period

To intervene effectively during the birthing process (considered a normal process), the nurse must understand not only the physiology of labor and delivery (see *Stages of labor,* pages 258 and 259) but also the impact of sociocultural and personal factors on the client's childbearing experience. The following clinical situations focus on the nurse's ability to provide care to the client and family during the birthing process.

Clinical situation

Della DeShon is a 24-year-old primigravida who recently arrived at the hospital. She says she was due yesterday, has had a bloody show, and is having mild contractions every 5 minutes. On examination, her vital signs are stable; the fetal heart tones (FHTs) are 140 beats/minute in the lower left quadrant; the presenting part is the vertex at station 0; and her cervix is dilated 3 cm and 100% effaced. The physician's written admission orders include 1,000 ml of dextrose 5% in water (D_5W) I.V. at 125 ml/hour; obtain an electronic fetal monitor tracing showing FHTs and uterine activity. (See *Electronic fetal monitoring,* page 261.)

Assessment

NURSING BEHAVIORS	NURSING RATIONALES
1. Review Mrs. DeShon's prenatal record, as follows:	**1.** The information obtained from the prenatal record contributes to baseline information and provides data pertinent to the management of labor and delivery.
• age	• Extremes of age are commonly related to birthing process complications.
• gravida, para	• Information about the client's previous pregnancies and labor and delivery experiences may be a predictive factor for the current labor and delivery.
• expected date of delivery (EDD)	• The EDD gives information about gestational age and may help the nurse anticipate problems such as a preterm delivery.
• complications	• The nurse must consider pregnancy complications, such as diabetes or preeclampsia, when planning for management of the client's labor and delivery.
• allergies	• The nurse should note any food or drug allergies. For instance, if the client is allergic to seafood, iodine-based antiseptics should not be used.
• medications	• Current drug therapy may influence analgesia and anesthesia options. The nurse should evaluate all the client's current medications for their potential effect on labor as well as for their compatibility with drugs that may be administered during the intrapartal period.

Measuring fetal station

Fetal station (also called degree of engagement) describes where the presenting part lies in relation to the level of the ischial spines. Measured in centimeters, fetal station advances from -5 cm to 0 (ischial spine level) to +5 cm. The head is considered engaged when it reaches 0.

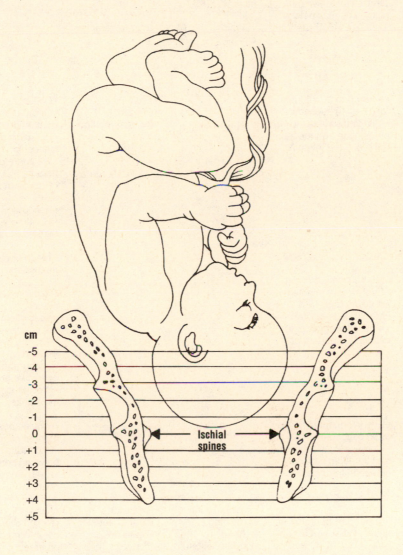

cm
-5
-4
-3
-2
-1
0
+1
+2
+3
+4
+5

Ischial spines

Source: Conrad, L.H. *Springhouse Notes: Maternal-Neonatal Nursing.* (3rd ed.). Springhouse, Pa.: Springhouse Corp., 1997.

MATERNAL-NEWBORN NURSING

• pregnancy progress

• laboratory data (prenatal).

• The progress of the pregnancy is documented on the prenatal record in routine assessments of the vital signs, weight gain, FHTs, and fundal height.

• These include urinalysis, hemoglobin and hematocrit levels, complete blood count, and Rh and blood typing.

Stages of labor

STAGE	CONTRACTION CHARACTERISTICS	MATERNAL PHYSICAL CHANGES	FETAL POSITION CHANGES	NURSING CARE
I. Dilation Starts with first true labor contraction and ends with complete cervical effacement and dilation	See contraction characteristics for individual Stage I phases below.	• Percent of effacement (0% to 100%) • Dilation (1 to 10 cm)	• Engagement • Descent • Flexion • Internal rotation	
Phases *Early (latent, inactive):* Cervix dilates 1 to 4 cm; longest, least uncomfortable phase	• Every 5 to 20 minutes for 15 to 40 seconds • Mild to moderate, increasing in frequency, duration, and intensity		• Descent • Flexion • Internal rotation	• Collect assessment data. • Orient client to environment and equipment. • Establish nurse-client relationship. • Welcome client's support person. • Provide comfort measures. • Encourage ambulation. • Measure vital signs and fetal heart rate per protocol. • Teach or review breathing methods.
Active: Cervix dilates 4 to 8 cm	• Every 2 to 4 minutes for 60 seconds • Moderate to strong • Most effacement and dilation in shortest period			• Reinforce breathing techniques. • Keep client informed of her progress. • Change client's position frequently. • Encourage client to void every two hours. • Provide ice chips and lip moisturizer.
Transitional: Cervix dilates 8 to 10 cm; shortest, most uncomfortable phase	• Every 2 minutes for up to 60 seconds • Increase in strength and duration; may decrease in frequency			• Provide positive reinforcement to support person. • Encourage client to rest between contractions. • Keep emesis basin nearby.
II. Expulsion Starts with complete cervical effacement and dilation and ends with delivery	• Strong • Upper part of uterus is active; lower part is passive	• Perineal bulging • Crowning of fetal head • Delivery of fetus	• Extension • External rotation • Expulsion	• Assist client to push. • Praise client, and keep her informed of her progress. • Maintain client's privacy.

Stages of labor *(continued)*

STAGE	CONTRACTION CHARACTERISTICS	MATERNAL PHYSICAL CHANGES	FETAL POSITION CHANGES	NURSING CARE
III. Placental stage Starts upon delivery of baby and ends with delivery of placenta and membranes	• Strong • Every 3 minutes	• Placental separation 5 minutes after delivery • Gush of blood • Descent of umbilical cord • Uterus rises in the abdomen and becomes globular • Placental expulsion		• Measure client's blood pressure. • Assess estimated blood loss. • Assess newborn. • Praise client, and provide information about client's and infant's status. • Administer oxytocin, as ordered.
IV. First hour post delivery	Not applicable	• Uterus contracted and usually midway between umbilicus and symphisis pubis • Lochia present • Perineum intact or site repaired		• Monitor client's vital signs, lochia, and fundus every 15 minutes. • Provide comfort measures, including warm blankets and perineal ice. • Introduce newborn to family, and encourage attachment behaviors.

2. Assess for signs of labor, as follows:

• Assess for contraction characteristics. (Mrs. DeShon's contraction characteristics indicate she is in the early phase of Stage I labor. During this phase, assess the contractions continuously with an electronic monitor or every 30 minutes by touch.)

2. Assessment routines for labor vary according to the setting, the available equipment, and the client's individual needs. The information included here is an example of assessments.

• Assessing contractions helps the nurse identify the client's stage and phase of labor and plan appropriate nursing care. The nurse should note the time the contractions began and their present frequency, duration, and intensity.

The fetal monitor continuously records uterine activity and FHT and displays this information in a number of ways: audible FHT, numerical FHT display, and a strip correlating FHT with the frequency, duration, and strength of contractions.

With external monitoring, the tocotransducer is placed over the fundus and the transducer over the fetal back; with internal monitoring, the monitoring catheter (pressure transducer) is placed inside the uterus to monitor contractions and an electrode is attached to the fetal scalp to monitor FHT.

Internal monitoring is more accurate. However, to insert the catheter and electrode, the membranes must be ruptured; in addition, the presenting part must be identified and must be low enough for safe attachment.

To monitor contractions by touch, the nurse places fingertips over the fundal area and evaluates the change in tone during several contractions and also times the duration and frequency of contractions.

• Assess the status of Mrs. DeShon's membranes.

The membranes may be intact, leaking, or ruptured. If the client is not sure of the status, test the vaginal secretions with nitrazine paper: Amniotic fluid, which is slightly alkaline (pH 7.2), will turn the paper dark blue. Also, ferning of the secretions indicates rupture of membranes. (The fern test is performed under a microscope.)

• Assess for bloody show.

• When the mucus plug is discharged, capillary bleeding may occur, making the discharge pink or bloody.

3. Assess Mrs. DeShon's vital signs on admission; then assess her pulse, respirations, and blood pressure every hour and her temperature every 4 hours, unless otherwise indicated.

3. The client's vital signs provide baseline information and contribute to overall assessment of maternal-fetal well-being. Pulse and blood pressure may be monitored more frequently.

4. Monitor FHTs, either continuously with an electronic monitor or every 30 minutes with a fetoscope or handheld ultrasound device.

4. The nurse should note FHTs routinely, as indicated throughout labor. FHTs should also be noted after rupture of membranes, and before and after medication is administered. (See *Early labor phase tracing*, page 262.)

5. Assess the results of the vaginal examination:

5. A vaginal examination is performed on admission and repeated as appropriate. During the early phase of Stage I labor, frequent examinations are not necessary.

• external examination

• Lesions (such as herpes lesions) and discharges noted during the external examination require further investigation and may alter the plan for delivery.

• internal examination (aseptic technique).

• The internal examination may indicate the degree of cervical dilation and effacement as well as fetal presentation, position, and station. The findings of Mrs. DeShon's vaginal examination confirm that she is in the early phase of Stage I labor.

6. Assess laboratory test results, as follows:

6. Laboratory tests are performed on admission to provide baseline information and to identify potential problems.

• urinalysis

• The client's urine may contain a small amount of glucose but should not contain protein or bacteria.

• complete blood count, hemoglobin, and hematocrit

• Blood test results reflect the client's general well-being and help identify problems, such as infection and excessive bleeding.

Electronic fetal monitoring

Electronic fetal monitoring (EFM) provides an objective means for evaluating fetal well-being and detecting fetal distress. This valuable assessment tool allows health care providers to obtain intermittent or continuous data about the fetal heart rate (FHR) and uterine activity during the antepartal and intrapartal periods. EFM may be performed with an internal or external method.

Nurses who care for clients on fetal monitors are expected to be able to test the equipment; obtain high-quality, legible tracings; interpret the tracings; take appropriate actions; communicate changes in fetal condition; and document observations and interventions. When analyzing EFM data, they must consider fetal gestational age, maternal medications, maternal temperature, hydration status, and other medical history data. The chart below lists indications for EFM and recommended monitoring frequency.

INTERPRETATION OF EFM TRACINGS

Use a systematic approach. First, determine baseline FHR from a tracing of at least 10 minutes, reading FHR between uterine contractions. Normal FHR is 120 to 160 beats per minute (bpm).

Next, assess for variability by checking for:
• changes that occur along the baseline
• presence of short-term beat-to-beat changes
• long-term FHR changes over time (more than 1 minute or three to five cycles). Less than a two-beat change indicates no variability; a three- to five-beat fluctuation, minimal variability; a six- to 10-beat fluctuation, average variability; an 11- to 25-beat fluctuation, moderate variability; and a fluctuation of more than 25 beats, marked variability. Also note any accelerations or decelerations. *Accelerations* are baseline FHR increases lasting less than 10 minutes; they are associated with a positive fetal outcome. *Decelerations* are decreases from the baseline lasting less than 10 minutes and may reflect fetal stress. They may be early, late, or variable.

Questionable FHRs require follow-up investigation.

DOCUMENTATION

When documenting a client's EFM strips, include the following information:
• baseline FHR
• short-term and long-term FHR variability
• accelerations
• decelerations
• fetal movements
• contractions

Use the sample chart entry below as a guideline for documentation. (*Note: STV* stands for short-term variability: *LTV* for long-term variability, and *UC* for uterine contractions.)

6/1/97   0700:   FHR baseline = 140. STV present, average LTV. 3 accelerations of 15 bpm x 20 secs., with 5 fetal movements/10 mins. No decelerations noted. U.C. q 5 mins. x 40 secs. duration with moderate intensity per palpation.

J. Lamp, RNC

INDICATIONS FOR EFM

• Any client whose obstetric or medical history puts her at risk, including clients with the following conditions:
—prolonged labor
—bleeding from placenta previa or abruption
—amnionitis
—preeclampsia
—diabetes mellitus
—meconium-stained amniotic fluid.

• The following intrapartal events:
—rupture of membranes
—oxytocin labor augmentation or induction
—administration of medications or anesthesia
—abnormal uterine activity patterns
—urinary catheterization
—vaginal examination
—ambulation.

RECOMMENDED MONITORING FREQUENCY

Low-risk clients:
• intermittently
• every hour during latent phase of labor
• every 30 minutes during active phase of labor
• every 15 minutes during second stage of labor

High-risk clients:
• continuously
• every 30 minutes during latent phase of labor
• every 15 minutes during active phase of labor
• every 5 minutes during second stage of labor

MATERNAL-
NEWBORN
NURSING

Early labor phase tracing

This tracing for Mrs. DeShon shows a normal fetal heart rate, with a baseline of 140 beats per minute. Short-term variability is present; long-term variability is average. No decelerations or accelerations appear. *Note:* Each dark vertical line marks 60 seconds.

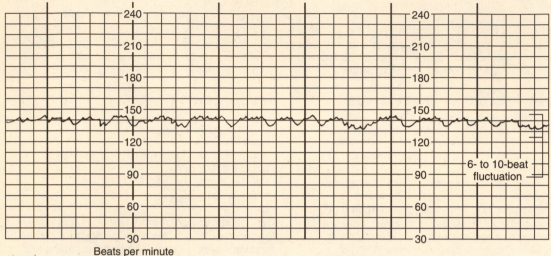

Beats per minute

This tracing shows latent-stage labor contractions, with a frequency of every 4 minutes and a duration of 30 seconds. Intensity is mild, with the acme at 30 mm Hg. Normal resting tone is 10 to 15 mm Hg.

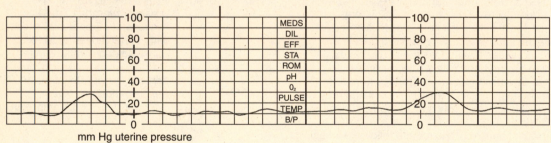

mm Hg uterine pressure

• vaginal cultures.

• Group B beta-streptococcal cultures may be obtained if the membranes ruptured more than 1 hour before onset of labor.

7. Assess Mr. and Mrs. DeShon's amount and type of childbirth preparation, including classes, relevant reading material, presence of a support person, and expectations.

7. Understanding the birthing process and developing useful coping techniques benefit the couple once labor begins. In general, the better prepared they are, the less fear they will have. Knowledge of the couple's preparations increases the nurse's effectiveness.

8. Assess Mr. and Mrs. DeShon's emotional status, particularly noting their verbal and nonverbal communication—willingness to talk, facial expressions, body language.

8. Changes in emotional status can be expected to accompany the labor experience and usually correspond to phases and stages of labor.

9. Assess for additional contributing data, as follows:

9. Additional admitting information supplements the data available to plan and implement care.

• edema

• Edema may indicate complications such as preeclampsia.

• rash

• A rash may indicate an infection.

• abdominal scars

• Abdominal scars should be investigated for possible involvement of the uterus.

• most recent intake of fluid or food

• Intestinal peristalsis decreases during labor. If the client has eaten recently, nausea and vomiting may occur; this factor must be considered if the client receives general anesthesia.

• prostheses, such as dentures, contact lenses, and glasses

• All prostheses must be removed before general anesthesia is administered.

• infant feeding plan.

• Breast-feeding can begin just after delivery.

Nursing diagnoses for various phases and stages of labor

• Pain related to uterine contractions and perineal stretching (Stage I labor)
• Risk for injury related to possible complications of delivery (Stage II labor)
• Risk for fluid volume deficit related to blood loss from delivery of the placenta (Stage III labor)
• Risk for injury (maternal, fetal) related to effects of analgesia and anesthesia (Stages I to IV)
• Altered family processes related to necessary adjustments in the new family unit (Stage IV labor)

Planning and goals

• Mrs. DeShon and her support person will express an accurate understanding of labor and delivery.
• Mrs. DeShon will ask questions to indicate her need for information.
• Mrs. DeShon will respond positively to the presence of a support person.
• Mrs. DeShon will be able to follow directions and assist with the birthing process.
• Mrs. DeShon and her fetus/infant will be free of complications during labor and delivery.
• Mr. and Mrs. DeShon will show signs of beginning attachment behaviors during Stage IV.

Implementation

NURSING BEHAVIORS

NURSING RATIONALES

1. Complete Mrs. DeShon's admission procedures as ordered.

1. The physician's admission orders are based on the client's individual needs. Perineal shaves and enema administration are no longer routine procedures.

2. Encourage Mrs. DeShon to void every 2 hours. Catheterize, as ordered and needed.

2. The nurse should assess the client's bladder throughout labor and encourage voiding to prevent trauma from distention, enhance comfort, and promote labor progress.

MATERNAL-NEWBORN NURSING

3. Monitor the I.V. site, solutions, and flow rate every hour.

3. Because she can take nothing by mouth, the client may receive I.V. fluids to prevent dehydration. Careful monitoring of I.V. fluid intake promotes safe administration throughout labor and delivery.

4. Provide comfort measures for Mrs. DeShon, as follows:

4. Cervical dilation, effacement, and contractions are uncomfortable. Narcotic analgesics are not administered in the early phase of labor because they may slow the labor process. Therefore, other comfort measures should be employed.

• Assist Mrs. DeShon with ambulation, if permitted.

• Walking may help relieve the client's discomfort and shorten labor. Activity need not be restricted even if the membranes have ruptured, provided the fetus's head is well applied to the cervix.

• If Mrs. DeShon is confined to bed, elevate the head of the bed, provide pillows for support, and encourage her to lie on her left side.

• Elevating the head of the bed, supporting the arms and legs, and maintaining a left-side-lying position help to prevent vena cava (supine hypotensive) syndrome.

• If necessary, encourage Mrs. DeShon to use the breathing and distraction techniques she has learned.

• Use of learned techniques should be delayed as long as possible: Once they are initiated, the client needs to concentrate and may tire more easily. She should not hold her breath during a contraction because the resulting overall tenseness may increase her discomfort.

• Encourage Mrs. DeShon to relax the pelvic floor muscles during the pelvic examination.

• Relaxing the pelvic floor muscles reduces resistance and makes the procedure more comfortable.

5. Provide emotional support, as follows:
• Orient Mrs. DeShon to her surroundings.
• Provide privacy, explain procedures, and answer questions.
• Reassess Mrs. DeShon's emotional status frequently.

5. The client will feel more secure if she is familiar with her surroundings, including how to call for assistance. The nurse promotes the client's trust by providing her with information and answering her questions throughout labor and delivery. Expected behaviors during the early phase of labor include excitement, willingness to talk, and slight anxiety.

Clinical situation
(continued)

Nursing care during the active phase of Stage I labor
Della DeShon's labor has progressed to the active phase, with strong contractions occurring every 3 minutes and lasting 45 seconds. At her most recent vaginal examination, her cervix was dilated 6 cm and 100% effaced; the vertex was at station +1. Her membranes have ruptured. The physician has ordered 50 mg of meperidine (Demerol) I.V. if needed.

Implementation
NURSING BEHAVIORS

NURSING RATIONALES

1. Monitor and record Mrs. DeShon's uterine contraction characteristics.

1. The nurse should assess contractions more frequently during the active phase to monitor labor progress and to plan the client's care.

Active labor phase tracing

This tracing for Mrs. DeShon shows a fetal heart rate of 150 beats per minute, with short-term variability and average long-term variability. An acceleration occurs with the first contraction. *Note:* Each dark vertical line marks 60 seconds.

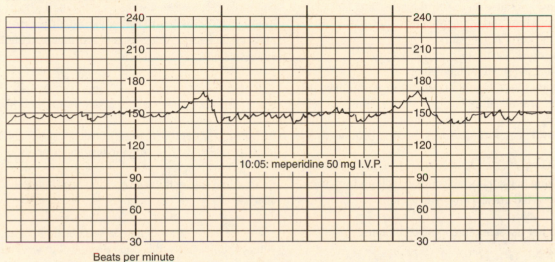

Beats per minute

This tracing shows active stage labor contractions, with a frequency of every 3 minutes and a duration of 45 seconds. Intensity is strong, with the acme between 50 and 60 mm Hg. Normal resting tone is 10 to 15 mm Hg. Note that the time of narcotic administration is documented.

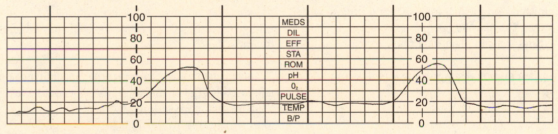

mm Hg uterine pressure

MATERNAL-NEWBORN NURSING

2. Obtain Mrs. DeShon's vital signs: Throughout her labor (unless otherwise indicated), take her temperature every 4 hours and assess her pulse, respirations, and blood pressure every 30 minutes.

3. Monitor and record FHTs, either continuously with an electronic monitor or every 30 minutes with a fetoscope.

4. Perform vaginal examinations only as necessary to determine cervical dilation.

2. Because active labor is more stressful physically, the client's risk of complications increases. Careful monitoring of vital signs helps detect complications early.

3. FHTs will indicate if additional care is needed. (See *Active labor phase tracing*.)

4. Although vaginal examinations are performed more frequently during active labor, the nurse should keep them to a minimum for client comfort and protection from infection.

5. Administer care related to rupture of membranes: Listen to FHTs, place a dry pad under Mrs. DeShon's buttocks, record the time of rupture and the appearance of amniotic fluid, and confine Mrs. DeShon to bed. If umbilical cord prolapse occurs, take the following action:
• Relieve pressure on the cord by elevating Mrs. DeShon's hips and lifting the presenting part away from the cord, if necessary.
• If the cord is exposed, apply moisture to it.
• Call the physician immediately.
• Prepare for emergency cesarean delivery if fetal distress is prolonged.

5. The membranes may rupture spontaneously or be ruptured artificially. After rupture, the nurse should immediately listen to FHTs for signs of distress. Umbilical cord prolapse may occur, especially if the presenting part is not engaged.

Signs and symptoms of fetal hypoxia include tachycardia (FHR above 180 beats per minute [bpm]), bradycardia (FHR below 100 bpm), an increase or decrease in fetal movements, and meconium-stained amniotic fluid.

6. Provide comfort measures for Mrs. DeShon, as follows:

6. The client's degree of comfort will affect her ability to cooperate and assist with the birthing process.

• Position her comfortably in bed, and perform sacral massage and assist with pelvic rocking.

• Sacral massage and pelvic rocking help relieve backache.

• Help her use learned coping techniques.

• Because active labor demands increased physical and emotional effort, the client may need to use coping techniques to deal with the discomfort.

• Apply a cool, moist cloth to her forehead.

• A cool, moist cloth can be refreshing.

• Administer pain medication (see *Pain management during the intrapartal period*) as ordered, keeping the bed side rails in place as a safety measure.

• Medication may be administered during active labor, with an assessment of FHTs before and after administration.

7. Provide emotional support for Mrs. DeShon.

7. During active labor, contractions become more uncomfortable. The client responds by becoming less talkative and more serious, self-centered, and anxious.

Clinical situation
(continued)

Nursing care during the transitional phase of Stage I labor

Della DeShon's labor has progressed so that her contractions are now very strong. She is perspiring profusely and she feels nauseated. Her cervix is dilated 8 cm, with the vertex at +1 station. These findings indicate she has reached the transitional phase of the first stage of labor. FHTs are within a normal range. She states she wants to push.

Implementation
NURSING BEHAVIORS

1. Monitor and record the characteristics of Mrs. DeShon's uterine contractions.

NURSING RATIONALES

1. As labor progresses, closer monitoring of the client is required. Assessments are the same as for active labor but are more frequent.

Pain management during the intrapartal period

Labor and delivery are accompanied by discomfort and pain. At some point during the pregnancy, the client and her health care provider should discuss the proposed pain-management plan. Options include psychoprophylaxis and hypnosis as well as analgesics and anesthetics. Pain perception and pain management are affected by the client's cultural background, knowledge of labor and delivery, coping skills, and anxiety level as well as the birthing environment and support person. For the high-risk client and fetus, pain relief involves individualized and cautious use of medications and anesthesia.

MEDICATIONS
In prescribing a medication for a woman in labor, the physician or midwife is aware that the fetus also is being treated. This factor affects the choice of drug as well as the route and time of administration. A drug that can slow the progress of labor will not be given until the labor is established, usually when the cervix is dilated 4 to 5 cm. Drugs that affect the establishment of respirations in the newborn will not be given if delivery and the drug's peak action time coincide. (See *Selected drugs commonly used in maternal-newborn nursing,* pages 325 to 329.)

ANESTHESIA
General anesthesia for a normal vaginal delivery is used selectively. It has the same implications for the pregnant woman as for any surgical client, with the additional concern that the fetus also can receive the anesthesia. Regional anesthesia acts only on the neuropathway that is being blocked. It may cause maternal hypotension, fetal bradycardia, and fetal lethargy.

Regional anesthesia administration and effects
Subarachnoid (spinal) block (A)
Local anesthetic injected through the dura directly into cerebrospinal fluid; provides anesthesia for delivery and episiotomy repair; may cause hypotension and postpartal headache.
Lumbar epidural block (B)
Local anesthetic injected outside of the dura in the epidural space; usually administered during the active labor phase and extends through delivery; provides anesthesia of contraction pain, perineal pain, and episiotomy repair; catheter may be left in place and may cause hypotension.
Pudendal block (C)
Local anesthetic injected near the ischial spines; provides anesthesia to the pudendal area for delivery and episiotomy repair
Nursing considerations
• Assist with the procedure.
• Encourage voiding.
• Monitor I.V. apparatus and maintain hydration.
• Monitor vital signs and fetal heart tones.
• Provide emotional support.
• Monitor progress of labor.
• Encourage pushing during the second stage of labor.
• Monitor closely for adverse reactions to the anesthetic agent.

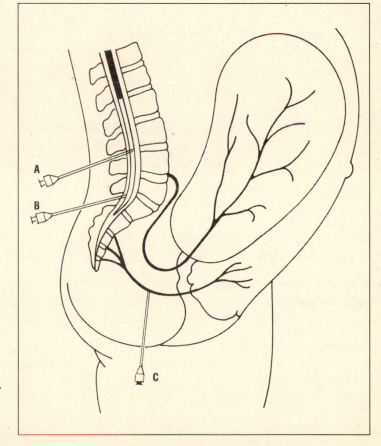

2. Monitor fetal status as follows:
• Assess and record FHTs, either continuously with an electronic monitor or every 15 minutes with a fetoscope, as indicated.
• Assess the amniotic fluid for meconium.

3. Perform a vaginal examination. (*Note:* A multigravida in transition requires closer reassessment.)

4. Assess for additional signs of transition: an increase in dark bloody show, nausea and vomiting, perspiration, skin irritability, and the urge to push.

5. Provide Mrs. DeShon with comfort measures during transition: a comfortable position in bed, assistance with learned coping techniques, moist cloths on the forehead and lips, dry bed pads, pelvic rocking, and a sacral massage if requested.

6. Do not allow Mrs. DeShon to push. Instead, encourage blowing or panting when she feels the urge to push.

7. Provide emotional support for the couple: Stay with them, and offer praise and encouragement.

2. Fetal status is assessed more frequently as labor intensifies. Meconium-stained amniotic fluid may signal fetal distress unless the fetus is in a breech position.

3. A multigravida in transition, with the presenting part descending, may progress rapidly through the second stage once dilation is complete.

4. Some or all of these signs commonly accompany the transitional phase.

5. Because transition can be demanding, the client may need to use more intense distraction techniques, including complicated breathing patterns. Besides a refreshing moist cloth for the forehead, another for the lips may be appreciated. The client may not want a sacral massage if her skin is irritated.

6. Pushing before the cervix is completely dilated may cause edema, obstruction, or laceration of the cervix. Blowing and panting make bearing down more difficult. The nurse should be alert for signs of hyperventilation.

7. Transition—considered the most difficult period of labor and delivery—can be overwhelming. The client does not want to be left alone and may fear losing self-control.

Clinical situation
(continued)

Nursing care during Stage II labor
Della DeShon, having completed the first stage of labor, appears relieved that she can now start to push with her contractions.

Implementation

NURSING BEHAVIORS

1. Monitor and record the characteristics of each contraction during Stage II labor.

2. Monitor and record fetal status, as follows:
• Assess FHTs every 15 minutes or after each contraction.
• Reassess for signs of distress.

3. Perform a vaginal examination to determine station. (*Note:* A multigravida requires more frequent reassessments.)

NURSING RATIONALES

1. As the time of delivery nears, closer monitoring is required.

2. A pattern of early decelerations may be noted, indicating head compression as the fetus proceeds through the birth canal. (See *Stage II labor tracing.*)

3. A multigravida usually progresses more rapidly through Stage II labor.

MATERNAL-NEWBORN NURSING

Stage II labor tracing

This tracing for Mrs. DeShon shows early decelerations, which indicate fetal head compression during contractions and pushing. *Note:* Each dark vertical line marks 60 seconds.

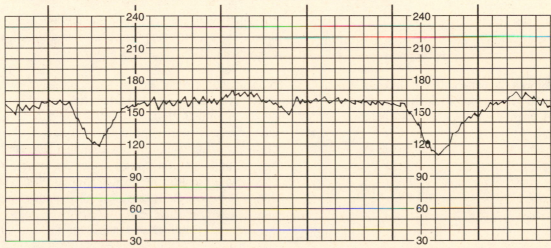

Beats per minute

This tracing shows contractions occurring every 2 minutes and lasting 60 seconds. Note that when the client pushes, uterine pressure can reach 80 to 100 mm Hg, or even higher.

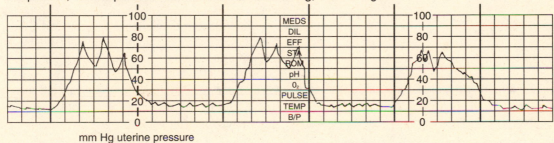

mm Hg uterine pressure

4. Be alert for other signs and symptoms of Stage II labor: increased bloody show, the urge to push, uncontrollable leg shaking, perineal bulging, crowning, and rectal bulging.

5. Teach Mrs. DeShon to use her abdominal muscles to push with the contractions.

6. Provide comfort measures, and encourage Mrs. DeShon to rest between contractions.

7. When crowning begins, prepare Mrs. DeShon for delivery, as follows:

4. As the fetus moves through the birth canal, the presenting part puts pressure on the surrounding tissues, and the woman may experience these signs and symptoms.

5. Using abdominal muscles to bear down with the contractions will assist in moving the fetus through the birth canal.

6. Besides the comfort measures used during transition, the client needs rest between contractions.

7. A primigravida usually takes longer than a multigravida to progress through Stage II labor. Thus, the nurse should prepare a primigravida for delivery when crowning begins and a multigravida during transition.

• Position her in the birthing bed, chair, delivery table, or position of choice, as indicated. If the delivery table is used, place the client's legs in the stirrups at the same time (and remove them at the same time after delivery).

• This technique helps prevent strain on the tissues.

• Cleanse the perineum.

• The perineum is cleansed with an antiseptic solution, using the principle of cleaning from a clean area to a soiled one.

8. Assist with the delivery by encouraging Mrs. DeShon to pant or blow as the head is delivered. If needed, provide forceps or equipment for episiotomy repair.

8. Panting or blowing decreases the possibility of forceful expulsion of the head. Forceps—most commonly low or outlet forceps—may be used to facilitate delivery. They are applied when the fetal head is below the ischial spines and are used to lift the head over the perineum. The physician may perform an episiotomy to facilitate delivery, to shorten Stage II labor, or to prevent lacerations. The midline incision is used whenever possible.

Perineal lacerations and episiotomy incisions are classified by degrees: first-degree are the most superficial and fourth-degree the most extensive. If the client has a third- or fourth-degree laceration or episiotomy incision, nothing should be administered rectally.

Cervical lacerations should be suspected if the client has excessive vaginal bleeding while the fundus remains firm.

9. Continue to provide emotional support, praise, and encouragement for the DeShons.

9. Once permitted to push, the client typically gains renewed energy, regains a feeling of control, and responds well to encouragement.

10. Allow the DeShons to touch their newborn as soon as possible.

10. Early family interaction enhances the bonding process. (For more information on the bonding process, see "Psychological responses during the postpartal period," page 286.)

Clinical situation
(continued)

Nursing care during Stages III and IV of labor and delivery
Della DeShon has delivered a 7-lb, 9-oz boy without complications. Both parents appear very happy and relieved.

Implementation
NURSING BEHAVIORS

NURSING RATIONALES

1. Administer oxytocic medication, such as oxytocin (Pitocin) or methylergonovine maleate (Methergine), during Stage III labor, as ordered.

1. When the placenta separates from the uterine wall, bleeding occurs. Oxytocics help control bleeding by contracting the myometrium and constricting the blood vessels.

2. Provide a blanket if Mrs. DeShon is chilled.

2. The client may feel chilled from loss of body heat, weight, and fluids, or simply from excitement.

3. Provide newborn care as follows:

• Maintain a patent airway.

• Stimulate the newborn's respirations.

• Record the newborn's Apgar score (evaluating heart rate, respirations, muscle tone, reflex irritability, and color) at 1 and 5 minutes after birth. (See *Apgar scoring system for neonates,* page 272.)

• Keep the newborn warm.

• Administer eye prophylaxis by applying an antibiotic ointment, as ordered. Erythromycin base (Ilotycin) is most commonly ordered.

• Complete the required identification procedures: footprints, fingerprints, and bracelets.

• Perform a preliminary cephalocaudal assessment.

4. Monitor Mrs. DeShon closely during Stage IV labor. Every 15 minutes, monitor her vital signs and perform a postpartal assessment, as follows:

• Note the consistency and position of the fundus. It should be firm and located in the midline, near the level of the umbilicus or lower. If it is not firm, massage it to stimulate contraction.

• Assess for bladder distention, and encourage Mrs. DeShon to void.

• Assess the amount and appearance of lochia.

3. The immediate care of the newborn is performed according to priorities.

• Suction may be needed to clear the airway. The nurse should suction the newborn's mouth first, then the nose, keeping the head in a dependent position for mucus drainage.

• Gently rubbing the newborn's back helps stimulate respirations.

• Apgar scoring provides an immediate assessment of the newborn's condition; each of five areas of observation receives a maximum score of 2. A total score of 7 to 10 is good; 4 to 6, fair; and below 4, poor.

• Because the newborn's temperature-regulating mechanism is immature, the nurse must keep the infant warm to prevent cold stress.

• The medication, used to prevent conjunctivitis and blindness that could result from a maternal infection (such as gonorrhea or chlamydia), should be administered within the first hour after birth or after initial parent-newborn bonding.

• Proper identification is a safety consideration.

• This brief assessment helps rule out obvious injuries and anomalies. A more complete assessment, including gestational age, is performed later.

4. Close monitoring during the first few hours after delivery is important in preventing and managing complications. Vital signs reflect the client's general well-being and alert the caregiver to possible complications. The frequent postpartal assessment reflects the client's immediate physical response to delivery.

• The fundus must remain firm to control bleeding.

• The bladder should be observed for filling. Voiding is encouraged because a full bladder may displace the uterus and prevent it from contracting properly.

• In Stage IV, lochia flow is heavy and bright red and may contain clots. A soaked perineal pad contains about 100 ml of blood; saturation of more than 1 perineal pad in 30 minutes indicates excessive bleeding.

MATERNAL-
NEWBORN
NURSING

Apgar scoring system for neonates

The Apgar test rates a neonate's condition at 1 minute after delivery and again at 5 minutes after delivery. The following scores denote the neonate's condition: 10, excellent; 7 to 9, adequate; 4 to 6, the neonate needs close observation; below 4, the neonate needs immediate care and further evaluation. *Note:* If the neonate's natural skin color is not white, alternative tests for color are applied, such as color of oral and conjunctival mucous membranes, lips, palms of hands, and soles of feet. Learn this useful mnemonic for remembering the signs in the Apgar scoring system: **A**—Appearance; **P**—Pulse; **G**—Grimace; **A**—Attitude (tone); **R**—Respirations.

SIGN	SCORE		
	0	1	2
Heart rate	Absent	Below 100 beats/minute	Above 100 beats/minute
Respiratory effort	Absent	Slow, irregular	Good, crying
Muscle tone	Flaccid	Some flexion of extremities	Active motion
Reflex irritability	No response	Grimace	Vigorous cry
Color	Blue, pale	Body pink, extremities blue	Completely pink

• Assess the perineum for intactness, hematomas, and hemorrhoids. Observe for approximation of perineal repair.

• A hematoma may form because of tissue trauma. The usual treatment consists of applying ice initially to minimize swelling, then applying heat. Hemorrhoids may have developed because of the trauma of labor and delivery.

5. Provide comfort measures for Mrs. DeShon: a comfortable position in bed, proper hygiene (bathing, changing linen and bed pads), and rest periods.

5. Ensuring the client's comfort contributes to her feelings of well-being.

6. Provide nourishment for Mrs. DeShon.

6. Labor and delivery require tremendous muscular activity and energy. The client may be hungry and thirsty after this experience.

7. Continue to provide emotional support to the new parents.

7. Continued emotional support from the nurse enhances beginning attachment behaviors and promotes family integration. (For more information on the bonding process, see "Psychological responses during the postpartal period," page 286.)

Evaluation

• Mrs. DeShon and fetus maintain physical parameters within normal limits throughout labor.
• Mrs. DeShon progresses through labor without complications.
• Mrs. DeShon responds positively to nursing coaching during labor and delivery.
• Mr. and Mrs. DeShon participate effectively during the delivery of their infant.
• Mrs. DeShon's delivery is uncomplicated, and she and the infant are healthy.
• Mr. and Mrs. DeShon appear comfortable with their baby and are displaying beginning attachment behaviors.

MATERNAL-NEWBORN NURSING

Dystocia and cesarean section delivery

Labor and delivery are normal processes; however, the nurse must be aware of complications that can significantly increase the risks involved. Dystocia—prolonged, difficult labor—is associated with one or more of the following problems: uterine muscle inertia or dysfunction from overstretching of the uterine wall, excess analgesic intake, or uterine anomalies; excessive fetal size; fetal anomalies; malpresentations; and contracted maternal pelvis. Anxiety and fear also can impede labor progress.

Indications for cesarean delivery include transverse lie or breech presentation, fetal distress, dystocia and failure to progress, prolapsed cord, abruptio placentae, placenta previa, and active vaginal herpes. However, cesarean delivery is not always related to a complication of labor and delivery; sometimes it is a planned, positive experience.

The following clinical situation focuses on care of the client experiencing dystocia, followed by cesarean delivery.

Clinical situation

Mae Flowers, gravida 3, para 2, has been in labor for 14 hours. Her membranes ruptured 6 hours ago. A pelvic examination reveals the same findings as those from an examination 2 hours earlier: Her cervix is dilated 6 cm and 100% effaced, and the presenting part is at -2 station. An I.V. infusion has been started. The fetal heart rate (FHR) is 152 beats per minute (bpm); variability is minimal to average, with intermittent decelerations. Her contractions have become less frequent and less intense (a hypotonic pattern), and Mrs. Flowers and her husband sense that something is wrong. The physician orders ultrasonographic studies and considers a cesarean delivery.

Assessment

NURSING BEHAVIORS

1. Assess Mrs. Flowers for signs and symptoms associated with dystocia: abnormal uterine contraction patterns, delayed cervical progress, and delayed descent of the presenting part.

2. Assess fetal heart tones (FHTs), fetal activity, and amniotic fluid to detect possible fetal distress. Assist with fetal scalp blood sampling for pH.

3. Assess Mrs. Flowers for signs of infection, such as by obtaining vital signs and a white blood cell count.

NURSING RATIONALES

1. Normal labor contractions increase in frequency, duration, and intensity. Dystocia is diagnosed in a primigravida if the latent phase lasts more than 20 hours or if cervical dilation does not progress more than 1.2 cm/hour in the active phase; in a multigravida, if the latent phase lasts more than 14 hours or if cervical dilation does not progress more than 1.5 cm/hour in the active phase. Delay in descent of the presenting part also indicates dystocia.

2. Prolonged labor compromising the fetal oxygen supply may cause fetal distress, indicated by abnormal FHTs, fetal hyperactivity, and meconium-stained amniotic fluid. Fetal scalp pH indicates the acid-base balance of the fetus. (See *Tracing showing fetal distress,* page 274.)

3. After rupture of the membranes, the fetus and uterus are vulnerable to infection, with the incidence of infection rising in proportion to the time between membrane rupture and delivery.

MATERNAL-NEWBORN NURSING

Tracing showing fetal distress

This tracing for Mrs. Flowers shows mild fetal distress caused by hypoxia. The baseline fetal heart rate (FHR) is 152 beats per minute. Long-term variability is minimal to average, with intermittent decelerations. When a fetal scalp blood sample is taken, there may be no change or the stimulus may increase the FHR; the acceleration could be more than or equal to 15 beats per minute above baseline for 15 seconds or more. Results show a scalp pH of 7.22, indicating a low-normal value; continue to monitor fetus. *Note:* Each dark vertical line marks 60 seconds.

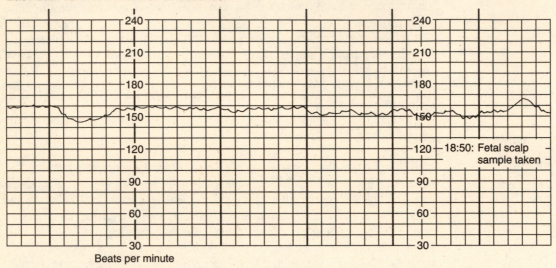

Beats per minute

This tracing indicates uterine dystocia. The hypotonic pattern shows decreasing frequency of contractions.

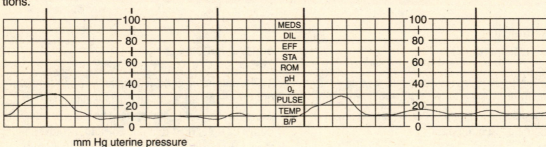

mm Hg uterine pressure

4. Assess Mrs. Flowers for adequate hydration.

4. Prolonged periods of taking nothing by mouth may lead to dehydration.

5. Observe Mr. and Mrs. Flowers's energy level and emotional state.

5. Little physical discomfort is associated with hypotonic contractions; however, prolonged labor can cause exhaustion and anxiety.

Nursing diagnoses

• Anxiety related to an unexpectedly prolonged labor and possible cesarean section
• Risk for infection related to the surgical procedure

Planning and goals

- Mrs. Flowers will not experience high levels of anxiety or exhaustion.
- The fetus will not develop signs of distress.
- Mrs. Flowers will not develop signs of infection.
- Mrs. Flowers will be well hydrated during labor and delivery.
- Mrs. Flowers will ask questions to indicate her need for information.
- Mrs. Flowers will verbalize understanding of the procedures related to a cesarean delivery.
- Mrs. Flowers will not develop postpartal complications.
- As appropriate, Mr. and Mrs. Flowers will verbalize acceptance of the need for cesarean delivery.

Implementation

NURSING BEHAVIORS	NURSING RATIONALES
1. Continuously monitor FHTs and Mrs. Flowers's uterine contractions.	**1.** Continuous monitoring provides a more accurate record of the FHT pattern and helps identify abnormal uterine contraction patterns.
2. Keep pelvic examinations to a minimum, and record Mrs. Flowers's vital signs every 2 hours.	**2.** These measures help prevent or detect infection. Minimizing pelvic examinations limits exposure of the fetus and birth canal to possible contamination. One of the earliest signs of infection is an elevated temperature.
3. Record Mrs. Flowers's intake and output. An I.V. bolus may be ordered.	**3.** Recording intake and output provides an accurate record and helps determine the adequacy of I.V. fluids. An I.V. bolus may increase maternal cardiac output.
4. Provide comfort measures, such as baths, freshened bed linen, back rubs, and position changes, as needed.	**4.** Keeping Mrs. Flowers comfortable will help her relax.
5. Prepare Mr. and Mrs. Flowers for ultrasonographic studies by explaining the procedure to the couple and answering their questions. Transport Mrs. Flowers to the radiology department, and remain with her during the procedure.	**5.** The client and her partner may be apprehensive. Adequate preparation for the ultrasonographic procedure provides support and helps calm their fears.
6. Administer an amnioinfusion, as ordered.	**6.** This will correct oligohydramnios and dilute the thick, meconium-stained amniotic fluid.

Clinical situation

(continued)

Preoperative nursing care for cesarean delivery

The ultrasonographic study results for Mae Flowers indicate cephalopelvic disproportion. The physician orders preparation for a cesarean delivery.

Implementation

NURSING BEHAVIORS	NURSING RATIONALES
1. Implement orders for routine preoperative care.	**1.** Refer to "Preoperative period" in Perioperative Nursing, on pages 123 and 124.

MATERNAL-NEWBORN NURSING

2. Shave Mrs. Flowers's abdominal-perineal area as ordered.

2. Hair, which harbors bacteria, is removed from the surgical site to reduce the risk of infection.

3. Insert an indwelling urinary catheter.

3. The anatomic relationship of the bladder to the uterus places the bladder at risk for trauma during uterine surgery. The indwelling urinary catheter is inserted to keep the bladder deflated, protecting it from trauma.

4. Administer a preoperative medication (such as an antianxiety agent), as ordered.

4. Antianxiety agents (such as benzodiazepines) are commonly used to calm the client and prepare her for anesthesia. Narcotics are not given to the client preoperatively because they may cause respiratory depression in the newborn if administered near delivery time.

5. Continue to monitor maternal-fetal status, assessing vital signs, uterine contractions, FHTs, and amniotic fluid.

5. Continual assessments ensure prompt detection of any potentially deleterious changes to the mother or the fetus.

6. Provide emotional support for Mr. and Mrs. Flowers.

6. When plans for delivery are changed, the client is likely to show signs of anxiety, anger, guilt, and feelings of failure. The nurse should spend time with the couple, responding appropriately to their needs. If possible and desired by the father, he should be allowed to attend the delivery.

Clinical situation
(continued)

Postoperative nursing care for cesarean delivery
Mae Flowers was delivered of a 10-lb, 12-oz boy by low-segment cesarean section. She and her new son are in good condition.

Implementation
NURSING BEHAVIORS

NURSING RATIONALES

1. Provide routine postoperative care for Mrs. Flowers.

1. Refer to "Postoperative period" in Perioperative Nursing, on page 125.

2. Perform a postpartal assessment of Mrs. Flowers, checking the breasts, fundus, abdominal dressing or incision, and lochia.

2. After a cesarean delivery, routine postpartal assessments are performed. A client who has had a cesarean delivery may not have as much lochia as one who has delivered vaginally.

3. Assess Mrs. Flowers for signs of infection, such as a temperature above 100.4° F (38° C) after the first 24 hours, foul-smelling lochia, and pain.

3. An infection may stem from a break in aseptic technique or from inflammation of the uterine lining.

4. Assess Mrs. Flowers for signs of hemorrhage, such as decreased blood pressure, rapid pulse and respirations, pallor, restlessness, perspiration, and excessive lochia.

4. Hemorrhage may result from surgical complications or from failure of the uterus to contract.

MATERNAL-NEWBORN NURSING

5. Assess Mrs. Flowers for signs of pelvic or femoral phlebitis.

5. Because of increased fibrinogen levels present during pregnancy and the prolonged recovery period, a client who has had a cesarean section delivery is considered to be at increased risk for phlebitis and thrombi.

6. Provide pain-relief measures as indicated and ordered for Mrs. Flowers: For incisional pain, administer an analgesic as ordered. For pain from flatus, turn Mrs. Flowers frequently, and assist her with ambulation.

6. The client may have incisional pain for several days after surgery. The client should walk as soon as possible to promote peristalsis, prevent complications, and restore feelings of well-being.

7. Teach Mrs. Flowers routine postpartal self-care and the importance of ambulation.

7. These measures help prevent infection and enhance circulation.

8. If Mrs. Flowers seems to need additional postpartal emotional support, provide appropriate referrals.

8. Women who have had cesarean deliveries may need additional support; some find support groups helpful for discussing their concerns with women who have had similar experiences.

Evaluation

- Mrs. Flowers is comfortable and remains in control.
- Mrs. Flowers does not develop an infection.
- Mrs. Flowers remains well hydrated throughout labor and delivery.
- Mr. and Mrs. Flowers state acceptance of the need for cesarean section delivery.
- Mrs. Flowers and her baby have an uncomplicated delivery and recovery.
- By the time of discharge, Mrs. Flowers can perform basic postpartal self-care and newborn care.
- By the time of discharge, Mrs. Flowers is ambulatory and expresses feelings of well-being.

POSTPARTAL PERIOD

Physiologic responses during the postpartal period

The postpartal period, or puerperium, begins with Stage IV labor and lasts approximately 6 weeks. During this period, the woman's reproductive organs return to their nonpregnant state. Knowledge of normal physiologic changes during the postpartal period enables the nurse to recognize deviations and provide early intervention.

The following clinical situation focuses on physical care during the early postpartal period.

Clinical situation

You are assigned to care for Della DeShon, a 24-year-old primigravida who delivered a 7-lb, 9-oz male infant 12 hours ago by spontaneous vaginal delivery over a midline episiotomy. Mr. DeShon was present to support his wife during labor and delivery, which were uncomplicated. Although the couple did not attend childbirth preparation classes, the recovery room nurse commented, "They worked together well as a couple and seemed very happy about the baby." The infant's Apgar score was 8 at 1 minute after birth and 9 at 5 minutes.

Assessment

NURSING BEHAVIORS	NURSING RATIONALES
1. Obtain baseline information about Mrs. DeShon's history and delivery: gravida and para, date and time of delivery, use of anesthesia and analgesia, and course of labor and delivery.	**1.** By comparing the client's data base with normative data on physiologic postpartal adaptation, the nurse can recognize problems quickly and intervene early.
2. Identify the components of Mrs. DeShon's support system besides the child's father.	**2.** The presence of significant others, including other children, relatives, and friends, provides support for the new mother and helps reduce fears and anxieties.
3. Obtain parenting information and information about the parents' value system and beliefs.	**3.** Individual care can be provided only when the nurse knows the parents' desires. Begin to develop a discharge plan of care.
4. Assess the infant's condition.	**4.** An immediate assessment of the infant's current status provides information needed to establish priorities of care.
5. Determine the family's plans for care of the infant.	**5.** The nurse should know whether the infant will be cared for by family members or whether other alternatives, such as adoption, are being considered.
6. Assess Mrs. DeShon's vital signs as follows:	**6.** Alterations in vital signs may indicate complications (see *Postpartal complications*). Vital signs should be evaluated in light of the client's history and clinical symptoms.
• temperature	• No systemic postpartal infection is indicated if the client's body temperature is within normal limits and other clinical signs of infection are absent. If stress or fatigue causes chills immediately after delivery, keep the client warm. Her temperature may rise to 100.4° F (38° C) after delivery but should stabilize to normal within 24 hours.
• blood pressure	• The client's blood pressure may increase immediately after delivery because of excitement and physical exertion but soon after should stabilize or fluctuate only minimally. A slight decrease may reflect blood loss and a decrease in circulating blood volume. A significant decrease may indicate bleeding, a reaction to medication, or delayed involution.
• pulse	• Postpartal bradycardia (a rate of 50 to 70 beats/minute) may occur during the first 6 to 10 days after birth because of decreased cardiac strain, decreased vascular bed, increased stroke volume, and contraction of the uterus. Tachycardia (rare) may indicate increased blood loss or a reaction to a difficult and prolonged labor and delivery.

Postpartal complications

COMPLICATIONS	CAUSES	SIGNS AND SYMPTOMS	NURSING INTERVENTIONS
Postpartal infection (one of the most common causes of maternal death)	Traumatic labor and delivery and postpartal hemorrhage make client more susceptible to invasion by such bacteria as nonhemolytic streptococci, *Escherichia coli,* and *Staphylococcus* species. Also, prolonged rupture of membranes may result in postpartal infection.	Depend on location and severity of infection and usually include fever, pain, swelling, and tenderness. Temperature of 100.4° F (38° C) or more after first 24 hours postpartal may indicate puerperal infection.	• Monitor for signs and symptoms and drainage (such as uterine); perform culture and sensitivity studies, as ordered. • Administer antibiotic therapy, as ordered. • Keep client comfortable and quiet. • Prevent spread of infection, such as by using universal precautions and isolation, if needed. • Force fluids and provide a high-calorie diet. • Keep parents and family informed of the mother's and infant's progress. • Promote maternal-infant contact as soon as possible. • Teach proper hygiene and asepsis. • Maintain follow-up care after discharge.
Perineal infection	Laceration and trauma of perineum facilitate the invasion of bacteria.	Localized pain, fever, swelling, redness, and seropurulent drainage	• Administer antibiotics and analgesics; recommend sitz baths or other heat applications.
Endometritis	Bacteria invade placental site and may spread to entire endometrium.	Temperature, chills, anorexia, malaise, boggy uterus, foul-smelling lochia, and cramps	• Administer antibiotics and ergonovine maleate, as ordered. • Recommend Fowler's position to promote drainage. • Force fluids.
Thrombophlebitis	Thrombus formation in deep or superficial vein in response to inflammation of vein wall.	• Chills and fever • Femoral: stiffness of affected area or part and positive Homans' sign • Pelvic: severe chills and wide fluctuations in temperature	• Assess the client for predisposing factors: obesity, advanced age, high parity, history of venous thrombosis, postoperative status, and varicosities. • Femoral thrombi: Rest and elevate leg; apply heat or ice to leg; administer antibiotics, analgesics, and anticoagulants, as ordered. • Pelvic thrombi: Encourage bed rest and force fluids; administer anticoagulants and antibiotics, as ordered.
Mastitis	Usually, *Staphylococcus aureus* from nose and mouth of infant invades lactational system if there are lesions or fissures of nipples. With stasis, breast milk is a good medium for growth of organism. Most commonly, mastitis arises 2 to 4 weeks' after delivery.	• Marked engorgement, pain, chills, fever, tachycardia • If untreated, single or multiple breast abscesses may form.	• Arrange culture and sensitivity studies of mother's milk. • Administer antibiotics and analgesics, as ordered. • Locally apply heat; assist with incising and draining abscesses. • Perform meticulous hand washing. • Encourage breast-feeding or use of manual breast pump, unless ordered otherwise.

(continued)

MATERNAL-NEWBORN NURSING

Postpartal complications (continued)

COMPLICATIONS	CAUSES	SIGNS AND SYMPTOMS	NURSING INTERVENTIONS
Postpartal hemorrhage (leading cause of maternal death worldwide)	• Uterine atony is principal cause. • Early postpartal hemorrhage occurs within first 24 hours after delivery and usually is caused by uterine atony, lacerations, mismanagement of Stage III labor, disseminated intravascular coagulation, or incomplete separation of placenta. • Late postpartal hemorrhage occurs from 24 hours up to 28 days after delivery and is caused by subinvolution of the uterus and retained placental fragments.	• Persistent or excessive blood loss • 500 ml or more of blood loss after delivery (500 ml weighs 1 lb) • Dark red—venous • Bright red—arterial • Boggy uterus • Spurts with clots may be caused by partial separation of placenta.	• Monitor blood loss. • Prevent improper management of Stage III labor. • Medical intervention is based on underlying cause. • Massage fundus if not firm. • Check vital signs every 30 minutes. • Check temperature every 4 hours. • Keep client's bladder empty. • Administer I.V. oxytocin as ordered (for example, 30 units Pitocin in 1,000 ml dextrose 5% in water may be ordered for rapid administration). • Use a face mask to administer oxygen 6 liters/minute. • Institute antishock therapy (see "Shock," pages 103 to 108). • Comfort client and family and inform them of treatments and progress to allay anxiety.

• respirations.

• Breath sounds for all lung lobes should be clear on auscultation. Respirations should be normal.

7. Assess the condition of Mrs. DeShon's breasts, as follows:

7. The client's breasts should be smooth and not tender. Depending on the postpartal day, the breasts may be soft, filling, full, or engorged.

• Check the fit and support provided by the client's bra.

• A well-fitted bra provides support for the breasts. The client who does not have a bra should be helped to obtain one from home.

• Check the nipples for fissures, cracks, soreness, and erectibility. Teach methods to prevent or relieve nipple trauma.

• Nipple problems may interfere with breast-feeding (see "The client who is breast-feeding," pages 306 to 310).

• Palpate the breasts for heat, edema, and engorgement.

• Heat and edema, which may be associated with mastitis, should not be present. Engorgement may occur on the third to the fifth postpartal day; the breasts become firm and tender from lymphatic or venous stasis. Engorgement typically subsides within 48 hours and is not accompanied by fever. (Preventive care makes engorgement unlikely, however.)

• Ask Mrs. DeShon if she has breast pain.

• Breast pain may accompany engorgement or may be associated with mastitis. Persistent pain should be evaluated by the physician.

• Evaluate Mrs. DeShon's milk production.

8. Palpate Mrs. DeShon's bladder for distention; her urine output may reach 3,000 ml/24 hours. Ask her if she has urinary frequency, urgency, or dysuria (pain).

9. Assess Mrs. DeShon's uterus and abdomen (uterine fundus), as follows:

• Once per shift, with Mrs. DeShon's bladder empty, check her uterine fundus for height, position, firmness, and tenderness. Chart your findings according to institutional policy (for example, U ↓ 3 or U ↑ 1). Massage the fundus if it is boggy (soft).

• If Mrs. DeShon appears to be at risk for involution problems, administer an oxytocic medication, such as 0.2 mg of oral methylergonovine maleate (Methergine), as ordered. Closely monitor Mrs. DeShon's blood pressure.

• Assess Mrs. DeShon's abdominal wall, and listen for bowel sounds. Expect the midline muscles to be weak and lax. Note any appearance of separation (diastasis recti).

• The client's breasts secrete colostrum for 2 to 3 days after delivery (true milk takes about 3 days to form).

8. Medication given at delivery may decrease the feeling of a full bladder. A full bladder may cause the uterus to relax by displacing it and interfering with its contractility. Marked diuresis normally occurs within 12 hours after delivery as reversal of the water metabolism of pregnancy causes the bladder to fill rapidly. Also, the stress of labor and delivery, and particularly of trauma, may cause edema and urethral spasm with pain.

9. The nurse assesses the client's uterine fundus not only to observe the progress of involution but also to detect early signs of complications that could prolong postpartal recovery. Involution occurs more quickly in a primigravida and in a woman who is breast-feeding (sucking stimulates the release of oxytocin).

• The uterus, normally situated in midline, can be palpated between the symphysis pubis and umbilicus. Immediately after delivery, the uterus should contract firmly to the size of a large grapefruit, then continue to decrease in size, reaching its nonpregnant state within 6 weeks. Decreased uterine size reflects decreased size of the myometrial cells.

Within 12 hours after delivery, the uterine fundus rises to 1 finger breadth (1 cm) above the umbilicus; on each succeeding day, it descends 1 to 2 finger breadths (1 to 2 cm). If it rises more than 1 finger breadth above the umbilicus, deviates from the midline, or feels boggy, the mother may have a distended bladder.

• Although no longer used routinely and capable of causing painful uterine contractions, an oxytocic medication may be ordered for a client at risk for involution problems from prolonged labor, hemorrhage, or uterine overdistention during pregnancy. Methergine may cause elevated blood pressure and should not be administered to a client who is receiving oxycodone hydrochloride (Percodan) for pain because the combination of drugs may cause hallucinations.

• Bowel sounds should be present in all four quadrants.

MATERNAL-NEWBORN NURSING

10. Assess Mrs. DeShon's lochia for color, amount, and odor, as follows:
• Lochia rubra is dark red and typically flows for 2 to 3 days after delivery (persistent lochia rubra indicates subinvolution or late postpartal hemorrhage). It should not contain clots. Lochia serosa is brownish pink (serosanguineous) and flows from approximately the 3rd to the 10th day. Lochia alba is whitish yellow and is seldom seen in the hospital.
• Flow is heavier in the morning than at night, when lochia pools in the vagina. The amount is usually scant to moderate.
• Lochia odor is musty but should not be foul.

11. Assess Mrs. DeShon's episiotomy (if present), using the REEDA scale: redness, edema, ecchymosis, discharge, approximation. Note any lacerations or hematomas, and evaluate perineal healing.

12. Assess Mrs. DeShon's anal area, noting any tenderness and the number and size of hemorrhoids.

13. Assess Mrs. DeShon's comfort and energy levels.

14. Weigh Mrs. DeShon and record her postpartal weight loss.

15. Check the results of Mrs. DeShon's laboratory tests, as follows:

• hemoglobin

• hematocrit

• white blood cell (WBC) count

10. As the placental site sloughs, the endometrium regenerates. The amount and character of lochia are assessed to detect hemorrhage and to evaluate the ability of the postpartal uterus to rid itself of debris, such as blood, decidual tissue, mucus, epithelial cells, and blood clots. A few small clots are normal. The passage of large amounts of lochia and large clots is associated with hemorrhage.

11. Causes of perineal trauma during delivery include tissue stretching and tearing and episiotomy. The REEDA scale provides a systematic approach to evaluating an episiotomy (or cesarean incision).

12. Tissue trauma and hemorrhoids may cause discomfort.

13. A wide range of emotional responses is normal: The client may be fatigued and uncomfortable or excited and exuberant.

14. Immediate postpartal weight loss averages about 10 to 12 lb; additional loss occurs from elimination of excess tissue fluids and from decreasing plasma volume. Most hospitals do not require a weight postpartally before discharge.

15. Pregnancy-related changes in blood values may continue for some time, varying with each client, but blood values usually return to normal by the end of the postpartal period.

• Hemoglobin should not be less than 2 g/dl below the client's level at admission.

• Hematocrit should be within 3% of the client's admission level. A 2-point drop in hematocrit reflects 1 pint of blood loss.

• Leukocytosis with an elevated WBC count of 15,000 to 25,000 is a normal body defense against postpartal infection and a normal response to the healing process.

• blood typing and Rh factor	• As ordered (for fetal protection in subsequent pregnancies), give Rh_o (D) immune globulin (RhoGAM) within 72 hours after delivery if the mother is Rh-negative and the infant is Rh-positive, if an indirect Coombs' test is negative (no Rh antibodies), or if a direct Coombs' test (on cord blood) is negative.
• rubella titer	• For fetal protection in subsequent pregnancies, rubella vaccination in the early postpartal period is recommended for women who have not been vaccinated or who have low rubella titers (1:8 or less).
• urinalysis.	• The client's urine should not contain glucose, protein, or bacteria. Red blood cells may result from a specimen contaminated with lochia or may represent true hematuria from a bladder infection. The specimen should be obtained midstream or by catheterization. The specific gravity should be near 1.020.

Nursing diagnoses
- Altered role performance related to the physiologic and psychological changes associated with the postpartal period
- Pain related to breast engorgement and the episiotomy
- Fatigue related to the emotional and physical stress of labor and delivery

Planning and goals
- Mrs. DeShon will recover without complications after delivery.
- Mrs. DeShon will participate in self-care activities.

Implementation
NURSING BEHAVIORS

NURSING RATIONALES

1. Implement measures to control Mrs. DeShon's pain from the episiotomy (including sitz baths, ice packs, and analgesic sprays) and hemorrhoids, if present (including sitz baths, witch hazel compresses [Tucks] or ointments, and stool softeners).

1. Pain, which can have multiple sources, may interfere with the mother's rest and comfort.

2. If Mrs. DeShon has afterpains, administer analgesics as ordered.

2. Painful postpartal uterine contractions are more common in multigravidas and in women who are breast-feeding (sucking stimulates oxytocin release and uterine contraction). Women who are breast-feeding may wish to receive a mild analgesic, which should be offered no later than 1 hour before breast-feeding.

3. Provide anticipatory guidance about breast discomfort from engorgement. Administer an analgesic, if ordered, and implement additional measures for comfort and pain relief, as follows:

3. Discomfort from engorgement is typically mild, but intervention may be necessary if discomfort interferes with the mother's rest or her ability to care for her infant. Preventive measures can reduce engorgement.

• If Mrs. DeShon is breast-feeding, teach her appropriate breast-feeding techniques (see "The client who is breast-feeding," pages 306 to 310).

• Education in breast-feeding techniques can help Mrs. DeShon achieve independence and success in her feeding efforts while minimizing discomfort.

MATERNAL-NEWBORN NURSING

• If Mrs. DeShon is not breast-feeding, discuss mechanical suppression of lactation. Advise her to avoid breast stimulation, to apply ice packs to her breasts and axillae, and to wear a well-fitted bra or binder.

• Nonpharmacologic methods of lactation suppression are used for 1 to 2 weeks. Breast stimulation should be avoided because it delays the milk suppression process. Application of ice packs to the breasts and axillae helps minimize engorgement and relieve discomfort. Wearing a well-fitted bra or a breast binder 24 hours a day is advisable.

• Teach Mrs. DeShon the signs of mastitis: fever, chills, tenderness, and a hard, palpable mass.

• These signs are common in primiparas and in breast-feeding mothers.

4. Implement measures to promote Mrs. DeShon's general comfort and perineal healing, as follows:

4. Personal hygiene measures, graded activity, and exercise promote postpartal physical and psychological comfort and well-being.

• Encourage Mrs. DeShon to shower or bathe often.

• Reversal of the water metabolism of pregnancy may result in profuse diaphoresis for 2 to 3 days after delivery, especially at night, as the client's body eliminates retained fluids.

• Teach Mrs. DeShon about the normal flow and characteristics of lochia.

• Knowledge of the normal flow and characteristics of lochia allows the client to identify abnormalities that should be reported to the nurse.

• Teach Mrs. DeShon to cleanse her perineal area from front to back, using a peri bottle, to change perineal pads after each voiding or defecation, and to remove or replace pads using a front-to-back maneuver.

• Routine cleansing of the perineal area after voiding and defecation is necessary to prevent postpartal infection, which can impede involution.

• Teach Mrs. DeShon the Kegel exercises.

• Tightening the pubococcygeal muscle improves support to the pelvic organs and promotes comfort.

5. Provide adequate sleep and rest for Mrs. DeShon, as follows:

5. The birth experience can be exhausting. In the excitement after delivery, however, the client may not be aware of her fatigue and may develop sleep hunger, which can interfere with postpartal adaptation.

• After evaluating Mrs. DeShon's needs, plan rest periods when she will not be disturbed, and organize nursing activities so they do not take place during those periods.

• Careful planning promotes the client's rest and helps her recognize the importance of scheduling activities to meet personal needs and those of her child.

• Encourage frequent rest periods, especially before the infant's feedings, and advise Mrs. DeShon to nap while the infant sleeps. Prepare her for getting needed rest at home.

• The new mother needs energy to adjust psychologically and physically to the new infant and to her new role.

6. Ensure adequate food intake for Mrs. DeShon by offering extra nourishment and between-meal snacks. Record her food intake.

6. Adequate food intake is the basis of successful recovery from the birth experience. A good appetite is the rule, and most new mothers talk a lot about food and eating. A poor appetite is one of the first signs that recovery is not proceeding normally.

7. Implement measures to promote the return of Mrs. DeShon's normal bladder functioning, as follows:

• Monitor fluid intake and output until the bladder is completely empty.

• Encourage her to void every 2 to 4 hours. Catheterize only if absolutely necessary.

• Help her walk to the bathroom if her condition is stable.

8. Implement measures to promote the return of Mrs. DeShon's normal bowel functioning, as follows:
• Encourage ambulation and fluid intake.
• Provide fresh fruit and other high-fiber foods.
• Administer stool softeners, as ordered.

9. Implement measures to promote the return of Mrs. DeShon's normal circulatory functioning, as follows:

• Encourage ambulation as soon as her condition permits.

• Examine her legs daily, comparing them for signs of thrombosis, such as edema, warmth, and tenderness. Measure leg circumference, and compare bilateral pulses.

• Daily, assess for Homans' sign (pain on passive dorsiflexion of the foot).

• If Mrs. DeShon is confined to bed more than 8 hours, remind her to do leg exercises.

• Teach Mrs. DeShon not to cross, rub, or massage her legs. Avoid using the knee gatch on her bed. If Mrs. DeShon is at high risk for circulatory problems, apply moist heat and elastic stockings or bandages to her legs, as ordered.

7. Bladder distention is common during the first 8 to 12 hours after delivery.

• Accurate intake and output records help identify the adequacy of bladder emptying.

• This allows the nurse to detect urine retention problems before they become severe and may prevent the need for catheterization.

• The client will be weak and will need assistance to ensure her safety.

8. During late pregnancy, pressure on the bowel decreases peristalsis, causing bowel sluggishness. Rectal and perineal soreness may also create difficulty with bowel elimination. Early ambulation stimulates bowel function, as does a high-fiber diet (including prune juice, dried fruit, bran, and raw fruit and vegetables). Stool softeners help prevent constipation and may relieve anxiety about the first stool being painful.

9. Women with high parity who have had a complicated labor and delivery are most at risk for circulatory impairment.

• Increased progesterone levels during pregnancy predispose the client to venous thrombosis and thrombophlebitis.

• The most common site for thrombosis is the woman's legs, which are compared because only one is usually involved. An affected leg will be larger and will have diminished pulses.

• Foot dorsiflexion, which causes the calf muscles to compress the tibial veins, is painful for a client with thrombosis.

• Alternate flexion and extension of the legs, rotation of the feet, and straight-leg raises promote circulatory return from the legs.

• These measures, which promote venous return from the legs, may be necessary for a client at risk for developing thrombophlebitis.

MATERNAL-NEWBORN NURSING

10. Reassess Mrs. DeShon for signs and symptoms of infection:
• fever
• foul-smelling lochia
• separation of the episiotomy incision, edema, discharge, or poor healing of the episiotomy
• urinary urgency, frequency, or pain
• abnormal abdominal or leg pain.

10. Premature rupture of the membranes, prolonged labor, and surgical intervention predispose the client to postpartal infection. In addition, the risk of maternal postpartal infection has increased with the advent of invasive diagnostic and treatment techniques (such as amniocentesis and fetal blood sampling) for high-risk pregnancies. Also increased is the incidence of gram-negative infections, which do not respond as well as gram-positive infections to the commonly used antibiotics.

Evaluation

• Mrs. DeShon does not experience thrombophlebitis, infection, or a fecal impaction.
• Mrs. DeShon can perform self-care activities, such as breast and perineal care and leg exercises.

Psychological responses during the postpartal period

During the postpartal period—a time of developmental transition—the new mother and father undergo significant psychological adaptations and role and identity changes. Family members, such as siblings and grandparents, also undergo significant identity changes. The following clinical situation focuses on psychosocial aspects of maternal and paternal adaptation to parenthood during the early postpartal period and on the beginning development of the new family unit.

Clinical situation

Della DeShon and her new son Sean, now 1 day old, are on the family care unit. Mr. DeShon visits frequently. Mrs. DeShon's physical recovery and Sean's transition period are proceeding without complications. Sean is alert and an avid, eager feeder. However, Mrs. DeShon, who is breast-feeding, is still somewhat nervous about caring for him. She comments, "I think we may be going home today. I'm not sure I'm ready to take care of Sean all by myself." Mr. DeShon states that he "will help as much as possible, but you know I don't know much about taking care of little babies."

Assessment
NURSING BEHAVIORS

NURSING RATIONALES

1. Assess the appearance of attachment behavior between Mrs. DeShon and Sean during the acquaintance phase (the period of mutual learning and orientation for the new mother and her infant).

1. Attachment refers to enduring bonds or relationships of affection between persons. Early mother-infant interaction in a warm and supportive environment is believed to facilitate beginning attachment behaviors.

2. Observe Mrs. DeShon periodically for appropriate maternal attachment behaviors, such as her attraction to Sean, close physical contact with him (including face-to-face contact and eye contact), inclination to nurture him, sensitivity to his needs, and pleasure in interacting with him.

3. Evaluate the persistence of any maladaptive attachment behavior, such as negative descriptions of the infant or indifference or inattentiveness toward the infant.

4. Assess the quality of Mrs. DeShon's puerperal restoration, as follows:
• taking in (the period when the mother takes in information about the infant): Mrs. DeShon's exploring behaviors (for example, touch, eye contact, the en face position), fingertip touching, integrating behaviors
• taking hold (Mrs. DeShon's initial efforts to become more autonomous and independent in caring for herself and for Sean)
• letting go (Mrs. DeShon's realization that the infant is a separate being).

5. Assess paternal-infant interaction between Mr. DeShon and Sean, including Mr. DeShon's attraction to his son.

2. Periodic reassessment of parent-infant interactions helps the nurse avoid attaching too much significance to any one behavior. Cultural and situational contexts should be considered during the assessment (for example, in some cultures, clients must appear stoic when in pain). After initial bonding, the acquaintance phase continues the attachment process. The infant contributes to a positive process by giving the mother cues that her mothering behaviors meet his needs. Clear behavioral cues from her infant and his predictable responses to her care help the mother feel effective and competent.

Infant behaviors that attract the mother include grasping, nursing eagerly, cuddling, and being easy to comfort or quiet when distressed. When an infant does not respond with such behaviors, the mother may have difficulty becoming attached to him. Similarly, if an infant exhibits unorganized behavior and unpredictable responses to mothering, this may confuse the new parents and interfere with a positive attachment process. Occasionally, a mother is unable to read her infant's cues accurately. As a result, she responds inappropriately to his behavioral cues.

3. Maladaptive attachment behaviors have been associated with child neglect and abuse.

4. The quality of puerperal restoration is important in planning nursing interventions keyed to the new mother's specific needs.

Taking in occurs during the first day or two after delivery. The mother, who may be somewhat passive and dependent, may not initiate contact with the infant. Instead, she is likely to be oriented to her own needs; despite her interest in the infant, she may not want to assume responsibility for his care. Food and sleep are important to the mother at this time (sleep hunger may occur).

The taking-hold period extends from the 2nd or 3rd day through the 10th day after delivery. The mother strives to become more autonomous and shows concern about her own bodily functions. She initiates responsibility for care of the infant, but she may be anxious about her abilities. During this period, the mother usually begins the total-hand-contact phase of maternal touch (if this behavior has not occurred earlier).

5. The nurse should understand the father's absorbing attraction to the new infant. A reciprocal attachment bond between father and infant is thought to develop from this early father-infant interaction.

MATERNAL-NEWBORN NURSING

6. Determine Mr. and Mrs. DeShon's goals, including their expectations of themselves and of Sean.

6. Understanding the new parents' goals enables the nurse to assist with clarifying them so they embody realistic expectations.

7. Assess Mr. and Mrs. DeShon's learning needs regarding maternal self-care and infant care.

7. Knowledge of maternal self-care and infant care promotes the parents' beginning skills in these areas and increases their self-confidence.

8. Assess the concerns Mr. and Mrs. DeShon may have about the resumption of sexual relations.

8. Resumption of the parents' sexual relationship may be impaired if they do not know what to expect.

9. Identify and reinforce the DeShons' strengths as a couple—for example, the quality of their communication with each other.

9. In this way, the nurse helps the parents recognize their ability as a couple to function competently and to cope with new tasks. This approach also avoids giving parents the impression that they are inadequate and that the professionals are the experts.

10. Assess cultural influences.

10. Postpartal rituals and routines may vary with the client's ethnic background and beliefs, including dietary customs, hygiene, and activity patterns.

11. Assess the interaction of siblings and grandparents.

11. Grandparents can help with family transition. Siblings may regress temporarily.

Nursing diagnoses
- Anxiety related to the development of parenting skills
- Family coping (potential for growth) related to the parents' recognition of their ability to handle new tasks

Planning and goals
- Mr. and Mrs. DeShon will exhibit behaviors commonly associated with positive attachment to a newborn.
- Mr. and Mrs. DeShon will demonstrate beginning parenting skills.
- Mr. and Mrs. DeShon will have adequate information to facilitate their sexual readjustment.
- Mrs. DeShon will verbalize understanding of self-care.
- Mr. and Mrs. DeShon will verbalize understanding of their postpartal follow-up schedule.

Implementation
NURSING BEHAVIORS

NURSING RATIONALES

1. Provide opportunities for the DeShons to express their feelings about Sean and their roles as parents.

1. By encouraging their self-expression, the nurse can help new parents accept their preoccupation with the infant as a normal part of parental development. Talking also helps the couple define realistic expectations for themselves, the infant, and their family.

2. Reinforce Mr. and Mrs. DeShon's positive attachment behaviors. Explain that father-newborn bonding is facilitated by touch, eye contact, awareness of physical similarities between father and newborn, and the newborn's positive response to the father's presence.

2. Reinforcement provides support for the couple in their new roles. *Note:* The nurse should seek consultation if attachment behaviors are maladaptive (for example, if one or both parents poke or pinch the infant); a team approach to intervention involving all nursing shifts is advisable, along with referral to appropriate community agencies for follow-up care.

3. Reinforce the DeShons' effective infant care skills, such as feeding, bathing, and diapering. Provide individual guidance (including teaching normal neonatal characteristics) and recommend parenting classes if appropriate.

4. To help Mrs. DeShon integrate the labor and delivery experience, encourage her to discuss it, giving her any information she needs to fill in the gaps.

5. As she increases her taking-hold behavior, encourage Mrs. DeShon to pace herself and to prevent fatigue or exhaustion by setting limits and modifying self-expectations.

6. Provide anticipatory guidance to Mrs. DeShon about the letting-go phase, particularly the potential for postpartal depression (baby blues). Reassure both parents that postpartal depression is a normal and usually temporary reaction to the parenting role transition.

7. Through individual teaching or a discussion group, provide guidance for Mr. and Mrs. DeShon concerning their resumption of intercourse, as follows:

• Explain that intercourse may initially be painful (dyspareunia) for Mrs. DeShon.

• For contraception, make sure the DeShons understand that they should use a condom, along with spermicide or a contraceptive foam. Provide information on all contraceptive methods.

3. Reinforcement increases the parents' confidence and helps them sort out problems. In particular, successful accomplishment of mothering tasks is extremely significant for the mother.

4. Discussion helps the mother realize that her labor and delivery are over and that the resulting infant is a separate individual. Filling in the gaps acknowledges her need to take in information about herself and her infant. For example, Mrs. DeShon may want to know how long she was in transition or how well she coped with the delivery phase. Reliving the delivery experience is important for psychological integration.

5. The nurse's reassurance and guidance are essential in reinforcing appropriate taking-hold behaviors. However, the nurse should not take over the mother's tasks; this can impair her ability to perform them and damage her confidence. Because much of this phase will take place at home after discharge, the nurse's encouragement now can have long-term helpful effects.

6. The letting-go phase (which usually occurs after the mother returns home) involves her full realization that the infant is a separate individual and she is a mother. She must adjust to the fact that, barring the child's death, she will never again be childless. This phase strongly influences the mother's degree of recognition of her parenting responsibilities.

7. Within 3 weeks after delivery, the episiotomy is usually healed, and lochia flow is scant. Therefore, sexual relations can be resumed safely by most couples at this time. However, the nurse should respect the couple's wishes in this matter; they should not be made to feel guilty or abnormal if they want to resume sexual relations earlier or later.

• The client may need to use vaginal lubrication for vaginal dryness resulting from altered hormones.

• Breast-feeding has no contraceptive value. The nurse must make sure the couple understands this.

MATERNAL-
NEWBORN
NURSING

• Explain to the DeShons that postpartal sexual responsiveness among couples varies and that maternal body changes affecting intercourse, such as ejection of breast milk at orgasm, are only temporary.

• Ejection of breast milk during orgasm occurs because sexual excitement stimulates oxytocin release. Some couples resuming intercourse after delivery are frustrated and distressed about changes in the mother's body image (and about the distraction of the baby's presence or crying). Adjustment to these changes is usually rapid.

8. Provide instructions for Mrs. DeShon's postpartal follow-up: telephone follow-up the first week, 2- and 6-week examinations, and referrals as indicated.

8. Follow-up examinations help ensure continued maternal-infant well-being. Referrals may involve physical assessment, nutritional guidance, psychological adjustment, counseling, family planning, and contraception instruction.

9. Review with the DeShons the signs of complications to report to the physician, such as infection, late postpartal hemorrhage, and psychological maladaptation.

9. Early discharge from the hospital places more responsibility on the client to know and report signs of complications.

Evaluation

• At discharge, Mr. and Mrs. DeShon can feed and care for Sean satisfactorily and verbalize satisfaction with their parenting skills.
• Mr. and Mrs. DeShon exhibit signs of positive attachment to Sean.
• Mrs. DeShon demonstrates skill in self-care.
• Mr. and Mrs. DeShon verbalize realistic expectations of their parenting roles and postpartal changes.
• Mr. and Mrs. DeShon verbalize awareness of their own abilities to adapt to the new baby and their new roles.
• Mr. and Mrs. DeShon verbalize knowledge of what alterations in sexuality they can expect and when they can resume intercourse.
• Mr. and Mrs. DeShon describe their postpartal follow-up schedule.

The adolescent parent

I. **Trends**
   A. Increase in percentage of infants born to adolescent mothers
   B. Increase in number of unplanned pregnancies outside of marriage
   C. Increase in number of adolescent mothers who choose to keep and raise the child as a single parent

II. **Factors associated with adolescent pregnancy**
   A. Early sexual maturity
   B. Early dating
   C. Ineffective contraceptive practices among sexually active teenagers
   D. Lack of explicit sex education at home and in school
   E. No effective way to predict those at risk of becoming pregnant on the basis of demographic characteristics (race, ethnicity, culture, religion) or attitudes

III. Physical consequences

    A. Greater risk of adverse pregnancy and neonatal outcomes (for example, pregnancy-induced hypertension and delivery of low-birth-weight infants), especially in mothers under age 15

    B. Fewer and less serious physical risks for adolescents who receive excellent prenatal care

IV. Psychosocial consequences

    A. Potential interference with achievement of new, more mature peer relations (pregnant adolescents are likely to be isolated from or in conflict with peers)

    B. Potential interference with acceptance of body image related to physical changes of pregnancy

    C. Potential interference with achievement of independence from parents and other adults

    D. Potential interference with the establishment of a satisfying personal and social lifestyle (interruptions in education may prevent the adolescent from achieving career and economic goals)

    E. Potential interference with progress in becoming a socially responsible adult (for example, a higher incidence of child neglect and abuse is associated with early pregnancy and parenting)

V. Nursing implications

    A. Antepartal period

      1. Assess the nature and extent of the client's support systems (such as the infant's father or the client's parents and friends)

      2. Assist the client in accomplishing the developmental tasks of pregnancy if she chooses to continue the pregnancy

      3. Help the client obtain high-quality prenatal care and pregnancy education geared to her special needs

    B. Intrapartal period

      1. Provide support during labor and delivery

      2. Arrange for significant support persons (such as the infant's father or the client's mother or grandmother) to be available during labor and delivery, if the client desires

      3. Acknowledge and protect the right of the adolescent parent to grant informed consent and to be informed about her health status and the status of her infant

    C. Postpartal period

      1. Promote the developmental tasks of parenthood if the adolescent chooses to keep the infant

        a. Determine the client's readiness and ability to assume caretaking responsibility for the infant (the client may lack knowledge of how to care for an infant because of physical, intellectual, and emotional immaturity)

        b. Support positive attachment behaviors

        c. Encourage significant others (such as the infant's father and the adolescent's parents) to participate in caring for the infant, based on the needs of the adolescent and her relationship with these individuals

      2. Teach infant care and early growth and development of the infant

      3. Assist the client in making plans to meet her educational and career goals

4. Support long-range development of parenting abilities and psychosocial development of the adolescent parents
   a. Assist the adolescent parents in developing effective problem-solving skills
   b. Make appropriate referrals to community and family services that assist adolescent parents

The normal newborn

The first 24 hours after birth are especially hazardous to the newborn, who is vulnerable to many problems in adjusting to extrauterine life. As a result, many institutions provide specialized neonatal care in an admission or transition nursery. The following clinical situation focuses on care of the normal newborn during this transition period and on parental guidance in caring for the newborn.

Clinical situation

You are the nurse responsible for admission and transition care of Sean DeShon, a neonate. He is 1 hour old on arrival in the nursery, having spent his first hour of life in the birthing room with his parents.

Assessment

NURSING BEHAVIORS

1. Admit Sean to the newborn nursery with a report from the delivery room nurse and a check of his identification. Place him under a radiant warmer.

2. Review the prenatal history.

3. Review Mrs. DeShon's labor and delivery record.

4. Determine Sean's general condition by assessing his cry (lusty or weak), muscle tone (flexed or floppy), color (pink, ruddy, pale, cyanotic, or jaundiced), and temperature.

5. Assess Sean's respirations as follows:
• breaths/minute (normal: 40 to 60); count respirations for a full minute
• respiratory effort (assess every 15 minutes for 2 hours, then every hour if necessary until it is stable)
• presence of grunting or nasal flaring
• breath sounds.

NURSING RATIONALES

1. These procedures establish baseline data. The warmer maintains the newborn's body heat until temperature regulation is established.

2. Various maternal factors (such as bleeding, preeclampsia, age, length of pregnancy, previous pregnancies, and incompatible Rh type) may affect the infant's health status at birth.

3. Perinatal situations or events that can affect neonatal status include length and difficulty of labor, use of forceps, administration of analgesics and anesthetics, type of delivery, care at time of delivery, and such problems as precipitous delivery or delivery with the umbilical cord around the infant's neck.

4. General inspection of the neonate allows the nurse to establish priorities quickly—for example, whether to complete a thorough assessment of the infant or to allow time for his temperature to stabilize.

5. Signs of neonatal respiratory distress signal the need for intervention. The most common signs include sternal retractions, persistent breathing at a rate exceeding 60 breaths/minute, facial grimacing, nasal flaring, dyspnea, and cyanosis (excluding palms and soles). Transient tachypnea may occur, especially in newborns delivered by cesarean section.

6. Take Sean's temperature; normal axillary temperature is 97.7° to 98.6° F (36.5° to 37° C). If necessary, reassess every 30 minutes until it is stable.

6. The neonate's temperature may be low on admission to the nursery (because of heat loss) but should stabilize within 12 hours. The axillary site gives the skin temperature rather than the core body temperature, alerting the nurse to cooling before cold stress becomes severe. Using the axillary site also eliminates any danger of rectal perforation. However, some institutions require taking a neonate's temperature rectally at least once, to assess rectal patency.

7. Take Sean's apical pulse (normal is 120 to 160 beats/minute), noting its rate and regularity as well as any murmurs.

7. The neonatal pulse rate is labile and follows the pattern of the infant's respirations, physical activity, temperature, and crying. Murmurs are common in newborns.

8. Take Sean's blood pressure, using a cuff of the correct size. (Normal newborn blood pressure mean is 74/47 mm Hg.

8. Blood pressure should be approximately equal in all extremities.

9. Assess the condition of Sean's umbilical cord, noting the number of cord vessels and evidence of meconium staining or bleeding.

9. Three vessels, two arteries, and one vein are normal. A single umbilical artery is associated with congenital anomalies. Meconium staining and bleeding are abnormal.

10. Assess the characteristics of Sean's stools and urine.

10. Excretory functioning is normally initiated within the first 24 hours after birth; most neonates void at birth or within a few hours. The first stool, meconium, should be passed within 24 to 48 hours.

11. Weigh and measure Sean.

11. A normal full-term white neonate averages 7 lb, 8 oz (3,405 g). Black, Asian, and Native American neonates may be somewhat smaller. The average length is 19 ½″ (49.4 cm). See "Assessment and characteristics of the normal newborn," pages 297 to 301, for head and chest measurements.

MATERNAL-
NEWBORN
NURSING

Nursing diagnoses
- Ineffective airway clearance related to mucus in the respiratory tract
- Risk for altered body temperature related to the neonate's immature temperature-regulating mechanism
- Risk for infection related to immunologic immaturity

Planning and goals
- Sean will adapt to extrauterine life without difficulty.
- Sean's body temperature and respirations will stabilize within normal limits.
- Adequate fluid and nutrient intake will be established for Sean.
- Sean's bowel and bladder elimination will be normal.
- Sean's skin will remain free of excoriation and inflammation.
- Mr. and Mrs. DeShon will demonstrate beginning skills in basic infant care.
- Mr. and Mrs. DeShon will have knowledge of normal newborn characteristics and will verbalize acceptance of the unique characteristics Sean exhibits.
- Mr. and Mrs. DeShon will verbalize knowledge of resources and services available to them after discharge and ways to contact those resources.

Implementation

NURSING BEHAVIORS	NURSING RATIONALES

1. Place Sean unclothed in a radiant warmer; attach a skin probe for a continuous temperature reading, or monitor Sean's axillary temperature every hour for the first 4 hours.

1. This environment helps stabilize body temperature and prevent further heat loss. When temperature stabilizes, monitoring every 4 hours should be sufficient. The skin probe senses the newborn's temperature, and the warmer regulates heat output accordingly.

2. Support Sean's respirations by maintaining a patent airway and taking the following precautions:

2. Maintaining a clear airway is essential to prevent respiratory distress from obstruction.

• Position Sean on his side to facilitate mucus drainage.

• Choking, gagging, and retractions indicate airway obstruction, probably from mucus.

• Monitor Sean constantly during reactivity periods (see "Assessment and characteristics of the normal newborn," pages 297 to 301).

• Signs of obstruction are common during the second period of reactivity.

• Aspirate mucus with a bulb syringe if necessary; suction Sean's mouth before his nostrils.

• Stimulation of the nostrils initiates the gasp reflex, which could pull mucus into the lower lungs.

3. Follow institutional precautions for promoting Sean's skin integrity and preventing skin infection:
• Provide skin care.
• Delay bathing until Sean's temperature is stable; if his temperature drops during his bath, return him to the radiant warmer; after his bath, reassess his temperature.
• Cleanse blood from his skin. (It is not necessary to remove all the vernix, which is protective and will disappear within 1 to 2 days.)

3. The overall goal is to promote skin integrity by keeping the skin clean and dry. Special attention should be given to creases, folds, and the genital area. The nurse should use mild soap and water unless otherwise ordered and should omit powder and oils, which may irritate sensitive skin.

4. Perform a complete physical assessment of Sean within 24 hours after birth (see "Assessment and characteristics of the normal newborn," pages 297 to 301). Assess him for hypoglycemia, hyperbilirubinemia, respiratory and circulatory distress, jaundice, pallor, abdominal distention and masses, failure to pass meconium within 24 hours after birth, and bile-stained vomitus.

4. This assessment allows evaluation of the neonate's maturity, characteristics, and physical and behavioral adaptations.

5. Perform a gestational age assessment.

5. Gestational age assessment can identify high-risk newborns. (See *Ballard gestational-age assessment tool.*)

6. Promote healing of the umbilical cord area, and provide cord care if needed. Report any oozing or hemorrhage to the physician.

6. Institutional policy for cord care should be followed; variations range from putting nothing on the cord to applying triple dye or alcohol. The clamp usually can be removed after 24 hours.

MATERNAL-NEWBORN NURSING

Ballard gestational-age assessment tool

To use this tool, the examiner evaluates and scores the neuromuscular and physical maturity criteria, totals the scores, then plots the sum in the maturity rating box to determine gestational age. Unlike portions of the Dubowitz neurologic examination, the Ballard neuromuscular examination can be done even if the neonate is not alert.

NEUROMUSCULAR MATURITY

NEUROMUSCULAR MATURITY SIGN	SCORE							RECORD SCORE HERE
	-1	0	1	2	3	4	5	
POSTURE								
SQUARE WINDOW (Wrist)	>90°	90°	60°	45°	30°	0°	—	
ARM RECOIL	—	180°	140° to 180°	110° to 140°	90° to 100°	<90°	—	
POPLITEAL ANGLE	180°	160°	140°	120°	100°	90°	<90°	
SCARF SIGN							—	
HEEL TO EAR							—	

TOTAL NEUROMUSCULAR MATURITY SCORE

PHYSICAL MATURITY

PHYSICAL MATURITY SIGN	SCORE							RECORD SCORE HERE
	-1	0	1	2	3	4	5	
SKIN	Sticky, friable, transparent	Gelatinous, red, translucent	Smooth, pink; visible vessels	Superficial peeling or rash; few visible vessels	Cracking; pale areas; rare visible vessels	Parchment-like; deep cracking; no visible vessels	Leathery, cracked, wrinkled	
LANUGO	None	Sparse	Abundant	Thinning	Bald areas	Mostly bald	—	
PLANTAR SURFACE	Heel-toe 40 to 50 mm: -1; <40 mm: -2	>50 mm; no crease	Faint red marks	Anterior transverse crease only	Creases over anterior two-thirds	Creases over entire sole	—	
BREAST	Imperceptible	Barely perceptible	Flat areola, no bed	Stippled areola; 1- to 2-mm bud	Raised areola; 3- to 4-mm bud	Full areola; 5- to 10-mm bud	—	
EYE AND EAR	Lids fused, loosely: -1; tightly: -2	Lids open; pinna flat, stays folded	Slightly curved pinna; soft, slow recoil	Well-curved pinna; soft but ready recoil	Formed and firm; instant recoil	Thick cartilage; ear stiff	—	
GENITALIA (Male)	Scrotum flat, smooth	Scrotum empty; faint rugae	Testes in upper canal; rare rugae	Testes descending; few rugae	Testes down; good rugae	Testes pendulous; deep rugae	—	
GENITALIA (Female)	Clitoris prominent; labia flat	Prominent clitoris; small labia minora	Prominent clitoris; enlarging minora	Majora and minora equally prominent	Majora large; minora small	Majora cover clitoris and minora	—	

TOTAL PHYSICAL MATURITY SCORE

SCORE

Neuromuscular _____

Physical _____

Total _____

MATURITY RATING

TOTAL MATURITY SCORE	GESTATIONAL AGE (WEEKS)
-10	20
-5	22
0	24
5	26
10	28
15	30
20	32
25	34
30	36
35	38
40	40
45	42
50	44

GESTATIONAL AGE (Weeks)

By dates _____

By ultrasound _____

By score _____

MATERNAL-NEWBORN NURSING

7. As ordered, give vitamin K (phytonadione [AquaMEPHYTON] 0.5 to 1.0 mg) I.M. to prevent blood loss from ineffective blood clotting and hemorrhagic disease of the newborn.

7. This measure prevents low prothrombin levels, which can result from inadequate synthesis of vitamin K during the first week of life. The injection is given in the upper thigh (vastus lateralis muscle).

8. Initiate Sean's intake of sterile water, formula, or breast milk, as indicated. Assess the newborn for sucking, swallowing, and gagging reflexes as well as for esophageal atresia.

8. The first breast-feeding may be given in the birthing or delivery room. Bottle-fed infants are given sterile water as a test feeding within 4 hours of delivery. Colostrum (the initial form of breast milk) is nonirritating and rapidly absorbed by the lungs, if aspirated; therefore, a water test feeding is not needed for the newborn who will be breast-fed.

9. Assist with tests and procedures ordered for Sean, including hemoglobin and hematocrit levels and a metabolic screening for phenylketonuria and other inborn errors of metabolism.

9. These tests indicate the neonate's degree of physiologic adaptation and may reveal potential problems. The metabolic screening is done after the neonate has ingested milk over a 24-hour period; if Mrs. DeShon is Rh-negative and Sean is Rh-positive with a positive Coombs' test, he is at risk for hemolytic anemia.

10. Once Sean is stable, transfer him to the normal newborn nursery or to the mother-baby unit.

10. The newborn is usually stable 5 to 10 hours after birth.

11. Support Mr. and Mrs. DeShon as they assume their parental roles and apply new parenting skills (for general information, see "Parental guidance in care of the newborn," pages 301 to 303). In particular, give them predischarge guidance in infant care, covering these areas: normal growth and development; newborn feeding (see "Neonatal nutrition," pages 303 to 306); bathing, holding, and diapering the infant; using a thermometer; normal respirations; signs and symptoms of illness; jaundice; infection; adjustments to breast-feeding; expected changes in stools and urine (color and number); care of the genital area, including circumcision care if appropriate; safety measures (such as an infant car seat); and community resources available for help.

11. The nurse helps new parents assume their roles by providing anticipatory guidance and individualized teaching based on the parents' needs. Parents should have basic infant-care skills and awareness of the unique characteristics of their infant. Inexperienced parents or those experiencing problems may need referral to appropriate community resources. Short hospital stays place more responsibility on the parents to know when to seek health care.

Evaluation

- Sean exhibits physiologic stability and adapts to extrauterine life without difficulty within 24 hours.
- Sean and his mother experience success during initial feedings.
- Sean's bowel and bladder functioning are normal.
- Sean's skin is clean and intact, with no redness or lesions.
- Mr. and Mrs. DeShon demonstrate basic skills in caring for Sean.
- Mr. and Mrs. DeShon exhibit appropriate parenting behaviors.
- Mr. and Mrs. DeShon describe normal neonatal characteristics and point out Sean's individual characteristics.
- Mr. and Mrs. DeShon verbalize appropriate resources.
- Mr. and Mrs. DeShon verbalize Sean's discharge plans and follow-up care.

Assessment and characteristics of the normal newborn

I.   **Transition period (adaptation to extrauterine life in the first hours)**
   A. Physiologic adaptations
      1. Normal respiration
         a. Spontaneous initiation of respirations with shift from fetal to neonatal pulmonary circulation and lung expansion
         b. Lung fluid cleared
         c. Normal respiratory rate of 40 to 60 breaths/minute
         d. Shallow, irregular, abdominal respirations with short periods of apnea and nose breathing
      2. Deviations and abnormal respiration
         a. Prolonged dyspnea, cyanosis
         b. Delay in clearing lung fluid
         c. Asphyxia at birth
         d. Increased use of intercostal muscles for breathing
         e. Nasal flaring
         f. Respiratory rate below 35 or over 60 breaths/minute when infant is at rest
      3. Circulatory changes—increased aortic and systemic pressure; decreased venous and pulmonary pressure; closure of foramen ovale, ductus arteriosus, and ductus venosus; residual cyanosis of hands, feet, and area around mouth for 1 to 2 hours from sluggish peripheral circulation; mottled skin
         a. Pulse rate
            (1) Normal: 120 to 160 beats/minute, increasing to 180 beats/minute briefly with crying or while very active, decreasing to 100 beats/minute during sleep
            (2) Abnormal or deviated: persistently greater than 160 beats/minute or less than 100 beats/minute
         b. Blood pressure—usually monitored only on admission unless newborn is in distress; averages 74/47 mm Hg during 1st week on Doppler ultrasonography
         c. Blood count—elevated red blood cell (RBC) count (5 to 6 million cells/mm^3); elevated hemoglobin (15 to 20 g/dl); elevated hematocrit (about 55%) [*Note:* These three values are necessary for adequate oxygenation in utero; values decline during first few months after birth]
         d. Physiologic jaundice—caused by increased breakdown of RBCs and impaired bilirubin conjugation, resulting in elevated serum bilirubin, visible when bilirubin level is 5 to 7 mg/dl or above; appears after first 24 hours after birth
            (1) Occurs in 40% to 60% of normal newborns between 2nd and 4th day, with average bilirubin level of 6 mg/dl at 60 to 72 hours
            (2) Averages may be higher in Asian newborns
            (3) Cord blood bilirubin level is less than 2 mg/dl
            (4) Adult bilirubin level is less than 1 mg/dl, reached by neonate around the 10th day
            (5) Abnormal level or deviation from normal would be pathologic jaundice—serum bilirubin level above 12 mg/dl developing during first 24 hours

e. White blood cells—normally leukocytosis at birth (10,000 to 30,000 cells/mm^3), diminishing during 1st week of life

4. Temperature changes—heat regulation and metabolism

    a. Heat losses from evaporation, conduction, convection, and radiation

    b. Heat production—chemical changes in brown fat (located between scapulae, nape of neck, axilla): triglycerides are converted into glycerol and fatty acids to produce heat if the infant is subjected to a cool environment

    c. Heat conservation by peripheral vasoconstriction and flexed fetal posture to reduce heat loss through body surface area

    d. Effects of cold stress—increased oxygen and calorie consumption from increased metabolism resulting from low body temperature; if not corrected, metabolic acidosis may result

    e. Normal newborn temperature should stabilize within 8 to 12 hours at 97.7° F (36.5° C)

B. Neurologic adaptations—normal reflexes indicate extent of normal functioning of central nervous system

C. Hepatic adaptations—temporary coagulation deficiency during first 2 to 5 days of life caused by the liver's initial inability to synthesize vitamin K (the liver plays an important role in blood coagulation and storage of iron during the first few months of life)

D. Gastrointestinal (GI) adaptations

1. Stomach capacity of 50 to 60 ml; empties in about 3 hours; initially, good digestion and absorption of protein and simple carbohydrates, poor absorption of fat, poor digestion of complex carbohydrates

2. GI tract sterile at birth but sufficiently contaminated within a few days for normal digestion and vitamin K synthesis

E. Renal adaptations

1. Over 90% of newborns void within 24 hours, with initial voiding shortly after delivery

2. High urine specific gravity (from urate concentration) and mucus initially causing urine to appear reddish and cloudy after first voiding; sometimes confused with blood in the urine

3. Normal voiding initially two to six times daily, with an average output of 60 ml/day; increasing in frequency and volume (as fluid intake increases) to 10 to 30 voidings daily and average output of 225 ml/day by end of 1st week

F. Immunologic adaptations

1. Normal newborn receives passive acquired immunity through transfer of maternal immunoglobulin antibodies to the fetus in utero

2. Provides temporary immunity of varying duration to tetanus, diphtheria, smallpox, mumps, measles, polio, and several other bacterial and viral diseases if the mother has sufficient immunity to them

G. Periods of reactivity (characteristics)

1. In the first period (30 minutes), the infant is awake and alert and may appear hungry; respirations are very rapid, possibly above 80 breaths/minute; heart rate is rapid; nasal flaring occurs; bowel sounds are absent; the infant soon goes to sleep and may sleep 2 to 4 hours; respirations and the pulse rate decrease; activity decreases; bowel sounds become present.

2. In the second period, the infant is awake and alert and may pass the first meconium; heart rate increases; the infant may have difficulty with mucus; the infant requires close observation during the first 12 to 18 hours because the length of the transition period varies from one infant to another

II. Physical characteristics

A. Head and face
1. Caput succedaneum (soft area of scalp), hematoma, or molding may be present in cephalic presentation
2. Suture lines easily felt
3. Anterior fontanelle open but neither bulging nor depressed; closes at 18 months
4. Posterior fontanelle small; closes by 3 months
5. Head circumference averages 33 to 35 cm (13″ to 14″); should measure 2 cm greater than chest
6. Face should be symmetrical
7. Milia on nose and forehead

B. Eyes
1. Closed much of the time but will open spontaneously if head is lifted
2. Vision present; infant can discriminate patterns, but vision not as acute as in adult
3. Eyes lack coordination (reassure parents this is normal during first few months)
4. Slate-gray color at birth; permanent color by 3 months
5. Red reflex present
6. Subconjunctival hemorrhage possibly present

C. Ears and hearing
1. Hearing present at birth; becomes acute several days later
2. Top of ear should be in line with an imaginary line extended through outer corner of eye to most prominent point of posterior occiput
3. Low-set ears frequently associated with renal and chromosomal abnormalities (such as Down syndrome)
4. Ear cartilage should be well-formed

D. Neck
1. Characteristic short neck
2. Head should move easily right to left and up and down
3. Infant can maintain head erect briefly

E. Lips, mouth, cheeks
1. Sucking blisters possibly on lips
2. Sucking pads in cheeks
3. Lips, palate, and gums intact
4. Epstein's pearls (small white cysts on gums or palate) possibly present
5. Short frenulum may cause unwarranted concern about the infant's becoming tongue-tied
6. Tongue—moves freely in all directions, proportionate to mouth

F. Clavicles straight and intact

G. Chest
1. Round and symmetrical
2. Circumference is slightly smaller than head
3. Breast engorgement common in males and females
4. Witch's milk sometimes secreted
5. Sternum neither depressed nor prominent

6. Bilateral chest expansion with no retraction, bilateral breath sounds present and clear

H. Abdomen
   1. Round and slightly protuberant; soft bowel sounds present
   2. Palpable liver edge; no palpable masses
   3. Diastasis recti abdominis is common in black newborns
   4. Cord has three vessels with no oozing or bleeding present

I. Genitals
   1. Male
      a. Slender penis with normal urinary orifice at tip
      b. Foreskin adheres to glans, but the prepuce usually is retractable over orifice—if retraction is not possible after 3 months, phimosis may be present
      c. Testes—descended or easily brought down into scrotum
      d. Scrotum—normal skin color; may be discolored in breech presentation
   2. Female
      a. Vaginal discharge (mucoid or slightly bloody) caused by maternal hormones; may be present but disappears spontaneously
      b. Labia majora covering labia minora
      c. Vaginal orifice and urinary meatus visible
      d. Clitoris normally large in newborn

J. Buttocks
   1. Symmetrical folds and buttock creases
   2. Patent anus
   3. Meconium passing during the first 24 to 48 hours

K. Extremities and trunk
   1. Extremities are short in relation to trunk
   2. Legs and arms usually flexed
   3. Legs equal in length; legs shorter than arms
   4. Flexor muscle tone good
   5. All joints having a full range of motion
   6. No webbing of fingers or toes (syndactyly)
   7. No extra digits (polydactyly)
   8. Absence of clubbing
   9. Normal palmar crease
   10. Nails extending beyond fingertips in term infants

L. Spine
   1. C-shaped
   2. Slight lumbar lordosis noticeable
   3. No masses or abnormal curvatures

M. Hips
   1. No hip click
   2. Abduct to more than 60 degrees
   3. Equal iliac crests

N. Skin
   1. Acrocyanosis (bluish discoloration of hands and feet, caused by sluggish circulation and chilling)
   2. Lanugo (downy hair) sometimes visible over shoulders
   3. Vernix caseosa (cheeselike substance) sometimes present in skin creases
   4. Erythema neonatorum toxicum (newborn rash) seen intermittently in some newborns

O. Neurologic and motor functioning
1. Normal reflexes present at birth
    a. Rooting and sucking
    b. Moro (startle)
    c. Palmar and plantar grasp
    d. Stepping or dancing
    e. Babinski's
    f. Tonic neck
    g. Prone crawl
    h. Trunk incurvation
    i. Blinking, sneezing, yawning (protective reflexes)
2. Motor functioning
    a. Symmetrical functioning and strength in all extremities
    b. Some brief jerking or twitching normal
    c. Head lag not greater than 45 degrees

III. Behavioral characteristics (Brazelton assessment)
A. Sleep states
1. Deep sleep—regular breathing; no eye movements; external stimuli may produce some startles with delay, but changes in state are not likely
2. Light sleep—eyes closed; rapid eye movements; startles, random movements, and external stimuli may cause change in state; respirations regular; frequent sucking movements
B. Alert states
1. Drowsy or semidozing—eyelids may be open or closed; reactive to sensory stimuli, but responses may be delayed; movements usually smooth; external stimuli may cause change in state
2. Wide awake—alert, bright look—appears to focus attention on source of stimulation; motor activity minimal
3. Active awake—eyes open, considerable motor activity—reactive to external stimuli with increased startles and motor activity
4. Crying—characteristically intense and difficult to break through with stimulation
C. Neonatal behavioral assessment scale designed by Brazelton to test certain behaviors in infants (for example, habituation, orientation, self-quieting abilities, motor activity, variations, and cuddliness or social behaviors); certain behaviors require a specific infant state for testing

Parental guidance in care of the newborn

I.   Assessment factors
A. Interview the parents to assess their parenting skills and understanding of their infant's needs
1. Establish their knowledge base (Some new parents may have a potential alteration in parenting from lack of knowledge of infant care. The nurse is in a unique position to meet the educational needs of these new parents.)

2. Identify specific concerns and needs related to infant care (Specific learning needs will vary based on the client's age, educational level, cultural background, experience, and expectations.)

B. Observe their responses to the infant and the infant's response to parenting

II. Intervention factors

A. Teach basic principles of infant care based on the parents' needs

1. Stress safety factors (for example, not leaving the infant alone on an unguarded surface)

2. Explore with the parents available equipment and facilities that will be used at home

3. Provide practice time for skill building

   a. Feeding (see "Neonatal nutrition," pages 303 to 306)

   b. Bathing and skin care (advise them to give the infant a sponge bath until the cord drops off and the area heals)

   c. Cord care

     (1) Clean the area with an alcohol wipe; keep clean and dry

     (2) Tub baths are appropriate after the cord area heals

   d. Skin care

     (1) Drying and peeling of skin are normal

     (2) Basic skin care should be with warm water and a mild soap; oils and lotion may irritate the skin or plug skin pores

     (3) Keep the infant warm during the bath

   e. Eyes and ears

     (1) Eyes and ears require no special care other than cleaning

     (2) Teach the parents to report redness, swelling, or discharge from the eyes

     (3) Cotton-tipped swabs should not be inserted into the nose or ears

     (4) Some parents are concerned about sneezing; explain that sneezing automatically clears nasal passages and does not mean the infant has a cold

   f. Genital and circumcision care

     (1) The area should be kept clean and dry

     (2) Encourage the parents to report oozing of blood or pus from the circumcised area

     (3) A newly circumcised infant should not lie on the abdomen

     (4) Teach parents normal variations in newborn stools and voiding

     (5) The genital area may become irritated despite proper care. Exposing the buttocks to air and light several times a day may help heal a diaper rash. Petrolatum, baby oil, or A and D ointment applied to the buttocks also offers protection from the irritating effects of urea and bacteria

   g. Dressing and care of clothes

     (1) Avoid overdressing; prickly heat rash may result, because the newborn does not perspire readily

     (2) Launder clothes separately with a mild detergent; fabric softeners cause rashes in some infants

   h. Handling the infant

     (1) Support the head and buttocks; the infant will be able to support the head independently in approximately 3 months

(2) Allow the parents to practice several holding techniques (cradle, upright, football)

(3) Place the infant in a side-lying position only; the prone position has been linked with sudden infant death syndrome

  i. Other

(1) Allow the parents to practice gentle nasal suctioning with a bulb syringe to remove mucus

(2) Teach the parents how to take the infant's temperature (rectal and axillary)

(3) Teach the parents how to recognize signs and symptoms of illness that should be reported. Provide instructions and telephone numbers in writing

B. Teach normal newborn characteristics and behavior, based on the individual needs of the new parents

C. Prepare the parents for discharge, and make follow-up appointments as indicated (for instance, with a well-baby clinic, pediatrician, community health nurse, or family service agency)

Neonatal nutrition

I. Breast-feeding

A. Mechanism of lactation

1. Colostrum is secreted in the first 2 to 4 days after delivery; breast-feeding during this time stimulates lactation and helps meet the infant's sucking needs; multigravidas may begin producing milk as early as 24 hours after delivery

2. High levels of progesterone and estrogen during pregnancy inhibit lactation by inhibiting the release of prolactin by the anterior pituitary

3. Delivery results in a rapid drop in progesterone and estrogen levels and promotes the release of prolactin

4. Prolactin stimulates the alveolar cells of the breasts and promotes milk production

5. Sucking by the infant induces the release of oxytocin, a posterior pituitary hormone, which causes myoepithelial cells lining the mammary ducts to contract; the let-down reflex occurs, resulting in the flow of milk

6. The let-down reflex (or milk-ejection reflex) may be stimulated by the infant through sucking or crying or by the mother through breast stimulation

7. The let-down reflex may be inhibited by maternal tension, pain, or fatigue or by breast engorgement

8. Lactation is a supply-and-demand process; when lactation is well established, sucking and emptying of the breasts is the most important factor in maintaining milk production

  a. The amount of milk increases with the infant's needs

  b. Breast size is irrelevant to successful breast-feeding because secretory tissue, not fatty tissue, produces milk

B. Problems associated with breast-feeding

1. Nipple pain is a common complaint; teach the client methods to prevent nipple trauma

2. The client may experience engorgement from venous and lymphatic stasis in the first 3 to 4 days (early engorgement) or from acini being filled with milk after that time (late engorgement); teach the client methods to relieve engorgement, including expression of milk

C. Needs of the lactating mother

1. Rest is crucial to the breast-feeding client; inadequate rest causes fatigue, which can diminish the milk supply

2. The client needs a well-balanced diet, similar to the recommended diet during pregnancy but with increases in calories, vitamins A and C, niacin, riboflavin, and iodine; if the recommended diet during pregnancy was adequate, the following plan during lactation should meet the mother's nutritional needs:

   a. Milk—4 cups daily

   b. Meat and meat substitutes—6 oz (2 or 3 servings) daily

   c. Vegetables and fruit—4 servings daily

   d. Bread and cereal—4 or 5 servings daily

   e. Fluids—6 to 8 cups besides milk

3. The client should avoid drugs unless prescribed by the physician; certain drugs—salicylates in large doses, bromides such as Bromo-Seltzer and other sleeping aids, oral contraceptives, and diazepam (Valium)—are excreted in breast milk and may adversely affect the infant

II. Bottle-feeding

A. Commercially prepared formula (usually prepared to meet nutritional standards established by the Committee on Nutrition of the American Academy of Pediatrics)

1. The mother who chooses to bottle-feed her infant can be assured that the infant's nutritional needs will be adequately met

2. Most commercial formulas (for example, Similac and Enfamil) use a nonfat cow's milk base; some commercial formulas attempt to closely approximate breast milk, including the low electrolyte and whey-casein ratio of human milk

3. Commercial formulas are digested more slowly than breast milk because of their larger curds.

B. Milk substitutes

1. Milk substitutes (for example, soybean-based formula) are used for infants with poor tolerance for milk-based formula

2. Nonfat milk is not recommended for infants under age 1 because it provides excessive intake of protein with inadequate amounts of calories, iron, vitamin C, and essential fatty acids

C. Preparation of formula at home

1. Clean technique is commonly recommended rather than strict sterilization (provided the client has an uncontaminated water supply and proper refrigeration)

   a. In the one-bottle method, use half the amount of commercial formula needed for one feeding; pour contents into a clean bottle and, if using a powder or concentrated variety, add the appropriate amount of tap water (some formulas come in ready-to-use form and do not require water); begin feeding within 30 minutes, and discard the unused portion after 1 hour

   b. In the whole-day method, prepare all formula at one time, using clean technique, and refrigerate

      c. Be sure to mix concentrates and powders with the recommended amount of water to prevent water intoxication, a serious consequence of diluting formula too much

    2. If using the aseptic method, wash, rinse, and boil all equipment for 10 minutes; mix cooled boiled water with the desired amount of formula and pour it into bottles; cap the bottles with nipples down; and refrigerate

    3. In terminal sterilization, mix formula with tap water and pour it into clean bottles; loosely cap the bottles; boil them in a sterilizer for 25 minutes; after cooling the bottles, tighten the caps and refrigerate the formula

III. Special considerations for infant feeding

A. Basic principles

    1. Wash hands thoroughly before beginning

    2. Wash the tops of cans before opening

    3. Wash and rinse all equipment thoroughly

    4. Cover and refrigerate partially used cans of milk or formula; use within 48 hours or discard

B. Common concerns of mothers

    1. Determining when the infant is hungry may be a concern initially, but the mother soon learns hunger cues from infant behavior, primarily crying

    2. Burping (removing air from the stomach) is best accomplished by holding the infant upright and gently stroking the back; vigorous pounding on the back is unnecessary

    3. Regurgitation, confused by many mothers with vomiting, represents overflow and relief of stomach distention in an infant who has been fed too much or has eaten too rapidly

    4. Hiccups will go away without doing anything to the infant

    5. Constipation is less common in infants fed breast milk or commercial formulas than in infants fed cow's milk. The quality of stool (soft and well-formed as opposed to dry and hard or loose and watery) is more important than quantity or frequency

C. Nutritional requirements of the newborn

    1. Easily digested nutrients include water, calories, carbohydrate, fat, vitamins, and minerals

    2. The newborn requires about 140 to 160 ml of fluid/kg of body weight/24 hours to meet fluid needs during the first 10 days of life

    3. The newborn requires 110 to 120 calories/kg of body weight/24 hours during the first 2 weeks, or 50 to 55 calories/lb/day (most prepared formulas provide 20 calories per ounce, as does mature breast milk)

    4. The recommended protein intake in the first month is 14 g/day

    5. Nutritional supplements usually are unnecessary during the first 6 months for infants fed on breast milk or commercial formulas, although some authorities recommend supplemental vitamin D for breast-fed infants; fresh cow's milk or evaporated milk formula may necessitate supplemental vitamin C and usually is not recommended for infants before age 6 to 9 months because it is allergenic

    6. Early addition of solid foods to the infant's diet usually is not recommended; these can be delayed for most infants for 4 to 6 months, at which time the infant is developmentally ready to accept and digest solid foods; commercially prepared baby foods without added salt or sugar are available

MATERNAL-NEWBORN NURSING

7. The nurse can help prevent infantile obesity by encouraging the parents to:
   a. Use a gauge other than the infant's weight as a measure of their success as parents
   b. Delay introduction of solid foods
   c. Avoid overfeeding the infant
   d. Promote activity in the infant
D. Feeding patterns
   1. The parents should allow the infant to establish the feeding pattern; because formula is digested more slowly, formula-fed infants usually feed less frequently (every 2 to 5 hours) than breast-fed infants (every 2 to 3 hours)
   2. Both breast- and bottle-fed infants will feed more often or require larger feedings with growth spurts; for example, at 10 to 14 days, 5 to 6 weeks, and about 3 months
E. Infant positioning
   1. The infant should be placed on the right side after feeding to promote digestion; placement on either side helps prevent aspiration of regurgitated matter or emesis, as does elevating the head of the bed
   2. The infant should not be placed in the prone position because this position has been linked to sudden infant death syndrome.

The client who is breast-feeding

Feeding her infant successfully is a major concern to a new mother such as Della DeShon; success in this area is important to her development of a positive self-concept as a new mother. Anticipatory guidance by a knowledgeable nurse, along with supportive hospital policies, can help make breast-feeding successful for the client who lacks experience. The following clinical situation focuses on nursing guidance of the new mother who is breast-feeding.

Clinical situation

Mrs. DeShon and infant Sean, age 4 hours, are rooming in. His initial feeding experience was brief and took place during the early bonding period, within an hour after birth. Now, you are the nurse present during this attempt by Mrs. DeShon to breast-feed Sean.

Assessment

NURSING BEHAVIORS	NURSING RATIONALES
1. Assess Mrs. DeShon's condition.	**1.** Although breast-feeding is recommended as soon as possible after delivery, the feeding may need to be postponed if the mother is heavily sedated, exhausted, or in pain.
2. Assess Sean's condition.	**2.** Breast-feeding is more likely to be successful if the infant is alert and awake. He must have an open airway and be able to maintain thermoregulation.

Nursing diagnoses
- Risk for maternal injury related to a lack of knowledge of proper breast-feeding techniques
- Altered maternal nutrition (less than body requirements) related to increased nutritional needs of the breast-feeding mother
- Altered infant nutrition (less than body requirements) related to adjustment to feeding

Planning and goals
- Mrs. DeShon will achieve basic understanding of the physiology of lactation and of breast-feeding techniques.
- Sean's fluid intake and nutritional needs will be adequately met through successful breast-feeding experiences.
- Mrs. DeShon will have knowledge of Sean's individual feeding pattern and behavior.
- Breast-feeding will be a mutually satisfying experience for mother and infant.

Implementation

NURSING BEHAVIORS

1. Prepare Mrs. DeShon for breast-feeding before Sean is ready for his feeding. Have her wash her hands, and give her as much privacy as she requests.

2. Help Mrs. DeShon into a comfortable position for feeding: side-lying or sitting. She can use a football hold (most often required by mothers who have delivered by cesarean section and mothers desiring to nurse twins simultaneously) or the traditional cuddle hold. Position Sean so his weight does not pull on the breast and so he can breathe (infants are obligatory nose-breathers). Turn him onto his side so that he is abdomen-to-abdomen with his mother.

3. Review the feeding reflexes with Mrs. DeShon, and show her how to elicit them, as follows:

- Teach her to help Sean grasp the nipple and areola.

- Assess the position of Sean's mouth on the breast. His upper and lower lips should flare outward.

- Teach her to squeeze a small amount of milk (colostrum) out of the breast to moisten the nipple.

NURSING RATIONALES

1. This approach reduces the mother's frustration as well as the waiting time between the infant's readiness to feed and the start of feeding. A restful, calm environment promotes the let-down reflex. Washing the mother's hands helps protect the infant from infection (neonatal resistance to infection is low).

2. Understanding these options enables the mother to experiment and find a comfortable position for her and her baby. Varying the position from one feeding to another changes the angle of the baby's mouth (jaws) on the nipple and may help prevent nipple soreness and promote drainage of all milk storage sinuses.

3. Rooting, sucking, swallowing, and gagging reflexes are present from birth. The mother's confidence is increased by eliciting them herself. For example, touching the cheek with the nipple stimulates the rooting reflex.

- To draw out milk, the infant needs to grasp the nipple and most of the areola, which keeps him from chewing on the nipple. Nipple rolling is helpful if the nipple is not prominent.

- Improper mouth position may impede complete emptying and promote breast engorgement and nipple soreness.

- The smell of milk and the moistened nipple may be necessary to get breast-feeding started. Nipple shields should not be used because they tend to confuse the newborn and prevent emptying of the sinuses.

MATERNAL-NEWBORN NURSING

4. Provide anticipatory guidance for Mrs. DeShon as follows:

4. Anticipatory guidance helps the mother achieve success and independence in her feeding efforts.

• Help Mrs. DeShon adjust to Sean's sucking cycle.

• The infant should not be forced to adopt a sucking rhythm that is not natural for him. Accepting her infant's feeding behavior also lets the mother know there is no single "right" behavior. Infants have different sucking behaviors—for example, suck-compress-swallow. Rest periods are interspersed throughout the suck-compress-swallow cycle.

• If Sean is sleepy and will not breast-feed, reassure his mother and explain that many infants do not breast-feed well during the first few days after birth.

• The infant will feed when he is hungry. Efforts to get breast-feeding started should be discontinued if the infant does not respond within 10 minutes. This will prevent frustration for the mother and the infant. The mother may become alarmed about her infant's lack of food intake or fear that he is rejecting her or her milk. To reassure her, the nurse can explain that a loss of 5% to 10% of the infant's body weight is common during the first few days after birth and that he has enough stored body fluids to meet his fluid needs until breast-feeding is established.

• Advise Mrs. DeShon to begin each breast-feeding session with the breast from which Sean finished the previous feeding.

• This promotes equal breast emptying and equal milk production in both breasts.

• Teach Mrs. DeShon to break nipple suction by inserting a finger into the infant's mouth beside the nipple.

• Pulling the infant from the breast may cause nipple damage.

• Teach Mrs. DeShon to burp Sean at intervals.

• The infant may be burped at a change of breast or at the end of feeding. Breast-fed infants do not swallow as much air as bottle-fed infants, but they still need to be burped, especially if they have been crying before or during a feeding.

• When Sean is finished feeding, position him on his right side.

• This positioning aids stomach emptying and prevents aspiration from regurgitation or spitting up.

5. Record the type of instruction given and the maternal-infant response to feeding.

5. Documentation of care according to institutional procedure promotes continuity of care and identifies areas where reinforcement is needed.

6. Allow Mrs. DeShon time alone to manage feedings by herself, with the call bell or signal within reach.

6. Self-initiated independent feeding periods instill confidence once the infant feeds successfully after a few minutes at the breast.

7. At Mrs. DeShon's request, provide for her attendance at breast-feeding classes on the maternity unit to explore common concerns, such as:

7. Group classes provide an opportunity for the new mother to discuss her progress and concerns with other breast-feeding mothers.

• scheduling

• Scheduling is self-regulatory or on demand: The infant indicates he is hungry by crying.

• time between feedings

• Most breast-fed infants nurse on demand every 2 to 3 hours at first; then, because feeding stimulates milk production and satisfies sucking needs, the time between feedings increases as the infant's feeding pattern is established.

• length of breast-feeding periods

• The mother should offer each breast for 10 to 15 minutes at each feeding, gradually increasing the time. The condition of the mother and the breast are useful as a guide to breast-feeding periods. Imposing time limits has not been found to reduce nipple soreness. Milk supply is regulated by demand or by breast emptying.

• measures to encourage milk let-down, such as a warm shower or application of warm compresses to the breasts, a warm drink, rest, increased fluid and protein intake, and breast massage before feeding.

• Anticipatory guidance provides the mother with self-care measures to alleviate potential problems.

8. Discuss nipple care with Mrs. DeShon, as follows:

8. These measures minimize nipple soreness and prevent dry, cracked nipples.

• washing nipples with plain water during a shower

• Hand washing is more important than washing the nipples. A natural antiseptic is provided by the oil-secreting nipples and the enzymes in milk.

• allowing colostrum to remain on the nipples after the feeding

• Colostrum promotes healing. Ointments and creams have questionable value.

• allowing nipples to air-dry.

• Plastic bra liners are not recommended because they retain moisture against the nipples. If leakage is a problem, an absorbent pad or large handkerchief may be used.

9. Teach Mrs. DeShon methods to relieve breast engorgement, as follows:

9. Breast engorgement during the first few days after delivery interferes with the let-down reflex. In addition, infant sucking typically becomes choppy rather than rhythmic.

• Massage the breasts before feeding and alternately during feeding.

• Breast massage promotes milk let-down.

• Express breast milk when Sean cannot be breast-fed.

• Emptying the breasts may be necessary if, for example, the mother cannot breast-feed because she is ill or at work. Although electric-pump expression is effective, manual expression is recommended because it closely resembles the action of the infant's mouth on the breast during feeding. Expressed milk can be refrigerated for up to 24 hours or frozen for up to 6 months; it should not be heated in a microwave oven.

MATERNAL-NEWBORN NURSING

10. Before discharge, provide Mrs. DeShon with literature on breast-feeding and, if necessary or requested, with telephone numbers for La Leche League, a pediatric nurse practitioner, or a lactation consultant.

10. Support and information for breast-feeding mothers should be continued after discharge because they enhance long-term success.

Evaluation

- Mrs. DeShon has a basic understanding of lactation and has beginning skills in breast-feeding Sean.
- Mrs. DeShon demonstrates correct use of a variety of breast-feeding positions.
- Sean exhibits correct attachment to the breast.
- Sean's nutritional needs are being met.
- Breast-feeding is a mutually satisfying experience for Mrs. DeShon and Sean.
- Sean's intake and output are normal.

The high-risk newborn

I. **Conditions that put the newborn at high risk**
   A. Prematurity
   B. Postmaturity
   C. Maternal diabetes mellitus
   D. Maternal substance abuse
   E. Infection
   F. Small-for-gestational-age (SGA) or large-for-gestational-age (LGA) status
   G. Hemolytic disease of the newborn (see *High-risk maternal and newborn problems,* pages 312 to 314)
   H. Obstetric complications
      1. Mechanical delivery interventions (for example, use of forceps)
      2. Abruptio placentae

II. **Problems associated with high-risk status**
   A. Greater neonatal morbidity
   B. Greater neonatal mortality

III. **Methods to prevent or mitigate high-risk newborn status**
   A. Antepartal identification of genetic, prenatal, intrapartal, and gestational risk factors
   B. Labor and delivery at facility equipped to manage high-risk newborns
   C. Prediction of risk from Apgar scores
   D. Complete physical examination, gestational age assessment, and evaluation for LGA and SGA status as soon as possible after delivery

The preterm newborn and family

The preterm (premature) newborn is one who is born before the end of the 37th week of gestation. (By comparison, the full-term newborn is born between weeks 38 and 42; the postterm newborn, after week 42).

To help identify preterm status, the newborn's birth weight and gestational age are plotted on a chart shortly after delivery. (See *Classification of newborns by intrauterine growth and gestational age,* page 315.) A preterm newborn may be of appropriate weight for gestational age, small for gestational age (below the 10th percentile), or large for gestational age (above the 90th percentile). Most preterm newborns weigh less than 2,500 g.

A high-risk newborn, the preterm newborn faces major problems resulting from physiologic immaturity. In the United States, where the incidence of prematurity ranges from about 7% for whites to 15% for nonwhites, improved management techniques and specialized neonatal care units with advanced technology have increased the survival rate for preterm newborns.

Risk factors for prematurity include low socioeconomic status or poor nutritional status of the mother; such maternal problems as anemia, diabetes mellitus, cardiac problems, and infections; and complications of pregnancy, labor, and delivery.

Preterm birth causes an unexpected emotional crisis for the infant's parents. The normal psychological adaptations to pregnancy may arouse feelings of guilt in the mother who delivers prematurely, regardless of her age, marital status, or degree of emotional maturity.

The following clinical situation focuses on care of the preterm newborn during the first few days after delivery and on the psychological needs of a preterm newborn's parents.

Clinical situation

Marietta Walters, 2 days old, was born at 28 weeks' gestation to a 20-year-old single mother. You are the nurse caring for Marietta in the neonatal high-risk nursery. She had an Apgar score of 5 at 1 minute after delivery and suffered three brief attacks of apnea during her first 24 hours of life. Her weight, 1,200 g (2 lb, 11 oz), is appropriate for her gestational age.

Assessment

NURSING BEHAVIORS

1. Review the maternal history (general, medical, and obstetric), noting age, socioeconomic status, labor and delivery events, and Apgar scores.

2. Assess Marietta's respiratory status, as follows:

• Assess Marietta's respiratory rate (average, 40 to 60 breaths/minute), depth, and regularity (usually shallow and irregular), and note any cyanosis, grunting, retractions, nasal flaring, and periods of apnea as well as periods when the respiratory rate is consistently below 30 or above 60 breaths/minute.

• Assess Marietta's breath sounds.

NURSING RATIONALES

1. Data from the maternal history contribute to baseline information and frequently point to risk factors associated with preterm delivery. Signs and symptoms of intrauterine hypoxia include meconium-stained amniotic fluid in cephalic presentation and abnormal fetal heart rate patterns related to asphyxia.

2. Immature respiratory system development and functioning increase the preterm newborn's risk of respiratory distress.

• The preterm newborn has weak respiratory muscles, a weak cough, and inadequate lung surfactant. Apnea is common in preterm newborns and typically results from respiratory distress syndrome. (See *Silverman-Anderson index of respiratory distress,* page 316.)

• Crackles, rhonchi, or inadequate breath sounds on auscultation may warrant further evaluation and treatment.

High-risk maternal and newborn problems

RISK FACTOR	POTENTIAL MATERNAL, FETAL, AND NEWBORN PROBLEMS	NURSING IMPLICATIONS
Maternal substance use		
Maternal alcohol abuse	• The mother may show evidence of nutritional deficiencies, acute withdrawal symptoms at time of delivery, ineffective coping and parenting skills, and family dysfunctioning. • The fetus or newborn is at high risk for fetal alcohol syndrome (FAS). Problems associated with FAS include intrauterine growth retardation (IUGR), mental retardation, and seizures. • Typically, the newborn has small eyes; a short, upturned nose; small, flat cheeks; and organ malformations.	• Teach pregnant and lactating clients not to consume alcohol. • Monitor the mother and the fetus or newborn for altered physiologic functioning. • Monitor the newborn closely for problems associated with increased risk of respiratory distress, cardiopulmonary arrest, and feeding problems resulting from congenital and developmental defects. • Avoid overstimulating the infant. • Help the parents recognize and accept anomalies. • Plan for long-term follow-up care.
Maternal narcotic abuse	• The mother may show evidence of nutritional deficiencies. She is at increased risk for pelvic inflammatory disease, malpresentations, third trimester bleeding, postpartal morbidity, and death. • The fetus or newborn is at risk for congenital anomalies from teratogenic effects of drugs taken during the first trimester. IUGR is common, and the risk of fetal or perinatal death is increased. Meconium aspiration at birth is also common. Withdrawal behaviors occur at birth and may persist for several months after delivery and initial withdrawal.	• Provide psychoprophylactic support of the mother for relief of discomfort during labor and delivery to minimize use of pain medications (these may cause fetal distress). • Assist with methadone maintenance therapy for the mother during pregnancy, and monitor for symptoms of risk to the fetus. • Observe for withdrawal behavior in the newborn (irritability, hyperactivity, hypertonia, sleep problems, feeding difficulties). • Medicate the infant as ordered to reduce withdrawal symptoms (phenobarbital or diazepam [Valium] is commonly used; methadone is not given to the infant). • Reduce environmental stimuli for the mother and the infant.
Maternal cocaine abuse	• The mother is at risk for abruptio placentae, preterm labor, seizures, pulmonary edema, respiratory failure, and cardiac problems. • The fetus is at risk for stillbirth and IUGR. • The newborn is at risk for poor state organization (quickly changing sleep-awake states); learning disabilities; decreased interactive behaviors; sudden infant death syndrome (SIDS); and central nervous system (CNS), cardiac, and genitourinary anomalies.	• Discourage breast-feeding (cocaine enters breast milk). • Assess maternal-infant attachment. • Make referrals, as appropriate, to social workers, parenting counselors, or support groups.
Maternal nicotine use	• The mother has a greater chance for spontaneous abortion, placenta previa and abruption, and premature rupture of membranes. Also, vitamin and mineral utilization may be poor from the vasoconstrictive effects of nicotine on uterine vessels. • The newborn is at risk for lower birth weight, preterm delivery, frequent respiratory infections and otitis media, and SIDS.	• Counsel pregnant clients to stop or reduce their smoking. • Teach clients about the effects of passive smoking on the fetus. • Inform lactating clients that nicotine can be transferred to the newborn through breast milk.

High-risk maternal and newborn problems *(continued)*

RISK FACTOR	POTENTIAL MATERNAL, FETAL, AND NEWBORN PROBLEMS	NURSING IMPLICATIONS
Gestational age and birth weight abnormalities		
Small-for-gestational-age (SGA) status	• These infants have a birth weight below the 10th percentile (excluding heredity factors). SGA infants are at increased risk for perinatal morbidity and mortality from asphyxia, meconium aspiration, hypoglycemia, and ineffective thermoregulation. • Common characteristics of SGA infants include decreased subcutaneous fat; loose, dry skin; normal head size but reduced size of chest and abdomen; thin, yellowish, dry umbilical cord; sparse scalp hair; and a wide-eyed look. IUGR is a condition of fetal undergrowth.	• Complete a gestational age assessment. • Maintain the infant's cardiopulmonary functioning. • Frequently monitor the infant for evidence of low blood glucose and hematocrit levels. • Assist with treatment of complications. • Teach the parents how to care for the infant; support development of a positive parent-infant relationship. • Be aware that knowledge deficits related to the special care of these infants and potential alterations in parenting are common nursing diagnoses for families of SGA infants; plan care accordingly.
Large-for-gestational-age (LGA) status	• The LGA newborn is macrosomic, with a birth weight above the 90th percentile. Excessive fetal growth is associated with maternal diabetes mellitus, genetic predisposition, multiparity, male sex, and hemolytic disease. Complicated delivery can result in birth trauma and injuries related to cephalopelvic disproportion and an increased cesarean section rate. The LGA newborn also is at risk for hypoglycemia, polycythemia, and hyperviscosity. Characteristics of macrosomia include excessive adipose tissue; a cherubic face; hypotonic extremities; reddened appearance; and difficulty feeding.	• Perform a careful gestational age assessment to promote early identification and treatment of LGA status. • Screen for hypoglycemia and polycythemia. • Provide newborn care similar to that required for the infant of a diabetic mother.
Preterm status (before 38 weeks)	• Immaturity of all body systems puts the preterm newborn at risk for respiratory distress syndrome, hypothermia, renal and digestive disorders (such as necrotizing enterocolitis), jaundice, infections, patent ductus arteriosus, apnea, intraventricular hemorrhage, retinopathy of prematurity, and delayed periods of reactivity.	• Provide higher-calorie and higher-protein formula and vitamin supplements, as ordered. Be aware that breast milk has many benefits for preterm newborns. • Maintain a patent airway and a neutrothermal environment. • Assess and report laboratory results. • Monitor oxygen administration; plan for long-term follow-up care. • Assess for sensory and neurologic defects. Provide sensory stimulation. • Organize care to allow rest periods.
Postterm status (after 42 weeks)	• Increased maternal risks of infection, dystocia, and bleeding are associated with tests to evaluate placental sufficiency and fetal status (such as the oxytocin challenge test). Labor may be induced, and the fetus may be delivered by cesarean section. The mother may feel emotionally drained during a prolonged pregnancy. She may fear for her own safety and the safety of her infant. • The infant is at risk for postmaturity syndrome (long, thin, emaciated infant with evidence of recent weight loss) and IUGR (from uteroplacental insufficiency). Some infants are small for their gestational age; others, large. The infant has an increased risk of congenital anomalies, seizure activity from hypoxia, cold stress, loss of subcutaneous fat, and poor development.	• Support cardiopulmonary functioning. • Provide warmth to balance diminished response to cold stress. • Monitor the infant's glucose levels and initiate early feeding if ordered and indicated. • Support development of the mother-infant relationship.

(continued)

High-risk maternal and newborn problems (continued)

RISK FACTOR	POTENTIAL MATERNAL, FETAL, AND NEWBORN PROBLEMS	NURSING IMPLICATIONS
Perinatal problems		
Neonatal infections	• High-risk newborns have an increased risk for acquiring a local or systemic infection, either through the mother or through environmental contamination during labor, delivery, and newborn care. • *Generalized sepsis* may cause lethargy, restlessness, poor weight gain, diarrhea, vomiting, CNS problems such as seizures and, in severe cases, death. Common causative organisms include *Escherichia coli* and Group B Beta *Streptococcus*. • *Hepatitis B* may be passed from the mother to the newborn at delivery. This viral disease may lead to death from cirrhosis or hepatocellular carcinoma before adulthood. • *Perinatal AIDS* causes frequent infections, diarrhea, failure to thrive, motor skill and speech delays and, ultimately, death. Enlargement of the liver, spleen, lymph nodes, and salivary glands is common.	• Minimize sources of environmental infection during labor, delivery, and newborn care. • Assist with identification, monitoring, and treatment of maternal infections during the prenatal, intrapartal, and postnatal periods. • Closely monitor I.V. antibiotics used to treat neonatal sepsis. Ampicillin and gentamicin are most commonly used. • Institute isolation procedures as needed. • Promote maternal-infant contact as soon as possible. • Administer hepatitis B prophylaxis to the newborn, as ordered. Hepatitis immunoglobulin is promptly administered (first 12 hours) to newborns of mothers with hepatitis B or who are carriers. The vaccine is recommended for all infants. • Screen at-risk mothers for human immunodeficiency virus (HIV) before delivery. Be aware that HIV testing is not reliable for newborns because maternal antibodies may be present in the newborn's blood for up to 15 months after birth. (However, new and more reliable tests are on the horizon.)
Isoimmune hemolytic disease of the newborn (Rh or ABO incompatibility)	• Rh incompatibility may occur when the pregnant woman who has Rh-negative blood is sensitized (has anti-Rh antibodies) and the fetus has Rh-positive blood. The anti-Rh antibodies cross the placenta and cause hemolysis of fetal red blood cells. The fetus or newborn is at risk for hemolytic anemia; cardiac decomposition; enlargement of heart, liver, and spleen; edema; ascites; hemorrhage; hypoglycemia; jaundice; kernicterus; irreversible brain damage; and neonatal death. • ABO incompatibility occurs when the pregnant woman has blood with anti-A or anti-B antibodies and the fetus has type A, B, or AB blood. The antibodies cross the placenta and cause hemolysis of fetal red blood cells. The fetus or newborn is usually mildly affected. ABO incompatibility rarely results in symptoms severe enough to be diagnosed and treated.	• Administer $Rh_o(D)$ immune globulin (RhoGAM), as ordered, to Rh-negative women who are at risk for developing isoimmunization. The physician may order RhoGAM based on results of laboratory tests (hemantigen, indirect Coombs' test) at about 28 weeks' gestation and within 72 hours of delivery to prevent anti-Rh antibody formation. • Prevent conditions that would further jeopardize the infant (respiratory distress, cold stress, acidosis, and infection). Assess the results of laboratory tests (Coombs', blood type, and bilirubin levels). Assess for jaundice within 24 to 36 hours after delivery. • Use phototherapy to reduce serum bilirubin levels, protecting the newborn's eyes with eye patches. Phototherapy may be provided by wrapping the newborn in or placing the newborn on a flexible fiberoptic mat. Observe for loose green stools and green urine. Provide additional fluids to compensate for fluid loss. Provide special skin care. Exchange transfusions may be necessary in severe cases. • Keep the parents informed and involved in the care of the newborn.
Meconium aspiration syndrome	Aspiration of meconium may lead to airway obstruction, increased alveoli inflation, and rupture of the alveoli, causing interstitial pneumonia.	• Provide supportive care for respiratory distress. • Minimize the possibility of asphyxiation and birth trauma during high-risk labor and delivery.

Classification of newborns by intrauterine growth and gestational age

WEIGHT PERCENTILES

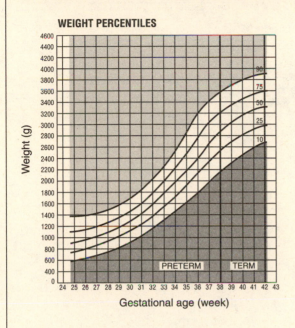

LENGTH PERCENTILES

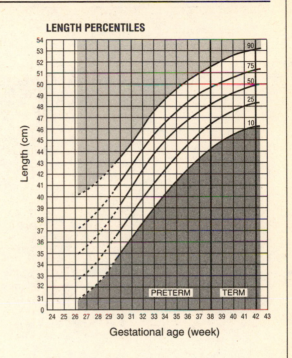

HEAD CIRCUMFERENCE PERCENTILES

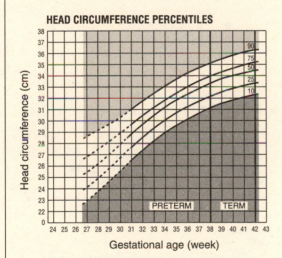

CLASSIFICATION OF INFANT*

	Weight	Length	Head circ.
Large for gestational age (LGA) (> 90th percentile)			
Appropriate for gestational age (AGA) (10th to 90th percentile)			
Small for gestational age (SGA) (< 10th percentile)			

*Place an "X" in the appropriate box (LGA, AGA, or SGA) for weight, for length, and for head circumference.

Adapted with permission from Battaglia, F.C., and Lubchenco, L.O. "A Practical Classification of Newborn Infants by Weight and Gestational Age," *Journal of Pediatrics* 71:159-163, 1967, and from Lubchenco, L.O., et al. "Intrauterine Growth in Length and Head Circumference as Estimated from Live Births at Gestational Ages from 26 to 46 Weeks," *Journal of Pediatrics,* 37:403-408, 1966.

MATERNAL-
NEWBORN
NURSING

Silverman-Anderson index of respiratory distress

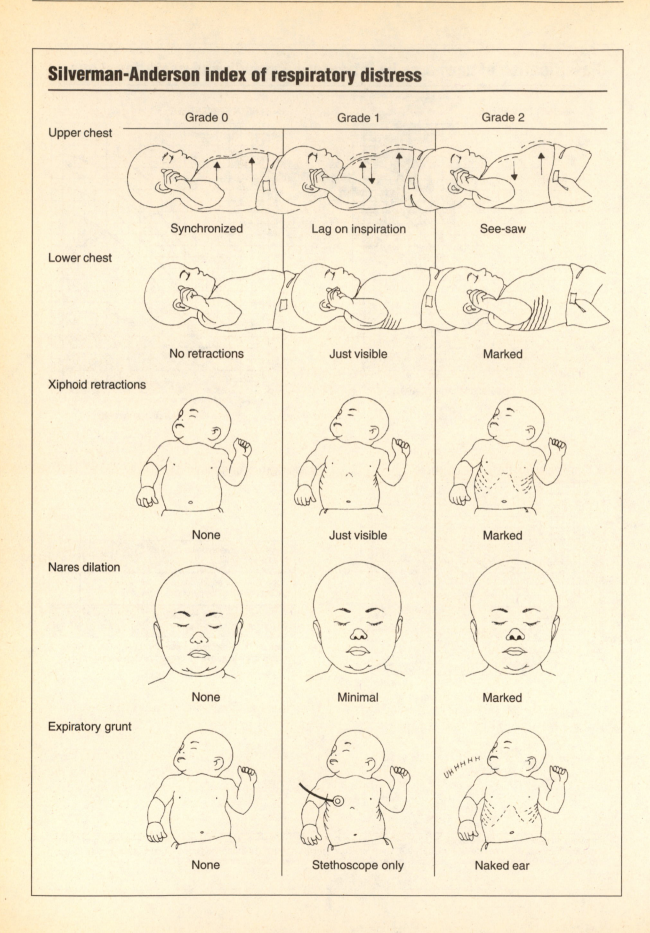

	Grade 0	Grade 1	Grade 2
Upper chest	Synchronized	Lag on inspiration	See-saw
Lower chest	No retractions	Just visible	Marked
Xiphoid retractions	None	Just visible	Marked
Nares dilation	None	Minimal	Marked
Expiratory grunt	None	Stethoscope only	Naked ear

3. Assess Marietta's body temperature.

3. The desired skin body temperature is 97° to 98° F (36.1° to 36.7° C). In the preterm infant, an immature temperature-regulating mechanism, decreased reserves of brown fat and glycogen, and a lack of subcutaneous fat cause fluctuations in temperature that may lead to cold stress.

4. Count Marietta's apical pulse rate (normal range: 120 to 160 beats/minute).

4. The preterm infant's pulse rate is usually rapid and irregular.

5. Assess Marietta's color (it is usually pink or ruddy, but acrocyanosis may be present).

5. Jaundice, cyanosis, and pallor are common in the preterm infant.

6. Assess Marietta's body movements and posture.

6. The infant's immature nervous system may cause jerky body movements. Any seizure activity is abnormal. The preterm newborn exhibits less flexion than a term newborn.

7. Assess Marietta's cry.

7. The preterm infant's cry may be weak and feeble.

8. Assess Marietta's patterns of elimination (voiding, stools). Check urine specific gravity.

8. The first meconium stool may be small because of weak peristalsis. Urine output is usually scanty for a few days after birth, but the first voiding normally occurs within the first 24 hours. Urine is dilute.

9. Evaluate Marietta's level of physiologic prematurity, noting any associated problems. (For this, the Dubowitz criteria may be useful.) Review the Ballard gestational age assessment tool.

9. This assessment helps the nurse develop a care plan based on individual variations among the physiologic parameters.

10. Assess Marietta for common problems of preterm infants, including respiratory distress syndrome, apnea, hypothermia, hypoglycemia, central nervous system hemorrhage, infection, and malnutrition.

10. These problems commonly occur in preterm infants of average gestational age.

11. Assess the mother's perception of her newborn's condition.

11. Delivery of a preterm infant presents a crisis for the parents. In particular, equipment and activities in the neonatal intensive care nursery may cause the mother to perceive the infant's condition as more critical than it actually is.

12. Assess the extent of accomplishment of parental tasks associated with preterm birth, as follows:

12. The nurse should support parental adaptation to the birth of a preterm infant.

• anticipatory grief and depression

• The parents may experience anticipatory grief related to fear that the infant will not survive. Grief and depression may persist until the infant is out of danger.

• confrontation and acknowledgment of failure to deliver a full-term infant

• The parents may have poor self-images as new parents because of the failure to carry the infant to term.

• initiation of bonding and attachment behaviors indicating that the parents are relating to their infant (for example, touch, eye contact, involvement in her care)

• Prolonged separation may interfere with bonding and attachment. For example, the touch sequence (fingertips-to-palm contact) may be delayed, and initiation of other behaviors may not occur for several visits. Also, parents may fear hurting the infant by handling her.

• learning about the newborn's special needs and growth patterns.

• The parents must understand and accept the special care needs and developmental patterns, different from those of full-term infants, that their preterm infant may require.

13. Assess the cultural, religious, financial, and family support systems available to the newborn's parents.

13. The preterm infant's parents, especially the mother, must have the support of other family members and, if necessary, of appropriate community resources.

Nursing diagnoses

• Altered nutrition (less than body requirements) related to immature feeding reflexes
• Impaired gas exchange related to immature lungs
• Ineffective thermoregulation related to an immature temperature regulatory center and lack of subcutaneous and brown fat
• Risk for infection related to immunologic immaturity
• Altered parenting related to lack of knowledge of infant care

Planning and goals

• Marietta will have minimal difficulty recovering from the effects of prematurity.
• Marietta's physiologic status will stabilize.
• Marietta will receive adequate fluid and nutrients.
• Marietta will not experience life-threatening complications.
• The mother will be referred for supportive services.
• The mother will accomplish psychological tasks and prepare for home care.

Implementation

NURSING BEHAVIORS

1. Support Marietta's respirations, as follows:
• Maintain a patent airway.
• Position her head so it is slightly elevated.
• Perform suctioning as needed.
• Assist with therapy for respiratory distress as needed.

NURSING RATIONALES

1. An immature respiratory system predisposes the infant to respiratory distress. Positioning the infant with the head slightly elevated helps maintain the airway. Avoid the prone position, which has been associated with sudden infant death syndrome. Gentle suctioning may also be needed to maintain airway patency. Additional measures are required if respiratory distress occurs.

2. To reduce apnea frequency, stimulate Marietta's respirations with a bag and mask or, if necessary, a ventilator.

2. Mechanical ventilation may be necessary if the infant becomes apneic (no breaths for 15 to 20 seconds) with bradycardia and cyanosis. A nonstimulating environment (gentle handling and suctioning) may also help reduce apnea frequency.

3. If Marietta becomes cyanotic, administer oxygen as ordered. Every 2 hours, check the environmental oxygen concentration (ideally less than 40%, or the minimum percentage needed to maintain pink mucosa color). Discontinue oxygen therapy as soon as possible. Monitor the partial pressure of arterial oxygen (PaO$_2$) via pulse oximetry. For the most accurate evaluation of oxygenation, draw arterial blood gas (ABG) samples.

3. Oxygen administration can relieve symptoms of respiratory distress. However, to prevent retinal damage, the fraction of inspired oxygen (FIO$_2$) should be kept at a level that maintains PaO$_2$ below 100 mm Hg. Vision loss may occur if retinal vascular development is halted by excessive oxygen concentration. FIO$_2$ is adjusted to keep PaO$_2$ at the desired level (50 to 80 mm Hg). Pulse oximetry is a noninvasive method for monitoring transcutaneous PO$_2$; it can be used continuously or intermittently. ABG analysis is an invasive PaO$_2$ monitoring technique.

4. Monitor Marietta's ABG values.

4. The infant's ABG values help determine the appropriate oxygen concentration. Normal values include a pH of 7.30 to 7.44, PaO$_2$ of 50 to 80 mm Hg, and partial pressure of carbon dioxide (PaCO$_2$) of 22 to 48 mm Hg.

5. Maintain Marietta's body temperature, as follows:
• Check the skin probe's position frequently.
• Keep her environment thermoneutral, and warm and humidify oxygen before administering it.
• Pad cold surfaces where she may be placed.
• Keep her incubator and radiant warmer away from drafts.

5. These measures minimize heat loss from body surface areas and prevent cold stress, which increases oxygen needs. Fluctuations in the preterm infant's temperature result from a lack of subcutaneous fat and brown fat as well as from immature central nervous system (CNS) mechanisms for regulating body temperature.

6. Provide adequate nutrition and calories, using the following techniques as ordered and appropriate:

6. Adequate nutrition helps prevent hypoglycemia, dehydration, and other metabolic problems.

• Give sterile water, as ordered, for Marietta's first feedings, 2 and 4 hours after birth.

• Sterile water allows assessment of feeding problems without danger of milk aspiration.

• Provide frequent, small oral feedings (usually 1 to 2 oz every 2 to 3 hours) of high-calorie formula, using soft nipples.

• This feeding pattern provides more calories in smaller fluid volumes.

• Provide gavage feedings (nasogastric or nasojejunal) if Marietta's feeding reflexes are inadequate.

• By preventing aspiration, gavage feedings prevent aspiration pneumonia. Poor muscle tone and weak feeding reflexes are apparent during feeding. Regurgitation is common.

• Provide I.V. supplementation as ordered.

• Initially, because the preterm infant's stomach is small and slow to empty, oral feedings may not meet her fluid and calorie requirements.

• Note any signs of fatigue or distress during Marietta's feedings.

• Preterm infants who are ill or who fatigue easily during feedings may require gavage or transpyloric feedings to conserve energy.

• Weigh Marietta daily.

• Weight gain is one measure of growth.

• Observe Marietta for signs of inadequate fluid intake, such as dehydration and low urine output.

• Inadequate hydration may lead to fluid and electrolyte imbalance.

7. Provide phototherapy, using a light or fiberoptic blanket.
• Cover Marietta's eyes.
• Use a radiance meter.
• Cover Marietta's ovaries (cover testes if the newborn is a boy).
• Provide skin care.
• Monitor Marietta's intake and output.

8. Implement measures to prevent and control infection, as follows:
• Provide the parents with guidance in hand washing and in handling the infant.
• Use aseptic technique when caring for Marietta.
• Isolate her from infants who may have infections, and follow infection control measures (especially hand washing and cleaning of equipment) in the nursery.
• If she develops an infection, administer antibiotic therapy as ordered.

9. Monitor Marietta for complications, assessing and recording any that develop, as follows:

• If hypoglycemia develops, test Marietta's capillary blood glucose with Dextrostix or Chemstrip every 4 hours until her glucose level stabilizes.

• As ordered, give Marietta oral or I.V. glucose. Monitor for glycosuria and osmotic diuresis.

• Monitor Marietta for signs and symptoms of hypocalcemia. Report serum calcium levels below 7 mg/dl, and observe for signs of tetany, such as jerking and tremors.

• If hypocalcemia occurs, administer 10% calcium gluconate I.V. as ordered. Monitor the infant (preferably with an electronic monitor) during administration.

10. Monitor Marietta for shocklike symptoms (pallor, cyanosis, apnea, bradycardia, seizure activity, and muscular rigidity) and signs of circulatory failure and CNS irritability. Assist with life-support therapies (for example, transfusion, oxygen, and medication for seizure activity), as ordered.

7. Phototherapy converts bilirubin to an enzyme that is excreted in urine and feces. Covering the newborn's body parts helps prevent damage from the light.

8. Physiologic immaturity, invasive procedures (for example, umbilical catheterization), and ventilation equipment place the premature infant at greater risk for infection. Most of the listed measures minimize the preterm infant's exposure to infectious agents; antibiotic therapy combats infection. Sepsis neonatorum (infection in the neonate) results most often from gram-negative organisms, such as *Escherichia coli*, *Proteus*, and *Klebsiella*, and gram-positive beta-hemolytic streptococci.

9. Early recognition of and intervention for complications in the preterm infant may help prevent long-term problems.

• Hypoglycemia is defined as a blood glucose level below 30 mg/dl during the first 72 hours. Signs include jitteriness, apnea, pallor, and lethargy. Unless detected and treated, hypoglycemia may cause CNS damage and death.

• Hyperglycemia (Dextrostix or Chemstrip value greater than 130 mg/dl) may cause osmotic diuresis and lead to dehydration.

• A preterm infant is at increased risk for neonatal tetany during the first 15 days after birth. Tetany is most common in preterm newborns who have suffered asphyxia or other forms of respiratory distress.

• Bradycardia may occur if calcium gluconate is administered too rapidly.

10. These signs and symptoms are associated with intraventricular hemorrhage, a common type of intracranial hemorrhage in the preterm infant. The infant may require respiratory support with a mechanical ventilator. Commercial pulmonary surfactants, such as colfosceril palmitate (EXOSURF Neonatal) and beractant (Survanta) may be given.

11. Explain the care plan to the mother.

11. This helps divert the mother's attention from the equipment and toward her newborn.

12. Encourage direct contact and development of caring skills.

12. This helps increase the mother's self-concept.

13. Encourage the mother to stimulate the infant's senses.

13. Stimulation promotes the newborn's development.

Evaluation

• Marietta exhibits physical and neurologic characteristics normal for her gestational age and weight.
• Marietta's respirations, pulse rate, and temperature stabilize within normal limits for her gestational age.
• Marietta's nutritional intake is adequate to promote growth, as evidenced by weight gain.
• Marietta is free of problems commonly associated with preterm delivery, such as respiratory distress syndrome, hypoglycemia, and increased intracranial pressure.
• The mother has accomplished psychological tasks.
• The mother knows how to use support services.

The newborn whose mother has diabetes mellitus

The neonate born of a diabetic mother requires special care related to having experienced, in utero, consistently high glucose levels and periodic acidosis; impaired fetal-placental circulation may also have occurred. The following clinical situation focuses on the care of a newborn whose mother is diabetic.

Clinical situation

Sam Baker, delivered by cesarean section at 36 weeks' gestation, is 2 hours old. His mother has had Type I (insulin-dependent) diabetes for 11 years. Sam weighed 10 lb, 3 oz at birth. You are the nurse assigned to care for the infant in the nursery.

Assessment

NURSING BEHAVIORS

NURSING RATIONALES

1. Assess Sam for signs of respiratory distress syndrome.

1. Respiratory distress syndrome may occur because the infant's lungs are physiologically immature and surfactant synthesis is poor. The infant of a diabetic mother is usually delivered early; the outlook for survival is best if delivery occurs after 36 weeks' gestation.

2. Note and record the infant's apical pulse rate.

2. Fluctuations in the infant's pulse rate may arise from physiologic immaturity.

3. Assess and record his temperature.

3. The infant's temperature may be labile because of physiologic immaturity. A thermoneutral environment should be maintained.

4. Assess Sam for neonatal complications of maternal diabetes mellitus, as follows:

• hypoglycemia (signs include lethargy, irritability, tremors, and a high-pitched cry)
—Test the infant's blood glucose every 2 hours until the glucose level is stable.
—Report values less than 40 mg/dl.

• hypocalcemia (primary sign: tremors)

• gestational age

• birth trauma from cephalopelvic disproportion (if delivered vaginally)

• congenital anomalies

• hyperbilirubinemia

• meconium aspiration

• electrolyte imbalance

• birth weight.

4. Infants of diabetic mothers are at risk for complications and require close observation for several days after birth.

• Fetal hyperinsulinism in utero occurs in response to high maternal blood glucose levels. After delivery, when maternal supply of glucose ceases, the infant continues to secrete large amounts of insulin and develops hypoglycemia (which may or may not be symptomatic) within 4 hours after birth. A plasma sample will be obtained and sent to the laboratory to confirm the glucose level.

• Diabetic mothers tend to have higher calcium levels at term that can cause secondary neonatal hypoparathyroidism—which may also be related to prematurity.

• Neonates born to diabetic mothers may be large for their gestational age (LGA); that is, their birth weight is at or greater than the 90th percentile for their number of gestational weeks.

• Because infants born to diabetic mothers are typically LGA, they commonly suffer birth trauma if delivered vaginally.

• The incidence of congenital anomalies (central nervous system, sacral, and lower-extremity deformities; tracheoesophageal fistulas; and congenital heart malformations) is higher in neonates born to diabetic mothers, especially if they are small for their gestational age.

• This finding is related to the infant's gestational age and immature liver functioning; the infant of a diabetic mother is usually delivered preterm.

• Aspiration of meconium with associated fetal distress is common in infants delivered vaginally to diabetic mothers.

• This finding may occur because of the infant's immature respiratory and renal system functioning.

• The infant's excessive size results from increased glycogen and protein synthesis and increased fat production. Other physical characteristics include a round, red, fat face; a chubby body; and macrosomia (enlarged viscera and heart and increased body fat).

5. Complete a physical assessment of Sam as soon as his condition permits, and report congenital anomalies or other disorders immediately. Assess Sam as follows:

• Evaluate the infant's physical maturity.

• Review test results to determine fetal maturity and maternalfetal status.

6. Assess Mrs. Baker for conditions other than diabetes (for example, preeclampsia).

5. Once the infant's condition stabilizes, he should be further assessed for such congenital anomalies as cardiac defects, which have a high incidence in infants of diabetic mothers.

• Although the infant may be physically large, he may function at a level closer to his gestational age.

• A lecithin/sphingomyelin ratio of at least 3:1 or phosphatid glycerol in the amniotic fluid is an index of lung maturity in the neonate born to a diabetic mother.

6. Maternal disorders may further jeopardize the infant's status.

Nursing diagnoses

• Risk for injury related to complications associated with the infant of a diabetic mother
• Altered parenting related to a delay in bonding

Planning and goals

• Sam will not experience the effects of hypoglycemia, hypocalcemia, or hyperbilirubinemia.
• Any congenital anomalies will be detected quickly, and appropriate treatment will be started promptly.
• Mr. and Mrs. Baker will verbalize understanding of the basis of the baby's health problems.
• Maternal-infant attachment will occur.

Implementation

NURSING BEHAVIORS

1. Monitor Sam's respirations frequently and have resuscitative equipment available for use if respiratory distress occurs.

2. Maintain a thermoneutral environment for Sam, and stabilize his temperature at 97.7° F (36° C). Use warming methods if necessary.

3. Feed Sam as necessary (oral or I.V. glucose, glucagon) to prevent or correct hypoglycemia.

4. Monitor Sam for hypocalcemia (serum calcium level less than 7 mg/dl).

• Give him 10% calcium I.V. as ordered.

NURSING RATIONALES

1. Respiratory distress commonly occurs in preterm neonates of diabetic mothers who have a cesarean section.

2. The neonate born to a diabetic mother needs the same care to maintain body temperature as a premature infant.

3. Hypoglycemia related to maternal diabetes may cause irreversible brain damage in the neonate. To treat mild hypoglycemia, the infant may be given 1 to 2 oz of 10% glucose in water. To prevent neonatal hyperinsulinemia and rebound hypoglycemia, a glucose bolus should be avoided.

4. This complication is associated with the infant's prematurity and the mother's diabetes.

• Calcium administered intramuscularly causes tissue necrosis.

MATERNAL-
NEWBORN
NURSING

• Monitor his cardiac status during calcium administration.

• Calcium administration may cause arrhythmias.

5. Promote maternal-infant attachment by keeping Mrs. Baker informed of Sam's status and by providing opportunities for mother-infant contact as soon as their conditions permit.

5. Prolonged separation may interfere with bonding and attachment.

6. Explain Sam's health problems to his parents; plan his follow-up care with Mrs. Baker.

6. The infant's problems reflect the response to maternal diabetes mellitus; they do not indicate that the infant is diabetic. However, the infant's risk of developing diabetes later in life is higher than average because diabetes mellitus can be hereditary.

Evaluation

• Sam's blood glucose, calcium, and bilirubin levels are stable and within normal limits.
• Any congenital anomalies are being investigated and managed appropriately.
• Mrs. Baker understands that her infant does not have diabetes mellitus; she also understands the importance of follow-up care for him.
• Maternal-infant attachment is progressing satisfactorily.

Selected drugs commonly used in maternal-newborn nursing

This chart presents information about drugs commonly prescribed in maternal-infant care, including the drug action, dosage, and common side effects. Nursing considerations focus on client comfort and teaching.

DRUG	DOSE	ACTION	SIDE EFFECTS	NURSING CONSIDERATIONS
Fertility agents				
chorionic gonadotropin, human [hCG] (APL, Pregnyl, Profasi, Profasi HP)	5,000 units to 10,000 units I.M. one day after the last dose of menotropins	Serves as a substitute for luteinizing hormone (LH) to stimulate ovulation of a prepared follicle	Headache, fatigue, irritability, restlessness, depression; pain at injection site	• When used with menotropins to induce ovulation, multiple births are possible. • Usually used only after failure of clomiphene in anovulatory patients. • In infertility, encourage daily intercourse from day before chorionic gonadotropin is given until ovulation occurs. • Be alert to symptoms of ectopic pregnancy. Usually evident between weeks 8 and 12 of gestation. • Reconstitute with 1 to 2 ml of supplied diluent just before use; use reconstituted solutions within 24 hours. • For I.M. use only; rotate injection sites to prevent muscle atrophy.
clomiphene citrate (Clomid)	50 mg P.O. q.d. for 5 days; a second course of 100 mg P.O. q.d. for 5 days may be used	Fertility agent; increases secretion of LH and follicle-stimulating hormone (FSH), thus stimulating follicular growth; induces ovulation 5 to 10 days after last dose	Decreased cervical mucus, nausea, vomiting, headache, vasomotor flushing, abdominal distention, ovarian enlargement, multiple gestation (5% incidence, mostly twins)	• Teach the client how to use a basal body temperature chart. • Encourage proper timing of sexual intercourse during ovulation. • Provide emotional support.
menotropins (Pergonal)	75 units each FSH and LH I.M. daily for 9 to 12 days, followed by 10,000 units chorionic gonadotropin I.M. 1 day after last dose of menotropins; repeat for one to three menstrual cycles until ovulation occurs	Mimics FSH in inducing follicular growth and LH in aiding follicular maturation	Nausea, vomiting, and diarrhea; ovarian enlargement with pain and abdominal distention; multiple births; ovarian hyperstimulation syndrome (sudden ovarian enlargement, ascites with or without pain, or pleural effusion)	• Close monitoring of patient response is critical to ensure adequate ovarian stimulation without hyperstimulation. • Tell patient that there is a possibility of multiple births. • In infertility, encourage daily intercourse from day before chorionic gonadotropin is given until ovulation occurs. • Pregnancy usually occurs 4 to 6 weeks after therapy. • Reconstitute with 1 to 2 ml sterile saline injection; use immediately. • Rotate injection sites to prevent muscle atrophy.

(continued)

MATERNAL-
NEWBORN
NURSING

Selected drugs commonly used in maternal-newborn nursing (continued)

DRUG	DOSE	ACTION	SIDE EFFECTS	NURSING CONSIDERATIONS
Antepartal drugs				
betamethasone (Celestone Soluspan)	12 mg I.M. 36 to 48 hours before delivery; repeat in 12 to 24 hours	Glucocorticoid; promotes fetal lung maturity; most effective when administered between 30 and 32 weeks' gestation	*Maternal:* increased risk of complications if the mother has pregnancy-induced hypertension (PIH), infection, peptic ulcer, or diabetes *Fetal:* hypoglycemia	• Administer by deep intramuscular injection. • Monitor the client for side effects such as hypotension. • Do not use estriol levels to assess fetal status.
ritodrine (Yutopar)	0.05 mg/minute; increase by 0.05 mg/minute q 10 minutes as needed; effective dose is usually 0.15 to 0.35 mg/minute	Tocolytic and beta-receptor agonist; relaxes uterine muscles	*Maternal:* hypertension, palpitations, tremors, nausea and vomiting, chest pain, headache, arrhythmias, hyperglycemia, pulmonary edema *Fetal:* tachycardia, hypoxia, fetal distress *Newborn:* hypoglycemia	• Do not use if clouded or discolored. • Use a piggyback set to infuse the solution. • Administer oral medication 30 minutes before discontinuing the I.V. medication. • Report a pulse rate greater than 120 beats/minute, a respiratory rate greater than 20 breaths/minute, a blood pressure of less than 90/60 mm Hg, and urine output of less than 30 ml/hour. • Continuously monitor uterine contractions and fetal heart rate (FHR). • Position the client on the left side to enhance circulation. • Assess for signs of pulmonary edema and fetal distress. • Monitor the newborn for hypoglycemia. • Keep antidote (propranolol) available.
terbutaline (Brethine)	0.01 mg/minute I.V.; 0.25 mg S.C.; 5 mg by mouth			
Intrapartal drugs				
butorphanol tartrate (Stadol)	2 mg I.M. or 1 mg I.V.	Opioid agonist-antagonist	*Maternal:* respiratory depression, nausea, vomiting, headache, floating sensation, depression *Fetal and newborn:* respiratory	• Do not use with morphine or meperidine. Additive effects may occur. • Monitor vital signs frequently and FHR continuously. • Institute safety precautions (promote bed rest, raise the side rails, monitor vital signs). • May precipitate withdrawal in opioid-dependent clients.
calcium gluconate	*Maternal:* 7 to 14 mEq calcium; repeat every 1 to 3 days as needed *Newborn:* 2.4 mEq/kg of body weight in divided doses	Replenishes or maintains the client's calcium level; administered to treat magnesium toxicity and hypocalcemia	Tingling, sensation of warmth, mild drop in blood pressure, respiratory or cardiac arrest, renal calculi, tissue necrosis	• Calcium gluconate is given I.V. as a 10% solution (0.45 to 0.48 mEq/ml); administer slowly per protocol. • Keep the client recumbent after administration. • Monitor the client's heart rate continuously on an electrocardiogram; assess for bradycardia and arrhythmias. • Observe for necrosis at the insertion site.

Selected drugs commonly used in maternal-newborn nursing (continued)

DRUG	DOSE	ACTION	SIDE EFFECTS	NURSING CONSIDERATIONS
Intrapartal drugs (continued)				
diazepam (Valium)	*For seizures:* 5 mg slow I.V.	Central nervous system (CNS) depressant and anticonvulsant; administered to treat seizures associated with PIH and preeclampsia	*Maternal:* hypotension, bradycardia, cardiovascular collapse, nausea, vomiting, lethargy, tremors; respiratory depression *Fetal or newborn:* loss of beat-to-beat variability, depression, hypotonia; respiratory depression	• Do not mix with other drugs. • Do not store in a plastic syringe. • Avoid extravasation. • Monitor vital signs and FHR. • Assess deep tendon reflexes continuously or every 5 to 15 minutes, as needed.
magnesium sulfate	2 to 4 g I.V. as a loading dose, followed by 1 to 2 g hourly as an I.V. infusion	CNS depressant and anticonvulsant; inhibits uterine contractions in preterm labor and prevents seizures in patients with severe preeclampsia or eclampsia	*Maternal:* Flushing, sweating, sedation, confusion, depressed reflexes, hypotension, respiratory depression, cardiac arrest *Fetal:* Decreased FHR *Newborn:* CNS depression; flaccid paralysis	• Maximum I.V. concentration is 200 mg/ml; maximum infusion rate is 150/mg/minute. • Use with an infusion pump. • Assess deep tendon reflexes and vital signs per protocol; report if severely depressed. • Assess the client's respiratory rate; report if fewer than 14 breaths per minute. • Assess hourly urine output; report if less than 30 ml/hour. • Continuously monitor fetal heart tones and contractions. • If magnesium sulfate is administered within 24 hours of delivery, observe the newborn for magnesium toxicity, including respiratory depression and hypotonia. Have calcium gluconate available as an antagonist. • As ordered, continue to administer drug for 24 hours after delivery.
meperidine hydrochloride (Demerol)	50 to 100 mg I.M. or 25 to 50 mg I.V. every 3 to 4 hours	Opioid analgesic	*Maternal:* bradycardia, tachycardia, hypotension, respiratory depression, nausea, vomiting, drowsiness, slowing of uterine contractions *Newborn:* CNS and respiratory depression if given near delivery	• Monitor vital signs and FHR continuously or per protocol. • Institute safety precautions: bed rest, side rails in place, and narcotic antagonist (naloxone) available. • Notify the physician or certified nurse-midwife if side effects occur. • Decrease sensory stimulation.
nalbuphine hydrochloride (Nubain)	10 to 20 mg S.C., I.M., or I.V. every 3 hours, p.r.n., or around the clock	Opioid agonist-antagonist	Respiratory depression, feeling of heaviness, disorientation, headache, nausea, vomiting	• Do not use with morphine or meperidine. • Additive effects may occur. • Monitor vital signs frequently and FHR continuously. • Institute safety precautions (promote bed rest, raise the side rails, monitor vital signs). • Do not administer to an opioid-dependent client; may precipitate withdrawal.

(continued)

MATERNAL-NEWBORN NURSING

Selected drugs commonly used in maternal-newborn nursing (continued)

DRUG	DOSE	ACTION	SIDE EFFECTS	NURSING CONSIDERATIONS
Intrapartal drugs (continued)				
naloxone (Narcan)	*Maternal:* 0.4 mg I.M. or I.V. *Newborn:* 0.1 mg/kg of body weight I.V.	Opioid antagonist; reverses effects of opioid analgesics	*Maternal:* nausea, vomiting, tremors, hypertension, tachycardia *Newborn:* irritability, tachycardia	• Use cautiously in a newborn or in a opioid-addicted mother. • Prepare for alternative resuscitation measures if the drug proves ineffective. • Monitor the mother's vital signs. • Monitor the newborn's vital signs frequently, especially respirations.
oxytocin (Pitocin)	*Induction:* 1 to 2 mU/minute in I.V. infusion; increase the rate as needed to induce normal contractions *After placenta delivery:* 10 U I.M. or I.V., according to protocol	Oxytocic; stimulates uterine muscle contraction, prevents uterine hemorrhage, initiates the let-down reflex or lactation	*Maternal:* tetanic contractions, hypertension, ruptured uterus, abruptio placentae, lacerations of the birth canal *Fetal:* hypoxia	• Use a piggyback set to infuse the solution. • Continuously monitor uterine contractions and FHR. • Assess blood pressure and intake and output. • Monitor the progress of labor.
promethazine hydrochloride (Phenergan)	25 to 75 mg I.M. or I.V.	Antihistamine, antiemetic, and sedative	Drowsiness, hypotension, dry mouth, photosensitivity	• Institute safety precautions (promote bed rest, raise the side rails, monitor vital signs).
Postpartal drugs				
methylergonovine maleate (Methergine)	0.2 mg per protocol (for example, 0.2 mg every 4 hours x 6 doses)	Oxytocic; stimulates uterine muscle contraction; administered post partum to prevent hemorrhage (contracts the muscles surrounding blood vessels at the placental site)	Transient chest pain, dyspnea, palpitation, tinnitus, hypertension, dizziness, headache, nausea and vomiting	• Monitor vital signs, especially blood pressure. • Assess the involution process. • Do not use to induce labor. • Store in tightly sealed, light-resistant containers.
Rh$_o$ (D) immune globulin (RhoGAM)	Dose determined by laboratory results (1= vial is a common dose)	Immune serum; prevents formation of antibodies; given to an RH- mother of an RH+ fetus or newborn	Inflammation at injection site, slight fever, allergic reaction	• Administer I.M. within 72 hours of delivery, as ordered. (Also may be administered at 28 weeks' gestation.) • Evaluate the need for repeated doses with each pregnancy. • Provide patient teaching.
rubella virus, vaccine, live	1 vial S.C.	Vaccine; provides passive immunity to rubella by inducing production of antibodies	Influenza-like symptoms, fever, joint pain, malaise, burning at injection site	• CDC has approved use of this vaccine in lactating clients. • Effectiveness of vaccine may be inhibited if given concomitantly with Rh$_o$ (D) immune globulin. • Advise the client to avoid pregnancy for 3 months after vaccine administration.

MATERNAL-NEWBORN NURSING

Selected drugs commonly used in maternal-newborn nursing (continued)

DRUG	DOSE	ACTION	SIDE EFFECTS	NURSING CONSIDERATIONS
Neonatal drugs				
beractant [natural lung surfactant] (Survanta)	4 ml/kg intratracheally; each dose is administered in four quarter-doses, with manual handbag ventilation between quarter-doses at a rate of 60 breaths/minute and sufficient oxygen to prevent cyanosis	Lowers the surface tension on alveolar surfaces during respiration and stablizes the alveoli against collapse; it mimics the naturally occuring surfactant	Adverse reactions, which may occur during the dosing procedure, include transient bradycardia, oxygen desaturation, pallor, hypotension, endotracheal tube reflux or blockage, hypertension, hypocarbia, hypercarbia, and apnea	• The drug should be adminsitered only by persons familiar with the care of clinically unstable preterm newborns. • Accurate determination of weight is essential to proper dosage. • Give within 15 minutes of birth. • Continuous monitoring of electrocardiogram (ECG) and transcutaneous oxygen saturation are essential; frequent arterial blood pressure monitoring and frequent arterial blood gas sampling are highly desirable.
colfosceril palmitate (EXOSURF Neonatal)	5 ml/kg intratracheally	Lowers the surface tension on alveolar surfaces during respiration and stabilizes the alveoli against collapse; it mimics the naturally occurring surfactant	Pulmonary air leak, hyperoxia, hypocarbia, pulmonary hemorrhage, endotracheal tube reflux or obstruction, oxygen desaturation	• The drug should be administered only by persons familiar with the care of clinically unstable preterm newborns. • Accurate determination of weight is essential to proper dosage. • Give within 15 minutes of birth. • Continuous monitoring of ECG and transcutaneous oxygen saturation are essential; frequent arterial blood pressure monitoring and frequent arterial blood gas sampling are higly desirable.
erythromycin ophthalmic ointment (Ilotycin)	0.5% ophthalmic ointment	Ophthalmic anti-infective; bacteriostatic prophylactic for ophthalmia neonatorum resulting from *Neisseria gonorrhoea* and ophthalmic *Chlamydia*	Local irritation, edema, inflammation	• Apply a thin line on the lower conjunctival sacs. • Apply within the 1st hour after delivery.
phytonadione [vitamin K₁] (AquaMEPHYTON)	0.5 to 1.0 mg I.M. in vastus lateralis	Vitamin; prevents hypoprothrombinemia caused by vitamin K deficiency	Minimal side effects, possible inflammation at the injection site	• May require 3 hours or more to stop active bleeding. • Assess need for transfusion. • Observe the injection site for inflammation and infection. • Assess for signs of hemorrhage. • Protect drug from light.

Child nursing

Introduction

This section reviews health problems of children from birth through late teens, focusing on conditions and disorders common to specific age-groups: the infant, the toddler, the preschooler, the school-age child, and the adolescent. Each entry provides an overview of the health problem and a typical clinical situation; these case studies demonstrate nursing concepts and skills essential to the care of hospitalized children.

The health problems covered in this section are those most likely to be found in test questions on the NCLEX-RN. The nursing diagnoses derived from the case studies are not exhaustive. Those listed represent the major focus of care for that clinical situation.

To enhance your understanding of this section, first review "Growth and development," pages 52 to 61.

THE INFANT (BIRTH TO AGE 12 MONTHS)

Tracheoesophageal fistula and esophageal atresia

Tracheoesophageal fistula and esophageal atresia are malformations in which the esophagus fails to develop as a continuous passage. The most common type of tracheoesophageal fistula (occurring in 80% to 95% of clients with this condition) is one in which the proximal esophagus ends in a blind pouch and the distal esophagus is attached to the trachea. The most common type of atresia (in 5% to 8% of clients) occurs with both the proximal and distal esophagus ending in a blind pouch unconnected to the trachea (see *Common types of tracheoesophageal fistula and atresia,* page 333).

Tracheoesophageal fistula and esophageal atresia occur in both sexes equally and do not seem to be caused by hereditary factors. A high percentage of affected infants are premature, and the birth weight of most is significantly lower than average. A history of maternal polyhydramnios (more than 2,000 ml of amniotic fluid) may exist, and half of affected infants have other anomalies, including heart defects, anorectal malformations, genitourinary anomalies, and vertebral anomalies.

Early diagnosis and treatment are essential to maintain nutrition and to prevent rapid death from respiratory obstruction.

Clinical situation

Baby Stevenson has been in the newborn nursery for about 3 ½ hours when he suddenly becomes cyanotic and begins coughing and choking. The nurse notices that he has excessive mucus in his mouth and that he has been drooling. Baby Stevenson is due to be fed the first bottle of glucose water in about 2 hours.

Assessment

NURSING BEHAVIORS

1. Observe for constant drooling and excessive mucus and secretions from the mouth and nose.

NURSING RATIONALES

1. When the blind pouch fills, saliva and mucus overflow into the mouth, increasing the possibility of aspiration.

Glossary

Atresia—complete closure of a tube or body opening

Cephalocaudal—having a head-to-tail direction, as in the development of an organism (for instance, infants gain control of the head before the trunk and extremities)

Cheiloplasty—plastic surgery performed to correct a deformity of the lips

Cognitive development—acquisition of increasingly complex knowledge, thought processes, reasoning, judgment, memory, and problem-solving skills

Congenital—existing at birth

Croup—inflammation of the larynx that commonly occurs in young children, usually at night, characterized by a barking, resonant cough

Development—increasingly complex functioning that progresses sequentially (for instance, the attainment of cognitive, psychosocial, motor, and communication skills)

Fistula—abnormal opening between two organs

Growth—quantitative increase in size resulting from an increase in the number or size of cells, or both

Meningocele—protrusion of the meninges outside the body through a defect in the vertebral column; the protruding sac is filled with spinal fluid

Myelomeningocele—meningocele that contains a portion of the spinal cord and spinal nerves in the sac

Neurogenic bladder—loss of bladder control from lesions or damage to the nervous system

Proximodistal—from the nearest to the farthest, as in the development of an organism (for instance, infants gain control of the arm before the hand)

Regurgitation—backward flow of fluid or solids from a cavity or tube (for instance, the backward flow of blood through a defective heart valve or stomach contents flowing into the throat and mouth)

Teratogen—substance that causes severely deformed fetal parts

Tetralogy of Fallot—congenital anomaly of the heart characterized by pulmonic stenosis, ventricular septal defect, overriding position or dextroposition of the aorta, and compensatory right ventricular hypertrophy

Transillumination—observation of a body part by shining a light through the part and viewing the quality and quantity of light on the other side

Stenosis—narrowing of the lumen of a tube or body opening

Ventriculoperitoneal shunt—diversion of cerebrospinal fluid from the cerebral ventricles to the peritoneal cavity, using a one-way flow valve and a tubing system

---

2. Assess for the 3 Cs: coughing, choking, and cyanosis.

2. The mucus and saliva overflow causes choking and coughing. When mucus is aspirated, cyanosis results from laryngospasm, the protective mechanism that prevents aspiration.

3. Assess for abdominal distention.

3. Severe abdominal distention will interfere with respirations.

4. Assess the infant's response to his first feeding.

4. The first feeding typically produces marked coughing, choking, and cyanosis.

5. Perform a complete cephalocaudal assessment of the infant (see "Assessment and characteristics of the normal newborn," pages 297 to 301).

5. A complete assessment is needed to evaluate the infant for additional anomalies.

Diagnostic evaluation
- A catheter cannot be passed through the nose or mouth into the stomach.
- Abdominal X-rays reveal air in the stomach.
- Fluoroscopy, using radiopaque fluid carefully introduced into the esophagus, reveals the atresia.

Common types of tracheoesophageal fistula and atresia

Esophageal atresia with fistula to the distal segment (86.5%)   **Esophageal atresia without fistula (7.7%)**

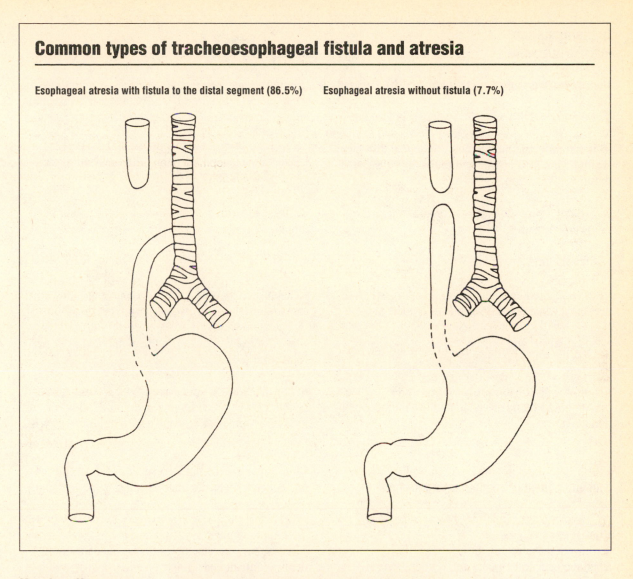

Nursing diagnoses	• Ineffective airway clearance related to abnormal opening between esophagus and trachea or obstruction to swallowing of secretions • Risk for aspiration related to mechanical obstruction • Risk for fluid volume deficit related to an inability to ingest fluids • Anxiety related to the parents' reaction to the infant's diagnosis and surgery
Planning and goals	• Baby Stevenson will maintain an adequate airway. • Baby Stevenson will not aspirate mucus into his lungs. • Baby Stevenson will not experience gastric reflux or aspiration pneumonia. • Baby Stevenson will feed without choking or developing cyanosis. • Baby Stevenson will regain and maintain fluid and electrolyte balance. • Baby Stevenson's incision will heal postoperatively without becoming infected. • The parents will bond with their infant. • Baby Stevenson will develop trust and not mistrust. • The parents will be able to care for their infant at home after surgery.

Implementation

NURSING BEHAVIORS	NURSING RATIONALES

Preoperative care (gastrostomy tube insertion)

1. Help to establish an early diagnosis before the first feeding. Note the 3 Cs, increased mucus and salivation from the nose and mouth, and abdominal distention. Withhold the first feeding and notify the physician if these symptoms appear.

1. Any neonate with the 3 Cs, increased secretions from the nose and mouth, and acute gastric distention should be suspected of having a tracheoesophageal fistula with esophageal atresia.

• Place the infant on his back, with the head of the bed elevated about 30 degrees.

2. Prevent aspiration and pneumonia by taking the following measures:

2. These measures help prevent aspiration and pneumonia.

• Withhold food and fluids.

• Place the client in semi-Fowler position, which eases breathing when the abdomen is distended.

• This prevents aspiration and prepares the infant for surgery.

• Aspirate nasal and oral secretions as well as secretions in the blind esophageal pouch.

• Removing secretions from the mouth and nose prevents aspiration.

• Drain the gastrostomy tube by gravity, leaving the tube unplugged and elevating it above the level of the abdomen.

• After diagnosis, a gastrostomy tube is surgically inserted through an abdominal incision to allow air entering the stomach to escape and to minimize gastric reflux into the trachea.

• Insert into the blind pouch an indwelling catheter with intermittent or continuous low suction.

• Intermittent or continuous suction with an indwelling catheter keeps the blind esophageal pouch empty.

Postoperative care

1. Prevent dehydration, as follows:
• Maintain accurate intake and output records.
• Monitor and record I.V. fluids hourly.
• Monitor and accurately record gastrostomy tube drainage.
• Note urine specific gravity.
• Weigh the infant daily.

1. These measures help assess and maintain the infant's fluid and electrolyte balance, thus preventing dehydration.

2. Prevent infection of surgical incision sites: Observe and care for wounds, and apply and change sterile dressings, as needed. If the infant has undergone a cervical esophagostomy, perform special skin care to prevent breakdown from continuous moisture.

2. The infant may require several surgical procedures (gastrostomy, thoracotomy, and cervical esophagostomy); thus, the nurse must carefully observe all incision sites for signs of infection and take appropriate measures to prevent it.

3. Maintain adequate respiratory exchange and prevent pneumonia, as follows:

3. This is part of routine postoperative care for a child with chest tubes.

• Maintain a patent airway by carefully suctioning the infant's trachea. Use the specially marked suction catheter.

• During surgery, the surgeon measures and marks a suction catheter at a distance slightly above the anastomosis site; the catheter's length is communicated to all caretakers. Using this catheter prevents trauma to the anastomosis site.

• Suction secretions from the mouth and nose, as necessary.

• Periodically check the chest tubes by auscultating both lungs for breath sounds, checking for loose connections and kinking and the drainage system for proper functioning.

• Place the infant under a radiant warmer with high humidity and oxygen.

• Keep the infant on his back, and elevate the head of the bed 30 degrees.

4. Administer antibiotics as ordered.

5. Maintain I.V. fluids as ordered.

6. On the 2nd or 3rd postoperative day, begin gastrostomy tube feedings. Continue the feedings, if tolerated, for 10 to 14 days.

7. Begin oral feedings with sterile water, observing the infant carefully to ensure that he can swallow without choking. Progress to small, frequent formula feedings; supplement these with gastrostomy tube feedings if the infant cannot consume enough orally to meet nutritional needs.

8. Begin to develop and nurture the infant's trust.

9. Begin mild sensorimotor stimulation, as follows:
• Offer the infant a pacifier to satisfy unmet sucking needs.
• Touch the infant frequently to provide tactile stimulation.
• Provide sensory stimulation with brightly lit musical mobiles.
• Talk to the infant when providing care.
• Position the infant comfortably, and regularly change his position during waking hours.

• This prevents aspiration of secretions.

• This ensures that the infant's lungs are fully expanded.

• This reduces tracheal drying and irritation.

• This position helps to prevent aspiration of secretions and makes breathing easier.

4. Antibiotics help prevent or combat infection.

5. I.V. fluid administration helps regain and maintain fluid and electrolyte balance.

6. The infant should be able to tolerate gastrostomy tube feedings by the 2nd or 3rd postoperative day. This delay helps avoid postoperative vomiting. Tube feedings maintain the infant's nutrition while bypassing the operative site to promote healing. Within 10 to 14 days, the anastomosis should heal completely; the surgeon may order an upper GI series to confirm healing.

7. Sterile water is given initially because it causes fewer problems than other solutions if the infant aspirates it or cannot swallow. Small, frequent formula feedings are gradually increased until they are sufficient to meet the infant's needs. The stomach will expand as the amount of food increases.

8. Trust is important to the neonate but sometimes is difficult to achieve in a hospital setting with many caregivers. Continuity of personnel helps ensure that the neonate's needs are met.

9. The infant is in an important stage of sensorimotor development. These activities stimulate the sucking reflex and the senses of touch, vision, and hearing.

CHILD NURSING

10. Support the parents during their infant's hospitalization, and assist them with bonding, as follows:
• Help the parents participate in caring for the infant (for instance, bathing, touching, and diapering).
• Provide visiting hours for working parents.
• Encourage the parents to verbalize their thoughts and feelings.

10. Hospitalization, especially in an isolation bassinet in the intensive care unit, may interfere with bonding and increase the parents' anxiety about caregiving and parenting skills. The parents also may grieve during this stressful period. Thoughtful encouragement and support from the nurse can help allay their anxieties and fears.

11. Prepare the parents for home care, as follows:

11. The parents need to know how to care for the gastrostomy tube and the operative site.

• Teach proper care of the gastrostomy tube and an esophagostomy if the infant has had a staged palliative procedure.

• If a staged repair is performed and anastomosis is delayed until age 18 to 24 months, the infant will be sent home with a gastrostomy tube and an esophagostomy.

• Teach the parents to recognize signs of wound infection, including swelling, redness, foul or oozing drainage, or elevated temperature.

• The infant typically is discharged 2 to 3 weeks after surgery; infection is possible even after discharge.

• Teach the parents to recognize signs and symptoms of esophageal stenosis: choking or coughing with feeding, refusal to eat, and painful swallowing.

• Recurring esophageal stenosis and dysphagia are common complications of scarring, which may develop at the anastomosis site.

• Teach correct positioning of the infant after feeding (on his back or right side, with the head of the bed slightly elevated).

• This position prevents regurgitation into the esophagus.

• Teach the parents to recognize signs of respiratory distress, including nasal flaring, retractions, and grunting.

• Respiratory distress may accompany dysphagia, or a fistula may develop at the operative site where the esophagus is separated from the trachea.

Evaluation

• Baby Stevenson receives enough nutrition—either in formula or breast milk—to maintain growth without choking, coughing, or aspirating.
• The parents bond with the infant and provide care without anxiety.
• The parents can list the signs of wound infection, esophageal stenosis, and wound infection.
• The parents maintain contact with the physician and continue follow-up care.

Myelomeningocele

The most severe spina bifida defect, myelomeningocele is a saclike cyst protrusion, usually located in the lumbosacral area, that contains meninges, spinal fluid, and a portion of the spinal cord with its nerves. This congenital neural tube defect, readily apparent at birth, is commonly encased in a thin membrane prone to tears and leakage of cerebrospinal fluid (CSF). The extent of neurologic dysfunction depends on the level of the vertebral column at which the defect occurs. Lumbosacral lesions tend to be associated with flaccid paralysis of the legs; neurogenic bladder and fecal incontinence; musculoskeletal deformities, including flexion or extension contractures; talipes varus or valgus; and hip dislocation or subluxation.

Hydrocephalus associated with Arnold-Chiari malformation (downward displacement of the cerebellar tonsils through the foramen magnum into the cervical spinal canal) occurs in approximately 90% of those with lumbosacral myelomeningocele. Surgical closure of the sac may be performed 24 to 48 hours after birth or may be postponed until the infant can more easily tolerate the procedure. Skin grafts are the usual method of closure.

Clinical situation

Terrence Lee is a 6-hour-old infant admitted from the newborn nursery with a lumbosacral myelomeningocele. The outer edge of the sac is partially covered by skin; the superior portion is covered by a thin membrane with visible fluid filling the sac. Terrence is lying prone, with legs flexed in a froglike position and both feet pointing downward and inward. He weighs 7 lb, 9 oz (3,430 g) and has an axillary temperature of 97.5° F (36.4° C), an apical pulse rate of 138 beats/minute, and a respiratory rate of 28 breaths/minute.

Surgery is planned for the next day. Terrence is to receive nothing by mouth and has an I.V. infusion flowing at a rate of 21 drops/minute (drip factor: 60 gtt/ml). Medical orders also include applying a sterile moist dressing of normal saline solution over the sac every 2 hours and performing urinary catheterization every 2 hours if the infant has not voided spontaneously.

Assessment

NURSING BEHAVIORS	NURSING RATIONALES
1. Perform a routine assessment of Terrence, as follows:	**1.** Routine assessment provides baseline data.
• Measure and record head and chest circumferences.	• A neonate's head circumference is usually about 1″ (2.5 cm) larger than the chest circumference. Either increased head circumference or unusual disproportion between the head and chest circumferences may indicate hydrocephalus before other neurologic symptoms appear.
• Assess the status of the anterior fontanel and the nature of Terrence's cry.	• A tense or bulging fontanel indicates increased intracranial pressure (ICP). Infants with neurologic damage commonly have a high-pitched cry.
• Assess the results of transillumination (light passed through the side of the sac to determine whether the sac is translucent).	• Transillumination is performed to detect solid matter within the sac. If the sac is translucent, Terrence may have a meningocele rather than a myelomeningocele.
• Assess for bladder distention, and determine Terrence's urine and fecal elimination patterns.	• A neurogenic bladder becomes distended with retained urine, which tends to be expressed in trickles because of overflow. The rectal sphincter will be relaxed.
2. Assess how Terrence's legs respond to tactile stimuli; observe leg movement.	**2.** Flaccid paralysis of the legs is associated with absence of sensation; areflexia occurs with lumbosacral lesions.

CHILD NURSING

Nursing diagnoses	• Risk for infection related to tearing of the meningeal sac
	• Impaired skin integrity related to limited body position alternatives
	• Altered urinary elimination related to neurogenic bladder
	• Risk for altered parenting related to lack of parental attachment with a child who has overt developmental defects

Planning and goals

• During hospitalization, Terrence will maintain:
—an intact myelomeningocele sac before surgery
—stable vital signs and neurologic status
—emrange of motion (ROM) and corrective positioning
—skin integrity
—urine elimination without bladder distention.
• Terrence's parents will:
—demonstrate at least three positive signs of attachment within 72 hours
—verbalize an understanding of preoperative and postoperative treatments
—speak to and stroke Terrence
—demonstrate appropriate care techniques (for example, monitoring neurologic status and performing Credé's maneuver and ROM exercises), which they will continue after discharge.

Implementation

NURSING BEHAVIORS	NURSING RATIONALES
1. Maintain Terrence in a prone position, with hips slightly flexed, in a heated isolation bassinet, with the head slightly lower than the hips; place a pad under the knees and a small roll under the ankles.	**1.** The prone position prevents tension on the sac and minimizes the risk of trauma. (*Note:* In marked hydrocephalus, the child's head may be elevated to reduce ICP further.) Thigh abduction (maintained by a pad beneath the knees) helps counteract hip subluxation, and ankle rolls help keep the feet in a neutral position.
2. Using aseptic technique, apply and change moist sterile dressings as ordered. With each dressing change, closely inspect the meningeal sac for leaks and irritation, and document the appearance of the sac and surrounding tissue.	**2.** Soaks are applied to prevent the sac from drying before surgery. Any tear in the sac could lead to a central nervous system infection.
3. Document Terrence's head circumference, anterior fontanel status, feeding behavior, nature of cry, and general behavior (such as irritability and lethargy) at least every shift.	**3.** An increased head circumference, a tense or bulging fontanel, feeding difficulty, a high-pitched cry, and behavioral changes (especially prolonged fussiness, irritability, and a sudden change in behavior) all suggest increased ICP, which may be related to hydrocephalus or an infection, such as meningitis.
4. Weigh Terrence daily, and maintain accurate intake and output records. Measure and record body temperature (axillary), pulse rate, and respiratory rate every 2 hours.	**4.** Excessive weight gain may indicate increased ICP from obstructed CSF flow or absorption or from urine retention in the neurogenic bladder; decreased weight indicates dehydration. Decreased urine output (with intervals greater than 2 hours between voidings) may indicate dehydration or urine retention in the neurogenic bladder. Decreased body temperature may indicate cold stress or gram-negative sepsis; increased body temperature may indicate infection.

5. Palpate Terrence's bladder, documenting whether or not it is distended. Perform clean intermittent catheterization (CIC) if Terrence has not voided in the past 2 hours; while performing the maneuver, assess and document urine passage. Place a diaper under the perineal area so any voided urine can be collected and the diaper weighed for an accurate output recording.

5. Infants with flaccid bladders have incomplete bladder emptying and risk vesicoureteral reflux resulting in hydronephrosis. CIC allows complete bladder emptying and is a procedure parents can learn.

6. Provide meticulous skin care to Terrence's rectal area, applying a generous layer of diaper ointment or petroleum jelly, clean the area with sterile water, and reapply ointment with each voiding.

6. The almost-constant passage of stool can irritate the skin and may lead to myelomeningocele sac infection.

7. Place Terrence on a sheepskin pad. Perform passive ROM exercises to foot, ankle, and knee joints every 2 hours (don't stretch against tight hip flexor or adductor muscles). Rub the skin with lotion and massage pressure areas (ankles, knees, elbows, face, and chin, in particular) at least every 2 hours. You may place Terrence on his side for short periods, with support to prevent him from putting pressure on the sac. Adapt position changes according to the size and nature of the sac, the need for constant hip abduction, and the capacity for immobilizing the infant in a side-lying position to ensure absolutely no pressure on the sac.

7. Because Terrence must be maintained in a prone position most of the time, pressure ulcers and skin breakdown are likely to occur. Massage improves circulation, and passive ROM exercises to the foot, ankle, and knee joints prevent contractures (stretching against tight hip flexor or adductor muscles can aggravate hip subluxation or bone fracture). Changing positions (prone to side to prone to opposite side) relieves pressure on the skin.

8. Every hour, monitor and document the I.V. infusion rate, the amount infused, and the appearance of the infusion site.

8. Terrence is not receiving food or fluids by mouth because surgery is to be performed early; therefore he is at risk for dehydration and overhydration. Monitoring the infusion rate ensures that he is receiving adequate fluid. Assessing the appearance of the infusion site helps in detecting extravasation.

9. Talk to Terrence regularly when caring for him; stroke his face and upper body with each contact; dangle a black and white geometric design from the side of the isolation bassinet at Terrence's eye level; provide a pacifier as necessary. Encourage the parents to speak to and stroke Terrence and maintain face-to-face posturing.

9. Because Terrence can't be cuddled like other infants, he should be exposed to other sources of sensory stimulation, such as speech and touch. Neonates are drawn to black and white colors and geometric designs; after 1 month, they begin to see other colors. A pacifier provides oral gratification, especially because Terrence is not receiving food or fluids. The parents may be unable to bond at this stage because of shock or disbelief, but they should be offered the opportunity and support of nursing staff to do so.

CHILD NURSING

10. If Terrence's mother can't visit him (because she hasn't recovered from the delivery, is in another hospital, or is depressed about the child's birth defect), take pictures of Terrence and see that she receives them. Also, write to her (preferably by hand), explaining equipment being used on Terrence and describing how he is responding to treatment. If possible, telephone his mother to allow her to ask questions and verbalize feelings.

10. If the opportunity for physical bonding does not exist, the mother needs evidence that she has given birth to a live infant. She also needs proof that something is being done to correct her child's problems and that he is being cared for by caring people.

11. Teach the parents postoperative care routines, including positioning, feeding, suture line care, bladder and bowel care, and checking for signs of complications.

11. The parents will need to develop these skills so they can provide appropriate care for their infant. After surgery, Terrence may be positioned on his sides but not on his back (the side-lying position may not be allowed if it would aggravate hip dysplasia or permit too much hip flexion); the infant may be held for feeding as long as no pressure is placed on the operative site. The physician may order soaks and antibiotic ointment for the suture line. Protocols for bladder and bowel care, passive exercise, and skin care remain the same after surgery. Complications to be especially alert for include infections and hydrocephalus. The postoperative evaluation will be the same as the preoperative (monitoring vital signs, head circumference, and behavior; observing site for inflammation; and so forth).

Evaluation

- Terrence has no leakage from the myelomeningocele sac or signs of inflammation.
- Terrence remains afebrile.
- Terrence maintains intact, unreddened skin preoperatively and postoperatively.
- Terrence is positioned with hips abducted; passive ROM exercise to the knees, ankles, and feet increase mobility and decrease downward and inward positioning of the feet.
- Terrence responds to visual, auditory, and tactile stimulation.
- Terrence's parents visit him twice daily. On the first visit, his mother declined to touch him but did face him; on later visits she progressed to touching Terrence's head lightly with her fingertips and speaking to him softly. After surgery, his mother seemed much less anxious and asked to feed Terrence. His father still hasn't touched Terrence (as of 3 days postoperatively) and has been nonverbal, except for saying, "I don't want to become too close to him—I am afraid we're going to lose him." During those visits, the father stands close to the mother, with his hand on her shoulder.

Clinical situation
(continued)

Terrence maintained the same head circumference until 2 days postoperatively, when a 0.5-cm increase was noted; a steady further increase in head circumference was noted over the next 3 days, along with weight gain associated with bulging fontanel; increased lethargy; difficulty feeding and decreased intake; and then a slight weight decrease. He was returned to surgery for a ventriculoperitoneal shunt to treat hydrocephalus (see *Ventriculoperitoneal shunt*). The postoperative nursing care plan was modified as follows:

Ventriculoperitoneal shunt

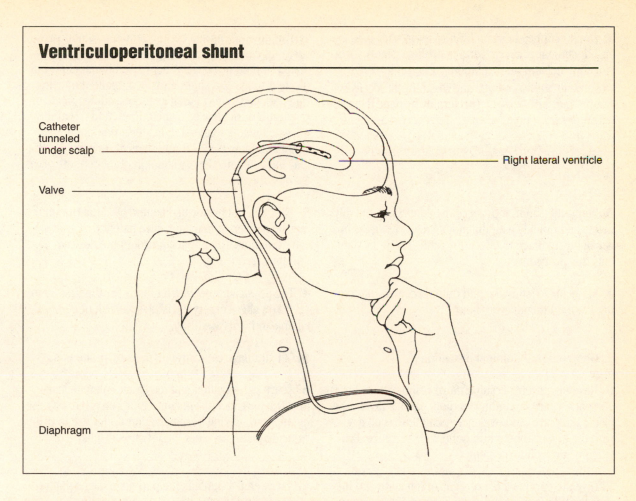

Catheter tunneled under scalp

Valve

Diaphragm

Right lateral ventricle

Planning and goals

• Terrence will have no symptoms of increased ICP (indicating shunt malfunction or infection).
• Terrence will have no pressure ulcers on his head.
• Terrence's parents will verbalize an understanding of the purposes of operative procedures, valve pumping, signs of increased ICP and infection (which they should promptly report), and the need for long-term follow-up treatment of problems related to myelomeningocele and hydrocephalus.
• Terrence's father will make progress in bonding with his child.

Implementation

NURSING BEHAVIORS

1. Place Terrence flat, with hips abducted, or on the unoperated side; change his position every hour.

NURSING RATIONALES

1. A flat position helps avoid too-rapid decompression of the intracranial fluid. Hip abduction continues to be necessary because of the neurologic deficit to the lower body. A side-lying position must be on the unoperated side to avoid pressure on the shunt valve. Changing position reduces the risk of hypostatic pneumonia and pressure sores.

2. Document head circumference every shift; assess and document vital signs and neurologic status (anterior fontanel and pupils; blood pressure; level of irritability; sucking reflex; listlessness; and seizure activity) every 4 hours.

2. The valve opens at a certain intraventricular pressure and closes when the pressure is sufficiently reduced by fluid drainage. A depressed fontanel may indicate a successful shunt if unaccompanied by other signs of dehydration (such as increased heart rate or respirations, decreased urine output, and irritability). A tense, bulging fontanel indicates a nonfunctioning shunt and increased ICP. Any signs of increased ICP may indicate infection or shunt malfunction, the greatest postoperative hazards.

3. Pump the shunt, if ordered, by depressing the valve firmly and quickly with the index finger; leave the finger lightly in place to check for refill. Teach the parents this procedure.

3. Although not performed routinely, shunt pumping may be needed to maintain valve patency or assess valve function. The physician orders the desired pumping frequency.

4. Maintain strict intake and output records, monitoring I.V. fluid intake every hour.

4. The physician may restrict fluids for the first 24 to 48 hours after surgery to reduce the risk of cerebral edema and increased ICP.

5. Observe for abdominal distention.

5. CSF drainage can cause an ileus or peritonitis.

6. Have the parents assume more responsibility for Terrence's care, including feeding, passive ROM exercises, skin care, and hygiene. Spend time each day with the father to help him bond with Terrence. Provide positive reinforcement.

6. Active participation and feedback enhance learning. The parents must become more involved with the infant's care during hospitalization if they are to provide adequate care after the infant is discharged.

7. Give the parents a list of signs of infection and increased ICP; include the physician's telephone number.

7. A written list reminds the parents of signs that require medical treatment.

8. Have the parents demonstrate their understanding of the long-term follow-up care that Terrence will need.

8. Terrence will need continuous medical evaluation of hydrocephalus and myelomeningocele; orthopedic evaluation and possible appliances; and urologic evaluation to maintain bowel and bladder control and prevent urinary tract infection. (Terrence may be a candidate for ureteroileostomy in the future.) The shunt will require periodic readjustment for growth or malfunction.

9. Tell the parents what to expect regarding Terrence's future development. For example, tell them that, as Terrence becomes stronger, they can help him develop head and shoulder control by placing him prone on the floor with toys in front of him, that he will develop strong arms and shoulders, and that he will creep and crawl using his arms and shoulders.

9. The parents won't be able to absorb much information at this point. However, they need a general idea of what to expect and how best to help their son at each stage of development.

Evaluation

- Terrence's vital signs remain stable; his fontanel remains soft to slightly depressed; and he is alert with a lusty cry.
- Terrence remains free from infection.
- Terrence's skin remains intact.
- Terrence's parents assume more responsibility for his care; they demonstrate an understanding of procedures, complication signs, and the need for long-term follow-up evaluation and treatment.
- Terrence's father demonstrates a marked change in attitude and a willingness to participate in Terrence's care.

Pyloric stenosis

Hypertrophic pyloric stenosis, obstruction of the stomach's pyloric orifice, is five times as common in boys as in girls. The cause is unknown, but heredity may be a factor.

Infants with pyloric stenosis are usually well for the first few weeks after birth. As the hypertrophy and hyperplasia progress, pyloric obstruction becomes apparent. Typically, the infant will regurgitate occasionally after feeding, then after every feeding. Vomiting quickly progresses to projectile vomiting, usually within 1 to 2 weeks. Moderate to severe dehydration occurs as vomiting increases. Surgery is the preferred treatment. Nonsurgical treatment is prolonged and has a higher mortality.

Clinical situation

Johnny Jacob, age 6 weeks, has been admitted to the hospital with a diagnosis of possible pyloric stenosis. Regurgitation and vomiting have gradually progressed to projectile vomiting at each feeding during the last 2 weeks. At present he can't retain formula and is mildly dehydrated. Johnny weighed 6 lb, 8 ½ oz (2,963 g) at birth, placing him at the 25th percentile. He now weighs 7 lb, 2 oz (3,232 g), placing him at the 5th percentile.

Assessment

NURSING BEHAVIORS

1. Observe Johnny for the classic signs and symptoms of pyloric stenosis: a palpable, olive-sized mass in the right upper quadrant; strong peristaltic waves moving left to right at feeding time; projectile, nonbile-stained vomiting during or 10 to 15 minutes after feeding (may be blood tinged); and weight loss or failure to gain weight.

2. Assess Johnny for signs and symptoms of dehydration: reduced weight; decreased urine output; sunken fontanel; absence of tears; sunken eyes; dry mucous membrane; rapid respiration; rapid, thready pulse; pale, cool skin; irritability; and lethargy.

NURSING RATIONALES

1. The sooner pyloric stenosis is recognized, the sooner it can be corrected. The pylorus hypertrophies, is palpable, and occludes the lumen at about 4 to 6 weeks. Peristalsis increases in the epigastrium to force formula into the duodenum. The obstruction is proximal to the ampulla of Vater where the bile duct enters the duodenum. Small amounts of fresh blood from irritation, inflammation, and edema may be present. Vomiting prevents the infant from gaining weight.

2. Body fluids are pulled from the soft tissue into the circulating blood volume. The pulse increases to maintain cardiac output, which is diminished because of the hemoconcentration. Fluid is pulled from the cerebrospinal fluid to replace blood volume.

3. Observe the infant's feeding behaviors. Assess for sudden projectile vomiting 10 to 15 minutes after feeding, followed by sucking on fingers and hands, and a voracious appetite (the infant feeds vigorously and desires and eagerly accepts a second feeding).

3. Because the infant vomits the food consumed, his hunger goes unsatisfied. The vomiting is probably not accompanied by nausea or pain. The infant's behaviors suggest chronic hunger rather than pain.

4. Assess Johnny's growth and development thus far, and compare with normal patterns for his age (see "Growth and development," pages 52 to 61).

4. This assessment helps determine whether the infant meets norms for his age and enables the nurse to plan care aimed at restoring and maintaining growth and development.

Diagnostic evaluation	• Upper GI X-rays reveal delayed gastric emptying and a small, threadlike pyloric lumen. • Serum chloride levels decrease and blood pH increases, reflecting metabolic alkalosis from prolonged vomiting. • Hemoconcentration results from extracellular fluid depletion.
Nursing diagnoses	• Fluid volume deficit related to vomiting • Altered nutrition: Less than body requirements, related to the infant's inability to retain ingested food • Risk for infection related to nutritional status and surgery • Anxiety related to the parents' knowledge deficit regarding the infant's care and postoperative feeding methods
Planning and goals	**Preoperative** • Johnny will: —regain fluid and electrolyte balance —not vomit after feeding —be free from infection —regain depleted body fat and protein stores —develop at the appropriate level. **Postoperative** These include preoperative planning and goals as well as the following: • Johnny will gain weight. • Johnny's parents will understand care to be continued at home, including: —feeding and positioning techniques —incision care —behaviors to expect and behaviors to report. • Johnny's parents will provide warm, loving care for him.

Implementation

NURSING BEHAVIORS

NURSING RATIONALES

Preoperative and postoperative care
1. Help establish the diagnosis before surgery by closely observing Johnny during feedings; document the amount, color, consistency, and contents of vomitus and when it occurs in relation to feeding; and record the number, amount, color, and consistency of stools.

1. Diagnostic data establish a baseline for treatment. Voracious appetite and avid sucking are typical of an infant with pyloric stenosis. The nature and characteristics of vomitus are significant in establishing the diagnosis. Typically, stools will be scant because of decreased intake, and the infant will be constipated because of fluid loss.

2. Take measures to restore the infant's fluid and electrolyte balance, and assess the adequacy of fluid intake. Begin by carefully monitoring and recording I.V. rate and volume every hour; calculate fluid and electrolyte replacement precisely to avoid circulatory overload. Then proceed as follows:

• Assess the I.V. site every hour for redness and swelling.

• Weigh the infant daily or as ordered (possibly once every shift if the infant is severely dehydrated).

• Strictly measure and record all oral and parenteral intake. Also measure and record output of vomitus, nasogastric (NG) tube drainage, stools, and urine (weigh diapers before and after applying them to determine urine output).

• Determine the specific gravity of the infant's urine at least once daily, or more often as needed.

3. Administer I.V. glucose and electrolyte replacements if the infant is not receiving food or fluids.

4. Minimize vomiting before and after surgery by using proper feeding techniques and, if ordered, by maintaining gastric decompression, as outlined below:

• Before surgery, feed the infant slowly, holding him upright. After surgery, provide small, frequent feedings, beginning with 1 oz (29.6 ml) every hour and gradually increasing the amount offered and the time between feedings. Begin with clear fluids containing glucose and electrolytes and progress to formula.

• Burp the infant before, during, and after feedings.

• Position the infant slightly on the right side in high Fowler's position, either in an infant seat or propped in the crib.

• Handle the infant minimally after feeding.

• Maintain gastric decompression by NG tube, if ordered: Document the amount, color, and consistency of secretions. Restrain the infant as necessary to prevent removal of the NG tube. Every 2 hours, remove restraints (one arm at a time) and exercise the infant's arms. Maintain NG tube patency.

2. In infants and children, I.V. fluid administration is assessed and regulated hourly to prevent circulatory overload. Surgery is usually delayed for up to 48 hours to allow for correction of fluid and electrolyte balance.

• This helps prevent infiltration of the I.V. site.

• Weight gain or loss is the most accurate measure of fluid balance.

• Measuring the infant's fluid intake and output is essential to an ongoing assessment of fluid balance.

• Because urine is concentrated, its specific gravity will increase with dehydration.

3. This helps regain and maintain fluid and electrolyte balance.

4. Special precautions to minimize vomiting are necessary preoperatively if the infant is receiving food and fluids and postoperatively until he can feed without vomiting.

• When the infant is fed slowly and held upright, the formula can pass more easily through the pylorus. Small, frequent feedings and clear fluids are better tolerated by the infant immediately after surgery.

• Because infants tend to suck their fingers between feedings and suck voraciously when feeding, they swallow large amounts of air.

• This position facilitates gastric emptying.

• This helps to prevent vomiting.

• An NG tube will maintain decompression preoperatively and may be required during the initial postoperative period of postanesthesia vomiting. Food and fluids are withheld when the tube is in place. An accurate record of gastric secretions helps determine the infant's health status. Restraints may be necessary to prevent accidental removal of the NG tube, which must remain patent to maintain decompression.

CHILD NURSING

5. Maintain the infant's skin integrity by providing mouth care before feeding (every 3 to 4 hours if the infant isn't receiving food or fluids) and after vomiting. Immediately change wet or soiled diapers, wash the buttocks with soap and water, and rinse and dry completely, paying special attention to reddened areas.

5. The oral mucous membrane is dry when the infant is dehydrated; frequent mouth care helps maintain the infant's skin integrity. The infant is also prone to skin breakdown from dehydration, urine concentration, and alkaline stools, all of which irritate the diapered area.

6. Wash hands well before handling Johnny, allow no contact with staff or visitors with infections, and use only clean or sterile supplies when providing care.

6. Infants with impaired nutrition are more susceptible to infection.

7. Promote Johnny's growth and development, as follows:

7. The listed measures provide stimulation and comfort to the infant, contributing to his normal growth and development.

• Give Johnny a pacifier to satisfy sucking needs.

• This comforts the infant and minimizes crying.

• Encourage the parents to participate in Johnny's hygienic care and feeding.

• Successful attachment depends on the mother's continued involvement.

• Hold and cuddle Johnny as much as possible (except after feeding).

• This provides the infant with comforting physical contact and reduces crying.

• Provide for short periods of gentle sensory stimulation (except after feeding).

• The infant's sensorimotor development depends on tactile, auditory, and visual stimulation.

• Follow bathing, sleeping, and feeding routines used at home.

• Schedules similar to those used at home maintain the infant's sense of trust.

Postoperative care

1. Prevent wound infections by maintaining sterile technique when changing dressings, keeping diapers well below the incision site, and assessing the wound daily for signs of peritonitis, such as distention, vomiting, and increased temperature.

1. The pylorus is located in the epigastrium. Once surgically exposed, it is separated down to the submucosa. Postoperatively, the nurse must observe for signs of peritonitis in case the submucosa was inadvertently nicked, allowing gastric contents to enter the peritoneal cavity.

2. Support the parents by encouraging them to verbalize concerns and anxieties, assuring them that pyloric stenosis is an anatomic anomaly and not a result of parental behaviors, and keeping them informed of the infant's progress.

2. The parents may feel guilty or responsible for the infant's condition, especially if they lack sufficient knowledge to understand its physiologic cause. As a result, the parents may be reluctant to verbalize their concerns or questions without the nurse's encouragement.

3. Teach the parents feeding and positioning techniques and incision care (as outlined above in preoperative and postoperative implementations 4 and 6 and postoperative implementation 1).

3. The parents need this information if they are to provide appropriate home care for the infant.

Recommended childhood immunization schedule*—United States, 1997

Vaccine	Birth	1 Mo.	2 Mos.	4 Mos.	6 Mos.	12 Mos.	15 Mos.	18 Mos.	4–6 Yrs.	11–12 Yrs.	14–16 Yrs.
							Age				
Hepatitis B†§	Hep B-1	Hep B-1								Hep B §	
			Hep B-2	Hep B-2		Hep B-3	Hep B-3	Hep B-3			
Diphtheria and tetanus toxoids and acellular pertussis ¶			DTaP or DTP	DTaP or DTP	DTaP or DTP		DTaP or DTP	DTaP or DTP	DTaP or DTP	Td	Td
Haemophilus influenzae type b **			Hib	Hib	Hib	Hib	Hib				
Poliovirus ††			Polio††	Polio		Polio	Polio	Polio	Polio		
Measles-mumps-rubella §§						MMR	MMR		MMR or MMR	MMR or MMR	
Varicella virus ¶¶						Var	Var	Var		Var	

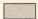 Range of Acceptable Ages for Vaccination

"Catch-Up" Vaccination

* This schedule indicates the recommended age for routine administration of currently licensed childhood vaccines. Some combination vaccines are available and may be used whenever administration of all components of the vaccine is indicated. Providers should consult the manufacturers' package inserts for detailed recommendations. Vaccines are listed under the routinely recommended ages. Bars indicate range of acceptable ages for vaccination. Shaded bars indicate catch-up vaccination: At 11–12 years, hepatitis B vaccine should be administered to children not previously vaccinated, and varicella virus vaccine should be administered to unvaccinated children who lack a reliable history of chickenpox.

† **Infants born to hepatitis B surface antigen (HBsAg)-negative mothers** should receive 2.5 μg of Merck vaccine (Recombivax HB®) or 10 μg of SmithKline Beecham (SB) vaccine (Energix-B®). The second dose should be administered 1 month after the first dose. **Infants born to HBsAg-positive mothers** should receive 0.5mL hepatitis B immune globulin (HBIG) within 12 hours of birth and either 5 μg of Merck vaccine (Recombivax HB®) or 10 μg of SB vaccine (Engerix-B®) at a separate site. The second dose is recommended at age 1–2 months and the third dose at age 6 months. **Infants born to mothers whose HBsAg status is unknown** should receive either 5 μg of Merck vaccine (Recombivax HB®) or 10 μg of SB vaccine (Engerix-B®) within 12 hours of birth. The second dose of vaccine is recommended at age 1 month and the third dose at age 6 months. Blood should be drawn at the time of delivery to determine the mother's HBsAg status; if it is positive, the infant should receive HBIG as soon as possible (no later than age 1 week). The dosage and timing of subsequent vaccine doses should be based on the mother's HBsAg status.

§ Children and adolescents who have not been vaccinated against hepatitis B during infancy may begin the series during any childhood visit. Those who have not previously received three doses of hepatitis B vaccine should initiate or complete the series at age 11–12 years. The second dose should be administered at least 1 month after the first dose, and the third dose should be administered at least 4 months after the first dose and at least 2 months after the second dose.

¶ Diphtheria and tetanus toxoids and acellular pertussis vaccine (DTaP) is the preferred vaccine for all doses in the vaccination series, including completion of the series in children who have received one or more doses of whole-cell diphtheria and tetanus toxoids and pertussis vaccine (DTP). Whole-cell DTP is an acceptable alternative to DTaP. The fourth dose of DTaP may be administered as early as 12 months of age provided 6 months have elapsed since the third dose and if the child is considered unlikely to return at age 15–18 months. Tetanus and diphtheria toxoids (Td), absorbed, for adult use, is recommended at age 11–12 years if at least 5 years have elapsed since the last dose of DTP, DTaP, or diphtheria and tetanus toxoids. Subsequent routine Td boosters are recommended every 10 years.

(continued)

Recommended childhood immunization schedule*—United States, 1997

(continued)

** Three *H. influenzae* type b (Hib) conjugate vaccines are licensed for infant use. If PRP-OMP (PedvaxHIB® [Merck]) is administered at ages 2 and 4 months, a dose at age 6 months is not required. After completing the primary series, any Hib conjugate vaccine may be used as a booster.

†† Two poliovirus vaccines are currently licensed in the United States: inactivated poliovirus vaccine (IPV) and oral poliovirus vaccine (OPV). The following schedules are all acceptable by ACIP, AAP, and AAFP, and parents and providers my choose among them: 1) IPV at ages 2 and 4 months and OPV at age 12–18 months and at age 4–6 years; 2) IPV at ages 2, 4, and 12–18 months and age 4–6 years; and 3) OPV at ages 2, 4, and 6–18 months and at age 4–6 years. ACIP routinely recommends schedule 1. IPV is the only poliovirus vaccine recommended for immunocompromised persons and their household contacts.

§§ The second dose of measles-mumps-rubella vaccine is routinely recommended at age 4–6 years or at age 11–12 years but may be administered during any visit provided at least 1 month has elapsed since receipt of the first dose and that both doses are administered at or after age 12 months.

¶¶ Susceptible children may receive varicella vaccine (Var) during any visit after the first birthday, and unvacccinated persons who lack a reliable history of chickenpox should be vaccinated at age 11–12 years. Susceptible persons aged ≥ 13 years should receive two doses at least 1 month apart.

Use of trade names and commercial sources is for identification only and does not imply endorsement by the Public Health Service or the U.S. Depatment of Health and Human Services.

Source: Advisory Committee on Immunization Practices (ACIP), American Academy of Pediatrics (AAP), and American Academy of Family Physicians (AAFP).

---

4. Tell the parents what to expect when the infant goes home. Make sure they are aware of follow-up appointments and the immunization schedule (see *Recommended childhood immunization schedule*).

4. The infant can be expected to sleep 16 to 20 hours a day. Parents should know which behaviors to report to the physician, including regurgitation or vomiting after feeding, constipation, and incision infection.

Evaluation

- Johnny ingests appropriate amounts of formula without regurgitating or vomiting.
- Johnny's parents can:
  —explain feeding and positioning techniques
  —describe incision care
  —list signs and symptoms of incision infection.
- Johnny will gain weight at the rate of 6 oz (170 g)/week and will again be at the 25th percentile for weight.
- Johnny's mother demonstrates a warm, caring relationship with Johnny.

Cleft lip and cleft palate

Cleft lip and cleft palate are developmental defects caused by a combination of genetic and environmental factors such as maternal exposure to teratogens. Cleft lip is a facial malformation resulting from failure of the premaxillary process to merge during the 7th and 8th weeks of gestation. (The malformation may be unilateral or bilateral and may range from a notch in the vermilion border of the lip to a separation extending to the floor of the nose.) Cleft palate results from failure of the palatal process to fuse from the 7th to the 12th week of gestation.

Cleft lip may be repaired surgically (cheiloplasty) immediately after birth or in early infancy (age 6 to 12 weeks) after a steady growth rate has been established. Cleft palate repair is usually postponed until between ages 1 and 2 and may require several stages of repair over a period of years. Long-term problems with cleft palate include impaired speech, malpositioned teeth and maxillary arches, impaired hearing from repeated otitis media, and recurring respiratory infections, all of which can result in impaired growth.

Clinical situation

Brad and Charlene Evans have admitted their 2-month-old son, Billy, for repair of a unilateral complete cleft lip. Billy also has a complete cleft palate. He weighed 7 lb, 2 oz (3,232 g) at birth and now weighs 8 lb, 2 oz (3,686 g)—a drop from the 50th to the 3rd percentile in weight. The parents have been using a Breck feeder (a syringe with rubber tubing attached) to feed Billy.

Assessment

NURSING BEHAVIORS	NURSING RATIONALES
1. Assess the parent-infant attachment as well as interaction between the parents.	**1.** Overt congenital anomalies can be difficult for parents to accept and thus may interfere with bonding.
2. Determine Billy's respiratory status.	**2.** Respiratory infections (upper and lower) are common in patients with a cleft palate, resulting from their difficulty in sucking and swallowing.
3. Observe the parents' feeding techniques and their degree of comfort with feeding.	**3.** The degree of comfort parents display with feeding can determine the amount of guidance and support they need to become more adept and how actively they should participate in preoperative and postoperative care.
4. Determine how well Mr. and Mrs. Evans understand preoperative and postoperative care routines for cleft lip repair and their level of anxiety about this surgery.	**4.** Too much anxiety will limit the parents' ability to learn.
5. Ensure that Billy's preoperative laboratory data (complete blood count [CBC], serum electrolyte levels, and urinalysis) are within normal limits.	**5.** Alterations in oxygenation and nutrition caused by feeding difficulties may lead to an increased white blood cell (WBC) count, abnormal serum electrolyte levels, and high urine specific gravity.
6. Assess changes in weight.	**6.** Height and weight percentiles for an infant or child should remain constant. Plotting weights on a percentile graph is the best way to assess the significance of any changes.

Nursing diagnoses

• Ineffective airway clearance related to cleft palate and increased postoperative edema of the upper airway
• Altered nutrition: Less than body requirements related to inability to suck effectively
• Risk for infection related to aspiration of food
• Knowledge deficit related to proper care of the child
• Parental role conflict related to infant's congenital defect

Planning and goals

Preoperative
• Billy will:
—maintain satisfactory respiratory and nutritional status
—be restrained and positioned as required postoperatively.
• Mr. and Mrs. Evans will:
—understand preoperative and postoperative procedures used in Billy's care
—participate in Billy's care to the extent they feel comfortable.

Postoperative
These include preoperative planning and goals as well as the following:
• Billy's suture line will remain intact and infection-free.
• Mr. and Mrs. Evans will help plan home care after cheiloplasty and ongoing care of cleft palate.

Implementation

NURSING BEHAVIORS	NURSING RATIONALES
Preoperative care	
1. Explain preoperative and postoperative procedures to Mr. and Mrs. Evans.	1. Fears about Billy's surgery and its effects on his future health care can be minimized if the parents know what to expect.
2. Position Billy only on his back with his head elevated (use an infant seat).	2. This will accustom Billy to the necessary postoperative position. An elevated head will help maintain a patent airway.
3. Document bilateral breath sounds at least every shift.	3. Billy's cleft palate and restricted positioning put him at risk for respiratory congestion and infection.
4. Weigh Billy each day, and record the weight; also measure and record Billy's fluid intake and output.	4. These actions help monitor the infant's fluid balance and nutritional intake.
5. Feed Billy in a sitting position on your lap, using a syringe feeder; burp him after every ounce. After feeding, place Billy upright in an infant seat. Allow Mr. and Mrs. Evans to feed Billy if they wish.	5. Feeding the infant while he is upright helps the nurse manage the infant's gagging or coughing. A cleft lip and cleft palate prevent good suction, which leads to increased air intake during feeding. An upright position after feeding helps the infant retain the formula and enables the nurse to wipe up secretions easily if he regurgitates. (Postoperatively, Billy won't be positioned on his side or stomach because of the possibility of trauma to the suture line.)
6. Apply elbow restraints to Billy periodically before surgery.	6. Billy will need elbow restraints after surgery to prevent tension on or trauma to the suture line. Preoperative exposure to the restraints may help Billy tolerate them better after surgery.
• Remove restraints every 2 hours, gently massage the skin around the elbows with lubricating lotion, then reapply restraints.	• Billy's attempts to flex his elbows can result in skin irritation and breakdown under the elbow restraints.

CHILD NURSING

Logan bar in position

• Demonstrate this procedure to Mr. and Mrs. Evans and have them provide return demonstration; permit the parents to perform this procedure, with supervision, when they are ready to do so.

• Assess for and document any signs of irritation or excoriation.

• Active participation and practice with feedback enhance learning. The parents' involvement will improve their caregiving skills and add a new dimension to their relationship with Billy.

• Assessment and documentation provide baseline data for later comparison to measure improvement or worsening of skin irritation and breakdown under the elbow restraints.

Clinical situation   Billy returns to the nursing unit after cheiloplasty. He is wearing a U-shaped metal bar placed on either side of the suture line (Logan bar) to prevent tension on or trauma to the sutures (see *Logan bar in position*).

Implementation
NURSING BEHAVIORS

NURSING RATIONALES

Postoperative care
1. Monitor and document Billy's temperature with a tympanic membrane sensor or an axillary thermometer every 4 hours, or every hour if the temperature exceeds 101° F (38.3° C).

1. Billy's temperature may be slightly elevated postoperatively secondary to tissue trauma and mild dehydration. A body temperature higher than 101° F may indicate infection.

2. Monitor and document Billy's pulse rate, respiratory rate, and bilateral breath sounds at least every 4 hours.

2. Hypostatic pneumonia can result secondary to anesthesia and restricted positioning. Aspiration pneumonia can occur secondary to special feeding techniques and cleft palate.

3. Aspirate the mouth and nostrils only when necessary, using a bulb syringe on the side opposite the suture line. If nasal packing has been inserted, do not disturb it.

3. Excessive secretions can cause aspiration and respiratory complications.

4. Position Billy only on his back or in an infant seat when in the crib. Maintain elbow restraints.

4. These measures help prevent direct contact with the suture line. Skin irritation and breakdown can occur under elbow restraints from efforts to flex the elbow, as discussed previously.

5. Feed Billy on demand; allow his parents to participate in feeding if they feel comfortable doing this.

5. Gratifying Billy's oral needs may prevent crying, which may put tension on the suture line. The parents' fear of traumatizing the suture line may supersede their desire to feed Billy.

6. Feed Billy in an upright position on your lap; place the tip of a syringe feeder on the side of the mouth opposite the suture line. Burp him after every ounce. Rinse his mouth with clear water after formula feeding. Place him in an infant seat after feeding.

6. The upright position makes it easier for the nurse to manage coughing or gagging that sometimes results from fluid being expressed through the cleft palate and entering the airway. Rinsing the mouth prevents formula particles from crusting on the suture line.

7. Using gauze or a cotton-tipped applicator, clean Billy's suture line after each feeding and at least every 2 hours with normal saline solution; apply solution with a rolling motion. Then apply antimicrobial ointment, as ordered. Do not remove the Logan bar.

7. Normal saline solution will help loosen any dried or crusted foods and secretions from the suture line. Ointment will provide a barrier to bacterial invasion (inflammation and sloughing may interfere with optimal healing of the suture line).

8. Hold and cuddle Billy as often as possible when not feeding, and encourage his parents to do the same (demonstrate a holding position that avoids contact with the Logan bar). Provide visual and auditory stimulation. Check diapers at least every hour.

8. Meeting the infant's needs for comfort and security promotes trust. Comfort measures may also reduce Billy's frustration, thus preventing undue tension on the suture line.

9. Review with Mr. and Mrs. Evans care of Billy's suture line after discharge, and discuss plans for follow-up care related to cheiloplasty and cleft palate.

9. If Billy is discharged before his sutures are removed, his parents will have to follow the same feeding and suture-line precautions discussed earlier, until the sutures can be removed.

10. Ask Mr. and Mrs. Evans to explain their understanding of how to care for Billy's cleft palate.

10. Cleft palate repair can be postponed to allow growth of the palate, jaw, and teeth, but it is usually done between ages 1 and 2 to avoid permanently impaired speech.

11. Clarify their understanding of available resources, such as children's medical services, social services, public health associations, and a local cleft palate parent group.

11. Families of children with cleft lip or cleft palate need the support and guidance of health care professionals.

Evaluation	• Billy remains afebrile, has clear breath sounds bilaterally, feeds without aspiration, and maintains admission weight.

• Billy remains afebrile, has clear breath sounds bilaterally, feeds without aspiration, and maintains admission weight.
• Billy's suture line remains intact and free from inflammation and sloughing.
• Billy has no skin irritation or breakdown under elbow restraints.
• Billy responds well to cuddling and ceases crying quickly after being held.
• Mr. and Mrs. Evans participate in feeding Billy and caring for the suture line before discharge.
• Mr. and Mrs. Evans verbalize an understanding of long-term cleft palate care and the potential problems with respiratory infection, dentition, and speech development.

Clinical situation
(continued)

Billy returns for cleft palate repair at age 16 months.

Assessment

NURSING BEHAVIORS	NURSING RATIONALES
1. Assess Billy's respiratory status.	**1.** A client with a cleft palate is particularly susceptible to respiratory infection, which would make Billy a poor candidate for anesthesia.
2. Observe Billy's physical, motor, speech, hearing, and psychosocial development.	**2.** Decreased nutritional intake and frequent respiratory infections (which could also reduce oral intake) usually result in below-average height and weight and may also impede motor development. A cleft palate typically interferes with speech development, and the frequent respiratory infections may lead to hearing impairment (from secondary otitis media). Psychosocial development should proceed normally; the child should have acquired a sense of trust by 16 months, along with a beginning sense of independence.
3. Assess feeding techniques used by the parents, noting Billy's receptivity to and participation in feeding. Anticipate ways in which the parents will have to modify these techniques and Billy's diet after surgery.	**3.** Although the child may currently be able to take soft solid foods from a spoon, he won't be allowed to eat solid foods after surgery for cleft palate repair. Anticipating modifications in diet and feeding techniques before surgery enables the nurse to plan appropriate postoperative client teaching.
4. Determine Mr. and Mrs. Evans's perception of preoperative and postoperative care routines for cleft palate repair and their anxieties about surgery.	**4.** Parental anxiety may spread to the child, whose consequent crying and fidgeting can damage the suture line postoperatively.
5. Check Billy's preoperative laboratory results (CBC, serum electrolyte levels, and urinalysis).	**5.** Abnormal values may contraindicate anesthesia and surgery.

Nursing diagnoses   Nursing diagnoses for cleft palate repair are essentially the same as those for cleft lip repair. The differences are related to the surgical site (inside the mouth) and to growth and developmental considerations based on Billy's current age.

Planning and goals   Planning and goals for cleft palate include many of the same behaviors that apply to cleft lip (such as use of elbow restraints and parent participation).

CHILD NURSING

Implementation

NURSING BEHAVIORS	NURSING RATIONALES
1. Determine how involved the parents want to be in Billy's care while he is hospitalized. Review necessary modifications to his diet and to the feeding techniques they have been using with Billy.	**1.** The parents have been responsible for feeding Billy for 14 months and probably have developed a technique and diet that work well. Billy will receive feedings best from them. Diet and feeding techniques require modification because the child cannot eat solid foods after surgery.
2. Position Billy on his abdomen.	**2.** This will ease drainage of secretions and help maintain an open airway.
3. Use bulb suctioning only to prevent aspiration or compromised breathing; position Billy on his side and insert the bulb syringe only into the side of the mouth.	**3.** After cleft palate surgery, the child may have difficulty adjusting to a new breathing pattern. This seldom requires more than positioning and support. Some children may need humidification of air for a short time postoperatively to prevent drying of secretions.
4. Assess and document bilateral breath sounds every shift, and document body temperature every 4 hours. Also check Billy's WBC count.	**4.** Crackles, rhonchi, and wheezing or an elevated body temperature or WBC count may indicate respiratory infection, a common occurrence (secondary to aspiration) in children with cleft palate.
5. Before and after surgery, feed Billy in such a way that no solid object can enter his mouth. Use a wide-bowl spoon such as a soup spoon. Provide fluids from a firm plastic cup (avoid straws and foam or glass cups). Do *not* offer a pacifier. Prevent Billy from sucking his thumb.	**5.** Any solid object in the mouth postoperatively may cause trauma to the suture line. A wide-bowl spoon is too wide to enter the mouth easily. Firm plastic cups are recommended because the client may bite off pieces of foam or glass. Sucking a straw, pacifier, or thumb may cause trauma to or tension on the suture line postoperatively.
6. Follow each feeding with at least 1 oz (29.6 ml) of water.	**6.** Water rinses the mouth of food particles, which may cling to the suture line if allowed to remain. This may lead to irritation and sloughing of the incision.
7. Clarify Mr. and Mrs. Evans's perception of the follow-up care Billy will need after discharge.	**7.** Follow-up care should include an interdisciplinary team consisting of a community health nurse, a plastic surgeon, a pediatrician, a speech therapist, an audiometrist, an orthodontist, a prosthodontist, and a social service worker.

Evaluation

- Billy remains free from infection and maintains an open airway.
- Billy's suture line remains intact.
- Billy has no skin irritation or breakdown under elbow restraints.
- Mr. and Mrs. Evans verbalize plans to continue follow-up care with an interdisciplinary cleft lip and cleft palate team.

Developmental dysplasia of the hip

Heredity and ethnic and sociologic factors contribute to developmental dysplasia of the hip (DDH). Swaddling of infants with hip adduction and extension increases the incidence of the disorder. DDH can be unilateral or bilateral and is seven times as common in girls as in boys. It is usually diagnosed during the initial pediatric assessment, although screening for DDH should be done at all visits for the first year of life. Treatment, which varies according to the child's age, is most successful when begun under age 2 months; it becomes difficult after age 4 and inadvisable after age 6. The goal, regardless of age, is to maintain abduction and prevent deformity. (See *Assessing developmental dysplasia of the hip,* page 356.)

Clinical situation

Sara Taylor, age 4 months, is admitted to the hospital with a medical diagnosis of bilateral congenital dislocated hip. Sara's pediatrician diagnosed the problem before she left the hospital after birth. The Pavlik harness she has worn since birth has proven to be an unsuccessful treatment. Sara is being hospitalized now to have a hip-spica cast applied.

Assessment

NURSING BEHAVIORS

1. Observe Sara for early signs and symptoms of congenital dislocated hip:

• extragluteal fold on the affected side

• inability to abduct the affected leg to the bed

• one knee significantly lower than the other (Allis' sign)

• broadening of the perineum (in bilateral dislocation)

• prominence of the greater trochanter

• Ortolani's and Barlow's signs.

NURSING RATIONALES

1. The head of the femur is not firmly seated in the acetabulum, which is shallow. This results in the signs described below.

• The femoral head is displaced upward and out of the acetabulum, "shortening" the femur and causing extra folds in the thigh of the affected leg.

• With the femoral head out of the socket, abduction is limited.

• The leg appears shorter on the affected side, but the femurs are actually equal in length.

• Displacement broadens the perineum. This is not evident when only one leg is affected.

• This also results from displacement.

• The examiner can feel the femoral head slip into the acetabulum when applying pressure from behind and sometimes can hear an accompanying click.

CHILD NURSING

Assessing developmental dysplasia of the hip

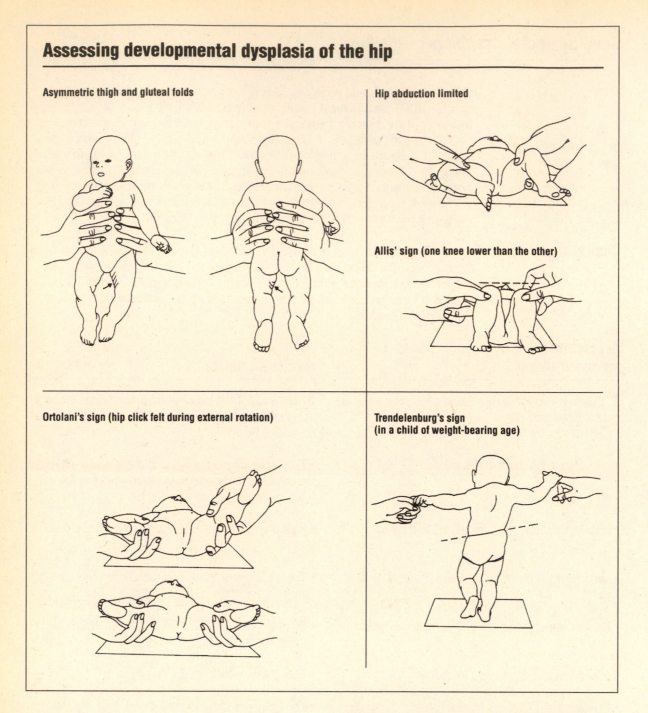

Asymmetric thigh and gluteal folds

Hip abduction limited

Allis' sign (one knee lower than the other)

Ortolani's sign (hip click felt during external rotation)

**Trendelenburg's sign
(in a child of weight-bearing age)**

Note: Signs of congenital hip dysplasia in a toddler include a shortened leg on the affected side (weight bearing and attempts to walk produce a characteristic gait with one leg shorter than the other), contractures of hip adductor and flexor muscles, and Trendelenburg's sign (when the child stands on the affected leg, the pelvis on the unaffected side tilts downward instead of upward). Developmental dysplasia of the hip may not be evident until the child begins to walk.

Cast care

I. Maintain hip abduction by applying a hip-spica cast; abduction holds the femoral head in the acetabulum

II. Observe for circulatory and nerve impairment
    A. Feel the cast for tightness
    B. Blanch toes or toenails every 1 to 2 hours initially
    C. Feel the toes for coldness, and observe for swelling, cyanosis, and pain
    D. Feel the cast for warm spots, especially over bony prominences
    E. Smell the cast for odors from pressure areas under the cast
    F. Observe respirations carefully for signs of impairment; neurovascular checks are vital because infants can indicate discomfort only through crying, fretfulness, and not eating

III. Maintain skin integrity under the cast
    A. Inspect the skin and cast regularly for crumbs
    B. Inspect cast edges
    C. Petal raw cast edges as soon as the cast is dry
    D. Keep exposed skin clean and dry

IV. Maintain cast integrity
    A. Turn the infant every 2 hours until the cast is dry; then change the infant's position frequently for comfort
    B. Handle a wet cast with the palms
    C. Check the infant's temperature frequently while the cast is drying
    D. Position the infant with hips lower than shoulders for toileting; use a plastic-backed disposable diaper under the cast rim to prevent soiling
    E. Clean the cast only with a damp cloth and a small amount of white cleanser; apply the cleanser only to soiled areas

V. Teach the parents cast care and ways to perform routine activities; for example, if the mother is breast-feeding, she can hold the infant on the hip and under the arm in the football position, or the infant can straddle the mother's legs in a face-to-face position

VI. Refer the family to an agency for disabled children

---

2. Compare Sara's growth and development with what is expected of a 4-month-old infant (see "Growth and development," pages 52 to 61).

2. This determines whether the infant meets age-related norms and helps the nurse plan care aimed at regaining and maintaining growth and development.

Nursing diagnoses
- Altered peripheral tissue perfusion related to interruption of arterial and venous blood flow from a tight hip-spica cast
- Risk for impaired skin integrity related to lack of mobility
- Impaired physical mobility related to cast limitations

Planning and goals
- Sara will maintain hip abduction.
- Sara will maintain adequate circulation and innervation of the legs while in the cast.
- Sara's skin integrity will not be impaired.
- Sara's parents will describe cast care and be able to provide care at home.
- Sara will continue to develop trust and not mistrust.

Implementation   Nursing care consists of maintaining casts and braces and organizing activities so that Sara can continue to develop and be able to compensate for any limited mobility (for specific nursing behaviors, see *Cast care,* page 357).

Evaluation   • Sara maintains adequate circulation and innervation of the legs while in the cast.
• Sara is interested in her environment and shows age-appropriate developmental behaviors.
• Sara's parents can describe the cast-care procedures they must follow when they bring Sara home from the hospital.

Congenital clubfoot

Congenital clubfoot (talipes equinovarus), a skeletal deformity of the ankle and foot in which the foot is pointed downward and inward, accounts for 95% of all clubfoot cases. Readily detected at birth, clubfoot can occur unilaterally (more common) or bilaterally. The deformity is twice as common in boys as in girls and occurs once in every 700 to 1,000 live births.

The child with congenital clubfoot requires nursing care similar to that for congenital dislocated hip. In infancy, the legs are immobilized with various casts and braces. Immobilization, which begins at or shortly after birth and extends into the toddler period, limits the child's ability to explore the environment. The child usually requires multiple hospitalizations for cast reapplications, brace adjustments, and perhaps orthopedic surgery.

Clinical situation   Joshua Adams, age 6 months, is being treated for congenital clubfoot.

Assessment

NURSING BEHAVIORS	NURSING RATIONALES
1. Differentiate clubfoot from intrauterine positional deformity.	**1.** A positional deformity involves muscles but not bones and thus can be passively manipulated. True clubfoot involves deformity of ankle and foot bones, thus preventing passive manipulation.
2. Compare Joshua's growth and development with what is expected of a 6-month-old infant (see "Growth and development," pages 52 to 61).	**2.** This determines whether the infant meets age-related norms and helps the nurse plan care aimed at regaining and maintaining growth and development.

Nursing diagnoses   Nursing diagnoses for congenital clubfoot are similar to those for congenital dislocated hip.

Planning and goals   • The infant will attain a normal anatomic position.
• The infant will maintain a normal developmental level.
• The infant's parents will understand and follow through on home care.

Implementation

NURSING BEHAVIORS	NURSING RATIONALES
1. Assist with treatment in three stages: • correcting the deformity by applying a series of casts, beginning soon after birth and continuing until marked overcorrection is achieved; casts may be re-applied on a weekly basis because of rapid growth in early infancy (a Denis Browne splint may be substituted for casts) • maintaining correction by having the child wear special clubfoot shoes • providing follow-up care to prevent recurrence; surgery may be necessary if the deformity does not respond to conservative treatment.	**1.** Because infants' bones are soft and malleable, early diagnosis and treatment of orthopedic anomalies is essential. Anatomically correct or overcorrected positioning is an effective noninvasive treatment.
2. Teach appropriate home-care techniques to the infant's parents.	**2.** The infant will require competent care at home to achieve full recovery.

Evaluation

• The child demonstrates age-appropriate developmental behaviors.
• The child learns to walk without an apparent limp or deformity.

Bronchiolitis

Bronchiolitis, an infection of the lower respiratory tract, produces inflammation and obstruction with thick mucus and edema. In some areas of the lungs, mucus plugs and bronchiolar edema completely obstruct the small bronchioles, resulting in atelectasis. Some of these obstructed bronchioles trap air in the alveoli, producing hyperinflation. Overall, the child experiences generalized hypoxia and progressive respiratory distress.

The infection is viral; respiratory syncytial virus is the most common causative agent. Bronchiolitis is most prevalent during late fall and winter. It occurs in children from birth to age 2. Affected infants have several days of low-grade fever, mild upper respiratory infection, and anorexia. These signs and symptoms are followed by a paroxysmal wheezing cough, dyspnea, irritability, and possibly cyanosis. Treatment is supportive, and includes oxygen administration and fluid and electrolyte replacement. (For a review of respiratory problems in children, see *Pediatric respiratory infections,* pages 361 and 362.)

Clinical situation

Bryan Bailey, a 6-month-old infant weighing 15.2 lb (6.9 kg), has just been admitted with a diagnosis of bronchiolitis. His temperature is 101.5° F (38.6° C); respiratory rate, 56 breaths/minute; and apical pulse, 166 beats/minute. His respirations are accompanied by nasal flaring, retractions, and expiratory grunting. Bryan is in a high-humidity tent with 30% oxygen and is receiving dextrose 5% in lactated Ringer's solution I.V. at 25 ml/hour. He may have clear liquids by bottle as tolerated. His parents are present.

Assessment

NURSING BEHAVIORS

1. Determine Bryan's respiratory status by overt observation, auscultation of breath sounds, and review of X-ray findings.

2. Assess Bryan's hydration status: monitor urine output (decreased in dehydration) and daily weight, including weight gain or loss; check for depressed anterior fontanel, tearing with crying, moist oral buccal membrane, and skin turgor.

3. Review results of ordered laboratory studies: nasal wash, arterial blood gas (ABG) and pH levels, and urinalysis.

4. Assess the parents' perception of Bryan's illness; note expressions of anxiety, guilt, and fear about the prognosis or management of the illness.

5. Prevent spread of RSV by using proper handwashing technique and by cleaning all objects possibly contaminated by respiratory secretions.

6. Assess Bryan's developmental level (see "Growth and development," pages 52 to 61).

NURSING RATIONALES

1. Respiratory status can be compromised because bronchiolar occlusion by mucus usually results in increased chest diameter and hyperresonant sounds (detected by percussion). Overt observation may reveal flaring of nostrils, retractions, expiratory grunting, and circumoral cyanosis. Auscultation reveals wheezing; fine, moist crackles; and diminished breath sounds. X-rays may reveal areas of emphysema or atelectasis. An inability to clear the alveoli of air on expiration leads to overdistention (emphysema). This air may be absorbed gradually, but if inspirations are ineffective by this point, the alveoli will collapse (atelectasis).

2. Infants with respiratory distress cannot take in adequate amounts of fluid and will lose up to 1 quart (1L)/day from tachypnea. Coughing spells may precipitate vomiting, another form of fluid loss.

3. Respiratory syncytial virus (RSV), the most common cause of bronchiolitis, can be identified by nasal wash culture in 3 to 7 days. The physician may order ribavirin, an antiviral drug administered by small-particle aerosol, if the culture is positive. ABG levels indicate the degree of hypoxia. Expect respiratory acidosis (decreased pH and increased $PaCO_2$) with hypoventilation. Increased specific gravity and positive ketone bodies may accompany dehydration.

4. Infants with bronchiolitis appear to be—and are—acutely ill, which increases parental anxiety. The parents' ability to remain in the acute care environment, to relate to Bryan, and to comprehend explanations is directly related to their anxiety level: The less anxious they are, the more they will be able to understand.

5. RSV is spread by direct contact with respiratory secretions, which can survive on objects and hands for up to 30 minutes.

6. This determines whether the infant meets age-related norms and helps the nurse plan care aimed at regaining and maintaining growth and development.

Pediatric respiratory infections

CONDITION (ETIOLOGY)	AGE OF PEAK INCIDENCE	PATHOLOGY	MANIFESTATIONS	MANAGEMENT
Acute epiglottitis (*Haemophilus influenzae*, type B)	2 to 7 years	Infection of epiglottis; can be severe, rapidly progressive, and fatal if untreated	• Abrupt onset • Sore throat, inability to swallow • Tripod positioning (the child remains upright, resting weight on the hands; the chin is thrust out, with the mouth open and drooling) • Froglike sound on inspiration • Marked restlessness and anxiety • High fever	• Don't try to visualize the epiglottis with a tongue depressor. • Prepare for intubation or tracheostomy. • Provide high humidity with oxygen and I.V. hydration. • Withhold food and fluids. • Administer antibiotics, as ordered.
Chlamydial pneumonia (bacterial)	Less than 6 months	Acquired as ascending infection before or during birth; nonspecific pathology, but severe disease is thought to be responsible for one-third of reported pneumonia cases in infants under age 6 months	• Persistent cough, tachypnea • Normal or mildly elevated temperature • Feeding difficulty • Failure to thrive • Possible accompanying condition: conjunctivitis	• Treat symptomatically (as above). • Administer erythromycin and sulfa drugs, as ordered.
Pneumococcal pneumonia (bacterial)	1 to 4 years	Involves all or almost all of one or more pulmonary lobes; transmitted by droplet spread	• Fever (102° to 105° F [38.9° to 40.6° C]) • Shaking, chills, headache • Tachycardia • Rapid, shallow respirations; hacking, nonproductive cough; pleuritic chest pain • Complications: otitis media, pleural effusion, empyema	• Administer penicillin G and antipyretics, as ordered. • Provide high humidity with oxygen and increased hydration. Suction as needed. • Percuss lung segments with postural drainage. • Use thoracentesis or closed chest drainage (or both) to treat pulmonary complications if needed.
Staphylococcal pneumonia (bacterial)	Infancy (70% of cases) to 2 years	Bronchopneumonia (begins in bronchioles; exudate consolidates in neighboring lobules)	• Mild symptoms of upper respiratory infection, which may progress to tachypnea and anxiety • Fever, shocklike state • Progressive dyspnea • Complications: empyema, tension pneumothorax, pyopneumothorax	• Treat symptomatically. • Administer semisynthetic penicillins (such as methicillin or nafcillin) because many staphylococcal organisms are penicillin-resistant.
Streptococcal pneumonia (bacterial)	Not age-specific (usually a complication of strep throat, upper respiratory tract infection, or contagious disease)	Interstitial pneumonitic pneumonia with disseminated infiltration	• Similar to those of pneumococcal pneumonia in most cases, but sometimes only mild symptoms • Complications: pleural effusion, empyema	• Treat symptomatically. • Administer penicillin G I.V. or I.M.

(continued)

Pediatric respiratory infections (continued)

CONDITION (ETIOLOGY)	AGE OF PEAK INCIDENCE	PATHOLOGY	MANIFESTATIONS	MANAGEMENT
Acute spasmodic laryngitis— spasmodic croup (viral)	3 months to 4 years	Inflammation of the larynx, leading to laryngeal muscle spasms and partial obstruction of the upper airway	• Predominantly nighttime attacks that last 1 to 3 hours • Inspiratory stridor with barklike, nonproductive cough • Restlessness, dyspnea, anxiety • Slight, if any, temperature elevation	• Provide cool mist. • Help relieve the child's and parents' anxiety.
Acute laryngo- tracheo- bronchitis (viral)	1 to 3 years	Inflammation and edema of the larynx, trachea, and bronchi with exudate	• Possible marked temperature elevation • Marked dyspnea, tachypnea, bilateral wheezing, diminished breath sounds, prolonged expiration • Tachycardia • Complications: secondary pneumonia, septicemia, cardiac failure	• To maintain an open airway, keep intubation equipment and tracheostomy set at the bedside; provide cool humidity with oxygen; suction as needed; and administer ordered medication (possibly epinephrine by aerosol or intermittent positive-pressure breathing) • Maintain hydration by giving I.V. fluids. • Take measures to reduce temperature.
Bronchitis (secondary to cystic fibrosis, asthma, or bronchiolitis)	Late infancy and early childhood	Inflammation of mucous membrane lining bronchi	• Wheezing if underlying asthma is present • Dry cough progresses to productive cough with purulent sputum • Moderate emphysema	• Provide high humidity and maintain adequate hydration. • Administer sympathomimetic bronchodilators (subcutaneous epinephrine or oral ephedrine) if ordered.
Atypical primary pneumonia (*Mycoplasma pneumoniae*)	5 to adulthood	Interstitial pneumonitis, bronchitis, bronchiolitis	• Fever, chills, headache, malaise, anorexia, myalgia, rhinitis, sore throat	• Treat symptomatically.
Bronchiolitis (usually respiratory syncytial virus)	Infancy and early childhood	Interstitial (alveolar walls) pneumonitis with inflammation of bronchial and bronchiolar mucosa	• Rapid or insidious onset after upper respiratory tract infection • Mild to marked temperature elevation • Slight to severe cough • Possible signs of obstructive emphysema • Symptoms similar to bronchiolitis	• Treat symptomatically (high humidity, increased hydration, antipyretics if needed).

Nursing diagnoses

• Risk for fluid volume deficit related to increased insensible fluid loss and poor intake
• Ineffective airway clearance related to increased tracheobronchial secretions and bronchial edema
• Ineffective breathing pattern related to mucus accumulation and respiratory tract edema

• Ineffective family coping (compromised) related to anxiety over infant's illness

Planning and goals
• Bryan will have a respiratory rate of less than 40 breaths/minute and be free from physical signs of respiratory distress within 24 hours.
• Bryan's daily fluid intake will be at least 100 ml/kg of body weight; urine output will be 350 ml/day.
• Bryan will have at least 1 hour of uninterrupted rest four times daily during hospitalization.
• Bryan will respond positively to visual, auditory, and tactile stimulation within 48 hours.
• Bryan's parents will increase the amount of physical contact they have with him each day, and their anxiety level will decrease.
• All personnel and visitors will use proper hand-washing technique after contact with Bryan or objects in his room.

Implementation

NURSING BEHAVIORS	NURSING RATIONALES
1. Take the following measures to ease Bryan's respirations:	**1.** These measures will help clear Bryan's airway.
• Suction the nose and mouth as necessary, but avoid suctioning the upper respiratory tract if secretions are not apparent.	• Suctioning irritates the mucous membrane, resulting in edema and mucus secretion. This, in turn, can narrow and obstruct the upper airway, further complicating Bryan's respiratory problems.
• Place Bryan upright in an infant seat, and closely observe him to ensure that he does not slump down.	• Sitting upright in an infant seat facilitates respirations. If the infant slumps down, his tongue can obstruct the posterior pharynx, interfering with adequate lung expansion.
• Administer nothing by mouth during an acute phase of dyspnea.	• This reduces the infant's risk of aspirating secretions and keeps him from overtiring.
2. Assess and document Bryan's respiratory rate and status at least every 2 hours. Observe for the following:	**2.** Signs of respiratory distress must be promptly recognized and treated before the infant sustains damage from hypoxia.
• restlessness, flaring of the nostrils, retractions, and cyanosis	• Restlessness is the first sign of hypoxia, followed by flaring of the nostrils and retractions. Cyanosis is a late sign. The infant's accessory muscles of respiration are still poorly developed. Retractions and grunting indicate increased respiratory effort.
• expiratory grunting	• Knowing whether grunting is inspiratory or expiratory can help determine the nature of a respiratory problem. An infant with bronchiolitis can inspire adequately but does not have enough expiratory force to move gas-exchanged air around the mucus plugs in the bronchioles.
• breathing pattern (abdominal, chest, or a combination)	• The infant's breathing pattern indicates the ease or difficulty of respiratory effort.

CHILD NURSING

• bilateral breath sounds.

• Bilateral breath sounds ensure adequate lung expansion.

3. Maintain a highly humid, cool environment with 30% oxygen content, as ordered.

3. High humidity helps loosen and liquefy thick secretions in the respiratory tract, facilitating their removal. Coolness helps reduce edema of the mucous membranes.

• Check the oxygen level every 2 hours, and reposition the canopy if needed.

• Checking the oxygen level ensures correct concentration. The canopy may shift, causing discomfort or loss of oxygen.

• Keep the bottom of the plastic canopy tucked securely under the mattress; open the canopy as infrequently as possible.

• Oxygen, heavier than air, settles to the bottom of the tent; opening the canopy from the bottom thus allows oxygen to escape.

• Wipe moisture from the canopy sides and top every 2 hours or more frequently if needed. Place extra layers of bedding on the mattress, and place a towel around Bryan's head and shoulders.

• High humidity causes moisture to condense on the canopy sides, making it difficult for the nurse to observe the infant's color and respiratory status. Moisture also condenses on the canopy top; the droplets that fall can cause chilling, which may further increase the infant's metabolic rate and oxygen needs.

• Remove Bryan from the tent for oral fluids and cuddling only if his respiratory rate is less than 36 breaths/minute and he displays no retractions, expiratory grunting, or cyanosis.

• Removing the infant from the oxygen tent is contraindicated if his respiratory rate exceeds 36 breaths/minute or he exhibits other signs of respiratory distress.

4. Maintain adequate hydration, as follows:

4. An infant with bronchiolitis is at risk for fluid imbalance.

• Weigh Bryan daily, and record the weight.

• Body weight changes are the best measure of fluid lost or gained.

• Record I.V. intake every hour to ensure that Bryan is receiving the prescribed rate of 25 ml/hour.

• I.V. fluids administered at 25 ml/hour provide 100 ml/kg of body weight to meet the infant's fluid needs. Remember, water lost via the lungs also must be replaced. Inadequate fluid intake can contribute to dehydration. Parenteral administration of too much fluid can increase the infant's blood volume, which may lead to cardiac overload, congestive heart failure, or pulmonary edema.

• Use a gram scale to weigh used diapers.

• This enables the nurse to measure and record urine output; 1 g is equivalent to 1 ml of urine output.

• Document Bryan's hydration status at least every shift.

• Documentation at each shift enables the staff to monitor the infant's hydration status, evaluate changes, and initiate treatment, if necessary.

• Check urine specific gravity at least once each shift.

• The specific gravity of normal urine in infants ranges from 1.003 to 1.030. Less than 1.003 represents dilution (overhydration); more than 1.030 represents concentration (dehydration).

5. Offer 60 ml of oral fluids (electrolyte solution or sterile water) every 2 hours; discontinue oral feedings if Bryan demonstrates a weak sucking reflex or an increased respiratory rate (more than 46 breaths/minute). If Bryan cannot tolerate oral fluids, notify the physician.

5. The infant needs additional fluids to supplement the insensible water lost through the lungs. However, in the acute phase of bronchiolitis, he will become exhausted even by the effort required for sucking. Clear fluids are preferable if the infant experiences feeding difficulty, gagging, or choking because he will have less risk of aspiration pneumonia. If the infant cannot tolerate oral fluids, the physician may increase the I.V. rate.

6. Explain to the parents the purpose of all equipment being used in Bryan's care. Tell them that bronchiolitis is common in infants, and reassure them that infants respond well to treatment. Outline the nursing plan of care and welcome the parents' presence at any time, but acknowledge that their anxiety may be overwhelming.

6. These explanations may help relieve the parents' anxiety about how ill the child looks and may lessen their fear of the unknown.

7. Organize nursing care to provide Bryan with at least 1 hour of uninterrupted rest between tasks.

7. Handling the child or disrupting his rest will further increase Bryan's metabolic rate and oxygen needs.

8. Provide Bryan with gentle auditory, visual, and tactile stimulation each time nursing tasks are performed. Allow the parents to provide tactile stimulation while Bryan is in the tent; involve them in selecting bright pictures that can be hung outside the tent for visual stimulation.

8. In the acute phase, which usually lasts 2 to 3 days, Bryan will not respond. However, the stimuli are comforting and promote a sense of security and trust.

Evaluation

- Bryan breathes without distress and has a healthy color.
- Bryan is taking adequate fluids to maintain normal hydration.
- Bryan smiles readily, reaches out for his mother, focuses on visual stimuli, and makes eye contact with the person speaking to him.
- Bryan's parents show decreased anxiety and are participating in his care.
- Bryan's infection is not transmitted to other children or staff.

Diarrhea

Diarrhea is an increase in the frequency, volume, and liquidity of stools. Acute diarrhea, the sudden onset of frequent loose or watery stools, usually results from an inflammatory response to an intestinal tract infection. Chronic diarrhea begins more slowly, with a gradual increase in the number of stools, whose consistency becomes loose and unformed. It usually results not from an infection but from an inflammatory reaction and allergic response or a malabsorption syndrome.

Diarrhea becomes a problem for children because water and electrolyte loss from the bowel can cause dehydration. Dehydration is classified as isotonic, hypertonic, or hypotonic, based on the relationship of electrolyte loss to fluid loss, or as mild, moderate, or severe, based on the percentage of body weight lost (mild, 2% to 4%; moderate, 5% to 9%; severe, 10% or greater). Hospitalization is usually required for severe diarrhea to replace fluids and electrolytes and to treat infection if present.

Clinical situation

Lisa Hunt is an 11-month-old infant admitted to the hospital with dehydration secondary to nausea and vomiting. Two days before admission, Lisa began having loose stools, which progressed from brown to green and became increasingly liquid. She began vomiting yesterday and Lisa hasn't tolerated anything by mouth since then. Mrs. Hunt states that Lisa's stools contained pus and mucus, and today she noticed some bright red blood. She also says that Lisa feels "feverish," is irritable, and cries shrilly before each bowel movement.

On admission Lisa's temperature is 100.8° F (38.2° C) and her weight is 18 ½ lb (8.4 kg). Before this illness, her weight was 21 lb (9.5 kg). Lisa's initial serum sodium level is 132 mEq/L; bicarbonate, 18 mEq/L; and pH, 7.28. Admission orders include no food or fluids by mouth; I.V. dextrose 5% in 0.25% sodium chloride infused at 62 ml/hour; rectal swab for culture and sensitivity tests; stool culture three times; and serum electrolytes every day.

Assessment

NURSING BEHAVIORS

1. Obtain a thorough client history, including food that Lisa ingested in the 24 hours before the onset of diarrhea, the family's source of water, and family pets; document whether or not other family members have Lisa's symptoms (see *Common fungal, parasitic, and bacterial infections,* pages 367 and 368, for more information).

2. Assess Lisa's hydration status by recording her weight; examining the oral mucous membrane; checking for tearing with crying; determining the amount, color, and frequency of her urine; and assessing skin turgor, temperature, and color. Also assess her behavior, sensory response, and neurologic signs (which may include twitching, numbness, and cramping in the extremities). Review laboratory reports of serum electrolyte levels.

NURSING RATIONALES

1. This information can help the staff determine the causative agent, which has a direct bearing on treatment and follow-up measures. Lisa's symptoms (especially abdominal cramping, watery diarrhea, and stools with pus, mucus, and blood) suggest shigellosis or salmonella. Salmonella tends to be transmitted from animals to humans, either directly or by food products, especially poultry and eggs. (Pet turtles have been a source of salmonella infection, and their importation and sale are now regulated by law.) Shigella causing bacillary dysentery, on the other hand, is transmitted from human to human or through water supplies, improper refrigeration, and sometimes flies.

2. The status of the anterior fontanel is a significant indicator of hydration. Lisa's weight loss of 2 ½ lb (1.1 kg) is greater than 10% of her body weight and thus classifies her as severely dehydrated. Lisa's initial serum electrolyte levels (sodium, 132 mEq/L; bicarbonate, 18 mEq/L; and pH, 7.28) indicate isotonic dehydration (balanced fluid and electrolyte loss) with metabolic acidosis. Lisa will probably exhibit physical symptoms of dehydration in each category listed, with the exception of neurologic signs, which would be found with electrolyte imbalance (hypertonic or hypotonic dehydration). Correcting Lisa's fluid loss and metabolic acidosis will require therapy to restore and maintain fluid balance. Accurate nursing assessment and documentation enable the physician to prescribe the correct fluid, administration rate, and appropriate electrolytes (especially potassium chloride).

Common fungal, parasitic, and bacterial infections

CONDITION	SIGNS AND SYMPTOMS	NURSING CARE
Fungal infections		
Ringworm Tinea capitis (head)	Scalp pruritus, scaly patches, erythematous scaling patch that clears centrally and spreads peripherally, scalp lesions (may spread to hairline and neck), temporary hair loss; usually contracted from household pets (puppies and kittens) or person to person	• Administer oral griseofulvin. • Administer ketoconazole for resistant cases. • Recommend frequent shampoos and haircuts. • Apply antifungal ointment (clotrimazole, haloprogrin, or miconazole) locally.
Tinea corporis (body)	Lesions (same as those in tinea capitis); contracted from household pets	• Administer oral griseofulvin. • Apply Whitfield's or tolnaftate ointment.
Tinea cruris (jock itch)	Skin response similar to that in tinea corporis; usually limited to crural fold and medial proximal thigh, but may involve scrotum	• Apply tolnaftate liquid locally. • Recommend wet compresses or sitz baths.
Tinea pedis (athlete's foot)	Pruritus, maceration, and fissures between toes; patches with pinhead-size vesicles on soles	• Administer oral griseofulvin. • Apply tofnaftate liquid or antifungal powder. • Apply compresses or soaks for 15 minutes, followed by steroid creams. • Tell the client to wear light socks and well-ventilated shoes.
Parasitic infections		
Pinworm (GI)	Intense perianal and (in women and girls) perivaginal pruritus; occasionally causes appendicitis	• Perform a cellophane tape test: Press the tape's sticky side tightly over the perianal area; then seal the tape on a slide and view with a microscope to identify the presence of and type of worm. • Prevent the infection from spreading: —Decontaminate the client's bed linens and clothing by washing in hot water, using strong soap and chlorine bleach. —Cut the client's fingernails short. —Teach the client to wash hands on arising and after toileting. —Administer mebendazole to children over age 2. —Administer piperazine or pyrvinium pamoate (Povan), as ordered. Note that Povan stains vomitus, stool, and urine red; do not mistake it for blood. • Treat other family members.
Roundworm (GI, pulmonary)	Anorexia nervosa, enlarged belly, weight loss, fever, intestinal colic; may progress to intestinal obstruction, appendicitis, perforation, obstructive jaundice, pneumonitis	• Teach the client hygienic measures, as with pinworm. Reinfection is common. • Administer pyrantel pamoate (Antiminth) or piperazine. • Collect and keep stool specimens warm to test for ova and parasites.

(continued)

Common fungal, parasitic, and bacterial infections *(continued)*

CONDITION	SIGNS AND SYMPTOMS	NURSING CARE
Parasitic infections *(continued)*		
Hookworm (GI, pulmonary)	Anemia, weight loss, pruritus, malnutrition, coughing, dyspnea	• Tell the client to avoid going barefoot and to wear gloves when gardening; tell a pediatric client not to play in dirt. • Administer mebendazole, piperazine, or pyrvinium. • Teach hygienic measures, as with pinworm and roundworm.
Pediculosis (lice) Capitis	Severe scalp pruritus, white eggs (nits) firmly attached to hair (visible upon close examination of scalp); excoriation on scalp may develop into secondary infection; children with long hair are usually affected	• Wear gloves and protective cap during examination and treatment. • Apply lindane shampoo (Kwell), pyrethrins solution, or permethrin cream. • Rinse hair and comb it with a fine-tooth comb dipped in vinegar to remove nits. • Decontaminate clothing and bed linen, as with pinworm and roundworm.
Corporis	Pruritus; erythematous macules, wheals, and excoriated patches (usually found on the upper back and pressure areas from tight clothing)	• Thoroughly launder clothing and bed linen, and iron seams. • Administer lindane, pyrethrins, or pesmethrin solution.
Bacterial infection		
Impetigo contagiosa (from *Staphylococcus* or *Streptococcus*)	Red macule initially; vesicles that coalesce and rupture easily, leaving superficial moist lesion; spreads easily in sharply marginated but irregular lesions; exudate dries to form heavy, honey-colored crusts; pruritus	• Apply Burrow's compresses of 1:20 dilution to remove crusts and debris. • Apply topical antibiotic ointment (Neosporin, Garamycin, or NeoPolycon). • Administer parenteral antibiotics.

3. Assess Lisa's behavior before and during each bowel movement, and examine the stools for abnormalities.

3. Abdominal cramping (demonstrated by crying, clutching the abdomen, and flexing the knees to the abdomen) and stools tinged with blood, mucus, and pus indicate that an organism, rather than a noninfectious inflammatory response or malabsorption syndrome, is causing the diarrhea.

4. Assess Lisa's developmental level, and compare it with expected norms for her age (see "Growth and development," pages 52 to 61).

4. This determines whether the infant meets age-related norms and helps the nurse plan care aimed at regaining and maintaining growth and development.

Nursing diagnoses
• Diarrhea related to bowel malabsorption and/or bacterial or viral toxins
• Fluid volume deficit related to frequent watery stools
• Risk for impaired skin integrity related to alkaline stools contacting the skin
• Knowledge deficit related to the parents' understanding of infection and measures to prevent its spread within the family

Planning and goals

- Lisa's infection will not be transmitted to others.
- Lisa will regain fluid and electrolyte balance.
- Lisa will have fewer stools per day.
- Lisa's skin will remain intact in the perianal area.
- Lisa's family will understand current treatments and the anticipated approach to her diet when she resumes oral intake.
- Lisa will maintain or regain her preillness developmental level.

Implementation

NURSING BEHAVIORS

1. Ensure that hospital personnel and visitors wash hands carefully, and follow hospital policies regarding universal precautions. Apply diapers snugly.

2. Obtain rectal swab and stool specimens, as ordered. Use a tongue blade to scrape stool from the diaper to a specimen cup, and include mucus in the specimen, if present. Promptly transport specimens to the laboratory, following hospital policy (for example, placing them in double containers).

3. Weigh Lisa every morning at 7 a.m.; know the previous day's weight beforehand.

4. Each hour, monitor and document the amount of I.V. fluid infused, the appearance of the infusion site, and urine output. Add sodium bicarbonate to I.V. fluid, as ordered.

5. Document Lisa's hydration status at least every 4 hours (include items listed under "Assessment"). Additionally, monitor for signs of overhydration (bounding pulse, dyspnea, moist crackles, increased blood pressure, pitting edema, marked weight gain, and urine specific gravity less than 1.003).

6. Maintain strict intake and output records, as follows:

NURSING RATIONALES

1. Enteric isolation is necessary until a stool culture confirms the causative organism; most organisms that cause diarrhea are contagious. Careful hand washing is the most effective means of preventing cross-infection between clients. Linens are usually double-bagged and laundered using special techniques. A snug diaper prevents liquid stool from leaking and keeps the client from placing her hands in stools that may be infected.

2. Proper care in obtaining and transporting specimens helps ensure an accurate test for the causative agent. Mucus should be included in the specimen because it can serve as another source for the culture. Double containers prevent contamination of personnel during transport. Prompt transport of specimens is important because organisms usually live for only a short period.

3. Weight is the most reliable measure of fluid loss or gain. The infant should be weighed at the same time each day, with the same scale, and by the same person, if possible, to ensure accuracy.

4. The infant totally depends on the I.V. infusion for hydration and nutrition. If I.V. fluids are not flowing into the appropriate vessels because of obstruction or infiltration, the infant will not receive adequate hydration and may experience discomfort and tissue damage. Sodium bicarbonate helps to correct metabolic acidosis.

5. Lisa's response to fluid therapy should be reflected in physical manifestations of hydration. Overhydration can occur rapidly or insidiously as a response to I.V. fluid therapy.

6. Accurate intake and output records enable the staff to monitor the client's fluid balance.

CHILD NURSING

• On a stool chart, record the time of bowel movements; the amount (in milliliters if stools are liquid), color, and consistency of stools; and Lisa's behavior before and during elimination. If the physician orders dipstick tests for pH, blood, or glucose, also record these results on the stool chart.

• Recording this information on a separate chart can help the staff determine the client's elimination patterns and response to therapy.

• Weigh each diaper on a gram scale. If stools are watery, apply a pediatric urine collector to differentiate urine and stool output.

• Weighing the diapers helps determine fluid loss more accurately (1 ml of urine weighs 1 g; thus, urine's weight in grams equals urine output).

• Record the amount, consistency, and color of any vomitus.

• This detects additional fluid loss from other sources.

7. Document urine specific gravity at least once every shift (along with urine pH, if ordered).

7. Urine specific gravity is one indication of the client's hydration status. Dehydration leads to decreases in circulating blood volume, glomerular filtration rate, and urine production. A higher concentration of solutes increases urine specific gravity. As fluid balance is restored, urine specific gravity should decrease.

8. Clean Lisa's perianal skin carefully after each bowel movement, and apply a clean diaper. Check the diaper at least every hour.

8. Intestinal contents are strongly alkaline, and contact with the skin can cause skin irritation and breakdown. Open skin lesions can lead to secondary infection.

9. Provide oral care every 2 hours with a gauze-covered tongue depressor moistened with water; apply petroleum jelly to the lips.

9. Dehydration, mouth breathing, and increased respiratory rate dry the oral mucous membranes and lips.

10. Record Lisa's temperature, pulse rate, and respiratory rate every 4 hours.

10. An elevated temperature increases the client's metabolic rate, as evidenced by increases in the pulse rate (approximately 10 beats/minute per degree Fahrenheit of elevation) and respiratory rate. An increased respiratory rate contributes to greater insensible water loss. An elevated temperature is common early in the course of shigellosis but later in diarrhea caused by *Escherichia coli*.

11. Explain the treatment regimen to Lisa's parents; prepare them for the expected approach to oral feedings.

11. Lisa will be kept off food and fluids until her stools decrease in frequency and contain less liquid. Oral intake usually begins with small amounts of oral rehydrating solution; if the solution is well tolerated, the number of stools doesn't increase and no vomiting occurs, the infant can progress to human milk and soft foods.

Cow's milk is usually withheld for at least a week until the intestinal tract can tolerate it (and lactose). It is reintroduced in a diluted preparation. The I.V. infusion will continue until the child's ability to tolerate oral intake is confirmed. Foods with high sodium content (such as broth and salted crackers) should be given with caution to avoid hypernatremia.

12. Offer Lisa a pacifier as desired.

12. Oral needs intensify in response to regression and food and fluid restrictions.

13. Provide age-appropriate sensorimotor stimulation; include auditory (musical toys, verbal conversation), visual (colorful toys, pictures, mobiles), and tactile (stuffed toys, stroking, books) stimuli.

13. Lisa is in the sensorimotor stage of development and, if able, should participate in activities that maintain this developmental stage.

14. Encourage Lisa's parents to remain with her as much as possible.

14. Lisa is at the age of separation anxiety (fear of abandonment). She needs repeated reassurance of the parents' love and presence.

15. Prepare the family for possible follow-up and discharge planning.

15. If shigellosis is diagnosed, the family must be told that the disease is communicable for several weeks, and they should receive written instructions for careful hand washing, disposing of Lisa's excretions, and cleaning toilet facilities. The family should also be taught how to avoid transmitting enteropathologic organisms, with an emphasis on proper hand washing and food handling. If stool specimens are needed from family members, provide written instructions for proper collection and delivery.

Evaluation

• Lisa's I.V. infusion remained patent, fluids were administered as ordered, and she experienced no further weight loss. Urine output increased by day 2.
• The number of stools decreased from 20 on day 1 to 4 on day 5.
• Although Lisa's perianal skin became markedly reddened, no open lesions or rash developed.
• Lisa plays peek-a-boo with her parents and staff members.
• Lisa's parents expressed a verbal understanding of the hospital treatment regimen.
• Lisa's parents received, discussed, and expressed understanding of written discharge instructions.
• Lisa's family is free from symptoms and remains so after her discharge from the hospital.

THE TODDLER (AGES 1 TO 3)

Anemia

The most common hematologic disorder in infants and children, anemia is a reduction either in the volume of red blood cells (RBCs) or in hemoglobin concentration. Causes include excessive blood loss, destruction (hemolysis), and diminished RBC production. Anemia diminishes the blood's capacity to carry oxygen and therefore reduces the amount of oxygen available to tissue. Its symptoms stem from tissue hypoxia and the body's compensatory response.

Iron-deficiency anemia, the most prevalent nutritional disorder in the United States, occurs most commonly in children between ages 6 months and 2 years and again during adolescence. In infants (whose iron stores are depleted between the 5th and 6th month) and children up to age 2, this anemia may develop because they do not receive enough iron in their diets to meet growth demands. In adolescents, it may develop as a result of a rapid growth rate, fad diets, and poor nutritional choices and eating habits.

Clinical situation   Kimberly, age 15 months, is diagnosed with iron-deficiency anemia. She is the firstborn child of Sue, age 18, and Jim, age 20. Although she is a fat baby, Kimberly is a picky eater who refuses most foods; if she didn't drink as much milk as she does, she would have very little food intake. She is pale and irritable, and has a grade II systolic murmur. Her pulse is rapid, 140 beats/minute (above normal for her age), and thready; her respiratory rate is 32 breaths/minute; and her hemoglobin level is 7.2.

Assessment

NURSING BEHAVIORS

NURSING RATIONALES

1. Assess for cardiac decompensation by checking apical pulse rate, blood pressure, and respiratory rate every 4 hours. Also observe Kimberly's skin color.

1. Until the hemoglobin level falls below 6 g, compensatory mechanisms effectively prevent most overt symptoms. Blood viscosity is less because the number of RBCs is reduced. This hemodilution results in decreased peripheral resistance, which increases the quantity of blood returned to the heart. The cardiac workload increases as the heart pumps faster to circulate the thinned blood. The heart may enlarge and have a functional systolic murmur. Increased cardiac output (from tachycardia and cardiac dilation) compensates for the decreased number of RBCs. However, with exercise, infection, emotional stress, or circulatory overload, cardiac failure may occur.

2. Obtain a detailed diet history from the parents, including food preferences and dislikes.

2. Infants should receive only breast milk or commercial formula with iron until age 1 year. As a rule, an infant should receive no more than 32 oz (960 ml) of milk per day. One quart of milk provides only 0.5 mg of iron, whereas 1 tbs of fortified baby cereal provides 2.5 to 5 mg of iron. Infants with iron-deficiency anemia should receive no more than 16 oz (480 ml) of milk per day because cow's milk causes blood loss from the GI tract.

3. Assess for chronic fecal blood loss by testing stools with a fecal occult blood test (Hemoccult) each shift.

3. Stool analysis for occult blood is performed to rule out chronic hidden blood loss as a cause of the anemia.

4. Observe for signs of infection, such as tugging at the ear (otitis media), runny nose, reluctance to swallow (sore throat), coughing, sneezing, and elevated temperature.

4. Children with chronic anemia are prone to infections.

5. Assess Kimberly's growth and development level (see "Growth and development," pages 52 to 61).

5. Toddlers with iron-deficiency anemia commonly have poor muscle development and are reluctant to explore their physical surroundings.

Nursing diagnoses
- Altered nutrition: Less than body requirements, related to inadequate iron in the diet
- Risk for infection related to poor nutrition and lowered resistance
- Activity intolerance related to weakness and fatigue from diminished oxygen transport
- Knowledge deficit related to the parents' understanding of nutritional requirements of toddlers

Planning and goals
- Kimberly will conserve energy and decrease tissue oxygen needs until her hemoglobin level and RBC count return to normal.
- Kimberly will not develop cardiac complications from the anemia.
- Kimberly's iron intake will increase sufficiently to replace depleted stores and to maintain RBC production.
- Kimberly will remain infection-free.
- Kimberly's parents will provide a nutritionally balanced diet that has enough iron.
- Kimberly will regain physical activity appropriate to her developmental stage.

Implementation

NURSING BEHAVIORS

NURSING RATIONALES

1. Have the parents plan care to decrease Kimberly's tissue oxygen demand. Encourage them to anticipate her needs and assist with feeding. Perform daily hygienic care (bathing, dressing, diapering) at one time, if possible, to provide for rest. Schedule and adhere to rest periods between peak activity periods. Assess Kimberly's activity tolerance, and provide for quiet play in a crib or on the parents' lap.

1. The child with anemia may be easily fatigued. The toddler is a particular challenge because he is geared to explore the environment yet lacks the energy to do so. Providing nonstrenuous activity helps conserve the child's energy by decreasing tissue oxygen demands.

2. Monitor Kimberly's cardiac function, as follows:
- Check the pulse rate, respiratory rate, and blood pressure at each visit.
- Immediately report tachycardia or tachypnea to the physician.
- Administer oxygen as necessary.

2. Anemia increases the cardiac workload and can lead to cardiac failure. If oxygen administration is needed, the child may require hospitalization to monitor cardiac status.

3. Prevent or minimize emotional stress, as follows:
- Encourage the parents to participate in daily hygienic care.
- Support the parents and keep them informed of Kimberly's progress and of her need to conserve energy.
- Anticipate the child's irritability, fussiness, short attention span, and low frustration tolerance.
- Prepare the child for venipunctures and fingersticks by performing them quickly and then holding, cuddling, and comforting her afterward.
- Perform painful procedures at times other than immediately before scheduled rest periods and meals.

3. Children with anemia demonstrate central nervous system effects of tissue hypoxia, including headache, light-headedness, irritability, low frustration tolerance, short attention span, dizziness, fatigue, emotional lability, slowed thought processes, apathy, depression, and lethargy. Emotional stress can intensify these symptoms.

CHILD NURSING

4. Observe Kimberly for signs and symptoms of infection (especially of the upper or lower respiratory tract), such as runny nose, cough, sneezing, reluctance or inability to swallow, and tugging or rubbing the ear. Additionally, take these preventive measures:

• Teach the parents and household visitors proper hand washing.

• Teach the parents the signs and symptoms of infection; urge them to call the physician immediately if present.

• Immediately report an elevated white blood cell (WBC) count to the physician.

5. Provide the child with a balanced iron-rich diet, as follows:
• Give iron-fortified cereals at breakfast.
• Reduce milk intake to less than 16 oz (480 ml)/day (32 oz [960 ml] after anemia is resolved). Substitute water in a bottle at naptime.
• Begin offering the child liquids in a cup.
• Use finger foods and small amounts of food at meal times.
• Support the parents during mealtimes and as milk is withheld from Kimberly.
• Discuss proper nutrition with the parents, and teach them to provide a balanced, iron-rich diet for Kimberly. Advise them to expect mealtimes to be difficult because of the child's decreased appetite, irritability, and developing independence.

6. Administer ferrous sulfate orally in three divided doses between meals, using an oral syringe to place the medication behind the gums. Provide Kimberly with citrus fruit or juice, and brush her teeth afterward.

7. Monitor the amount, color, and consistency of Kimberly's stools. Advise the parents to expect greenish black stools and to notify the physician if constipation becomes a problem.

8. Inform the physician if Kimberly experiences vomiting or other gastric symptoms; expect the physician to increase the dose and to order administration with meals rather than between meals.

4. Children with anemia are prone to infection because of lowered resistance.

• General hygiene measures such as hand washing are important in preventing infection.

• Reporting signs and symptoms of infection facilitates prompt treatment.

• An elevated WBC count may indicate infection; reporting an elevated count ensures prompt treatment.

5. In many cases, the parents of milk-fed anemic infants believe the myth that milk is the perfect food, not realizing that it is actually low in iron. They may also believe that fat infants are healthy infants. Parent education may have to begin with dispelling these myths.

Providing water at naptime reduces milk intake and prevents nursing bottle caries; a cup helps wean the child from the bottle and from milk. Finger foods promote autonomy and normal development and decrease milk intake. Parents need support because they may feel responsible for their child's illness.

6. Ferrous sulfate, an iron supplement, is given between meals when free hydrochloric acid levels are greatest. Citrus fruit or juice helps reduce iron to its most soluble form. The nurse uses an oral syringe because liquid ferrous sulfate stains the teeth black and the client is too young to use a straw. Brushing the teeth afterward reduces staining.

7. Greenish black stools indicate that ferrous sulfate is being administered properly.

8. Administering ferrous sulfate with meals can reduce vomiting and other gastric symptoms. Increasing the dose ensures that the client is receiving an adequate amount when free hydrochloric acid levels are low.

9. Monitor Kimberly's reticulocyte count.

9. An increased reticulocyte count starting 3 to 4 days after beginning ferrous sulfate indicates that rapid RBC proliferation is correcting the anemia. (In some cases, iron therapy may continue for up to 1 year to replenish iron stores.)

10. If iron dextran (Imferon) is given I.M., inject it deep, using the Z-track method; document the injection time and site; alternate injection sites.

10. The Z-track method is recommended to minimize skin staining and irritation at the injection site.

Evaluation

• Kimberly does not develop cardiac decompensation.
• Kimberly's reticulocyte count indicates rapid RBC proliferation; RBC and hemoglobin levels are within normal range.
• Kimberly demonstrates physical and emotional development appropriate for an autonomous toddler.
• Kimberly's parents understand that they must provide her with a balanced, iron-rich diet.
• Kimberly is free from infection at discharge.

Hirschsprung's disease

In Hirschsprung's disease, also known as congenital aganglionic megacolon, a portion of the colon lacks ganglionic cells and the peristaltic waves needed to pass feces through that segment of the colon. The result is chronic constipation as stool accumulates proximal to the aganglionic segment, which is narrowed. However, the child may pass small ribbonlike stools through the narrow segment despite the internal sphincter's failure to relax.

Hirschsprung's disease is more common in boys than in girls and is usually diagnosed between ages 6 and 18 months. The child typically presents with a distended abdomen, poor appetite and fussy eating habits, and a history of inability to pass stool without an enema, a suppository, or manual removal. Treatment is generally surgical; the procedure varies with the extent of bowel segment affected. (For more information about bowel obstructions, see *Causes of lower bowel obstruction,* page 376.)

Clinical situation

Noah, age 14 months, is admitted to the hospital for surgery to resect a portion of his colon. A rectal biopsy earlier showed a lack of ganglionic cells extending into the midportion of the descending colon. On admission, Noah has a distended abdomen, which causes shortness of breath unless he is upright. His mother reports that he is irritable, has a poor appetite, and averages one bowel movement a week. Except for his enlarged abdomen he appears thin, and he has a fecal odor to his breath. Since his last admission, he has been on a low-residue diet. Noah's mother knows he may need a temporary colostomy.

CHILD NURSING

Causes of lower bowel obstruction

CONDITION	CHARACTERISTICS	MEDICAL DIAGNOSIS AND TREATMENT	NURSING CARE
Intussusception (telescoping of the intestine into an adjacent portion)	• Incidence: rare in 1st month after birth; most common between ages 3 and 12 months • Paroxysmal abdominal pain • Currant-jelly stools (mixture of blood and mucus) • Vomiting • Abdominal distention, tenderness, and a palpable mass • Dehydration and fever progressing to shock	• Air enema (may reduce intussusception; also used in diagnosis) • Surgery to remove hypoxic bowel section and reconnect remaining healthy bowel sections	• Restore and maintain fluid and electrolyte balance. • Prevent vomiting and aspiration. • Carefully assess progression of the client's stools (normal brown indicates resolved intussusception). • After surgery, maintain stomach decompression until the client passes the first stool.
Appendicitis (inflammation of the appendix; the most common cause of abdominal surgery in children)	• Abdominal pain, localized tenderness, and fever • Initially, generalized pain around the umbilicus, then localized pain in the right lower quadrant • Changes in behavior, anorexia, or vomiting (common early signs) • White blood cell (WBC) count of 15,000 to 20,000/mm³ • Constipation or diarrhea • Possible perforation (indicated by sudden pain relief) or peritonitis (indicated by increased pain, rigid abdomen, obvious guarding of the abdomen, high fever, and elevated WBC count) if untreated	• Surgical removal of the appendix • Management of peritonitis, shock, dehydration, and infection • Chest X-ray to differentiate appendicitis from pneumonia (pneumonia may cause referred pain in the right lower quadrant and thus may be misdiagnosed as appendicitis) • Barium G.I. series and ultrasonography to differentiate appendicitis from other abdominal problems	• Do not administer enemas or laxatives or apply heat to the abdomen. • When the appendix is not perforated, perform the same postoperative care as for any abdominal surgery. • When the appendix is perforated (and Penrose drains are in place), place the client in semi-Fowler's position or on the right side after surgery. • Change dressings frequently, and provide meticulous skin care at the operative site.
Imperforate anus (absent anal opening or opening obliterated by thin, translucent membrane)	• One of the most common congenital anomalies caused by abnormal development • Absence of anus noted when taking the first rectal temperature in the neonatal unit • Absence of meconium • Possible meconium in urine, indicating an associated rectourinary fistula	• Digital and endoscopic examination • Abdominal X-ray with opaque marker at the anal dimple and with the infant in the inverted position—the air will outline a blind rectal pouch • Surgery to reconstruct the anus and perform a colon pull-through or sigmoid colostomy with anastomosis and pull-through 1 year later	• After anorectal repair, place the infant in a side-lying or prone position, with the hips elevated to keep pressure off the sutures. • Feed the infant when peristalsis returns.

Assessment

NURSING BEHAVIORS	NURSING RATIONALES
1. Assess Noah's nutritional status and fluid balance.	**1.** Children with Hirschsprung's disease tend to be thin, undernourished, and anemic, even though their abdomens are distended. Some children may require I.V. hyperalimentation.

2. Assess bowel patterns for constipation. Obtain a complete history from the mother.

2. In true constipation, the rectum will contain stool; however, in Hirschsprung's disease, the rectum will be empty.

3. Assess and monitor Noah's abdominal distention.

3. Abdominal distention can impair the client's respirations.

Diagnostic evaluation
• Rectal examination reveals no stool in the rectum.
• Abdominal X-rays show the narrowed segment near the anus and colon dilation proximal to the narrowed segment.
• Rectal biopsy shows reduced or absent ganglionic cells.

Nursing diagnoses

Preoperative
• Constipation related to aganglionic bowel segment
• Risk for infection related to retained feces
• Altered nutrition: Less than body requirements, related to poor appetite

Postoperative
• Pain related to surgery
• Fluid volume deficit related to decreased oral intake and nasogastric (NG) tube drainage
• Knowledge deficit related to the parents' understanding of colostomy care

Planning and goals

Preoperative
• Noah will have adequate nutrition to provide for growth and weight gain.
• Noah's bowel will be emptied preoperatively and prepared for a colostomy.
• Noah's parents will understand the procedures involved in preoperative bowel preparation, the surgical procedure and desired outcome, and changes in body function.

Postoperative
• Noah will regain and maintain fluid and electrolyte balance.
• Noah will heal postoperatively without infection.
• Noah will have adequate nutrition to provide for growth and weight gain.
• Noah will participate in activities to develop autonomy.
• Noah's colostomy will function normally.
• Noah's parents will understand and participate in colostomy care.
• Noah and his parents will return home able to cope with Noah's altered body functions.

Implementation

NURSING BEHAVIORS

NURSING RATIONALES

Preoperative care

1. Prepare Noah's bowel for surgery by administering antibiotics and saline colonic enemas until the bowel is clear; seek his mother's help, if she agrees, because she has been administering the enemas at home.

1. The bowel is prepared for surgery with enemas and antibiotic installation through an NG tube. The enemas and antibiotics reduce bacterial flora. This preparation is not necessary in the neonate, whose bowel is sterile.

2. Insert an NG tube.

2. An NG tube helps prevent abdominal distention and maintain gastric decompression. Antibiotics may be instilled to prepare the GI tract further.

CHILD NURSING

3. Monitor output of feces, urine, and NG and rectal tube drainage (if such tubes are in place).

3. This continually assesses fluid loss and therefore fluid balance.

4. Monitor and record abdominal circumference at least every shift. Mark the abdomen with a pen to indicate where you took the measurement.

4. Abdominal distention crowds the diaphragm and interferes with respirations.

5. Weigh Noah at the same time each day, using the same scale.

5. Accurate weight measurements can help in monitoring the client's fluid balance and nutritional state.

6. Place Noah in an infant seat or prop him with pillows in semi-Fowler's position.

6. This position improves respirations.

7. Teach Noah's parents about the surgical procedure (temporary colostomy with or without pull-through anastomosis to anus) and about required preoperative care. Space the explanations to prevent anxiety and confusion from too much information. Show parents pictures of a colostomy and discuss surgery and postoperative care.

7. Anxiety may be reduced if the parents know what to expect. Parents often cannot visualize colostomy without pictures.

Postoperative care

1. Weigh Noah at the same time each day, using the same scale.

1. Accurate weight measurements can help in monitoring the client's fluid balance and nutritional state.

2. Monitor and record abdominal circumference at least every shift. Use a pen to mark where the measurement is taken.

2. Abdominal distention crowds the diaphragm and interferes with respirations.

3. Withhold food and fluids until bowel sounds return, the NG tube is removed, and the colostomy or anastomosed bowel can tolerate feedings; begin with small, frequent meals.

3. Bowel decompression will continue postoperatively until bowel sounds return.

4. Change stomal dressings with each bowel movement. Pin the diaper below the stoma. Use a urine collection bag as an ostomy appliance.

4. Changing dressings prevents contamination of the surgical site and promotes healing. Pinning the diaper below the stoma avoids contaminating the stoma with urine. A urine collection bag works well as an ostomy appliance in young children, who usually do *not* require irrigations.

5. Involve the parents early in dressing changes and irrigations, if ordered, to help them gradually accept their child's altered body functions.

5. The parents should begin participating in care soon after surgery because they will be caring for the stoma at home.

6. Evaluate Noah's pain level; include parents' assessment of child's behavior. Provide pain relief measures, such as medications, distraction, and relaxation techniques.

6. Bowel surgery is painful. Parents know their child's behavior and commonly can assess their child's pain level.

Evaluation

- Noah has a comfortable recovery.
- Noah returns home free from stomal infection.
- Noah has an average of at least one bowel movement each day and is free from abdominal distention.
- Noah begins to enjoy mealtimes and eats without discomfort.
- Noah is gaining weight and continues to develop autonomy.
- Noah's parents are performing stoma care and irrigations as instructed.

Acute acetaminophen poisoning

Because toddlers and preschoolers are mobile, active, and curious, they are particularly vulnerable to accidental ingestion. Among the drugs that children ingest most commonly, acetaminophen (Tylenol) ranks number one. Although aspirin poisoning has decreased, it still occurs in young children. Like acetaminophen, aspirin is readily available in most homes and taken freely by adults, whom children imitate. Also, children's aspirin and acetaminophen are brightly colored, with an appealing flavor. Other substances that children commonly ingest include soap, plants, cleaning agents, detergents, vitamins, and other drugs.

In acetaminophen poisoning, hepatic damage results from a metabolite of acetaminophen. Normally, the liver enzyme glutathione combines with and neutralizes the metabolite, which is then excreted in the urine. With ingestion of large acetaminophen doses, the metabolite overwhelms glutathione, causing hepatic necrosis. Acetaminophen poisoning is treated by administering acetylcysteine (Mucomyst), which substitutes for glutathione.

Clinical situation

Holly, age 20 months, is admitted to the pediatric unit from the emergency department with a diagnosis of acute acetaminophen poisoning. Apparently, she crawled from her crib during a nap, climbed onto a stool in the bathroom, and took a bottle of acetaminophen from the medicine cabinet. About 2 hours ago, her mother found her slightly diaphoretic, playing with the empty bottle of adult Tylenol. Her mother is not sure how many tablets Holly swallowed.

Assessment

NURSING BEHAVIORS	NURSING RATIONALES
1. Observe Holly for signs and symptoms of stage I acetaminophen poisoning. (See *Stages of acute acetaminophen poisoning*, page 380.)	**1.** Initial symptoms of acetaminophen poisoning are mild. Therefore, the diagnosis is confirmed by serum acetaminophen levels.
2. Assess and plot Holly's serum acetaminophen levels. Monitor hepatic and kidney function studies.	**2.** Serum levels are drawn 4 hours after ingestion and frequently thereafter for the first 24 hours. Liver and kidney function studies reveal the severity of acetaminophen toxicity.
3. Evaluate Holly for other illnesses.	**3.** The mild initial clinical findings may be confused with signs and symptoms of common childhood illnesses.

CHILD NURSING

Stages of acute acetaminophen poisoning

The stages of acute acetaminophen poisoning are outlined here. During the first stage, acute illness develops and is followed by a subclinical progression of hepatic damage resulting in later abnormal laboratory findings and the return of clinical findings. The last stage represents possible long-term outcomes from the poisoning.

STAGE	ONSET	SIGNS AND SYMPTOMS
I	1 to 24 hours after ingestion	• Anorexia • Nausea • Vomiting • Malaise • Pallor • Diaphoresis
II	24 to 48 hours after ingestion	• Latency period, with resolution of stage I signs and symptoms • Early manifestations of subclinical hepatic dysfunction, such as right upper quadrant pain and tenderness, oliguria, elevated serum bilirubin level, increased prothrombin time, and increased hepatic enzyme levels
III	72 to 96 hours after ingestion	• Peak liver function abnormalities • Possible reappearance of stage I signs and symptoms
IV	4 days to 2 weeks after ingestion	• Beginning of resolution of hepatic dysfunction (full hepatic recovery may take 3 months) • Possible complications: disseminated intravascular coagulation, renal failure, pancreatitis

4. Assess the parents' knowledge of acute poisoning in children as well as methods of childproofing the home.

4. Most cases of acute poisoning occur in children under age 4.

Nursing diagnoses
- Fluid volume excess related to hepatic toxicity
- Risk for fluid volume deficit related to vomiting
- Activity intolerance related to weakness and fatigue
- Knowledge deficit related to the parents' understanding of how to childproof the home

Planning and goals
- Holly will regain normal liver function.
- Holly will regain fluid and electrolyte balance.
- Holly will regain her normal energy level.
- Holly's parents will learn about emergency measures to take for a child with acute acetaminophen poisoning.
- Holly's parents will learn how to childproof their home.
- Holly's parents will not experience guilt.

Implementation

NURSING BEHAVIORS	NURSING RATIONALES
1. Take immediate measures to remove acetaminophen from Holly's stomach. For instance, perform gastric lavage or give ipecac syrup, as ordered. Administer activated charcoal, as ordered, to absorb any drug remaining in the stomach.	**1.** Because Holly's acetaminophen ingestion may have gone undiscovered for some time, a significant amount of acetaminophen may have been absorbed.
2. Administer acetylcysteine in soda, fruit, or juice or through a nasogastric (NG) tube, as ordered.	**2.** Children can receive 18 doses of acetylcysteine over 72 hours. Acetylcysteine smells like rotten eggs and many young children refuse to drink it, even when it is mixed with other liquids. Therefore, administering it by NG tube may be less traumatic.
3. Record all fluid intake and output. Monitor Holly's fluid balance.	**3.** Hepatic failure may lead to fluid retention and decreased urine output. Vomiting and anorexia also may decrease urine output, further complicating fluid balance assessment.
4. Monitor Holly's activity level and level of consciousness (LOC).	**4.** Hepatic coma, as indicated by reduced activity level and altered LOC, is the most severe stage of hepatic toxicity.
5. Teach Holly's parents about poison control measures, including keeping ipecac syrup in the home, placing the telephone number for the poison control center near the telephone, and viewing the home from a toddler's eye level to find hazards.	**5.** Poisoning is an emergency. Advance preparation can lead to earlier intervention, resulting in milder toxicity.
6. Instruct Holly's parents on poisonous agents and preventive measures, as follows:	**6.** Accidental poisonings are common among children in the client's age group (see *Common poisoning agents,* page 382).
• Tell them to store all medications, including aspirin, cold remedies, and other over-the-counter (OTC) drugs, out of the child's reach and sight. List several examples of OTC drugs because many people don't consider them to be medications.	• Parents tend to underestimate their child's curiosity and intrusive activities and overestimate the child's ability to understand and follow verbal instructions. Therefore, they need specific guidelines for preventing future accidents.
• Caution the parents not to store drugs in containers without safety caps if small children are part of the household.	• Many adults transfer drugs to containers without safety caps because they have difficulty in removing the caps.
• Have the parents teach their children not to take nonfood items without supervision.	• This helps prevent accidental ingestion of nonfood items.
• Instruct the parents to read the labels of cold remedies for ingredients, recommended dosages, and contraindications.	• Most cold and cough medicines contain aspirin or other salicylates and should not be given to children under age 6.
7. Support the parents and Holly during hospitalization, as follows:	**7.** Parents usually feel guilty about the accident and will need support and positive suggestions for preventing similar occurrences.

Common poisoning agents

SUBSTANCE INGESTED	ASSESSMENT	TREATMENT
Salicylates (such as aspirin)	• Determine if ingestion is acute or chronic. • Assess for signs and symptoms of salicylate poisoning, including deep respirations, decreased level of consciousness, dehydration, metabolic acidosis, blood loss, and tinnitis. • Assess the parent's knowledge of proper aspirin adminsitration. • Assess the child's serum salicylate levels.	• Remove aspirin from the child's stomach by giving ipecac syrup or administering gastric lavage, as ordered. • Adminster activated charcoal, as ordered, to absorb drug in the stomach. • Administer electrolyte solutions and sodium bicarbonate, as ordered, to correct metabolic acidosis. • Offer adequate calories and fluids to meet the child's increased metabolic demands.
Lead	• Identify high-risk groups by screening for pica (an abnormal desire to eat substances, such as lead paint or hair, not normally eaten) and an environment high in lead. (Universal blood screening is recommended for children ages 6 months to 6 years.) • Observe for signs and symptoms of encephalopathy: hyperactivity, aggression, impulsiveness, lethargy, irritability, clumsiness, learning difficulties, short attention span, convulsions, mental retardation, and coma. • Observe for signs and symptoms of anemia: fatigability, irritability, decreased hemoglobin level, and exercise intolerance. • Observe for signs of renal damage: excretion of glucose, protein, amino acids, and phosphate.	• Administer chelating agents, such as EDTA and dimercaprol, which cause lead to be removed from blood and soft tissues, deposited in bone, and excreted in urine. —EDTA and dimercaprol are given in a series of *deep* I.M. injections, in rotating sites; multiple injections may result in painful fibrotic tissues. —EDTA adverse effects include hypocalcemia (resulting in tetany and seizures) and nephrotoxicity (resulting in decreased urine output). • Eliminate lead from the environment; a few chips of paint the size of a thumbnail contain 100 mg of lead—200 times the safe daily dose. Other sources of lead are unglazed pottery, colored newsprint, and painted food wrappers.
Hydrocarbons (petroleum distillates, such as kerosene, gasoline, turpentine, lighter fluid, furniture polish, metal polish, cleaning fluid, and insecticides)	• Recognize early signs and symptoms of toxicity: gagging, choking, coughing, nausea, vomiting, lethargy, drowsiness, weakness, and respiratory symptoms (from inhalation of vapors), including cyanosis, retractions, and grunting.	• Maintain a patent airway. • Give nothing by mouth. • Call the poison control center. • Take the child to the emergency department for immediate treatment. • Do not give emetics.
Corrosives (oven and drain cleaners, dishwasher detergents, and other strong detergents and cleaning agents)	• Observe for signs and symptoms of toxicity: severe, burning pain of the mouth, lips, tongue, throat, and stomach; white, swollen oral mucous membranes; swollen tongue and pharynx; violent vomiting with blood; shock; anxiety; and agitation.	• Maintain a patent airway. • Administer steroids as ordered. • Give nothing by mouth except as ordered. • Give analgesics as needed. • Do not give emetics; vomiting will redamage tissue.

• Encourage the parents to visit frequently and, if possible, arrange for them to sleep in the child's room.

• Allow the parents to express their feelings about circumstances surrounding the poisoning. Avoid placing blame on either parent.

• This helps lessen the child's separation anxiety, which is at its peak at this stage.

• The parents may feel guilty about the poisoning, blaming themselves for their child's illness. A candid discussion enables the nurse to help them resolve these feelings and refocus their attention on promoting the child's recovery and future health.

| • Explain all procedures and treatments to the parents. | • The parents' anxiety usually lessens when they know what to expect. |

Evaluation

- Holly regains fluid and electrolyte balance and normal liver function, and returns home free from complications.
- Holly's parents do not feel guilty about the poisoning.
- Holly's parents have made their home childproof.

Congenital heart disease

Congenital heart disease occurs in approximately 8 to 10 of every 1,000 live births and is the major cause of death in the 1st year (besides prematurity). Congenital heart defects are of two types (based on alteration in blood flow): *acyanotic,* in which deoxygenated blood is not mixed in the systemic circulation (the child is not blue), and *cyanotic,* in which deoxygenated blood is mixed in the systemic circulation (the child usually is blue or dusky). They may be further categorized by normal, decreased, or increased pulmonary blood flows.

Signs and symptoms of acyanotic defects vary, depending on the size and location of the defect and whether pulmonary vascularity is increased, among other factors. Most acyanotic defects can be corrected surgically or by cardiac catheterization. Signs and symptoms of cyanotic defects result from blood flowing from the right side of the heart to the left. This leads to hypoxemia, polycythemia, and sluggish circulation, symptoms that can be reduced in severity by palliative surgery. (For more information, see *Signs and symptoms of congenital heart defects,* page 384 and *Common congenital heart defects,* pages 385 and 386.)

Clinical situation

Joey, age 2 ½, is admitted to the hospital for cardiac catheterization. He was diagnosed in infancy as having tetralogy of Fallot, the most common cyanotic heart defect, and underwent his first catheterization at that time (see *Normal heart and tetralogy of Fallot,* page 387). This procedure is performed to determine pressure readings and the degree of oxygen saturation in the chambers and major vessels and to release a radiopaque contrast medium that allows fluoroscopic visualization of the heart.

Joey is currently being reevaluated and will have corrective surgery as soon as it can be scheduled. He is small for his age and appears dusky, with cyanotic lips and nail beds, although he is not in acute distress.

Assessment

NURSING BEHAVIORS	**NURSING RATIONALES**
Precatheterization	
1. Assess Joey's pulse rate, respiratory rate, and temperature. Obtain accurate height and weight. Ask the parents if Joey has allergies to dye.	**1.** The staff will need baseline measurements of the client's vital signs to identify arrhythmias and complications after catheterization. Height determines selection of catheter size.
2. Assess the parents' understanding of cardiac catheterization, and answer any questions they have about the procedure.	**2.** Although the physician will explain the procedure after obtaining an informed consent, reinforcement from the nurse can help alleviate the parents' fear and anxiety.

Signs and symptoms of congenital heart defects

The following signs and symptoms are the most common indicators of congenital heart disease in infants and children.

INFANTS	CHILDREN
Dyspnea	Dyspnea
Difficulty feeding	Poor physical development
Stridor and choking spells	Decreased exercise tolerance
Pulse rate over 200 beats/minute	Recurrent respiratory infections
Recurrent respiratory infections	Heart murmur and thrill
Failure to gain weight	Cyanosis
Heart murmurs	Squatting
Cyanosis	Clubbing of fingers and toes
Cerebrovascular accident	Elevated blood pressure
Anoxic attacks	

3. Assess Joey's developmental level (see "Growth and development," pages 52 to 61).

3. Assessing the client's developmental level helps the nurse choose the best approach for explaining the procedure to a toddler and may reveal developmental delays caused by decreased circulation.

Postcatheterization
1. Assess Joey's physiologic status, including vital signs, until stable. Check the operative site for bleeding and swelling. Compare general circulation with that in the affected extremity.

1. Possible complications of cardiac catheterization include arrhythmias, cardiac perforation (most common in infants), hemorrhage, arterial obstruction, reaction to contrast medium, infection, phlebitis, and hypoxia.

2. Assess Joey's hydration status (weight; amount, color, and frequency of urine; and skin turgor, color, and temperature).

2. Because the client has not received food or fluids since 4 to 6 hours before catheterization, dehydration may be a problem.

Nursing diagnoses
- Altered tissue perfusion (cardiopulmonary) related to polycythemia, increased blood viscosity, and stasis
- Activity intolerance related to oxygen supply and demand
- Anxiety related to illness, cardiac catheterization, and hospitalization
- Pain related to myocardial hypoxia and cardiac catheterization
- Altered growth and development related to inadequate oxygenated blood to meet metabolic needs
- Risk for injury related to operative procedure, blood loss during catheterization, and reaction to contrast medium

Planning and goals

Precatheterization
- Joey will undergo cardiac catheterization with minimal fear and anxiety.
- Joey will be physically prepared for cardiac catheterization.
- Joey's parents will understand the procedure.

Postcatheterization
- Joey will not develop infection in the cutdown (insertion) site or any other complications of cardiac catheterization.

Common congenital heart defects

MAJOR ACYANOTIC DEFECTS

An **atrial septal defect** is an abnormal opening between the right and left atria. Basically, three types of abnormalities result from incorrect development of the atrial septum. An incompetent foramen ovale is the most common defect. The high ostium secundum defect results from abnormal development of the septum secundum. Improper development of the septum primum produces a basal opening known as an ostium primum defect, commonly involving the atrioventricular valves. Generally, left-to-right shunting of blood occurs in all atrial septal defects.

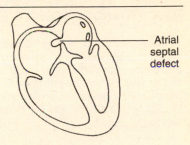

Atrial septal defect

Coarctation of the aorta is a narrowing of the aortic lumen that results in a preductal or postductal obstruction, depending on its position in relation to the ductus arteriosus. Coarctations occur with great variation in anatomic features. The lesion obstructs the blood flow through the aorta, thus increasing left ventricular pressure and cardiac workload.

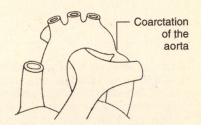

Coarctation of the aorta

The **patent ductus arteriosus** is a vascular connection that, during fetal life, short-circuits the pulmonary vascular bed and directs blood from the pulmonary artery to the aorta. Functional closure of the ductus normally occurs soon after birth. If the ductus remains patent after birth, the direction of blood flow in the ductus is reversed by the higher pressure in the aorta.

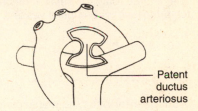

Patent ductus arteriosus

A **ventricular septal defect** is an abnormal opening between the right and left ventricle. Ventricular septal defects vary in size and may occur in either the membranous or the muscular portion of the ventricular septum. Because of higher pressure in the left ventricle, blood shunts from the left to the right ventricle during systole. If pulmonary vascular resistance produces pulmonary hypertension, blood shunting is then reversed (from the right to the left ventricle), resulting in cyanosis.

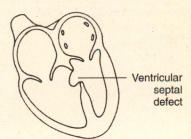

Ventricular septal defect

MAJOR CYANOTIC DEFECTS

A **complete transposition of great vessels** is an embryologic defect caused by a straight division of the bulbar trunk without normal spiraling. As a result, the aorta originates from the right ventricle; the pulmonary artery, from the left ventricle. An abnormal communication between the two circulations must be present to sustain life.

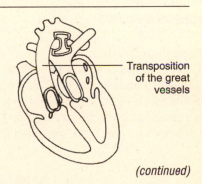

Transposition of the great vessels

(continued)

Common congenital heart defects (continued)

MAJOR CYANOTIC DEFECTS (continued)

Tetralogy of Fallot is a combination of four defects: pulmonic stenosis, ventricular septal defect, overriding aorta, and hypertrophy of the right ventricle. It is the most common cyanotic defect in clients who survive beyond age 2. The severity of symptoms depends on the degree of pulmonary stenosis, the size of the ventricular septal defect, and the degree to which the aorta overrides the septal defect.

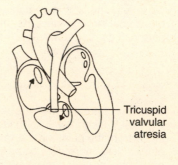

Pulmonic stenosis

Overriding aorta

Ventricular septal defect

Right ventricular hypertrophy

Tricuspid valvular atresia is characterized by a small right ventricle, a large left ventricle, and, usually, diminished pulmonary circulation. Blood from the right atrium passes through an atrial septal defect into the left atrium, mixes with oxygenated blood returning from the lungs, flows into the left ventricle, and is propelled into the systemic circulation. The lungs may receive blood through one of three routes: a small ventricular septal defect, patent ductus arteriosus, or bronchial vessels.

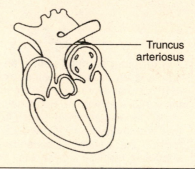

Tricuspid valvular atresia

Truncus arteriosus, normal septation of the embryologic bulbar trunk into an aorta and pulmonary artery does not occur. This single arterial trunk overrides the ventricles and receives blood from them through a ventricular septal defect. The entire pulmonary and systemic circulation is supplied from this common arterial trunk.

Truncus arteriosus

Implementation

NURSING BEHAVIORS

Precatheterization
1. Prepare Joey physically for catheterization after obtaining parental consent (see "Preoperative period," in Perioperative Nursing, pages 123 and 124):
• Arrange for an electrocardiogram, if ordered.
• Arrange for chest X-rays and other tests, as ordered.

NURSING RATIONALES

1. Most of these actions are performed to determine the child's precatheterization status; comparing baseline values to postcatheterization values helps detect complications. Withholding food and fluids minimizes postcatheterization vomiting. A sedative helps calm the client before surgery. The procedure will be canceled if infection is present. For femoral access, skin in the diaper area must be intact. Marking pedal pulses will help locate them after catheterization.

Normal heart and tetralogy of Fallot

NORMAL HEART

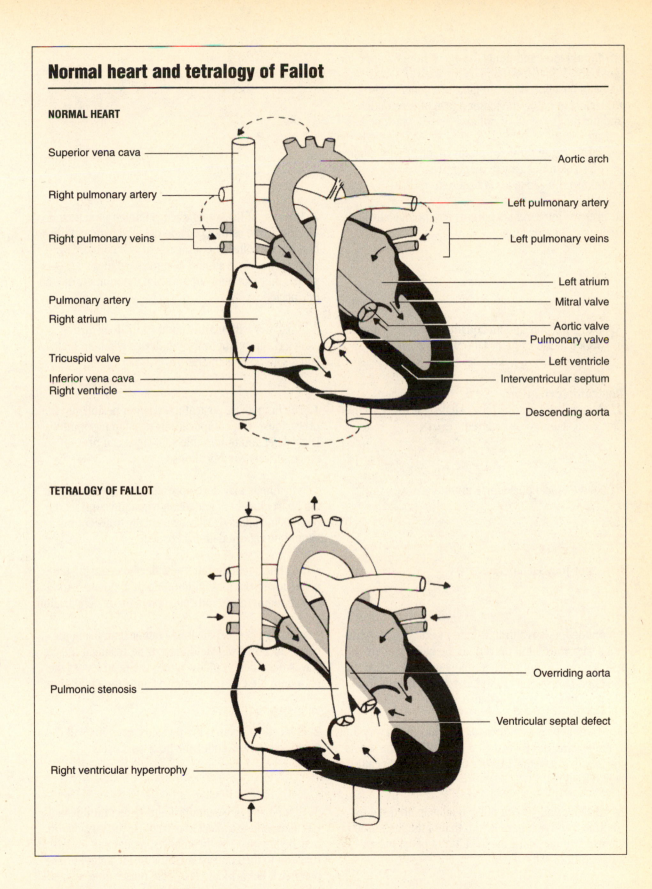

Superior vena cava

Right pulmonary artery

Right pulmonary veins

Pulmonary artery

Right atrium

Tricuspid valve

Inferior vena cava

Right ventricle

Aortic arch

Left pulmonary artery

Left pulmonary veins

Left atrium

Mitral valve

Aortic valve

Pulmonary valve

Left ventricle

Interventricular septum

Descending aorta

TETRALOGY OF FALLOT

Pulmonic stenosis

Right ventricular hypertrophy

Overriding aorta

Ventricular septal defect

• Withhold food and fluids for 4 to 6 hours before surgery.
• Obtain baseline vital sign measurements.
• Check skin color, the temperature of extremities, and the quality of all peripheral pulses. Mark pedal pulses.
• Assess for signs and symptoms of infection including impaired skin integrity in diaper area.
• Administer a sedative, as ordered.

2. Prepare Joey and his parents psychologically for cardiac catheterization.

2. Because of the young client's limited understanding, the nurse cannot provide detailed explanations to him but can offer encouragement and comforting words. The nurse should also prepare Joey's parents so that they can help support him emotionally during this period.

3. Send a pacifier and an aquathermia pad or warming device to the catheter laboratory.

3. A pacifier will provide comfort for Joey during catheterization. The warming device will help maintain a safe body temperature.

Postcatheterization
1. Measure and record Joey's vital signs every 15 minutes until stable or as ordered:

1. The immediate postcatheterization period can be precarious, with complications developing rapidly. Early detection of unstable vital signs can prevent more serious complications.

• Take the apical pulse for 1 minute.

• Arrhythmias may develop when the catheter enters the heart chambers and again when the contrast medium is introduced. They are usually transient but should be reported and recorded.

• Monitor Joey's temperature.

• The child's temperature may decrease during the procedure from air conditioning or exposure. An elevated temperature indicates infection or dehydration.

• Monitor Joey's respiratory rate by counting respirations with your hand in front of the child's mouth to feel airflow. Do not place a pillow under his head until the child is responsive and has fully recovered from the precatheterization sedative.

• Counting chest expansions (rather than using the child's airflow) will yield inaccurate results if the airway is occluded. A pillow under the head forces the chin onto the chest; this may occlude the child's airway.

2. Examine pressure dressings for bleeding every time you measure and record vital signs. Check the sheets for blood and wetness under the limb used in catheterization.

2. If bleeding occurs, the pressure dressing will cause the blood to flow under the body part used.

3. Measure and record pulse quality in all distal extremities, and compare it with that of the limb used in catheterization. Mark the location of pedal pulses with a ballpoint or felt-tip pen.

3. Comparing pulse quality helps detect diminished circulation in the affected extremity. The circulation may be impaired by thrombosis, hematoma, or vessel reaction to the contrast medium or the catheter. The pen mark helps locate the pedal pulses after surgery, when the pulses may be weaker and more difficult to detect.

CHILD NURSING

4. Assess Joey's overall skin color as well as the color and temperature of extremities.

4. This also helps detect diminished circulation in the affected extremity, which may indicate arterial obstruction.

5. Provide Joey with small sips of water, gradually increasing the amount as tolerated.

5. Large sips or gulping may produce vomiting, especially when femoral vessels are used as the cutdown site. Vomiting increases intra-abdominal and intrathoracic pressure, which in turn creates pressure on the cutdown site, possibly leading to severe bleeding.

6. Keep Joey in bed for 3 to 4 hours after catheterization. Immobilize the affected leg or arm, keeping it as straight as possible. Provide a calm, quiet environment.

6. Immobility reduces the likelihood of bleeding at the catheterization site. A calm, quiet environment prevents undue excitement and promotes rest and recovery. The parents may hold the child, keeping the affected limb in the correct position.

7. Keep Joey comfortably warm; avoid overheating or chilling him.

7. Overheating causes peripheral vasodilation, and chilling may cause vasoconstriction. Either of these conditions can precipitate bleeding at the catheterization site.

8. Prepare the parents and child for discharge. Teach them to keep the cutdown site clean and dry and to cover it with a bandage.

8. The parents will need instructions for home care while their child awaits corrective surgery. The listed measures help prevent infection at the cutdown site.

Evaluation

- Joey undergoes cardiac catheterization without complications or major psychological trauma.
- Joey's cutdown site remains free from infection.
- Joey returns for corrective surgery of tetralogy of Fallot when scheduled.

Clinical situation
(continued)

Joey returns to the hospital in 3 weeks for corrective surgery of tetralogy of Fallot. He is admitted the day before surgery.

Some children with tetralogy of Fallot require palliative surgery to increase arterial oxygen and saturation and to alleviate symptoms of chronic hypoxia. Older infants and children may undergo the Blalock-Taussig procedure, an anastomosis of the subclavian artery to the pulmonary artery.

The four defects of tetralogy of Fallot are ventricular septal defect, pulmonic stenosis, overriding aorta, and right ventricular hypertrophy. Corrective surgery involves closure of the ventricular septal defect, resection of infundibular stenosis, and pericardial patch to increase the right ventricular outflow tract. The ventricular hypertrophy will diminish over time in response to surgical correction of anatomic defects.

CHILD NURSING

Assessment

NURSING BEHAVIORS	NURSING RATIONALES

Preoperative care

1. Assess for symptoms of cyanotic heart disease, such as small stature, moderate to severe exercise intolerance, and the following:

1. Small stature stems from difficulty eating and breathing at the same time. Chronic hypoxia also causes easy fatigue and diminished growth. Hypoxia, dyspnea, and exercise intolerance may be insidious and not apparent until the toddler stage. The healthy toddler is quite active, whereas the child with a cyanotic heart defect may prefer to sit and watch.

• chest pain that becomes severe with increased exercise

• Chest pain occurs because the heart muscle does not receive enough oxygen.

• tetrad spell (or hypoxic episode) with exercise— shortness of breath, increased cyanosis, chest pain, and squatting

• The tetrad spell is characteristic of the child with a cyanotic heart defect. Squatting in the older child (the knee-chest position in infancy) is an automatic response to tissue hypoxia. It decreases venous return by partially occluding the femoral veins, thus lessening the workload of the right side of the heart and increasing arterial saturation.

• clubbing of the fingers and cyanosis

• Clubbing of the fingers, a characteristic of cyanotic heart defects and chronic tissue hypoxia, is believed to result from soft-tissue fibrosis and hypertrophy from anoxia. An increase in the capillary bed occurs to increase blood supply to the fingertips.

• a history of frequent and severe respiratory infections

• Pulmonary vascular congestion and blood pooling make the lungs susceptible to bacterial and viral infections.

• a history of choking, coughing, cyanosis, and fatigue with feeding as an infant.

• The infant is too fatigued from hypoxia, tachycardia, and dyspnea to consume all of the formula or to close the mouth around the nipple.

2. Monitor and record Joey's vital signs: apical pulse for 1 minute (for evidence of tachycardia), respiratory rate (for evidence of dyspnea and tachypnea), blood pressure, and temperature.

2. The body attempts to compensate for decreased arterial oxygen saturation by increasing the heart rate (resulting in tachycardia) and the force of the contraction (resulting in cardiomegaly). In tetralogy of Fallot, the right ventricle enlarges as it pumps blood against the increased resistance caused by pulmonic stenosis. With the large ventricular septal defect and overriding aorta, the right ventricle is also pumping blood systemically with the left ventricle.

Children with tetralogy of Fallot do not go into congestive heart failure (CHF) before surgery, because pulmonic stenosis prevents pulmonary hypertension and the right ventricle enlarges to compensate. The heart appears boot-shaped on X-ray because of the enlarged right ventricle.

3. Assess for signs and symptoms of cerebrovascular accident (CVA), a major complication of cyanotic heart anomalies: loss of consciousness, confusion, paralysis, drooling, convulsions, inability to swallow, and other symptoms associated with adult CVA.

3. Chronic hypoxia causes the kidneys to release erythropoietin, which stimulates bone marrow to produce more red blood cells that can carry more oxygen. The result is polycythemia, with a hemoglobin level as high as 20 to 30 g/dl and a hematocrit of 60% to 80%—almost double the normal values. Polycythemia results in increased blood viscosity and blood stasis without the added benefit of increased arterial blood oxygenation because venous and arterial blood are still being mixed systemically. The increased viscosity and stasis cause CVA. It may also give the child pink skin tones, masking the cyanosis.

4. Assess Joey's hydration status.

4. Adequate hydration is critical because dehydration increases hemoconcentration and blood viscosity.

5. Assess Joey's developmental level (see "Growth and development," pages 52 to 61).

5. This assessment helps the nurse determine the best approach for preoperative preparation.

Postoperative care
This includes all of the preoperative assessment behaviors as well as the following:
1. Assess for CHF (see "Congestive heart failure," page 442).

1. After corrective surgery, the child with tetralogy of Fallot almost always experiences CHF because the enlarged right ventricle continues to contract with the same force postoperatively as it did preoperatively. With the ventricular septal defect closed and the pulmonic stenosis corrected, the blood leaves the right ventricle under great pressure, causing pulmonary hypertension and increased pulmonary blood volume.

2. Assess chest tubes for correct function.

2. Correct chest tube function ensures lung expansion.

3. Assess the operative site for infection.

3. Early treatment of infection at the operative site can prevent more serious complications.

Nursing diagnoses See the nursing diagnoses for cardiac catheterization, page 384.

Planning and goals **Preoperative**
• Joey will be physically and psychologically prepared for surgery.
• Joey's cardiac workload will decrease.
• Joey's fluid and electrolyte balance will be maintained.
• Joey will not develop a respiratory infection.
• Joey's nutrition needs will be maintained to meet growth needs.

Postoperative
These include preoperative planning and goals as well as the following:
• Joey's airway will remain patent.
• Joey's operative site will remain free from infection and eventually heal.
• Joey's chest tubes will remain intact and provide for lung reexpansion.
• Joey will exhibit normal developmental behaviors for a toddler.
• Joey's parents will understand his need to become increasingly independent.
• Joey's parents will know how to contact available community resources.

Implementation

NURSING BEHAVIORS	NURSING RATIONALES
1. Prepare Joey for surgery by performing routine preoperative care (see "Preoperative period" in Perioperative Nursing, pages 123 and 124).	**1.** This ensures that the child is in optimum condition for surgery: free from infection, with fluid and electrolyte balance, adequate kidney function, and sound nutritional status.
2. Assist with Joey's feeding and hygiene. Schedule plenty of rest periods for the child, and provide quiet play activities in bed, with the child in semi- or high-Fowler's position. Help Joey assume a knee-chest or squatting position during a tetrad spell.	**2.** These nursing actions reduce the child's physical activity and thus help lessen cardiac workload.
3. Maintain fluid and electrolyte balance.	**3.** This prevents complications of dehydration and increased blood viscosity.
4. Prevent respiratory infection.	**4.** The child with a cyanotic heart defect is prone to respiratory infections because of increased pulmonary vascularity.
5. Maintain nutrition for growth needs.	**5.** Even though the child with a cyanotic heart defect may tire during feeding, he needs adequate nutrition in this rapid growth period.
6. Provide chest tube care.	**6.** This ensures proper function, prevents infection and kinking, and maintains patency.
7. Reduce the stress of hospitalization for the toddler, as follows: • Encourage Joey to express feelings of protest. • Arrange for his parents to stay in his room if possible. • Have the parents bring a security toy or object from home. • Accept Joey's regressive behaviors, and explain them to reassure the parents. • Follow home schedules for bedtime, bath time, and meals as closely as possible. • Encourage the parents to participate in daily care when possible. • Relieve Joey's pain with medication and comfort measures.	**7.** Separation is the major cause of stress for the hospitalized toddler. Hospitalization also curtails developing autonomy by altering rituals and routines and limiting mobility and exploration. Pain and bodily injury force the toddler to be dependent. The toddler reacts to these threats with protest, physical resistance, increased aggression and negativism, and regression to an earlier stage. The nurse should strive to remove or reduce barriers to development by accepting regressive behavior (without promoting it) and by helping parents cope with the increased aggression, protest, and regression. The parents' participation in daily care reduces separation anxiety and reacquaints the child with familiar routines. Pain may be a new experience for the child, and he may be unable to verbalize it; thus, when the child seems restless or uncomfortable, the nurse should provide pain medication and comfort measures.
8. Prepare Joey and his parents for discharge, as follows:	**8.** The postoperative recovery period is 1 to 5 days for most pediatric heart surgery clients, but commonly longer for children with tetralogy of Fallot, who invariably develop CHF postoperatively.

• Tell the parents to let Joey increase physical activity gradually, as tolerated; remind them that it may take him 6 months to 1 year to achieve a normal activity level.

• Advise the parents that Joey should receive prophylactic penicillin before dental procedures, including teeth cleaning.

• The parents may be hesitant about allowing the child to return to his usual physical activities. In tetralogy of Fallot, return to normal activity is delayed because of CHF.

• Children with congenital heart anomalies are susceptible to endocarditis.

Evaluation

• Joey returns home free from symptoms of tetralogy of Fallot and CHF.
• Joey regains a toddler's normal developmental level.
• Joey remains free from respiratory infections and endocarditis.
• Joey's blood viscosity returns to a normal range.
• Joey develops no complications from heart and chest surgery.
• Joey's parents allow him to become increasingly independent.
• Joey's parents apply for financial aid from their state's disabled children's agency.

Nephrotic syndrome

Nephrotic syndrome (also known as idiopathic nephrotic syndrome or minimal-change nephrotic syndrome) develops when large amounts of plasma protein are lost in urine because of increased glomerular permeability. The syndrome usually occurs most often in preschool-age children. About 80% of those affected display no other signs of systemic or renal disease; about 60% are boys. The cause of nephrotic syndrome is unknown, and the pathogenesis is not clearly understood. The increased glomerular permeability to plasma protein results in massive proteinuria, hypoproteinemia, hypovolemia, edema, and hyperlipidemia. Treatment is usually symptomatic and supportive.

Clinical situation

Ned, age 3, is admitted to the hospital with obvious edema, labored breathing, skin pallor, and lethargy. His urine specimen on admission was dark-colored and frothy, with a specific gravity of 1.040 and 4+ proteinuria. The medical diagnosis is nephrotic syndrome. Physician's orders include complete bed rest, regular diet, and prednisone.

Assessment

NURSING BEHAVIORS

1. Assess for edema from head to toe, and obtain a thorough history regarding onset of symptoms.

2. Assess urine for volume, color, specific gravity, protein, and red blood cells (RBCs).

NURSING RATIONALES

1. The generalized edema of nephrosis tends to develop slowly, starting with facial puffiness (especially around the eyes) and progressing over a period of weeks to abdominal swelling, respiratory difficulty, and labial or scrotal swelling.

2. Volume is usually diminished, color dark, specific gravity greatly increased, protein level high, and RBC level low.

CHILD NURSING

3. Evaluate Ned's respiratory rate and rhythm, check breath sounds, and assess for orthopnea.

3. The fluid shift—from the intravascular to the interstitial compartment—results from altered colloidal osmotic pressure caused by loss of plasma protein in urine. Ascites also develops, resulting in upward pressure on the diaphragm, which interferes with pulmonary expansion. The fluid shift can also result in pleural effusion, which interferes with lung expansion.

4. Note Ned's behavior, activity level, and appetite.

4. Lethargy, irritability, decreased activity tolerance, and fatigability are characteristic of children with nephrosis, and anorexia is common. Markedly elevated blood pressure and blood urea nitrogen levels, although rare, can cause altered sensorium.

5. Assess Ned's developmental level (see "Growth and development," pages 52 to 61).

5. This assessment helps determine whether the child meets age-related norms. Some regression in response to illness and hospitalization can be expected.

Nursing diagnoses
- Risk for infection related to altered immune response and steroid therapy
- Altered urinary elimination related to impaired renal function
- Ineffective breathing pattern related to pulmonary edema, ascites, and decreased lung expansion
- Impaired skin integrity related to edematous skin surfaces rubbing together
- Fluid volume excess related to hypoproteinemia

Planning and goals
- Ned will remain free from secondary infection.
- Ned will have increased urine output, decreased proteinuria, decreased body weight, decreased edema, decreased respiratory effort, and increased appetite within 10 days.
- Ned will maintain or regain age-appropriate development.

Implementation

NURSING BEHAVIORS

NURSING RATIONALES

1. Document Ned's vital signs (including blood pressure) every 4 hours.

1. Increased blood pressure may indicate renal failure. Increased temperature and pulse rate could be related to a secondary infection.

2. Prevent visitors and staff members with respiratory symptoms or other infections from coming in close contact with Ned.

2. Children with nephrotic syndrome are susceptible to secondary infection because the plasma proteins lost in the urine are immunoglobulins.

3. Maintain Ned on complete bed rest in an upright position until edema subsides.

3. Bed rest decreases tissue oxygen demands. An upright position decreases upward pressure of the ascitic abdomen on the diaphragm.

4. Turn Ned every 2 hours, and provide support (sheepskin pad, special skin care) to extremely edematous areas such as the scrotum.

4. The skin is the first line of defense in preventing infection. Taut, edematous skin will break down quickly. Skin surfaces should be cleaned and separated with clothing, powder, or padding.

CHILD NURSING

5. Keep strict intake and output records. Document voiding times and the volume, color, and specific gravity of urine. Test urine with a dipstick after each voiding, and document the presence or absence of proteins and RBCs.

5. Corticosteroids are the primary treatment for nephrosis. Within 7 to 21 days of starting treatment, urine excretion should increase and proteinuria should disappear. Careful monitoring helps evaluate the client's response to therapy.

6. Assess and document edema status at least every shift: Accurately measure body weight and abdominal girth, and assess the periorbital area, abdomen, sacrum, pretibial area, and extremities.

6. Physical measurements identify the degree of fluid accumulation or fluid shift.

7. Offer Ned small amounts of a no-salt-added diet at frequent intervals.

7. Severe salt and fluid restrictions are usually unnecessary unless the child shows signs of renal failure. Although increased protein may be desirable, children with nephrotic syndrome are anorexic and do not usually accept a high-protein diet.

8. As Ned's energy level permits, offer age-appropriate toys, such as large blocks, crayons and coloring books, illustrated books, music boxes, and large puzzles.

8. This enhances normal growth and development and prevents boredom.

9. Before discharge, prepare the parents for providing home care, as follows:

9. The child will require careful monitoring for a long time; this syndrome is marked by remissions and exacerbations.

• Tell the parents to report weight gain, headaches, nausea, fever, and other signs of infection.

• These signs may signal a relapse.

• Teach them how to test urine for protein. (Parents should participate in urine testing in the hospital and continue testing at least twice weekly at home.)

• Protein in urine is an early indicator of exacerbation; the child should receive medical attention before extensive edema occurs.

• Inform them of prednisone's adverse reactions, including cushingoid response and masking of usual infection signs. Warn them not to stop therapy suddenly.

• Steroid therapy may continue for weeks or months, so parents should be aware of possible adverse reactions. If the drug is stopped suddenly, the child will develop signs of shock and vascular collapse, requiring emergency care.

• Tell them what kind of behaviors to expect from Ned in response to illness and hospitalization.

• Regressive behaviors, especially increased dependence and clinging behaviors, may persist for several weeks.

Evaluation

• Ned remains free from secondary infection.
• Ned responds positively to steroid therapy.
• Ned shows more interest in his surroundings and participates willingly in age-appropriate activities before discharge.

CHILD NURSING

THE PRESCHOOLER (AGES 3 TO 6)

Asthma

The leading cause of acute and chronic illness in children, asthma is a reversible respiratory disorder of bronchial obstruction and irritation after exposure to stimuli. Attacks may be triggered by many different stimuli, including allergens, environmental pollutants, exercise, weather change, infections, medications, and emotions.

Most asthmatics have extrinsic (immunoglobulin E [IgE]–mediated) disease, although exercise- or infection-induced (non-IgE-mediated) disease is not uncommon. The patient experiences shortness of breath, wheezing, or chest tightness as the airway becomes narrow, edematous, and inflamed. Mucous membranes hypersecrete, and the smooth muscle of the bronchi and bronchioles contract and spasm. Most asthmatics experience their first attack before age 4.

Asthma should be considered in any child with a history of a recurrent dry, hacking, nonproductive cough who also has a viral illness or has been exposed to animals, environmental pollutants (including cigarette smoking), exercise, or cold. Children with atopic dermatitis have a particularly high incidence of asthma. Establishing the diagnosis is important to ensure that the child is not mistreated with over-the-counter cold medications.

Clinical situation

Molly Harlow, age 4, arrives at the clinic with her parents. She is in obvious respiratory distress. This is her fourth respiratory infection in the past 6 months. She is afebrile and has a respiratory rate of 38 breaths/minute with audible wheezing on expiration. She has a productive cough of clear, thick mucus; her parents give a history of coughing at night even when no infection is present. She is acyanotic, but is pale and restless. The physician orders humidified oxygen by face mask at 4 L/minute and albuterol 0.5% by nebulized aerosol every 30 minutes. Asthma is the diagnosis. The physician also orders blood gas studies, a chest X-ray, and sputum eosinophil count.

Molly's blood gas results show a decreased partial pressure of arterial oxygen (PaO_2) before oxygen administration and an elevated partial pressure of arterial carbon dioxide ($PaCO_2$). Her chest X-ray is consistent with asthma, and her sputum is positive for eosinophilia. When her current attack subsides, she is to begin cromolyn sodium by inhaler, be scheduled for pulmonary function studies, and have skin testing for allergens.

Assessment

NURSING BEHAVIORS

1. Assess Molly's respiratory status, including rate and depth of respirations, use of accessory muscles, and presence and timing of wheezing or other adventitious breath sounds. Assess frequency and nature of cough and any sputum produced.

NURSING RATIONALES

1. Forced respiratory expiration through a narrowed airway results in air being trapped, leading to hyperinflation of the alveoli. Consequently, the person breathes deeply in an attempt to inspire adequate air. Wheezing is heard as air is forced through the narrowed bronchioles and bronchi. As the condition worsens, wheezing becomes both inspiratory and expiratory. Cessation of all wheezing can be a sign of impending respiratory failure.

CHILD NURSING

2. Assess Molly's general appearance and behavior.

2. As breathing becomes more compromised, the child may appear pale with a malar flush and red ears. The child may want to sit upright or in a tripod position. Often the child is tired but may be restless and anxious.

3. Evaluate results of laboratory tests, and report abnormal findings.

3. Asthma results in respiratory acidosis, with an increase in pH and $PaCO_2$ and a decrease in PaO_2. Sputum cultures and the complete blood count differential will show the presence of eosinophil. Chest X-rays may demonstrate hyperinflation, pulmonary infiltrates, and atelectasis.

4. Assess Molly's exposure to possible "attack triggers," including activities she was doing at the onset of the attack.

4. Exposure to animals, wood, or cigarette smoke, new foods, medications, activities, or a change of weather may precipitate an attack.

5. Assess the parents' knowledge of asthma: its causes, diagnostic workup, and management.

5. Parents need to understand the importance of prompt treatments and of establishing a definitive diagnosis, as the diagnostic tests can be expensive and time-consuming.

Nursing diagnoses
- Ineffective breathing pattern related to bronchial irritation and obstruction, as evidenced by prolonged inspiration, expiratory wheezing, sputum production, and decreased PaO_2
- Impaired gas exchange related to hyperinflation of alveoli and narrowed airway, as evidenced by increased $PaCO_2$, decreased PaO_2, and paleness
- Risk for fluid volume deficit from inability to consume adequate fluids and insensible water loss
- Fear related to diagnostic procedures, as evidenced by crying and avoidance of professional caregivers
- Risk for caregiver role strain related to role demands of financial resources required to care for a child with chronic respiratory disease

Planning and goals
- Molly's respiratory rate will decrease to 24 breaths/minute, and normal breath sounds will be present throughout all lung fields.
- Molly will attain normal respiratory oxygenation on room air.
- Molly will take adequate fluids by mouth and will not require I.V. hydration.
- Molly will be relaxed, and her skin will have pink tones with no malar flush or red ears.
- Molly will respond positively to the nursing staff and receive comfort and support from her parents during invasive procedures.
- Molly's parents will express understanding of the current treatment and planned future diagnostic workup.
- Molly's parents will discuss concerns regarding the care of a child with asthma.

CHILD NURSING

Implementation

NURSING BEHAVIORS	NURSING RATIONALES

1. Monitor Molly's respiratory status in response to medications, as follows:
• Auscultate lungs for rate, depth, and adventitious sounds.
• Assess for changes in the amount and quality of cough and sputum.
• Assess use of accessory muscles and energy expended on breathing.
• Position Molly upright to assist with breathing.
• Assist Molly with use of inhaled medications.

1. Pharmacologic treatment of asthma is either prophylactic with anti-inflammatory medications or therapeutic with bronchodilator medications. Oral and inhaled steroids and nonsteroidal anti-inflammatory drugs (cromolyn sodium and nedocromil sodium) are used to prevent asthma attacks. Beta$_2$-adrenergic agonists (albuterol, metaproterenol, and terbutaline) are the preferred drugs in treating an acute asthma attack. Methylxanthines, primarily theophylline, are now considered the third line of defense in the treatment of asthma. Children too young to use a metered-dose inhaler (MDI) can take inhaled medications by adding a spacer that allows the caregiver to deliver the medication through the MDI. Parents and older children need to be cautioned not to abuse the inhaled medication.

2. Monitor Molly's level of oxygenation through oxygen saturations, blood gas analysis, and laboratory values.

2. Blood gas values and blood electrolytes will indicate the effectiveness of treatment in correcting respiratory acidosis.

3. Offer Molly small sips of fluids, but avoid cold beverages. Record her intake and output.

3. Promoting adequate fluid intake is important, but cold beverages should be avoided because they could trigger bronchospasm. Recording intake and output helps in evaluating the effectiveness of treatment.

4. Have Molly's parents stay with her during invasive procedures. Offer simple explanations of all procedures to be done.

4. Molly can understand concrete descriptions of tests but may still need the comfort of her parents to reduce anxiety.

5. Explain all procedures to Molly's parents. Assess their understanding of asthma, and explain the diagnostic tests that may need to be performed after this acute attack.

5. To establish a diagnosis, the physician may order diagnostic studies to rule out other possible causes of respiratory distress, such as cystic fibrosis, aspirated foreign body, or tracheoesophageal (TE) fistula. Pulmonary function studies will help establish a baseline of respiratory function. Skin testing may be done if allergens are suspected as triggers for attacks.

• Teach the purpose and use of a peak expiratory flow meter (PEFM).

• PEFMs have color zones that are helpful in guiding treatment of asthma at home. They also can aid in early identification of respiratory infections.

• Teach allergen control of the home.

• Specific allergens identified by skin tests need to be removed, if possible, or minimized by plastic covers, thorough and frequent cleaning, or avoidance by the child. Humidity should be kept below 50% to remove dust mites. Exposure to animals should be limited.

• Teach Molly's parents to perform chest physio-therapy (CPT).

• CPT—including breathing exercises, use of inhalers, and physical exercise—helps promote respiratory function through physical and emotional conditioning.

• Help parents plan activities to encourage normal child development.

• Asthmatic children should be encouraged to participate in all age-appropriate activities, including sports, particularly those that require an even-level expenditure of energy, such as distance running or swimming.

Evaluation

• Molly breathes easily and with normal breath sounds.
• Molly breathes room air and has normal blood gas values.
• Molly takes fluids freely and has a normal hydration status.
• Molly has pink cheeks and normal skin tones.
• Molly describes tests to be done to establish the diagnosis.
• Molly's parents outline a plan for coping with upcoming tests and measures to decrease Molly's exposure to allergens.
• Molly's parents correctly describe asthma and treatment for Molly.

Leukemia

Leukemia is the most common form of cancer in children, with peak onset between ages 3 and 5. The 5-year survival rate varies from 50% to 90%, depending on the type of leukemia. Its main feature is a rapid increase in the number of immature white blood cells (WBCs). Diagnosis is confirmed by bone marrow examination and various other blood studies and examinations. Leukemic cells have the same properties as malignant cells of solid tumors: high metabolic rate, infiltration of surrounding tissue, and migration to other body parts.

Because of leukemic cells' high metabolic rate and rapid proliferation in the bone marrow, other blood components are deprived of nutrients and are crowded out of the existing space. The result is progressive anemia from decreased erythrocyte levels and bleeding problems from decreased thrombocyte levels. Though increased in number, the leukemic WBCs cannot fight infection.

The leukemic cells tend to migrate first to the highly vascular organs of the reticuloendothelial system—namely, the spleen, liver, and lymph glands. Infiltration of the central nervous system results in signs of increased intracranial pressure (ICP) and meningeal irritation. Finally, all organs are involved, and the child is deprived of metabolic nutrients, resulting in generalized wasting. (See *Signs and symptoms of leukemia,* page 400.)

Leukemias are treated with chemotherapy. The type of chemotherapeutic agent depends on the type of leukemia. Nursing care is symptomatic and supportive, both for the leukemia and for the various adverse reactions to chemotherapeutic agents.

Clinical situation

Kenny, age 4, is admitted to the hospital for suspected acute lymphocytic leukemia. He has been treated for the past few weeks for a bad cold and several sore throats. His physician noted that he had many bruises and petechiae over his body without a history of injuries. Kenny has lost weight during the past 2 months, is not hungry, and seems more tired than usual. His mother states that he has been a healthy child until now and just can't seem to get over this cold.

CHILD NURSING

Signs and symptoms of leukemia

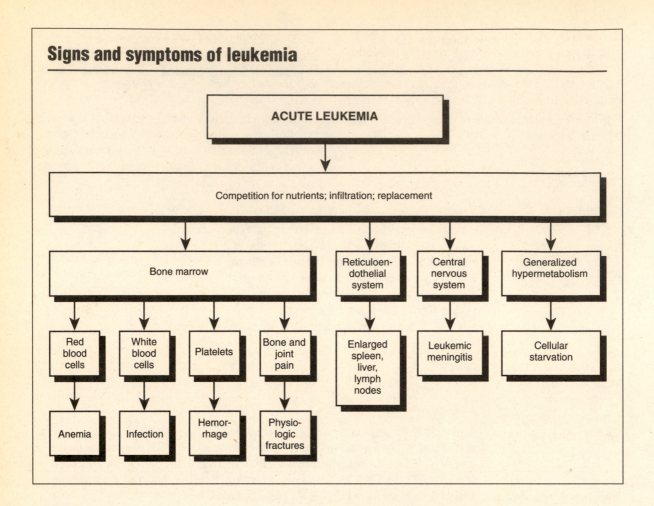

Assessment

NURSING BEHAVIORS

1. Assess for bleeding tendencies, as follows:
• Document the location and color of bruises and petechiae.
• Check the mouth and gums for bleeding and ulcers.
• Complete a neurologic assessment, observing for signs of increased ICP.
• Check urine and stools for occult blood.
• Interview the parents for a history of nosebleeds.

NURSING RATIONALES

1. Invasion of the bone marrow by leukemic cells deprives platelet precursors of metabolic nutrients, resulting in thrombocytopenia. The platelets are an essential component of the clotting mechanism, and they maintain capillary integrity.

2. Assess for infection, as follows:
• Measure and record temperature, pulse rate, and respiratory rate.
• Perform a cephalocaudal examination to locate signs of infection from cuts, scratches, or abrasions. Examine the common sites and sources of infection first.
• Listen to Kenny's breath sounds.
• Note whether the child swallows with pain.
• Inquire about pain or burning with urination.
• Examine the condition of Kenny's teeth and gums.

2. Neutropenia renders the body incapable of warding off even the slightest infection. Breath sounds help reveal respiratory infection. Painful swallowing may indicate sore throat or tonsillitis. Dental caries may be a source of infection.

3. Assess Kenny's activity tolerance, and find out the child's scheduled nap times at home.

3. Activity and exercise intolerance will develop as anemia worsens.

4. Assess the parents' understanding of leukemia and its progression.

4. To be fully informed and prepared, the parents must understand the disease, the normal blood values of all components, and the reasons for innumerable venipunctures, bone marrow aspirations, and fingersticks.

5. Observe the parents to identify patterns of coping with crisis.

5. Leukemia in a child is catastrophic for parents. Assisting them through grief and anticipatory mourning is a major goal.

6. Assess the child's developmental level on admission (see "Growth and development," pages 52 to 61).

6. The numerous painful diagnostic procedures and the long hospital stay are likely to cause regressive behavior.

Nursing diagnoses
• Risk for infection related to bone marrow suppression
• Altered nutrition: Less than body requirements, related to pain and anorexia
• Impaired tissue integrity (skin and mucous membranes) related to decreased function of blood components
• Pain related to the cancer and the effects of chemotherapy
• Altered family processes related to having a child in treatment for a life-threatening illness

Planning and goals
• Kenny will not experience chronic or acute blood loss.
• Kenny will regain his infection-free state and will not develop another infection while hospitalized.
• Kenny's skin integrity will be maintained.
• Kenny's energy will be conserved and tissue oxygen needs will decrease.
• Kenny and his parents will learn to cope with the problems of his disease.
• Kenny will be pain-free.

CHILD NURSING

Implementation

NURSING BEHAVIORS	NURSING RATIONALES
1. Teach the parents how to assess and care for Kenny, including how to observe for signs of chronic and acute blood loss (see "Shock," pages 103 to 108). Tell them to take necessary measures to prevent hemorrhage, such as padding the child's crib and living area and keeping sharp objects out of the child's reach.	**1.** Observing for blood loss and taking measures to prevent hemorrhage helps prevent anemia in the child. Treatment for acute leukemia lasts up to 3 years. Kenny will have intermittent hospitalizations; however, he will be treated primarily on an outpatient basis.
2. Monitor Kenny for infection, and take measures to prevent it, as follows: • Remove broken toys and other sharp objects from the room. • Use aseptic technique during all invasive procedures. • Monitor Kenny's temperature every 4 hours. • Screen all staff and visitors for signs of infection. • Advise all staff and visitors to use good hand-washing technique. • Make sure Kenny maintains a well-balanced diet.	**2.** Infection is the leading cause of death in children with leukemia. Infection prevention, including good nutrition, is the best defense against this complication.
3. Conserve Kenny's energy to reduce cardiac demands.	**3.** This relieves generalized hypoxia from the anemia.
4. Do not give aspirin to Kenny; control pain by taking these steps:	**4.** Aspirin may further suppress the platelets and interfere with clotting.
• Schedule analgesia to get maximum pain relief and optimal mental functioning.	• The physician may prescribe acetaminophen (Tylenol) or a low-dose narcotic.
• Advise the parents to have Kenny sit in a reclining chair or a beanbag chair at home.	• A reclining chair or a beanbag chair allows frequent repositioning to control pain.
5. Provide nursing care measures for the adverse reactions accompanying radiation therapy and chemotherapy, as follows.	**5.** Radiation and chemotherapy cause severe adverse reactions (see "Chemotherapy," page 607, and "Radiation therapy," page 613).
For anorexia • Allow Kenny to select his own food. • Give Kenny any food he wants. • Take advantage of hungry periods with snacks. • Add nutritious supplements (such as custards, puddings, and milk shakes) to his diet.	• Chemotherapy may cause anorexia. These nursing measures improve the child's nutritional intake during this period.
For nausea and vomiting • When possible, administer chemotherapeutic drugs when the child's stomach is empty, and administer an antiemetic 20 minutes before vomiting can be expected.	• These measures reduce the likelihood of vomiting.

For mouth ulcers

• Have the child use a soft, rubber toothbrush.

• This prevents bleeding at the ulcer site.

• Provide frequent mouthwash with normal saline.

• Saline mouthwash prevents infection and cleans the palate, making food more appetizing. Commercial mouthwashes containing lemon glycerine and hydrogen peroxide are too drying.

• Provide a bland, moist, soft diet; avoid hot and cold foods and beverages.

• Bland foods prevent irritation of mouth ulcers.

• Administer a local anesthetic—for example, lidocaine hydrochloride (Xylocaine Viscous Solution)—before meals.

• This makes swallowing and chewing more comfortable.

For rectal ulcers

• Do not use rectal thermometers or suppositories.

• This prevents damage to the vulnerable rectal area.

• Give sitz baths or tub baths as often as necessary for comfort.

• Baths relieve rectal pain and discomfort and promote healing.

• Expose the affected area to air or warm heat.

• This promotes healing.

• Apply A and D Ointment before a bowel movement.

• Ointment lubricates the anorectal area, facilitating passage of stool.

• Provide dietary fiber and fluids. Give stool softeners, as ordered.

• Prevent constipation from chemotherapy.

For hemorrhagic cystitis

• Give the child 3 qt (3 L) fluid/day.

• The chemotherapeutic drug cyclophosphamide (Cytoxan) is an alkylating agent that irritates the bladder mucosa. Fluids dilute the urine, reducing the irritation.

• Observe Kenny for burning pain on urination.

• Burning pain indicates a urinary tract infection.

• Encourage frequent voiding; arouse Kenny at night to void.

• An empty bladder reduces the amount of time that the bladder is exposed to the alkylating agent in urine.

For alopecia

• Tell Kenny and his parents that alopecia will probably be less severe during a second treatment with the same drug.

• Hair will begin to grow back in 3 to 6 months but may be slightly different in color and texture. An older child or adult can wear a wig.

• Keep the scalp clean and dry.

• This prevents infection.

• Obtain a baseball cap or favorite hat for Kenny to wear.

• Many young children prefer caps and hats to wigs.

• Tell Kenny's parents to keep his head covered when exposed to the sun, wind, or cold.

• Scalp skin is vulnerable to sunburn, and exposed scalp increases heat loss.

For moon face

• Return Kenny to his peer group as soon as possible.

• Moon face results from steroid use. It develops slowly, so a quick return to peer group will decrease the impact of a changed appearance.

• Evaluate weight gain carefully.

• This helps detect fluid retention from steroids.

6. Support the child and parents through the grief process (see "Grieving," pages 72 and 73, in Part III).

6. Kenny and his parents will be experiencing differing levels of anticipatory grief and loss. They will profit from support during this time.

7. Inform the parents of expected adverse effects of medication, as follows:

7. This information helps them differentiate drug adverse effects from exacerbation of symptoms and thus may relieve their anxiety.

• Tell the parents which adverse effects need medical attention: mouth and rectal ulcers, hemorrhagic cystitis, peripheral neuropathy, infection, and dehydration.

• Parents need specific instructions on which adverse effects require medical attention.

• Inform the parents that drug adverse effects do not indicate a return of leukemia.

• Relieving the parents' anxiety enables them to support Kenny emotionally.

• Listen to the parents, remain supportive, and be available to answer their questions.

• These actions help the parents cope with anticipatory grief.

Evaluation

• Kenny remains free from infection.
• Kenny enters a period of remission.
• Kenny is free from chemotherapy and radiation adverse effects.
• Kenny and his parents regain strong family unity.

Hypospadias

Hypospadias (opening of the urethra on the ventral surface of the penis) occurs in approximately 8 of every 1,000 male neonates. The defect may be accompanied by a downward curvature of the penis (chordee) resulting from penile constriction by a fibrous band of tissue. The objectives of surgical correction are to facilitate voiding while standing, to provide a more normal physical appearance of the male genitalia, and to facilitate reproductive capability later. The timing of hypospadias repair depends on the placement of the defective urethral opening. However, the current trend is repair in one surgical procedure before 18 months. Repair can be a relatively simple procedure if the urethral opening is near the glans penis and chordee is absent. If the urethral opening is nearer the middle of the shaft, more than one surgical procedure may be necessary to lengthen the urethra progressively. Circumcision should be avoided in neonates with hypospadias—their foreskin can be used in reconstructive surgery.

Clinical situation   David Johnson, age 4 ½, is hospitalized for hypospadias repair. At birth, David's urethral opening was on the ventral surface of his penis, approximately ¾" (2 cm) from the tip of the glans; significant chordee was present. He had surgery as an infant for release of the chordee and at age 3 had the first stage of what is hoped to be a two-stage repair.

Assessment

NURSING BEHAVIORS	NURSING RATIONALES
1. Determine David's perception of the surgery to be performed and of postoperative dressings, drains, and so forth; ask him to tell you about his previous hospital experiences.	**1.** Surgery involving male genitalia is apt to be extremely threatening to a preschooler, who strongly fears mutilation. Eliciting the client's perception is important because memories of his previous surgery may significantly affect David's reaction to this hospitalization and surgery.
2. Document David's term for his penis.	**2.** Many preschoolers have their own vocabulary for genitalia.
3. Assess David's developmental level, and compare it with norms for his age (see "Growth and development," pages 52 to 61).	**3.** This helps the nurse plan care aimed at regaining and maintaining growth and development.

Nursing diagnoses
- Altered urinary elimination related to an anomalous urethra
- Risk for infection related to surgical repair
- Impaired verbal communication related to the young client's limited vocabulary
- Body image disturbance related to a displaced urethra and penile reconstruction

Planning and goals
- David will participate in role playing before and after surgery.
- David will demonstrate a basic understanding of postoperative procedures and catheter drainage.
- Postoperatively, David will remain free from infection, and any bladder or urethral catheter will remain patent.
- David will develop positive feelings about his sexuality as he ages.

Implementation

NURSING BEHAVIORS	NURSING RATIONALES
1. Provide concrete explanations and demonstrations to prepare David for upcoming surgery, as follows:	**1.** Explanations and demonstrations must be concrete so that the child does not reach inaccurate conclusions.
• Take David to the operating suite and recovery room to acquaint him with surgical equipment and personnel. If a visit can't be arranged, use photographs or illustrations.	• The opportunity to touch and handle equipment in its proper setting and to see operating room personnel will make them less threatening when the child is brought to the operating room for surgery.
• Provide hospital equipment and dress (mask, caps, gowns, anesthesia face mask, and so on) as well as dolls for role playing.	• The child's role playing, using puppets and dolls as well as hospital dress and equipment, helps the nurse determine his perception of events and evaluate the effectiveness of teaching up to this point.

• Use an anatomically correct doll to demonstrate anticipated postoperative catheters and dressings, and encourage David to play with the doll and comment. As part of the demonstration, include reassuring statements—for example, "It's hard to see the doll's penis (or David's term for his penis), but it's still there, covered by the bandage."

To make sure your demonstration is accurate, check with the surgeon to find out which type of catheter and dressing will be used.

• This concrete demonstration can effectively allay the preschooler's fears of mutilation and castration. An anatomically correct doll should be used with children having genital surgery.

• Avoid using such terms as *cut off*.

• The child at this age interprets words literally and is intensely afraid of mutilation.

• Discuss preoperative medication last, particularly if it will be administered by injection.

• This delay gives the child as little time as possible to worry about an injection.

2. Postoperatively, maintain hourly urine output records, documenting the urine's color and consistency; irrigate the catheter as necessary, according to the physician's orders.

2. Urine should appear normal after surgery. Hematuria or cloudiness may indicate unexpected bleeding or exudate, which could occlude the drainage.

3. Assess and document the appearance of the penis visible under the dressing.

3. Some postoperative edema is expected. Excessive redness or swelling may indicate infection.

4. Avoid scolding David if he exposes his dressing and catheter to others.

4. Exposure is an expected behavior for a preschooler who has genital surgery. It reassures the child that his penis is still present.

5. Inform the parents that David may be preoccupied with his penis after discharge and that this is normal behavior. Encourage them not to criticize David or draw attention to the behavior.

5. Parents may become embarrassed about their child's preoccupation with his penis. In most cases, this preoccupation gradually lessens when the parents display a matter-of-fact attitude about it.

6. Discuss with David's parents the importance of providing positive reinforcement in as many areas as possible to promote self-esteem.

6. David's penis may have an abnormal appearance, which could result in serious body-image problems in later years (particularly in adolescence). For this reason, the parents should promote a positive self-image in David in as many other areas as possible.

Evaluation

• David actively participates in role playing before surgery and administeres shots to doctor and nurse dolls.
• David asks many questions when the doll with the simulated catheter and dressings is used for demonstration.
• Postoperatively, David experiences no untoward temperature elevation; voids sufficient quantities of clear, yellow urine; and has no unusual drainage or inflammation of the operative site.
• David's parents are receptive to advice about promoting David's self-esteem.

THE SCHOOL-AGE CHILD (AGES 6 TO 12)

Rheumatic fever

Rheumatic fever, an autoimmune disease affecting the connective tissue, occurs primarily in those between ages 5 and 20. Occurring most commonly during cold, humid weather, the disease, which declined in the United States during most of this century, recently has increased in the Western part of the country and remains a major problem in Third World countries. Evidence suggests that rheumatic fever is preceded by a group A beta-hemolytic streptococcal infection, such as scarlet fever, strep throat, otitis media, impetigo, and tonsillitis. Antibodies against the streptococcus develop and remain after the organism is eradicated. About 2 to 6 weeks later, the antibodies mistake the child's connective tissue for the streptococcus and begin to attack it. The symptoms, caused by inflammation, are manifested in the endocardium, skin, joints, and central nervous system. The most serious problem is carditis, which damages the heart valves. Treatment is largely symptomatic and supportive.

Clinical situation   Larry, age 6, is being cared for at home with a fever of 101.8° F (38.8° C). His knees are swollen, red, and painful. His mother states that the physician thinks he has rheumatic fever. She also says that Larry missed 3 days of school about a month ago because of tonsillitis. The initial medical diagnosis is rheumatic fever.

Assessment

NURSING BEHAVIORS

1. Assess for *major* manifestations of rheumatic fever, including carditis (endocarditis, myocarditis, pericarditis, pancarditis), murmur, cardiomegaly, congestive heart failure, polyarthritis, chorea, subcutaneous nodules, and erythema marginatum (red rash with clear margins). Then assess for *minor* manifestations, revealed by clinical findings (history of rheumatic fever or rheumatic heart disease, arthralgia, fever), laboratory findings (increased erythrocyte sedimentation rate, C-reactive protein, leukocytosis, anemia, prolonged PR and QT intervals on electrocardiogram), and supportive evidence (recent scarlet fever, positive throat culture for group A beta-hemolytic streptococci, increased antistreptolysin-O [ASO] titer, and streptococcal antibodies).

2. Assess the location and intensity of Larry's pain and specific joints involved.

NURSING RATIONALES

1. Because no single diagnostic test can identify rheumatic fever, these major and minor manifestations (the modified Jones criteria) are used to diagnose the disease. Either two major manifestations or one major and two minor manifestations with supporting evidence of recent streptococcal infection indicate a high possibility of rheumatic fever. Two elevated ASO titers are the most objective tests supporting streptococcal infection. Normal values are 0 to 120 Todd U. Values of 333 or above indicate recent streptococcal infection.

2. The pain of polyarthritis and arthralgia may be so severe that the weight of clothing and sheets is intolerable.

3. Assess for chorea, its severity, and precipitating factors.

3. Chorea, also known as Sydenham's chorea or St. Vitus' dance, is characterized by sudden, aimless, irregular movements of the extremities; involuntary facial grimaces; speech disturbances; emotional lability; and muscle weakness. It is aggravated by anxiety and attempts at fine motor activity and is relieved by rest and sleep. Chorea may occur weeks or months after the illness or, in some cases, in children not diagnosed with rheumatic fever. Fortunately, chorea is transitory and disappears without residual effects.

4. Assess for lingering streptococcal infection.

4. Streptococcus can be cultured in fewer than half the children with rheumatic fever.

5. Assess the child's developmental level and his progress in school (see "Growth and development," pages 52 to 61).

5. This assessment helps the nurse determine whether the child will need tutoring while confined at home. Maintaining schoolwork is a major goal at this age.

Nursing diagnoses
- Decreased cardiac output related to mitral or aortic valve scarring
- Pain related to inflamed joints
- Diversional activity deficit related to bed rest and activity restrictions
- Altered nutrition: Less than body requirements, related to anorexia
- Knowledge deficit related to the parents' understanding of care of their ill child

Planning and goals
- Larry will have minimal demand placed on his heart.
- Larry will be relieved of pain in his joints.
- Larry will be relieved of fever, anorexia, malaise, and fatigue.
- Larry will regain and maintain nutrition adequate to meet growth needs.
- Larry will continue to preform age-appropriate developmental tasks.
- Larry will not experience carditis as a complication of rheumatic fever.
- Larry will not experience subsequent streptococcal infection or rheumatic fever.

Implementation
NURSING BEHAVIORS

NURSING RATIONALES

1. Teach parents to maintain complete bed rest for Larry, as follows:
- Assist with feeding.
- Bathe the child in bed or carry him to the tub and back.
- Explain the need for bed rest, using simple anatomic drawings of how the heart works.
- Place a footboard on the bed or use high-top athletic shoes to prevent footdrop.
- Supply a commode if the child has moderate to severe carditis.

1. The goal of bed rest is to reduce cardiac workload. However, because many children rest better when they are not rigidly confined to bed, consultation with the physician and estimation of the degree of carditis are essential to determine the necessary level of confinement. Because of his desire to succeed and please, the school-age child usually cooperates when the reason for bed rest is explained to him.

2. Assess for symptoms of carditis by monitoring and recording vital signs (temperature, apical pulse, respirations, blood pressure) during nursing visits. Teach parents to monitor temperature, pulse, and respirations.

2. Typically, the child has a low-grade fever (100° to 102° F [37.8° to 38.8° C]) in the late afternoon and early evening. Symptoms of carditis include a sudden high fever (104° F [40° C]), tachycardia, pallor, and a feeling of severe illness.

3. Place a cradle over the bed to support sheets, and handle swollen joints gently, using your palms rather than fingers. Do not encourage range-of-motion (ROM) exercises.

4. Administer aspirin, ibuprofen, or acetaminophen as ordered.

5. Provide small, frequent meals and high-protein snacks as tolerated or desired. Let Larry select any foods available at home, but discourage fat-rich foods that may lead to obesity.

6. Schedule activities to provide time for schoolwork, play, and rest. Provide a quiet environment for homework and lessons, and contact Larry's school for tutorial services if needed. Schedule frequent rest periods, and allow time for quiet play in bed.

7. Encourage Larry's teacher and schoolmates to visit or write. Help the child collect and display get-well cards and letters.

8. Begin administering prophylactic penicillin, and teach Larry and his parents the importance of long-term penicillin therapy, as follows:
• Advise the parents to seek medical care at the first signs of streptococcal infection (scarlet fever, strep throat, otitis media, impetigo, or tonsillitis).
• Reassure Larry and his parents that except for carditis, all symptoms are transitory and have no residual effects.
• Advise Larry and his parents that he should take penicillin throughout life before dental work (major or minor), certain medical procedures, and oral surgery to prevent bacterial endocarditis. (Women should also take penicillin before childbirth.)

3. A cradle supports the weight of bed sheets, preventing further pain to already painful joints. Palms exert less pressure (and thus cause less pain) than fingers. ROM exercises are unnecessary because the arthritis is nondeforming and quite painful.

4. Aspirin and ibuprofen are the preferred drugs to relieve pain, fever, and inflammation. Acetaminophen has only analgesic and antipyretic properties.

5. The school-age child, in a period of slow growth, has a small appetite and prefers snacks to meals. Making his own choices gives him a sense of control at a time when he feels powerless. Obesity is a potential problem for children who require prolonged bed rest.

6. The typical school-age child is a high-level achiever who fears failure. One of the child's areas of achievement and success is schoolwork. Scheduling time for homework and lessons allows the client to keep up with schoolmates; falling behind them would be a failure. The morning is best for schoolwork because of the afternoon fevers. As for play, the child enjoys competitive games, especially when he wins.

7. The school-age child is quite attached to his teachers. Usually, the teacher is the first close adult other than family members with whom he develops a relationship. His schoolmates of the same sex are important in the early "gang" period as he practices the interpersonal and social skills of adults, such as negotiation, cooperation, compromise, communication, and competition. A collector who likes to classify things, he will want to save and display his get-well cards and letters, tangible evidence of how much he is liked.

8. Subsequent attacks of rheumatic fever dramatically increase the chances that the child will develop carditis. Each episode of carditis increases the likelihood of valvular damage. The valves damaged most commonly are the mitral, aortic, tricuspid, and pulmonary, in that order. Thus, the client needs long-term penicillin therapy to prevent or aggressively treat streptococcal infections at the outset.

CHILD NURSING

Evaluation

• Larry recovers without evidence of valvular damage from endocarditis.
• Larry complies with penicillin therapy to prevent endocarditis.
• Larry's parents involve siblings and friends in quiet play and schoolwork to relieve the boredom of bed rest.
• Larry maintains normal growth patterns without becoming overweight.

Insulin-dependent diabetes mellitus

Diabetes is a disorder of carbohydrate metabolism characterized by insufficient insulin to allow glucose to cross the cell membrane. Type I diabetes mellitus, known as juvenile-onset or insulin-dependent diabetes, develops in childhood.

Type II, also called adult-onset or non-insulin-dependent diabetes, occurs in adults. Type I diabetes commonly has a rapid onset (several days); signs and symptoms include polydipsia, polyuria, polyphagia, and weight loss. The Type I diabetes client is also prone to sporadic episodes of ketoacidosis and hypoglycemia. Type II also is marked by polydipsia, polyuria, and polyphagia but occurs over a much longer period and may not include weight loss. The psychological and emotional demands of growth and development and the generally increased but unpredictable activity levels of children complicate management.

Infants' rapid metabolism and growth and their potential for acute illnesses will require careful monitoring of insulin needs. Their frequent childhood infections and, in late infancy, their food preferences make management difficult. Recognition of hypoglycemia and ketoacidosis is difficult in infants and toddlers.

Toddlers' erratic activity patterns, decreased growth rate, and finicky eating behaviors will affect insulin needs. Toddlers have difficulty understanding why their parents purposely hurt them with fingersticks and injections.

Preschoolers may be ready to learn about the disease and to participate in care. Preschoolers also may resist daily injections; management of resistant behavior may be more difficult at this age than at any other.

School-age children may have both cognitive and motor ability to participate actively in managing diabetes (that is, injecting insulin, planning diet and exercise, and testing blood). They also may use their disease effectively to achieve secondary gain such as pretending to be ill so they can stay home from school. Increased participation in active sports can present problems in balancing diet, insulin, and activity.

Teenagers should be capable of self-management; however, the rapid growth and metabolic changes they undergo make management quite complex. Also, the chronic disease plays havoc with identity formation. Teenagers need the opportunity to express their grief and anger at being burdened with something they didn't ask for. Group discussions, health clinics specifically for diabetic adolescents, and juvenile diabetic camps are effective. See the Adult Nursing section for a review of diabetes pathophysiology.

Clinical situation

Denise Burton, age 8, is admitted from the intensive care unit after being treated for diabetic ketoacidosis. Three months earlier, she was medically diagnosed as having insulin-dependent diabetes mellitus. Denise experienced vomiting and diarrhea for 3 days before becoming ketoacidotic and decided to stop administering her insulin because "there was no food for the insulin to work on."

Assessment

NURSING BEHAVIORS	NURSING RATIONALES
1. Administer a multiple-choice pretest to Denise and her parents to determine their understanding of diabetes and its management.	**1.** Pretests are important in identifying the learning needs of the client and her family. They are available from the American Diabetes Association.
2. Have Denise complete an assessment protocol that includes such questions as "What are your feelings now about having diabetes?" and "If you could change anything in your life, what would it be?"	**2.** A child's success in managing diabetes is directly related to self-esteem and the ability to accept responsibility for self-care.
3. Assess family interaction with and response to Denise in relation to diabetes management.	**3.** This helps plan for parental understanding of and participation in their child's diabetes management.

Nursing diagnoses
- Altered nutrition: Less than body requirements, related to vomiting, diarrhea, and insulin insufficiency
- Knowledge deficit related to the parents' and child's understanding of the disease and its management
- Fluid volume deficit related to ketoacidosis

Planning and goals
- Denise will:
—accurately test her urine for ketones and record results at least once during hospitalization
—accurately test her blood for glucose level at least once daily
—state the onset, peak, and duration of action of neutral protamine hagedorn (NPH, or isophane insulin) and regular insulins
—accurately and safely draw up and administer her own insulin at least two times during this hospital stay
—demonstrate an understanding of appropriate body sites for insulin administration and rotation scheduling.
- Denise and her parents will state appropriate actions to take in case of illness or change in normal activity schedule.
- Denise will state at least three signs or symptoms of hyperglycemia and hypoglycemia.
- Denise will describe appropriate action to take during an insulin reaction.
- Denise's parents will recognize her need for independence.
- Denise and her parents will understand the principles of her diet.

Implementation

NURSING BEHAVIORS	NURSING RATIONALES
1. Discuss with Denise and her parents the relationship of dietary intake to blood glucose levels. Explain the significance of taking three meals and three snacks per day, and describe the effects of concentrated sweets.	**1.** Denise and her parents need to understand the relationship between regularly scheduled food intake and insulin's onset, peak, and duration of action. This eating pattern most accurately reflects a child's activity pattern. It may be adjusted so that a large snack is given before increased physical activity. Generally, concentrated sweets should be avoided because their simple sugars are absorbed rapidly from the GI tract, resulting in rapidly elevated blood glucose levels. More complex sugars (such as those con-

tained in starches and bread) are absorbed more slowly; thus, they raise blood glucose levels more slowly and more consistently. Milk is strongly recommended because its sugars are the most slowly absorbed and yield the most sustaining effect.

2. Have Denise demonstrate how to test blood for the glucose level, using the prescribed method, and how to record results.

2. Home blood glucose monitoring is a significant part of successfully managing type I diabetes. Blood glucose monitoring is preferred over urine glucose monitoring.

3. Have Denise demonstrate how to test urine for ketones and how to record results.

3. Urine should occasionally be tested for ketones when blood glucose levels are high.

4. Teach Denise and her parents about NPH and regular insulin, including their onset, peak, and duration of action and their effects. Explain the reasons for administering two doses daily.

4. Insulin enables the body cells to absorb glucose. Without insulin, glucose accumulates in the blood, resulting in hyperglycemia. NPH is an intermediate-acting insulin. Onset is 1 to 2 hours after administration; peak, 6 to 8 hours after administration; duration, 12 to 24 hours. (*Note:* The effective duration of intermediate-acting insulin has been found to be different in children than in adults.) Regular insulin is a rapid-acting insulin. Onset is 30 minutes to 1 hour after administration; peak, 2 to 4 hours after administration; duration, 6 to 8 hours. This combination effectively covers activity periods for most children.

To maintain a relatively consistent blood glucose level, the insulins are administered twice daily, with approximately two-thirds of the total daily dosage given about $1/2$ hour before breakfast and one-third given $1/2$ hour before dinner.

5. Have Denise draw up her morning NPH and regular insulin in a single syringe and administer the dose to herself.

5. Self-administration of insulin, particularly when two insulins are mixed, is not a simple task. Denise was diagnosed only a few months ago and may not feel entirely comfortable with the procedure. However, 8-year-olds have the fine-motor skill, binocular vision, and cognitive ability necessary to assume this responsibility.

Watching Denise draw up and administer a dose allows the nurse to evaluate the child's comfort and proficiency with the procedure and to provide clarification, answer questions, and correct problems she may be having.

6. Have Denise demonstrate appropriate insulin injection sites and her plan for rotating them.

6. Acceptable sites for those subcutaneous injections include the thighs, abdomen, arms, back, and buttocks. Site rotation is essential to enhance insulin absorption and to prevent lipoatrophy.

Hyperglycemia and hypoglycemia: Causes, manifestations, and interventions

CAUSES	SIGNS AND SYMPTOMS	NURSING INTERVENTIONS
Hyperglycemia		
• Too much food • Too little insulin	• Fatigue • Flushed face • Fruity breath • Polyuria • Polyphagia • Polydipsia • Irritability • Abdominal cramping • Nausea and vomiting	• Assess blood glucose levels at least four times daily. (Blood glucose monitoring is a more accurate measure of control than is urine glucose monitoring.) • Blood glucose levels above 250 mg/dl indicate a need to test for urinary ketones. • Parents and children can learn self–blood glucose monitoring using one of the many commercially available systems.
Hypoglycemia		
• Too little food • Too much insulin • Too much exercise	• Tremulousness • Headache • Numbness of tongue or mouth • Irritability, anxious behavior • Dizziness • Cold, clammy sweating • Sudden onset	• Inform the parents and child that they should always have sugar cubes or candy readily available. For mild hypoglycemia, tell the child to consume complex sugars (milk, crackers, or fruit); for moderate hypoglycemia, simple sugars (a sugar cube, orange juice, or cola) followed by more complex sugars; for severe hypoglycemia, glucagon followed by a simple sugar in 15 to 20 minutes. • Tell the child to have an extra meal 1 to 2 hours before engaging in extra activity (such as cheerleading practice).

7. Discuss with Denise and her parents the causes and manifestations of hyperglycemia and hypoglycemia, as well as appropriate interventions for each condition. (For a complete listing, see *Hyperglycemia and hypoglycemia: Causes, manifestations, and interventions.*)

7. Severe hyperglycemia may be caused by illness, growth, or emotional upset as well as by excessive glucose intake or decreased insulin levels; growth and emotional upset are the most significant in the type I diabetic client. Manifestations of hypoglycemia may be highly individualized in the type I diabetic client. In many cases, the first sign may be a behavioral problem, obstinacy, or simply not acting like oneself. Because Denise was diagnosed only a few months ago, she may not have experienced an insulin reaction yet and thus may not know her particular manifestations of hypoglycemia.

Evaluation

• Denise accurately monitors urine and blood glucose levels.
• Denise accurately and safely administers insulin in dosages appropriate for her diet and activity.
• Denise can state the signs of hyperglycemia and hypoglycemia and knows how to intervene appropriately.
• Denise shows verbal evidence of a positive self-image.
• Denise and her parents explain reasons for three meals and three snacks a day and give at least three examples each of simple sugars and complex sugars.
• Denise's parents support her efforts at independence and offer but do not force appropriate help.

CHILD NURSING

Tonsillitis and otitis media

Tonsillar tissue, the lymphoid tissue encircling the pharyngeal cavity (Waldeyer's ring), consists of several pairs of tonsils. Their function is to filter pathogenic organisms. With repeated exposure to the organisms, the tonsils become enlarged and infected. Tonsillectomy, as a routine surgical procedure, is considered unnecessary by many experts. However, for some clients, removal is the best approach to eliminate the tonsils as a chronic source of infection. The palatine tonsils at the back of the posterior portion of the nasopharynx are the groups of tissues excised in a tonsillectomy and adenoidectomy.

Inflammation of the tonsillar tissue results in edema, obstructing the passage of air and food through the naso-oral cavity. Because of the proximity to the eustachian tube, normal drainage is impaired by edema of the adenoids, and chronic otitis media is common. Myringotomy, surgical incision of the eardrum with insertion of myringotomy tubes, allows exudate to drain from the middle ear. Tonsillectomy, adenoidectomy, and myringotomy are commonly performed simultaneously but may be performed separately, depending on the severity of otitis media.

Clinical situation

Craig, age 9, is admitted for day surgery for tonsillectomy, adenoidectomy, and bilateral myringotomy with insertion of tubes. Craig has experienced recurrent bouts of tonsillitis and secondary otitis media since infancy. He is an only child with no previous hospitalizations.

Assessment

NURSING BEHAVIORS

1. Note and document Craig's breathing style (nasal or oral), breath odor, and speech tone; also document presence of a cough.

2. Assess Craig's hearing acuity by addressing him without letting him see your face.

3. Review the results of laboratory tests, including bleeding time, clotting time, hemoglobin level and hematocrit.

NURSING RATIONALES

1. A child with enlarged adenoids compensates for airflow obstruction by breathing through the mouth. Because the child tends to hold the mouth open at all times, an offensive breath odor is common. Speech has a nasal twang, and enunciation is impaired. A persistent, nagging cough is common.

2. Recurrent otitis media typically results in unrecognized hearing impairment. (Chronic serous otitis media is the most common cause of conductive hearing loss in young children.)

3. The tonsillar area is highly vascular. Any problem that might interfere with adequate coagulation could be life-threatening postoperatively. A decreased hemoglobin level (less than 10 g/dl) poses an anesthesia risk because it reduces the blood's oxygen-carrying capacity.

Nursing diagnoses

- Pain related to postoperative sore throat
- Risk for fluid volume deficit related to postoperative vomiting and bleeding
- Ineffective breathing pattern related to an obstructed airway from enlarged tonsils and adenoids
- Knowledge deficit related to home care after surgery
- Risk for injury related to postoperative hemorrhage and aspiration.

Planning and goals	• Craig will be prepared for surgery. • Craig will experience no postoperative hemorrhage. • Craig will consume and retain at least 2 oz (60 ml) of oral liquids hourly in the first 6 postoperative hours. • Craig's parents will repeat discharge instructions on diet, activity, and follow-up care.

Implementation

NURSING BEHAVIORS	**NURSING RATIONALES**
1. Provide anticipatory guidance on preoperative and operative routines.	**1.** The typical 9-year-old child understands explanations and tries to cooperate. Anticipatory guidance helps prepare the client for surgery and may relieve some of his anxiety.
2. Provide anticipatory guidance on postoperative events, such as positioning, sore throat, and the importance of drinking liquids. Engage Craig in preoperative role playing (for example, drinking noncitrus, nonred juices from a medicine cup and pretending that the throat is sore).	**2.** After surgery, the child will have a sore throat (relieved by drinking liquids). He will be positioned on his abdomen or side to promote drainage of secretions. He may spit up some dark blood, and dark red fluid may drain from his ears. Anticipatory guidance and role playing can effectively prepare the child for these postoperative events.
3. Postoperatively, position Craig on his side or prone, with his upper knee flexed and his head tilted forward slightly.	**3.** This position promotes drainage of blood or vomitus from the mouth.
4. After surgery, assess for signs of hemorrhage: frequent swallowing and throat clearing, a pulse rate above 120 beats/minute, and vomiting of bright red blood.	**4.** Trickling of blood from the surgical site and continuous swallowing are the most obvious early signs of hemorrhage after a tonsillectomy or an adenoidectomy. An increased pulse rate is a sign of hemorrhage. Bright red blood in vomitus indicates fresh bleeding.
5. Provide an ice collar to ease Craig's discomfort, if ordered by the physician and accepted by the child.	**5.** Although coolness relieves a sore throat, the child may find this device more frustrating than beneficial. If the ice collar is not well received, it can lead to fussiness and crying, which creates tension on the surgical site.
6. As soon as Craig is fully awake, offer cool liquids (½ to 1 oz [15 to 30 ml] every 15 minutes); avoid citrus juices.	**6.** Initially, the client should be given fluids in small amounts at frequent intervals. The child's throat will be quite sore, and the sight of a large quantity to swallow may discourage him. Also, after general anesthesia, ingesting a large volume of fluid could result in nausea and vomiting. Citrus juices may be irritating to the child's throat because of their high acidic content.
7. Do not give Craig straws or red liquids.	**7.** Sucking through a straw creates a vacuum, which may cause bleeding. Red liquids may be confused with bleeding.
8. Provide anticipatory guidance on home care, as follows:	**8.** Parents should be provided with printed information to supplement any verbal instructions given to the

CHILD NURSING

• Encourage Craig to eat soft foods for the first few days and to avoid highly seasoned foods.

• Firm or spicy foods may traumatize the surgical area or cause enough irritation to induce forceful coughing.

• Discourage Craig from forceful coughing and throat clearing.

• Forceful coughing and throat clearing may cause bleeding from the vessels closed by cautery.

• Tell the parents to administer mild analgesics (such as acetaminophen) for persistent pain.

• Aspirin should not be given because it may interfere with clotting.

• Urge the parents to report the following signs and symptoms immediately: bright red bleeding, severe earache, temperature above 100° F (37.8° C), and persistent coughing.

• These are signs and symptoms of possible hemorrhage or infection.

• Caution them to cover Craig's ears or gently insert earplugs before he shampoos, showers, or plays in water.

• Fluids can enter the middle ear through the myringotomy tubes; the entrapped moisture creates an environment for bacterial growth.

• Advise Craig and his parents that *minimal* bleeding may occur 7 to 10 days after surgery, when the scab is shed from the tonsillectomy site. Tell them to call the physician if more than a teaspoonful of bright red blood appears.

• The parents should be prepared for this possibility so they will not panic if it occurs.

• Inform Craig and his parents that he can resume regular activity in 1 to 2 weeks and that he should avoid vigorous running and jumping until then.

• The child usually limits his activity willingly for the first few days. As throat discomfort fades, however, an adult will probably have to structure the child's activities.

Evaluation

• Craig expresses an understanding of preoperative teaching.
• Craig has no postoperative bleeding.
• Craig consumes and retains fluids postoperatively.
• Craig's parents express an understanding of discharge instructions.

Sickle cell anemia

Sickle cell anemia, also called sickle cell disease, occurs in about 1 of 400 African Americans and, rarely, in whites. The disease is inherited as an autosomal recessive trait. In sickle cell anemia, the hemoglobin, in the presence of low oxygen tension, crystallizes quickly, causing the red blood cells (RBCs) to bend into a crescent (or sickle) shape (see *Sickling phenomenon,* page 418). The sickle cells accumulate, obstructing capillary flow throughout the body. The thickened blood results in capillary stasis, obstructed blood flow, and thrombosis. Ischemia and necrosis occur distal to the thrombosis, causing further oxygen depletion and sickling. The body hemolyzes the fragile sickle cells, quickly producing severe anemia (sickle cell crisis).

child, who is usually discharged late on the day of surgery and still groggy from anesthesia.

Symptoms of sickle cell crisis vary among episodes because of the various organs involved. Sickle cell anemia usually is not apparent until after age 4 months, by which time fetal hemoglobin (HbF) has been replaced with sickle hemoglobin (HbS). Persons with *sickle cell trait* have normal and abnormal hemoglobin and are usually asymptomatic.

Clinical situation   Nickie, age 11, is admitted to the hospital for sickle cell crisis, his fifth hospitalization for this condition. An infection has precipitated each crisis. This time, he is admitted through the emergency department with severe abdominal, knee, and leg pain. His mother states that he came home from school yesterday with a sore throat and was vomiting. She called the pediatrician, who prescribed antibiotics. At the time of admission, Nickie's temperature is 100.2° F (37.9° C).

Assessment

NURSING BEHAVIORS	NURSING RATIONALES
1. Assess for signs and symptoms of sickle cell crisis: loss of appetite; pallor; weakness; abdominal, leg, and arm pain; joint swelling; and jaundice (especially of sclerae).	**1.** These are signs of a thrombocytic crisis, which occurs when the sickle RBCs occlude the capillaries in the long bones, mesentery, spleen, and liver. The sickle cells begin to hemolyze, ultimately resulting in jaundice and loss of appetite. The sudden anemia arising from hemolysis produces pallor and weakness.
2. Review the nursing history taken on admission to identify possible precipitating factors: infection, dehydration, trauma, strenuous physical exercise, extreme fatigue, and exposure to extreme cold or high altitudes. Teach the parents to avoid these situations if possible and to treat infection, dehydration, and trauma quickly and aggressively.	**2.** These factors, singly or in combination, may precede a sickle cell crisis.
3. Assess for infarctions in other areas and organ systems, such as gastric and intestinal ulcer, kidney infarction and hematuria, cerebrovascular accident (which can cause hemiplegia and blindness), and pulmonary infarction (which can cause dyspnea and chest pain).	**3.** Sickle cell crisis that progresses to the organ systems can be life-threatening or may result in a long-term chronic disability. Symptoms may vary from one thrombocytic crisis to another, depending on which organs experience the greatest infarctions.
4. Assess the location and intensity of Nickie's pain.	**4.** Medical and nursing staff use this information to determine the best treatment for pain and to evaluate the effectiveness of treatment measures for thrombocytic crisis.
5. Assess for signs of circulatory collapse, including pallor, cyanosis, decreased blood pressure, increased pulse rate, and altered level of consciousness.	**5.** Large amounts of blood pool in the liver and spleen, resulting in hypovolemia. As blood pressure decreases and the pulse rate increases, the child will exhibit progressive signs and symptoms of hypovolemic shock.
6. Assess for symptoms of chronic anemia, including fatigability, exercise intolerance, muscle weakness, and short attention span.	**6.** When healthy, children with sickle cell anemia typically have a lower-than-normal hemoglobin concentration and may be considered mildly anemic. This, of course, depends on the severity of the disease.

CHILD NURSING

Sickling phenomenon

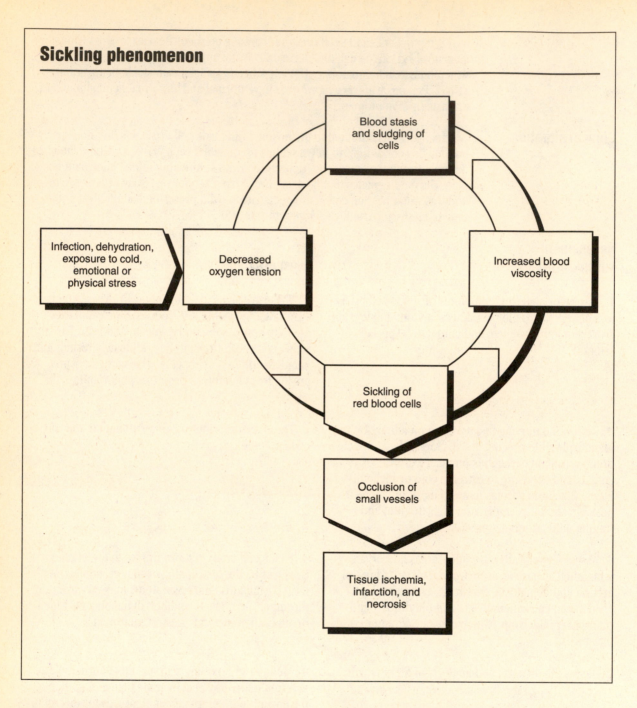

Blood stasis and sludging of cells

Increased blood viscosity

Sickling of red blood cells

Occlusion of small vessels

Tissue ischemia, infarction, and necrosis

Decreased oxygen tension

Infection, dehydration, exposure to cold, emotional or physical stress

7. Assess Nickie's immunization history, including *Haemophilus influenzae* and hepatitis B vaccines. Also assess his history of prophylactic penicillin administration.

8. Assess Nickie's level of growth and development (see "Growth and development," pages 52 to 61).

7. Full immunization is an important measure in preventing infection. Prophylactic penicillin is recommended until age 6 to prevent pneumococcal infection.

8. This assessment helps the nurse determine whether the client meets age-related norms. Sexual maturation is delayed in sickle cell anemia.

Nursing diagnoses	• Altered tissue perfusion (peripheral) related to small-vessel occlusion by thrombi during sickle cell crisis • Impaired physical mobility related to pain from infarcts of multiple organs during sickle cell crisis • Functional incontinence related to forced fluid intake • Altered nutrition: Less than body requirements, related to decreased appetite and pain • Knowledge deficit related to the parents' understanding of factors that precipitate sickle cell crisis
Planning and goals	• Nickie's progressive sickling process will be halted. • Nickie's thrombocytic crisis will not progress to circulatory collapse. • Nickie will regain adequate levels of blood oxygen concentration. • Nickie will be free from infection. • Nickie will not experience the chronic disabling effects of thrombocytic crisis, such as stroke and hemiplegia. • Nickie will perform age-appropriate developmental tasks. • Nickie's parents will know and avoid factors that precipitate sickle cell crisis.

Implementation

NURSING BEHAVIORS

1. Monitor cardiac function for circulatory collapse and cardiac decompensation. (For more information on circulatory collapse and cardiac decompensation, see "Anemia," pages 371 to 374.)

2. Plan care to decrease Nickie's tissue oxygen demand; administer oxygen, as ordered.

3. Prevent or minimize emotional stress.

4. Administer blood (usually packed RBCs), as ordered.

5. Avoid situations that lead to hemoconcentration, as follows:
• Offer fluids frequently; provide soups, gelatin, frozen juice desserts (Popsicles), and puddings as fluid.
• Administer and monitor I.V. infusions, as ordered.
• Give the parents written instructions on minimum hourly intake requirements.
• Prepare Nickie and his parents for enuresis (bed wetting).

6. Control the pain of sickle cell crisis.

7. Monitor for cerebrovascular infarct.

NURSING RATIONALES

1. Blood pools in the liver and spleen during sickle cell crisis, so the client is hypovolemic. The heart rate increases to compensate. Without intervention, decompensation occurs.

2. Oxygen prevents additional sickling (but does not reverse sickling that already exists).

3. Emotional stress increases the sickling phenomenon.

4. Blood transfusions relieve generalized tissue hypoxia. Exchange transfusions may be performed.

5. Hemoconcentration from dehydration increases blood stasis and may cause another thrombocytic crisis. Encouraging or forcing fluids may not be sufficient, in which case I.V. fluids are administered. Involving the parents in their child's care reduces their feelings of powerlessness. Increased fluid intake combined with renal diuresis results in enuresis.

6. Children have a right to pain relief, which in this situation is essential to prevent further sickling.

7. The clumped sickle cells obstruct cerebral vessels, resulting in infarct.

CHILD NURSING

8. Prevent infection and observe for it.

8. Infection can cause sickling.

9. Provide emotional support and encouragement to Nickie and his parents.

9. A child with sickle cell anemia experiences many life-threatening episodes as he matures. Each episode brings grief for the entire family.

Evaluation

- Nickie will return home with a hemoglobin level of at least 10 g/dl and without symptoms of sickle cell crisis.
- Nickie will continue to perform age-appropriate developmental tasks.
- Nickie's parents will monitor his health status, avoid situations that precipitate a crisis, and seek early aggressive medical care for infections or signs of crisis.

THE ADOLESCENT (AGES 13 TO 19)

Scoliosis

Scoliosis, a lateral curvature of the spine, occurs more commonly in girls than in boys. About 10% of preadolescent children have some degree of scoliosis. The curvature progresses insidiously and may be quite prominent before the condition is diagnosed. It becomes more obvious at prepuberty, a time of rapid growth (see *Defects of the spinal column*).

Treatment consists of straightening the vertebrae by surgical or nonsurgical means. The conservative (nonsurgical) approach, implemented first, involves various braces and casts that are uncomfortable to wear and difficult to camouflage, although some newer braces that are worn only at night or are more easily concealed are receiving better acceptance by children. When surgery is indicated (a spinal fusion and Harrington or Dwyer instrumentation), the nursing care is the same as for spinal fusion of an adult with application of a body cast (see *Cast care*, page 357).

Clinical situation

Kathy, age 13, is diagnosed as having scoliosis. She will be fitted for and placed in a Milwaukee brace (see *Milwaukee brace*, page 422). She is not uncomfortable but appears anxious. She asks no questions and remains quiet and withdrawn during the visit. Kathy's mother is talkative and provides the information for the initial nursing history and assessment. She noticed that Kathy's clothes didn't fit correctly, that her hemlines were uneven, that one shoulder seemed lower than the other, and that one bra strap was pulling shorter than the other. Kathy's pediatrician recommended that she see an orthopedist. Spinal X-rays revealed a mild to moderate lateral curve to the right.

Assessment

NURSING BEHAVIORS

NURSING RATIONALES

1. Assess for curvature, as follows:

1. This is a general assessment to screen for scoliosis. In some communities, the screening procedure is performed by physical education teachers, who routinely see teenagers in gym clothes.

- Have Kathy undress except for underpants; provide privacy and respect her modesty.

- Preteens and teenagers are modest. Respecting their modesty and providing privacy build trust.

Defects of the spinal column

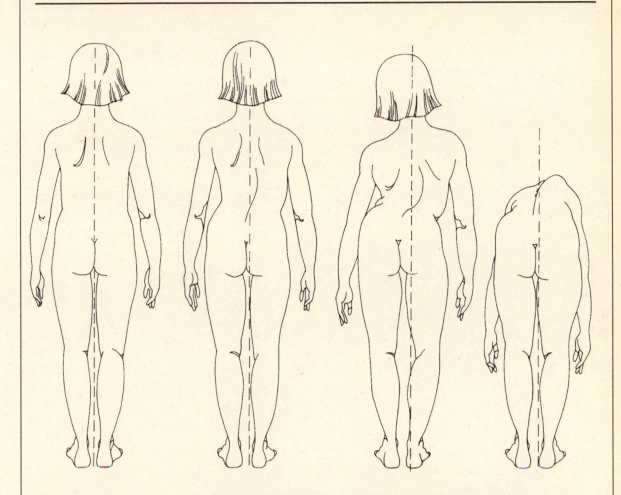

The normal spine in the upright position is vertically aligned, not twisted.

Mild to moderate spinal curvature (the upright spine has a marked serpentine twist) may benefit from corrective bracing or surgery.

The rib hump, a hallmark of severe scoliosis, is accentuated when the client bends forward. Severe curvature is generally treated with surgery.

• Look for forward thrusting of the head.

• Anteriorly, look for an asymmetrical rib cage.

• Determine whether the nipples align horizontally.

• Observe whether the shoulders and hips align horizontally.

• Ask Kathy to hold her arms at her sides; compare the level of the elbows with the iliac crest.

• Spinal curvature thrusts the head forward.

• Asymmetry is usually seen anteriorly and posteriorly.

• Breasts will not align horizontally in scoliosis.

• One hip will be higher with scoliosis.

• The elbows normally fall above the iliac crest. In scoliosis, the elbows will be at the level of the iliac crest or closer to the crest on one side.

Milwaukee brace

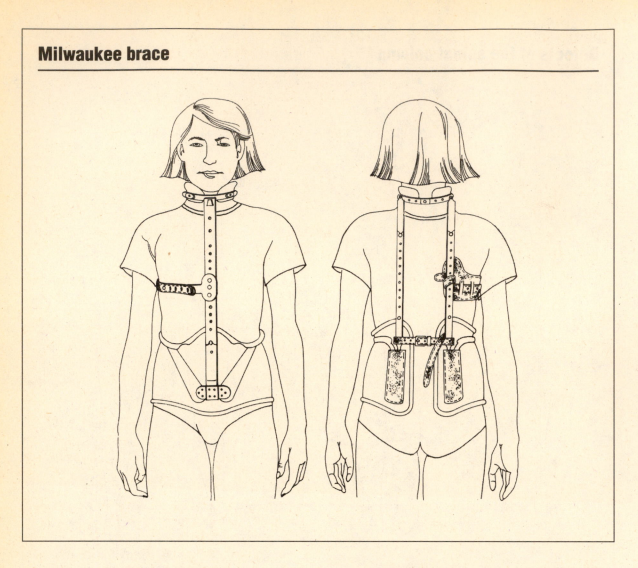

• Ask Kathy to bend forward and touch her toes.

2. Assess Kathy's developmental level (see "Growth and development," pages 52 to 61).

• Viewed from the rear, the scapula will be prominent on one side and hollow on the other, with a rib hump and asymmetrical flanks.

2. Teenage girls have difficulty adjusting to the changes in body image that the curvature and the brace bring. They also have difficulty accepting the long-term aspects of bracing and correction—they want and expect immediate results.

Nursing diagnoses
• Body image disturbance related to altered posture
• Chronic pain related to muscle spasms and soreness caused by the brace
• Powerlessness related to loss of control of body growth, structure, and posture
• Risk for noncompliance with the bracing regimen related to its lengthy duration
• Altered growth and development related to physical disability

Planning and goals
- Kathy's scoliosis will be arrested.
- Kathy and her parents will comply with bracing and traction.
- Kathy will accept the brace and activity restrictions.
- Kathy will physically adjust to the brace and help select clothing to wear with it.
- Kathy will develop a positive self-image and continue with developmental tasks of adolescence.
- Kathy's parents will understand and support Kathy's independence.

Implementation

NURSING BEHAVIORS

1. Teach Kathy and her parents how to apply the brace, as follows:

- Mark the proper strap holes with a ballpoint pen.

- Adjust the brace so that it doesn't rub against the iliac crest.

- Tell Kathy to wear a soft cotton T-shirt under the brace.

2. Instruct Kathy and her parents on activity restrictions, as follows:

- Tell them emphatically that the brace must be worn 23 hours a day, 7 days a week, without exception.

- Tell them that Kathy can remove the brace for no more than 1 hour a day—for bathing, showering, or swimming only.

- Advise them to structure Kathy's lifestyle around more sedentary and less physical activities, concentrating on what Kathy can do rather than what she can't do.

3. Help Kathy develop a positive self-image, as follows:

- Discuss types of clothing that can help camouflage the brace (for example, loose-fitting sweatshirts); at the same time, encourage Kathy not to feel ashamed about wearing the brace in front of family and friends.

NURSING RATIONALES

1. The brace will be removed once daily for hygiene. Initially, Kathy may need help in removal and replacement.

- The brace should always be worn in the same strap holes.

- Frequent follow-up visits may be necessary to obtain the proper fit.

- This prevents the leather and plastic from rubbing the skin. Sweat tends to deteriorate the leather.

2. Both Kathy and her parents must willingly comply with activity restrictions. A clear understanding of treatment rationales will improve the likelihood of compliance.

- Noncompliance with this regimen may prolong the time that Kathy must wear the brace or, worse, may necessitate surgery (spinal alignment and fusion). Removing the brace for special occasions sets a dangerous precedent that can become habitual.

- Kathy must be actively swimming or bathing. Sitting without the brace is nontherapeutic and should be avoided.

- Positive reinforcement of what the adolescent can accomplish is an effective motivating technique.

3. A Milwaukee brace alters the wearer's body image and diminishes independence at a time when teenagers are typically trying to find their identity and forge their independence.

- Dressing like her friends will help Kathy maintain self-esteem. However, the sooner she exposes the brace to family and friends, the sooner their questions will be out of the way.

CHILD NURSING

• Encourage Kathy to resume activity as soon as possible after the brace is applied; initially, assist with walking.

• After the brace is applied, the client will probably feel taller (she actually is a little taller) and may complain of awkwardness and fear of falling. Walking helps overcome these fears.

4. Encourage Kathy's independence and participation in decision making about her wardrobe, diet, daily hygiene, and schoolwork.

4. A teenager who is developing independence has a right to participate in decisions that affect her health, physical appearance, and cognitive development.

5. Offer positive, honest comments about Kathy's physical appearance with the brace in place.

5. Honest, positive comments about Kathy's appearance will help build self-esteem.

6. Assist Kathy's parents in accepting her independence by explaining the developmental tasks of adolescence. At the same time, remind them that they must be firm with Kathy if she balks at wearing the brace. Reemphasize that the only alternative to bracing is major surgery.

6. The parents face a seemingly contradictory task: accepting and promoting their daughter's emerging independence while insisting that she wear the brace. Further, the parents may feel sorry for Kathy and be tempted to allow her to remove the brace for special occasions. In these circumstances, the parents usually benefit from the nurse's guidance and support.

Evaluation

• Kathy and her parents comply with the bracing regimen, and the scoliosis does not progress.
• Kathy has a positive self-image.
• Kathy continues to develop independence.
• Kathy's parents support her need for independence while allowing her to be dependent when appropriate.
• Kathy maintains her friendships with peers, who accept her in a brace.
• Kathy returns for scheduled follow-up visits.

Cystic fibrosis

Cystic fibrosis of the pancreas (also known as fibrocystic disease of the pancreas and mucoviscidosis) is a generalized dysfunction of the exocrine glands characterized by thickened and tenacious secretions that occlude glandular ducts, causing dysfunction in many organ systems. It is a chronic, life-shortening disease, inherited as an autosomal recessive trait, that occurs in 1 of every 2,500 to 3,000 live births and primarily affects white children. Cystic fibrosis results from a genetic mutation of chromosome 7. Prenatal and carrier testing is now available.

The thickened, tenacious secretions of the mucous glands lining the respiratory tract plug the airways, resulting in progressive chronic obstructive pulmonary disease (COPD). In the GI tract, the thickened secretions may cause meconium ileus in the neonate and intestinal obstruction in the older child. Plugged pancreatic ducts lead to fibrosis of the pancreas, which ultimately reduces the amount of digestive enzymes reaching the stomach and small intestine. Bile also is thickened, resulting in cirrhosis of the liver and, eventually, portal hypertension. Diagnosis is confirmed by the sweat chloride test: sodium chloride levels are abnormally elevated in children with cystic fibrosis.

Major characteristics of cystic fibrosis are COPD and malnutrition. Treatment is aimed at improving respiratory function and nutrition and preventing respiratory infection. The average life expectancy is 27 years with respiratory involvement the leading cause of death.

Clinical situation   Phillip, age 16, was diagnosed as having cystic fibrosis of the pancreas at age 16 months and has been hospitalized for the condition many times. This time he is in acute respiratory distress, with an upper and lower respiratory tract infection. He has a fever of 101.8° F (38.8° C), a respiratory rate of 38 breaths/minute, and a pulse rate of 128 beats/minute. His skin is dusky, and the nail beds are cyanotic. Phillip has a barrel chest and supraclavicular and intercostal retractions. He is orthopneic, highly anxious, and restless. He is receiving oxygen by face mask.

Assessment

NURSING BEHAVIORS

1. Assess the level of Phillip's respiratory distress and infection, noting respiratory rate and depth; skin color; breath sounds; amount, color, and consistency of sputum; temperature; and clubbing of fingers and toes.

2. Assess Phillip's cardiac status, noting blood pressure and apical pulse rate, rhythm, and quality.

3. Assess Phillip's nutritional status, estimating the thickness of subcutaneous tissue and comparing his weight and height with growth chart measurements.

4. Assess Phillip's fluid and electrolyte balance.

5. Assess the family's ability to cope with the acute episode and their continuing ability to cope with chronic cystic fibrosis.

6. Assess Phillip's developmental level (see "Growth and development," pages 52 to 61).

NURSING RATIONALES

1. The child with cystic fibrosis has a chronic lung infection with acute episodes. The diminished respiratory excursion; dark, moist lungs; and mucoprotein provide ideal media for constant infection. Clubbing of fingers and toes stems from chronic hypoxia.

2. COPD will progress to cor pulmonale (right-sided heart failure), the usual cause of death in cystic fibrosis.

3. Diminished amounts of pancreatic enzymes result in malnutrition and malabsorption. The child will appear small for his age, thin and wasted, with little, if any, subcutaneous fat. He will have a distended abdomen, a voracious appetite, and pale, transparent skin and will be easily fatigued, displaying malaise, irritability, and lethargy.

4. Prevention of dehydration is important because dehydration thickens mucoid secretions.

5. This clarifies their need for support or counseling.

6. This assessment helps the nurse determine whether the client is meeting age-appropriate developmental tasks.

Nursing diagnoses
- Risk for infection related to malnutrition and thickened lung secretions
- Altered nutrition: Less than body requirements, related to an inability to digest food
- Activity intolerance related to an imbalance between oxygen supply and demand
- Ineffective airway clearance related to thick, tenacious mucus in tracheobronchial passages
- Altered family processes related to treatment demands and repeated hospitalizations
- Ineffective breathing patterns related to acute respiratory distress and chronic pulmonary obstruction

CHILD NURSING

Planning and goals

- Phillip will regain and maintain adequate ventilation.
- Phillip's fluid and electrolyte levels will return to normal.
- Phillip will be free from acute respiratory infection.
- Phillip's nutrition will be adequate to meet his needs.
- Phillip will continue to achieve age-appropriate developmental tasks.
- Phillip and his parents will continue to cope with chronic cystic fibrosis.

Implementation

NURSING BEHAVIORS

1. Monitor Phillip's vital signs every 2 to 4 hours or more often if indicated.

2. Perform aerosol therapy and postural drainage 2 to 4 times daily, starting the first session soon after Phillip awakens and the last one just before he goes to sleep. Schedule postural drainage before meals.

3. Observe and document the amount, color, and consistency of sputum from postural drainage and coughing episodes. Keep in mind the following special considerations for different age-groups:
- Children age 2 and under can't expectorate and will need suctioning.
- Older children may need encouragement to spit if they consider spitting socially unacceptable.
- Teenagers will suppress the cough and not expectorate for fear of offending someone of the opposite sex. They will also have bad breath from the chronic respiratory infection.

4. Administer antibiotics, as ordered, to combat the infection.

5. Administer pancreatic enzymes, as ordered, with meals and snacks; if the child can't swallow a capsule, open it and put the powder in a small amount of cold applesauce. Give a smaller amount if the child has constipation, a larger amount if he has diarrhea.

6. Administer vitamins A, D, E, and K in water-miscible form.

NURSING RATIONALES

1. This will detect respiratory distress, increasing infection, and cardiac problems.

2. Aerosol treatments—usually combining antibiotics, bronchodilators, and recombinant human DNASE—are followed by chest physiotherapy (CPT), positive expiratory pressure, or autogenic discharge. In CPT, all the pulmonary lobes (anterior, posterior, and lateral) should be percussed and vibrated to loosen and free the thick mucoid secretions. Postural drainage is performed before meals to prevent vomiting.

3. Documentation provides evidence of how well the infection is clearing. The most common infecting organisms are *Staphylococcus,* which colors the sputum yellow, and *Pseudomonas,* which colors the sputum green.

4. Thick mucoid secretions in the respiratory tract depress the cilia cells, resulting in potential infection and bronchial obstruction and ultimately progressing to COPD (with barrel chest) and cor pulmonale.

5. Pancreatic fibrosis diminishes pancreatic enzyme levels; these enzymes are necessary for digestion (lipase digests fat, amylase digests carbohydrates, and trypsin digests protein). Applesauce is high in cellulose and slows enzymatic action until the enzymes are in the stomach. The cold also slows enzymatic action.

6. Phillip can't use fat-soluble vitamins because he lacks enough bile to emulsify fat and enough lipase to digest it.

7. Administer adequate enzymes or lactulose, as ordered, to prevent constipation. Document the amount, color, consistency, and frequency of stools.

8. Encourage Phillip to follow a diet that supplies 100% to 150% of recommended daily allowances. Offer high-food-value snacks preceded by pancreatic enzymes.

9. Maintain Phillip's fluid and electrolyte balance. Monitor and report sodium and chloride laboratory values (the normal sodium value in sweat is 40 mEq/L or less; in cystic fibrosis, it rises to 60 mEq/L or more). Add salt supplements, if needed, in hot weather.

10. Help the family find continued financial and emotional support, as follows:

• Refer the family to public health nursing services for follow-up care after discharge.

• Refer the family to the Cystic Fibrosis Foundation for aid, and enroll the parents in a support group.

• Prepare the parents to help Phillip cope with probable sterility.

• Enlist the school nurse's aid with CPT, diet, and medication.

• Refer the family for genetic counseling; include parents, siblings, aunts, and uncles.

11. Assist Phillip in maintaining an age-appropriate developmental level, as follows:

• Encourage independence within the limits imposed by his condition.

• Allow Phillip to participate in decisions regarding care. Explain procedures, treatments, and routines directly and candidly. Approach him as an adult—do not condescend to or berate him.

7. Bowel obstruction is common because of inspissated stool. Rectal prolapse occurs in many young children and must be reduced quickly but gently before the anal sphincter impairs circulation.

8. If weight maintenance is problematic, a high-calorie, high-fat diet may be ordered. Many clients prefer high-food-value snacks to meals.

9. Dehydration, however slight, will cause even thicker mucous secretions in the respiratory tract as well as constipation in children with cystic fibrosis. The chloride level in sweat is two to four times normal, resulting in sodium and chloride depletion in hot weather.

10. Maintaining the health of a child with cystic fibrosis can deplete the family's financial reserves and drain their emotions.

• Public health nursing services can help the family identify and use community resources.

• The Cystic Fibrosis Foundation and other groups provide continued support for families as they cope with the disease's chronic progression.

• The thickened semen occludes the ducts so that sperm are contained in the testes; the result is testicular fibrosis and azoospermia. However, Phillip will not be impotent. (Women with cystic fibrosis are not sterile but do have difficulty conceiving because sperm cannot penetrate the thickened mucus plug in the cervical os.)

• The school nurse provides continuing care during school hours.

• Cystic fibrosis is inherited as an autosomal recessive trait.

11. Phillip is different from his peers and needs guidance in identifying ways in which he is the same. This will help him through the teen years, when peer relationships are most important.

• This promotes a feeling of control over his situation and helps him regain and maintain self-esteem.

• This will help him regain a sense of control.

• Encourage him to maintain contact with peers.

• Continued contact with other teenagers influences his identity formation.

• Encourage Phillip to continue schoolwork as his physical ability allows.

• Schoolwork provides opportunities for achievement and success and helps thwart feelings of failure.

• Encourage him to examine and discuss his feelings about illness and hospitalization.

• Expressing these feelings provides an outlet for his frustrations and may enable him to cope more effectively with his condition.

• Respect Phillip's privacy and modesty when providing care and in daily interactions with him.

• Privacy and modesty are important to teenagers, and they will respond more favorably to adults who respect their rights.

• Accept Phillip and his feelings.

• Acceptance reaffirms his importance and self-esteem.

12. Evaluate and reinforce the family's understanding and implementation of dietary needs, medication administration, and respiratory therapy.

12. This reassures the family that they can depend on continued professional care and provides opportunities to clarify misunderstandings about or intentional differences in the care they should provide at home.

Evaluation

• Phillip returns home with respiratory infection controlled.
• Phillip's nutritional intake results in slow, steady weight gain and meets his growth needs.
• Phillip and his parents perform aerosol therapy and CPT accurately and as frequently as necessary to prevent respiratory infection.
• Phillip and his parents regularly attend the Cystic Fibrosis Foundation support group.
• Phillip's parents state they will continue to seek medical care for respiratory infections or weight loss and will have Phillip see his physician routinely for preventive care.
• Phillip engages in age-appropriate behaviors.

Drugs commonly used in pediatric nursing

NAME OF DRUG	DOSE	ACTION	SIDE EFFECTS	NURSING CONSIDERATIONS
acetamino-phen (Tylenol)	*Children over 11 years:* Mild pain or fever: 325 to 650 mg P.O. every 4 to 6 hours. Maximum dosage should not exceed 4 g daily. *Children 11 years and under:* use the following P.O. dosing guidelines: 11 years, 480 mg/dose; 9 to 10 years, 400 mg/dose; 6 to 8 years, 320 mg/dose; 4 to 5 years, 240 mg/dose; 2 to 3 years, 160 mg/dose; 12 to 23 months, 120 mg/dose; 4 to 11 months, 80 mg/dose; up to 3 months, 40 mg/dose.	Nonnarcotic analgesic and antipyretic	• Rash • Urticaria • Severe liver damage with toxic doses	• This drug is contraindicated for repeated use in anemia, or renal or hepatic disease. • This drug has no significant anti-inflammatory effect. • Consult a physician before administering this drug to children under age 2. • This drug is only for short-term use; consult a physician if administering to a child for more than 5 days. • This drug may interfere with certain laboratory tests for urinary 5-hydroxyindolacetic acid. It also may produce false-positive decreases in blood-glucose levels in home monitoring systems using glucose reagent strips.
amoxicillin/ clavulanate potassium (Augmentin)	*Children weighing less than 88 lb (40 kg):* 20 to 40 mg/kg/day, given in divided doses every 8 hours. (Those weighing 88 lb or more may receive the adult dosage.)	Broad-spectrum bactericidal analog of ampicillin (Clavulanic acid increased amoxicillin effectiveness by inactivating beta-lactamases, which destroy amoxicillin.) Effective against lower respiratory tract infections, otitis media, sinusitis, infections of the skin and skin structure, and urinary tract infections	• Nausea • Diarrhea • Leukopenia • Hypersensitivity • Anaphylaxis	• Assess the child's history for allergic reactions to penicillin. • Obtain specimens for culture and sensitivity tests before drug therapy begins. • Periodically assess the child's complete white blood cell count.
cromolyn sodium (Intal)	*Children age 5 and over:* Two metered sprays from an inhaler four times daily at regular intervals. *Children ages 2 and over:* 20 mg/ 2 ml aqueous solution through a nebulizer four times daily at regular intervals.	Inhibits the release of histamine and slow-reacting substance of anaphylaxis; primarily used to control perennial asthma and as adjunct to therapy after an acute attack	• Dizziness • Headache • Irritation of the throat and trachea • Coughing • Esophagitis • Wheezing • Nausea • Dysuria and urinary frequency	• The drug is contraindicated in acute asthma or status asthmaticus. • Discontinue if the client develops eosinophilic pneumonia. • Use only after an acute episode has been controlled, the airway is clear, and the client can inhale.

(continued)

CHILD NURSING

Drugs commonly used in pediatric nursing *(continued)*

NAME OF DRUG	DOSE	ACTION	SIDE EFFECTS	NURSING CONSIDERATIONS
digoxin (Lanoxin)	Initial dose: Varies depending on child's age and weight. Maintenance dose: for premature infants, 20% to 30% of the initial dose, in two divided doses every 12 hours. For full-term infants and children, 25% to 35% of the initial dose, in two divided doses every 12 hours.	Strengthens and slows myocardial contraction	• Anorexia, nausea, vomiting • Blurred vision, photophobia, diplopia • Arrhythmias • Hypotension • Fatigue, muscle weakness, agitation • Headache	• Digoxin (rather than digitoxin) is usually administered to children because its more rapid onset and excretion reduces toxicity more quickly. • The therapeutic serum level is 0.8 to 2.0 ng/ml. • Carefully calculate divided oral doses. • Count the child's apical pulse rate for 1 minute. • Withhold the drug if the apical pulse rate slows. • Observe the child carefully for signs of toxicity.
theophylline (Bronkodyl)	Varies, depending on the administration route and form used	Relaxes bronchial, smooth-muscle, and pulmonary blood vessels	• Restlessness, dizziness, headache, seizures, muscle twitching • Increased respiratory rate from palpitations, flushing, and marked hypotension • Nausea, vomiting, anorexia	• The drug interacts with erythromycin and cimetidine to decrease clearance of theophylline by the liver, which increases the serum drug level and leads to toxicity. • The desired serum drug level is 10 to 20 mg/ml; toxicity occurs at levels greater than 20 mg/ml. • Use cautiously in young children, whose metabolism rates vary widely. • Monitor the child's vital signs and urine output.

Adult nursing

Introduction

This section reviews nursing care of adult clients with physiologic health problems, which are organized by body system for easy reference. As in other sections of this book, the text follows the nursing process format to help you solve the nursing problems presented. Selected clinical situations (case studies) represent their high incidence among hospitalized clients or demonstrate nursing care principles essential to safe practice. These situations, in our experience, are those most likely to appear on NCLEX-RN. The nursing diagnoses accompanying each situation are appropriate for the data presented and represent those likely to be discovered during assessment. They are not meant to be all-inclusive for that client or that health problem.

Before you begin reading this section, consider reviewing entries on the nursing process, acid-base balance, fluid and electrolyte balance, shock, immobility, and perioperative nursing.

Glossary

Adrenergic—nerve fibers in the sympathetic nervous system that release norepinephrine

Alopecia—hair loss

Ankylosis—fixation or immobility of a joint, usually from cartilage destruction

Ataxia—poorly coordinated muscle movement

Cellulitis—diffuse, often infectious inflammation of skin and underlying tissue, characterized by pain, redness, edema, and heat

Endogenous—coming from within the body

Extracorporeal—occurring outside the body

Hemiparesis—muscle weakness in half of the body

Hypercapnia—elevated partial pressure of carbon dioxide (PCO_2) in the blood

Intermittent claudication—periodic pain and lameness in a limb, brought on by activity and relieved by rest, commonly found in arterial peripheral vascular disease

Ischemia—decreased blood supply to a body part caused by an obstruction or constriction in a blood vessel

Leukopenia—abnormally low white blood cell count (below 5,000)

Mydriatic—drug that dilates the pupil

Nystagmus—rapid, involuntary rolling or vertical movement of the eyeballs

Oliguria—abnormally low urine output (less than 500 ml/day) such that metabolic wastes cannot be excreted

Osteomyelitis—infection of the bone and bone marrow

Palliative—designed to relieve symptoms rather than cure a condition

Paresthesia—abnormal sensation (such as numbness, tingling, or burning) that lacks an objective cause

Stomatitis—inflammation of the oral mucous membrane

Tetany—twitching, cramps, and muscle spasms caused by hypocalcemia

CARDIOVASCULAR SYSTEM

Angina pectoris

Angina pectoris—chest pain that results from myocardial ischemia—is the most common symptom of coronary artery disease (CAD), the term for cardiac conditions that result from myocardial ischemia, usually secondary to atherosclerosis.

Invasive interventions for CAD include percutaneous transluminal coronary angioplasty (PTCA). Under fluoroscopy, a balloon-tip catheter is placed in the coronary artery at the site of the defect, and the balloon is inflated to compress the plaque. If this proves unsuccessful, the client will require a coronary artery bypass graft (CABG), which uses either the saphenous vein or the internal mammary artery to bypass the occluded site. This surgery requires use of a heart-lung machine; postoperatively, the client will be cared for in the intensive care unit.

The following clinical situation focuses on client teaching to help the client cope with angina pectoris.

Clinical situation

Robert Brown, age 55, is a lumber company manager who has had several attacks of substernal chest pain, which his physician has diagnosed as angina pectoris. Mr. Brown has a wife and three children.

Assessment

NURSING BEHAVIORS	NURSING RATIONALES
1. Assess Mr. Brown's pain pattern (see *Ischemic pain patterns*).	**1.** Although anginal pain patterns vary among clients, the same pattern usually recurs in a given individual. The most common pain pattern develops to the left of the sternum and radiates down the left arm to the little finger.
2. Identify situations (for example, physical exertion, emotional arousal, overeating) that precipitate Mr. Brown's anginal episodes.	**2.** Physical exertion, such as exercise, increases demands on coronary circulation. Coronary arteries cannot transport enough oxygenated blood to the myocardium because of narrowed lumina. Emotional arousal stimulates the sympathetic nervous system, which, in turn, causes the heart to beat faster. Narrowed coronary artery lumina impede prompt delivery of oxygen to the heart. To aid digestion, blood circulating to the gastrointestinal tract increases, decreasing supply to the heart.
3. Assess Mr. Brown's lifestyle for stress related to such areas as job, family, and social relationships.	**3.** Persistent sympathetic nervous system stimulation causes the heart to beat faster.
4. Determine whether cold either causes or increases chest pain.	**4.** Cold temperatures stimulate vasoconstriction of the blood vessels.
5. Determine what relieves Mr. Brown's pain.	**5.** Immediate relief of a stressful situation decreases demand on the heart. Warmth causes vasodilation, which increases the blood supply to the heart.

Ischemic pain patterns

Ischemic pain experienced during a myocardial infarction radiates in various directions, as illustrated here.

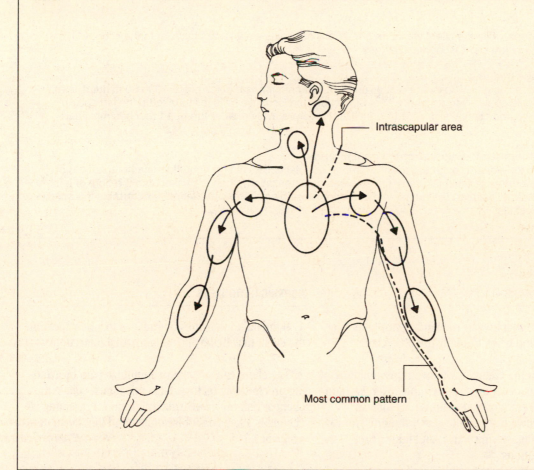

Intrascapular area

Most common pattern

---

6. Determine whether Mr. Brown smokes and, if so, how much.

6. Smoking causes arterial spasms.

7. Assess Mr. Brown's intake of high-fat foods as well as his overall caloric intake.

7. Obesity and elevated serum cholesterol contribute to atherosclerosis.

8. Analyze electrocardiogram (ECG) results and compare with baseline data in Mr. Brown's medical record. (See *Diagnosing angina,* page 436.)

8. A reduction in oxygenated blood flow to the heart may cause ECG changes—usually changes in the ST segment or T-wave.

Nursing diagnoses
- Altered health maintenance related to inadequate knowledge regarding ischemic condition and dietary and drug management
- Activity intolerance related to ischemic attacks

Planning and goals
- Mr. Brown will comply with the treatment regimen.
- Mr. Brown will alter his lifestyle to reduce chest pain episodes.

Diagnosing angina

Diagnostic tests used to evaluate the client with angina pectoris include the electrocardiographic (ECG) stress test, radioisotope imaging, and cardiac catheterization with coronary angiography.

Stress test
An ECG is done while the client walks on a treadmill or pedals a stationary bicycle. In the client with angina, the ECG may show ischemic changes.

Radioisotope imaging
The client receives an I.V. injection of thallium-201. Scanning, which takes place 10 to 60 minutes later, may show "cold spots"—areas where poor blood flow and ischemic cells fail to take up the isotope. In *stress imaging,* the client walks on a treadmill and receives thallium after the heart reaches maximal stress.

Cardiac catheterization and coronary angiography
A catheter is threaded through the client's femoral or antecubital vein (in right-sided catheterization) or through the femoral or brachial artery (in left-sided catheterization), then is passed into the right or left side of the heart. Dye then is injected into coronary vessels and X-rays are taken to determine the condition of the vessels.

Implementation

NURSING BEHAVIORS

1. Teach Mr. Brown how to recognize symptoms (his pain pattern) and when to notify the physician.

2. Discuss with the client how to avoid precipitating factors (such as heavy meals, strenuous exercise, and highly charged emotional situations), as follows:
• Teach Mr. Brown ways to alleviate symptoms; for example, by resting, staying warm, and taking prescribed medications.
• Teach him to reduce stress by identifying stress-producing factors or situations and changing them when possible.
• Identify the activity level that doesn't cause angina.
• Urge him to space activities (meals, snow shoveling, lawn mowing, sex) that might precipitate angina if performed over a short time.

3. Review with Mr. Brown how to take his medications and how to cope with their side effects, as follows:
• Teach Mr. Brown to take vasodilators, such as nitrates, as prescribed. Instruct him to prevent postural hypotension by changing positions slowly.
• Teach Mr. Brown to take beta blockers, such as propranolol (Inderal), as prescribed. Teach him to monitor his pulse rate for bradycardia, and tell him to stop taking the drug and notify his physician if his rate falls below 60 beats/minute.

NURSING RATIONALES

1. If the pain intensifies or radiates to a new location, the client may be having a myocardial infarction.

2. The client can prevent or minimize pain by avoiding precipitating factors. Ischemic attacks place the client at risk for myocardial infarction. Preventing ischemia is a key goal of treatment and long-term management.

3. The client must have thorough knowledge of his medication regimen.
• At the first sign of ischemia and before engaging in activities that cause anginal pain, the client should take short-acting sublingual nitroglycerin (3 tablets 5 minutes apart as needed) or translingual spray. Longer-acting oral agents are used to provide sustained vasodilation.
• Beta blockers reduce the client's heart rate, thereby decreasing cardiac workload, oxygen demands, and ischemia.

• Teach Mr. Brown to take calcium channel blockers, such as nifedipine (Procardia) and diltiazem (Cardizem), as prescribed.

• These drugs decrease myocardial workload by impairing calcium ion transport, decreasing contractile (inotropic) force and rate (chronotropic).

4. Encourage the client to stop or reduce smoking, if applicable.

4. Tobacco consumption causes arterial spasms.

5. Explain the need for dietary changes (for example, elimination of high-cholesterol, high-calorie foods), if ordered.

5. Weight loss reduces heart strain in an overweight client; reduced cholesterol intake may prevent further atherosclerosis, in which the arteries become clogged with fatty deposits.

Evaluation

• Mr. Brown describes lifestyle changes he is making to help prevent anginal episodes.
• Mr. Brown understands the purpose of vasodilators; can state the dosage, administration method, and common side effects of the drug prescribed for him; and has agreed to comply with the medication regimen at home.

Myocardial infarction

Myocardial infarction (MI) is the death of myocardial tissue from decreased blood flow to myocardial cells. It is the leading cause of death in coronary artery disease; as many as 40% of all clients die before reaching the hospital after onset of infarction. Early treatment (in 3 to 6 hours of onset), including bed rest, oxygen therapy, antiarrhythmic therapy, and thrombolytic therapy, greatly diminishes the risk of death. The following clinical situation focuses on nursing care for a client with MI.

Clinical situation

Rita Harris, age 54, is the assistant director of nursing at a large hospital. Married and the mother of three children, Mrs. Harris has a history of angina pectoris. Today her pain is severe and radiates down the left arm. After being admitted to the hospital with a diagnosis of MI, she is placed on an electrocardiogram (ECG). (*Note:* After an uncomplicated MI, the client receives care in a coronary care unit for the first 2 or 3 days, then is transferred to a stepdown or general unit for 5 to 7 days. The goal should be to have the client discharged from the acute-care setting by day 7.)

Assessment
NURSING BEHAVIORS

NURSING RATIONALES

1. Assess the client's vital signs, checking blood pressure and pulse rates bilaterally. Be particularly alert for a rapid pulse rate and decreased blood pressure. Note the client's temperature.

1. A rapid pulse rate and decreased blood pressure indicate cardiogenic shock (see "Shock," pages 103 to 108). Fever may develop within the first 24 hours as a generalized response to inflammation.

2. Assess the location, radiation, quality, and precipitating factors of the chest pain.

2. Myocardial oxygen deprivation results in chest pain. MI produces a crushing or stabbing pain more severe than anginal pain and radiating over a larger area. Rest and nitroglycerin fail to relieve it.

3. Obtain a current ECG rhythm strip.

3. ECG recordings document ischemia during chest pain episodes and can identify rhythm changes consistent with MI.

4. Ask Mrs. Harris to describe her lifestyle. Inquire about stress related to work, family, and social relationships.

4. Stress stimulates the sympathetic nervous system, thereby increasing the heart rate.

5. Identify the client's support persons (family members, friends, coworkers), and enlist their aid in comforting Mrs. Harris, if she wishes.

5. Emotional support from family, friends, and colleagues can be therapeutic for a client in crisis.

6. Determine what family members know about the client's problem, and assess their anxiety level.

6. Identifying their need for information helps the nurse develop interventions to reduce the family's anxiety.

7. Review laboratory data for the following serum enzyme changes: creatine kinase (CK; rises within 6 hours) and lactate dehydrogenase (LD; onset 12 to 48 hours). Also review white blood cell (WBC) count.

7. Myocardial tissue necrosis will result in elevated serum enzyme levels and WBC values. CK-MB-isoenzyme is specific to the myocardium; LD is specific to myocardial cells.

Nursing diagnoses	• Pain related to myocardial ischemia and tissue death • Anxiety related to current health crisis • Activity intolerance related to ischemia • Constipation related to immobility and morphine administration
Planning and goals	• Mrs. Harris will not develop preventable complications. • Mrs. Harris and her family will understand the care she requires and will learn to cope with lifestyle changes necessitated by her condition.

Implementation
NURSING BEHAVIORS

NURSING RATIONALES

Inpatient management
1. Evaluate Mrs. Harris's level of pain by having her rate her pain on a 1-to-10 scale. Administer analgesics (typically morphine sulphate), as ordered. Evaluate medication effectiveness.

1. Morphine relieves acute pain and also has a sedative effect. Pain relief is a priority because pain increases the work of the heart and leads to increased ischemia.

2. Place Mrs. Harris on continuous cardiac monitoring. Obtain rhythm strips at least every shift, or as indicated.

2. Myocardial tissue death may cause arrhythmias. The client is at risk for ventricular fibrillation, which may follow premature ventricular contractions and ventricular tachycardia.

3. Monitor Mrs. Harris's vital signs and heart and breath sounds. Note possible complications of MI.

3. Blood pressure may rise from stress or fall from cardiogenic shock. A weak, rapid pulse also may indicate shock. The respiratory rate may rise from anxiety or may decrease from morphine administration. Crackles (rales) may indicate pulmonary edema. A third heart sound (S_3) and fourth heart sound (S_4) may indicate impending congestive heart failure.

4. Administer oxygen, as ordered. (Usually, oxygen is given by nasal cannula at 2 to 6 liters/minute.)

5. Maintain the I.V. line as ordered for fluid therapy, or maintain a heparin lock for medications.

6. Monitor Mrs. Harris's fluid intake and output every hour until she is stabilized, then every 8 hours. Weigh her daily. Observe for dependent edema and jugular vein distention.

7. Maintain Mrs. Harris on bed rest in semi-Fowler's position (most likely for the first 24 to 48 hours; then progressive ambulation is started).

8. Take measures to prevent complications of immobility, as follows:

• Change the client's position every 2 hours except at night.

• Provide a bedside commode.

• Administer stool softeners and mild laxatives.

9. Teach Mrs. Harris to avoid the Valsalva maneuver when turning in bed or when having a bowel movement.

10. Apply elastic (TED) support stockings to the client's legs (usually up to the thighs); instruct Mrs. Harris not to cross her legs or wear constrictive clothing. Show her how to do ankle pushes.

11. As Mrs. Harris convalesces, observe her tolerance for sitting up, standing, and walking (caution her to move slowly); monitor her blood pressure, pulse rate, and ECG rhythm for changes.

4. Oxygen administration improves oxygen supply to the myocardium, thereby decreasing ischemia.

5. An I.V. line may be used to administer thrombolytic agents (such as streptokinase or alteplase [tissue plasminogen activator, or t-PA]) within 3 to 6 hours after an MI. The client may need I.V. medications, such as lidocaine, to treat arrhythmias; nitroglycerin to treat ischemia; and a digitalis glycoside, dobutamine, and other drugs to treat heart failure, cardiogenic shock, and other complications.

6. These measures help determine the client's fluid balance status. If she is dehydrated, her urine output and weight may drop. Edema, jugular vein distention, and increased weight may indicate volume overload.

7. Bed rest reduces the client's oxygen demand. Semi-Fowler's position lowers the diaphragm, improves lung expansion, and eliminates pooling in the pulmonary vessels.

8. Bed rest predisposes the client to complications of immobility.

• Frequent position changes decrease the potential for complications related to immobility.

• Using a bedside commode may reduce straining during a bowel movement.

• These medications will prevent straining during defecation, thereby lightening the heart's workload.

9. Holding one's breath, a component of the Valsalva maneuver, increases intrathoracic pressure, thereby decreasing blood flow to the heart and elevating venous pressure.

10. TED support stockings decompress superficial blood vessels, thereby preventing thrombus formation. Crossing the legs or wearing constrictive clothes can impede circulation. Ankle pushes promote venous return in the legs.

11. Increasing the client's activity is desirable, but it can cause arrhythmias and postural hypotension.

ADULT NURSING

12. Maintain an atmosphere conducive to mental and physical rest by helping Mrs. Harris with hygiene, ensuring a quiet and calm environment, remaining with her as much as possible, and organizing activities to provide uninterrupted rest and sleep periods.

12. Mental and physical rest reduces the heart's workload as well as the client's anxiety.

13. Observe Mrs. Harris for anxiety, depression, and denial.

13. These psychological reactions, common after an MI, must be recognized so that staff members can implement or make arrangements for psychosocial interventions.

14. Explain treatments and unfamiliar hospital routines and settings to Mrs. Harris and family members. Encourage them to ask questions, to express their anxieties and fears about MI, and to identify noteworthy stressors in their lives. Refer them to appropriate community resources for additional help, if necessary.

14. Anxiety stimulates the sympathetic nervous system, which, in turn, stimulates the heart; if family members are highly anxious or overly stressed, the client's anxiety may intensify, aggravating the heart problem. Receiving clear explanations of treatments and procedures usually helps alleviate anxiety for family members as well as for the client. In discussing their fears and stressors, the client and family provide information useful in identifying resources that can offer reassurance and relieve stress.

15. Teach Mrs. Harris to avoid overexertion by spacing activities and by increasing her activity level gradually.

15. The amount of exertion that precipitates angina varies for each client, depending on the severity of the client's condition. Maintaining a sensible balance between rest and activity helps prevent overexertion.

16. Review any prescribed dietary instructions, including reduced caloric and cholesterol intake (see *Recommended diet to lower cholesterol*).

16. Low-calorie foods promote weight reduction, which lessens heart strain. A reduced cholesterol intake helps lower the amount of cholesterol deposits in arteries and other blood vessels.

17. Assist Mrs. Harris and her family in coping with restrictions imposed by MI.

17. Activity and dietary restrictions can diminish the client's sense of independence and may cause resentment among other family members if these restrictions curtail their own activities. The family may need the nurse's guidance in learning to make the most of necessary lifestyle changes.

18. Explain dosages and effects of anticoagulant medications, as follows:

18. Anticoagulants can produce severe adverse reactions; client and family teaching is essential to prevent serious harm.

• With heparin therapy (rapid onset, short-acting effect), observe for signs of bleeding, such as blood in urine or stool, bleeding gums, bruises, and wounds. Discontinue heparin therapy at the first sign of bleeding. The common antidote is protamine sulfate. *Note:* Check prothrombin time (PT) or international normalized ratio (INR) to assess the effectiveness of oral anticoagulant therapy. Normal PT is 11 to 12.5 seconds; the therapeutic range for PT is 1.5 to 2 times the normal PT. The recommended target range for an INR for a client on warfarin (Coumadin) is 2 to 3 (in

• Understanding thoroughly the effects of heparin ensures its effective use and prevents adverse reactions.

Recommended diet to lower cholesterol

Clients can significantly reduce elevated cholesterol levels by following sound nutritional guidelines. As with any sensible diet, total caloric intake may vary widely among individuals but should not exceed the amount needed to achieve and maintain a desirable weight. Nutritionists generally recommend the following percentages of total caloric intake (with primary sources in parentheses):
• Carbohydrates (fruits, vegetables, legumes, whole grains), 50% to 60%
• Protein (dairy products, eggs, meats, fish), up to 20%
• Fat (total fat intake should be less than 30%)
—Saturated fat (beef, bacon, cheese, coconut oil), less than 10%
—Polyunsaturated fat (corn, cottonseed, and safflower oils), up to 10%
—Monounsaturated fat (peanut, olive, and canola oils), 10% to 15%.
The client with a high cholesterol level should limit fat intake to less than 300 mg/day; this can be accomplished by including plenty of low-cholesterol foods in the diet and by avoiding such high-cholesterol foods as organ meats, eggs, and shellfish—all of which contain significant amounts.

LOW-CHOLESTEROL FOODS	HIGH-CHOLESTEROL FOODS
• Fish (except shellfish), skinless chicken and turkey, lean meats • Egg whites (2 whites = 1 whole egg in recipes), cholesterol-free egg substitutes • Skim or 1% fat milk and buttermilk (liquid, powdered, or evaporated); nonfat and low-fat yogurt and cottage cheese (1% or 2% fat); low-fat, farmer, and pot cheeses (2 to 6 g of fat/ounce); low-fat or "light" cream cheese and sour cream; sherbet and sorbet • Fresh, frozen, canned, and dried fruits and vegetables • Whole-grain breads and cereals (oatmeal, whole wheat, rye, bran, multigrain); rice; pasta; angel food cake, low-fat crackers and cookies, homemade baked goods using unsaturated oils sparingly • Baking cocoa; unsaturated vegetable oil; olive, canola, safflower, sesame, soybean, and sunflower oil; margarine, shortening, mayonnaise, and salad dressing made with unsaturated oil	• Shellfish, fatty cuts of beef, lamb, pork, spareribs, organ meats, cold cuts, sausage, hot dogs, bacon, sardines, roe • Egg yolks • Whole milk (4% fat; regular, evaporated, or condensed), cream, half and half, imitation milk products, most non-dairy creamers, whipped toppings; whole-milk yogurt and cottage cheese (4% fat); all natural cheeses (blue, roquefort, camembert, cheddar, swiss), cream cheeses, sour cream; ice cream • Vegetables prepared in butter, cream, and other sauces • Homemade breads in which eggs are a major ingredient; egg noodles; commercially baked goods (pies, cakes, doughnuts, croissants, pastries, muffins, biscuits, crackers, cookies) • Chocolate; butter; coconut, palm, or palm kernel oil; lard; bacon fat; dressings made with egg yolk; coconut

Source: National Cholesterol Education Program; National Heart, Lung, and Blood Institute; National Institutes of Health (NIH Publication No. 92-2920, April 1992).

clients with mechanical heart valves or those who have recently experienced an MI, an INR of 2.5 to 3.5 is desired).

• With dicumarol and warfarin therapy (slow onset, longer-acting effect), watch for signs of hemorrhage. Tell the client to stop the medication at the first sign of bleeding and to call the physician. *Note:* Check PT to assess effectiveness of oral anticoagulant therapy (normal PT: 11 to 12.5 seconds; therapeutic range PT: 1.5 to 2 times normal PT).

• Because of the longer action of these drugs, an antidote, such as vitamin K (Mephyton), may be needed to prevent hemorrhage. The client should not take aspirin (it prolongs PT) and should avoid liver and dark vegetables (these are high in vitamin K).

ADULT NURSING

Home care management and rehabilitation

1. Assist Mrs. Harris with continued progressive activity, using the amount of metabolic equivalents (METS) exerted by each activity.

1. In phase I (the inpatient phase) of cardiac rehabilitation, the client's activities are low (1 to 3 METS). In phase II (early rehabilitation usually begun after discharge), the client begins a supervised walking program, with the goal of 2 miles in less than 60 minutes. In phase III, the client participates in an ongoing long-term cardiac rehabilitation exercise program.

2. Give Mrs. Harris appropriate instructions on resuming sexual activity and returning to work. Review psychosocial concerns that may arise.

2. After an uncomplicated MI, clients usually can resume sexual activity in 4 to 8 weeks (once they can comfortably climb one or two flights of stairs) and can return to work in 8 to 9 weeks. Depression is common for up to 1 year after an MI. Relationship problems may develop if the spouse is overprotective.

Evaluation

• Mrs. Harris can explain how and when to take her medications and understands their possible side effects.
• Mrs. Harris and her family describe how they plan to increase her activities gradually and to balance her activity with rest periods.
• Mrs. Harris experiences no complications.

Congestive heart failure

Congestive heart failure (CHF) results when the right or left ventricle cannot contract effectively enough to supply tissues and organs with adequate blood; the blood then backs up in the atria and in veins leading to the atria. The major causes of left ventricular failure include hypertension, diseased mitral or aortic valves or both, and arteriosclerotic heart disease. The major causes of right ventricular failure include right ventricular infarction, diseased tricuspid or pulmonary valves or both, and pulmonary disease. The following clinical situation focuses on nursing care of the client with CHF.

Clinical situation

Karl Campbell, age 55, had a severe myocardial infarction. Despite treatment, he experienced distended neck veins, nausea and vomiting, oliguria, and extreme weakness. He is medically diagnosed as having CHF. Mr. Campbell has a wife and three children, two of whom are in college. He works as an auto mechanic.

Assessment
NURSING BEHAVIORS

1. Assess for signs and symptoms of left ventricular failure: dyspnea, orthopnea, cyanosis, paroxysmal nocturnal dyspnea (respiratory distress caused by fluid in the lungs and occurring after sleeping in a reclining position), irritability, restlessness, confusion, extreme weakness and fatigue, oliguria, and anuria.

NURSING RATIONALES

1. Because the left ventricle cannot effectively pump the blood entering it, the blood backs up in the pulmonary veins, causing pulmonary congestion and respiratory distress symptoms. Irritability, restlessness, and confusion result from an insufficient blood supply to the cerebrum (hypoxia). Extreme weakness and fatigue result from decreased circulation of systemic cells, which do not receive adequate oxygen. Urinary problems reflect decreased circulation to the kidneys, which leads to renal failure.

2. Assess for signs and symptoms of right ventricular failure: distended neck veins, abdominal pain in the right upper quadrant, anorexia, nausea, vomiting, bloating, cool and cyanotic extremities, and dependent (ankle or sacral) edema.

2. Decreased right ventricular effectiveness increases the pressure in the vena cava (resulting in distended neck veins) and in the hepatic veins (causing congestion in the liver that produces abdominal pain in the right upper quadrant). Anorexia, nausea, vomiting, and bloating indicate GI tract congestion. Cool and cyanotic extremities suggest venous congestion. Dependent edema occurs from increased hydrostatic pressure in the capillaries, which leads to swelling at the lowest point of a body part.

3. Help Mr. Campbell identify stressors in his life.

3. Because stress increases the heart's workload, the client needs physical and mental rest.

4. Determine what Mr. Campbell and his family know about his heart problem.

4. This assessment provides baseline information for health teaching.

5. Assess Mr. Campbell's relationships with family members, friends, and coworkers.

5. The client will need support and understanding from these people during his convalescence.

6. Assess Mr. Campbell's anxiety level and those of other family members.

6. Anxiety among family members can intensify any stress or anxiety already felt by the client. A thorough assessment enables the nurse to plan appropriate interventions that will benefit all family members.

Diagnostic evaluation	• *Chest X-ray:* shows cardiac enlargement and increased pulmonary congestion • *Arterial blood gas studies* (normal arterial blood oxygen saturation, 95% to 100%): decreased levels suggest CHF • *Pulmonary function test* (determines vital capacity): reduced vital capacity is a signpost of CHF • *Echocardiogram:* uses ultrasound to determine structure of the ventricles • *Radionuclide angiography:* measures left ventricular ejection fraction to determine the severity of ventricular damage • *Other diagnostic tests (liver enzymes, blood urea nitrogen, creatinine):* may be ordered depending on symptoms
Nursing diagnoses	• Fluid volume excess related to impaired cardiac output • Activity intolerance related to impaired oxygenation to tissues • Altered health maintenance related to lack of knowledge about diet and lifestyle changes
Planning and goals	• Mr. Campbell and his family will understand how to cope with lifestyle changes necessitated by his condition. • Mr. Campbell will not develop preventable complications. • Mr. Campbell will understand how to continue his therapy at home.

Implementation

NURSING BEHAVIORS

NURSING RATIONALES

1. Promote complete mental and physical rest for Mr. Campbell.

1. Mental stress and physical exertion make the heart work harder.

Sodium-restricted diets

Mild (2 to 3 g/day)	• Use table salt sparingly in cooking (1/2 tsp or less daily); do not use to season foods after cooking. • Avoid preserved and processed foods high in sodium (such as pickles, olives, bacon, chips, canned soups).
Moderate (1 g/day)	• Do not use table salt for cooking or seasoning. • Avoid all preserved and processed foods, if possible. If canned products and baked goods can't be avoided, be sure they are sodium-free. • Consume milk and meat in moderation.
Strict (500 mg/day)	• Do not use table salt for cooking or seasoning. • Do not eat preserved or processed foods. • Limit consumption of milk, meat, and eggs.
All levels	• Read all food and beverage labels carefully. • Avoid all foods and ingredients unusually high in sodium (such as soy sauce, bouillon, and baking soda).

Adapted from William, S. *Nutrition and Diet Therapy* (7th ed.). St. Louis: Mosby, Inc., 1993.

2. Administer oxygen as ordered.

2. This will increase the oxygen supply to the cells.

3. Keep Mr. Campbell in high Fowler's position, and place the feet lower than the sacrum.

3. High Fowler's position helps decrease venous return, increase lung expansion, and prevent pulmonary edema. Keeping the feet lower than the sacrum causes fluid to collect in the ankles and legs, thereby reducing sacral edema and skin breakdown.

4. Apply thromboembolytic disease (TED) support stockings to the legs. Remove the stockings several times daily, provide thorough skin care to the legs and feet, and apply lotion to prevent dryness.

4. TED stockings support the veins in edematous legs, preventing skin breakdown and decreasing venous stasis.

5. Take measures to prevent complications of immobility.

5. Bed rest predisposes the client to complications from immobility (see "Immobility," pages 119 and 120).

6. Monitor Mr. Campbell's fluid intake to maintain urine output at 30 ml/hour. Space fluids to prevent thirst.

6. Excess fluid intake increases the heart's workload; insufficient intake can lead to dehydration and renal failure.

7. Monitor fluid and electrolyte balance hourly, especially if Mr. Campbell is receiving diuretics.

7. Diuretics can cause dehydration.

8. Put Mr. Campbell on a sodium-restricted diet (see *Sodium-restricted diets*). If he has nausea, vomiting, or diarrhea, provide bland, low-residue foods. Refer him to a registered dietitian as needed.

8. Reducing sodium intake helps decrease fluid retention. A bland low-residue diet relieves distress from nausea, vomiting, and diarrhea.

9. Use strategies to prevent thrombophlebitis.

9. See "Postoperative period," page 125, for specific strategies and rationales.

10. Observe Mr. Campbell for a productive cough, copious white- or pink-tinged sputum, crackles, dyspnea, orthopnea, and extreme anxiety.

10. These are symptoms of pulmonary edema, a common complication of CHF (see "Pulmonary edema").

11. Administer a diuretic, such as furosemide (Lasix), as ordered (initially as an I.V. bolus, then orally). If the physician prescribes a potassium-depleting diuretic, also administer potassium supplements and make sure Mr. Campbell's diet includes potassium-rich foods. As part of diuretic therapy, weigh the client daily, and monitor serum potassium levels.

11. Diuretics reduce fluid volume, which helps lighten the heart's workload. The client's weight reflects fluid loss or gain, a reliable indicator of the therapy's effectiveness. (*Note:* A pint of water weighs 1 lb.)

12. For rapid digitalization, administer a digitalis glycoside, such as digoxin (Lanoxin) or digitoxin (Crystodigin), as ordered (initially as an I.V. bolus, then orally). Before administering the drug, measure Mr. Campbell's pulse rate, and notify the physician if it is not higher than 60 beats/minute.

12. Digitalis glycosides strengthen heart muscle contractions (thereby improving cardiac output) and slow impulse conduction (thereby decreasing the heart rate). Because of the latter effect, the client's pulse rate should be higher than 60 beats/minute before drug administration. Side effects of digitalis glycosides include anorexia, nausea, vomiting, headache, heart block, arrhythmias, and yellow vision.

13. Administer vasodilators such as angiotensin-converting enzyme inhibitors, nitrates, and calcium channel blockers, as ordered.

13. Use of these drugs in clients with CHF is increasing. By reducing vascular resistance, vasodilators improve stroke volume and cardiac output.

14. Before discharge, prepare Mr. Campbell for self-care at home. Make sure he understands the importance and major effects of digitalis glycosides, diuretics, and potassium supplements. Show him how to measure his pulse rate, and tell him to notify the physician and withhold digitalis glycoside therapy if the rate falls below 60 beats/minute. Urge him to report dyspnea or pulmonary edema immediately.

14. Diuretics may lower the client's serum potassium levels; low levels potentiate the action of digitalis glycosides. An overdose of a digitalis glycoside can cause heart block. Dyspnea and pulmonary edema—symptoms of left ventricular failure—warrant immediate intervention.

15. Help Mr. Campbell identify current and potential financial resources.

15. Worrying about his hospitalization and medication costs (and perhaps his children's college tuition) will only intensify the client's stress and anxiety, especially if he will not be returning to work right away. By helping him explore potential resources (medical insurance, college scholarships, financial aid from community agencies), the nurse may alleviate many of the client's financial concerns.

Evaluation

- Mr. Campbell accurately describes his dietary restrictions and medication regimen, understands their purpose, and plans to abide by them.
- Mr. Campbell did not experience any complications.
- Mr. Campbell knows which symptoms to report to the physician.

ADULT NURSING

Pulmonary edema

Acute pulmonary edema—excess fluid in the lungs, either in the alveoli or in the interstitial spaces—can result from congestive heart failure, myocardial infarction, circulatory overload, lung injuries (for example, shock and pulmonary embolism), and allergic reactions. The following clinical situation focuses on emergency nursing care of a client with pulmonary edema.

Clinical situation

Dora Chandler, age 72, developed congestive heart failure as a complication of myocardial infarction. She has severe dyspnea and blood-tinged, frothy sputum. Hospital staff members have noted her anxiety, and she recently told a nurse that she felt panicky. Her medical diagnosis is pulmonary edema.

Assessment

NURSING BEHAVIORS	NURSING RATIONALES
1. Assess for severe dyspnea and orthopnea.	**1.** Increased hydrostatic pressure in the pulmonary capillaries forces fluids into the alveoli, resulting in acute breathing difficulty.
2. Observe Mrs. Chandler for a cough that produces frothy, white, or blood-tinged sputum.	**2.** These signs confirm pulmonary edema.
3. Auscultate breath sounds for expiratory wheezing and bubbling.	**3.** Wheezing and bubbling indicate fluid in the airways.
4. Note extreme anxiety and panic.	**4.** Difficult breathing causes a feeling of suffocation that can lead to panic.
5. Observe Mrs. Chandler for tachypnea, tachycardia, and perspiration.	**5.** Inadequate oxygen–carbon dioxide exchange causes tachypnea and increases the client's pulse rate and blood pressure.

Nursing diagnoses

- Impaired gas exchange related to pulmonary congestion
- Fluid volume excess related to left ventricular failure
- Anxiety related to the feeling of suffocation

Planning and goals

- Mrs. Chandler's pulmonary congestion and fluid volume will decrease.
- Mrs. Chandler will experience no preventable complications.
- Mrs. Chandler's physical and psychological comfort will improve.

Implementation

NURSING BEHAVIORS	NURSING RATIONALES
1. Ensure that Mrs. Chandler has complete bed rest, and remain with her when possible.	**1.** Bed rest and the nurse's reassuring presence will help reduce the client's anxiety.
2. Place Mrs. Chandler in high Fowler's position with the feet dependent.	**2.** High Fowler's position promotes blood pooling in the extremities, thereby decreasing venous return to the heart.

3. Administer oxygen, as ordered.

3. Oxygen relieves hypoxia.

4. Administer morphine sulphate, as ordered.

4. Morphine sulphate decreases anxiety, increases comfort, and vasodilates, promoting venous pooling and thus decreasing venous return to the heart.

5. Administer furosemide (Lasix), as ordered (I.V. bolus initially; then oral administration).

5. Furosemide is a rapid-acting loop diuretic. Diuresis begins within 10 minutes and peaks in 30 minutes, thereby relieving pulmonary congestion.

6. Administer vasodilators, such as I.V. nitroglycerin or angiotensin-converting enzyme inhibitors, as ordered.

6. By reducing vascular resistance, these drugs decrease afterload and improve cardiac output.

7. Administer aminophylline by slow I.V. infusion, as ordered, and observe Mrs. Chandler for arrhythmias.

7. Aminophylline decreases pulmonary artery pressure and reduces bronchospasms associated with pulmonary edema. The drug should be administered with caution, however—side effects include tachycardia, palpitations, and arrhythmias.

8. Administer digoxin (Lanoxin) I.V., as ordered.

8. Digoxin strengthens ventricular contractions and increases left ventricular output.

9. Insert an indwelling urinary catheter, and monitor fluid intake and output hourly.

9. Hourly analysis of the client's fluid intake and output reveals the diuretic's effectiveness.

10. Monitor Mrs. Chandler for falling blood pressure, increasing heart rate, and decreasing urine output.

10. These signs indicate the failure of compensatory mechanisms and the need for more aggressive treatment.

11. Monitor fluid and electrolyte balances hourly.

11. Rapid-acting diuretics can cause fluid and electrolyte imbalances. Because of the potential for hypokalemia, simultaneous use of furosemide and digoxin increases the risk of digoxin toxicity.

Evaluation
- Mrs. Chandler's pulmonary congestion and fluid volume decrease.
- Mrs. Chandler does not develop pneumonia.

Varicose veins

Varicose veins—dilated and tortuous saphenous veins in one or both legs—result from incompetent valves that incompletely empty during muscle contraction. Predisposing factors include hereditary weakness of venous walls or valves, pregnancy, obesity, occupations that require prolonged standing (such as police officer, cook, dentist, and operating room nurse), and age, with its accompanying loss of tissue elasticity. The following clinical situation focuses on nursing care of a client undergoing surgical correction for varicose veins.

ADULT NURSING

Clinical situation

John Gold, a 55-year-old dentist, has been experiencing leg cramps after standing all day on the job. His physician diagnosed the condition as bilateral varicose veins. Dr. Gold is scheduled for a bilateral ligation and stripping of the greater and lesser saphenous veins. He will be hospitalized overnight.

Assessment

NURSING BEHAVIORS	NURSING RATIONALES
1. Assess for large, tortuous leg veins.	**1.** Bilateral dilation and twisting elongation of the superficial veins confirm diagnosis. The deeper veins remain normal.
2. Assess the degree of leg cramps and fatigue. Suggest that cramps and fatigue are usually relieved by elevating the legs.	**2.** Elevating the legs decreases venous dilation and stasis in the superficial veins; blood flows toward the heart.
3. Assess Dr. Gold's lifestyle, occupational requirements, and predisposing factors (such as obesity).	**3.** Prolonged standing associated with certain occupations and obesity may contribute to the development of varicose veins.

Diagnostic evaluation

• *Retrograde filling test (Trendelenburg's test):* Ask the client to raise his legs about 65 degrees (to empty the veins). Apply a tourniquet to occlude superficial veins. Tell the client to stand; then remove the tourniquet. With incompetent venous valves, the vessels will fill quickly from the top of the leg downward.
• *Phlebography:* A radiopaque substance injected into the saphenous veins permits blood flow and valvular action to be seen on X-ray.

Nursing diagnoses

• Altered peripheral tissue perfusion related to venous insufficiency
• Knowledge deficit related to management of varicosities

Planning and goals

• Dr. Gold will develop no postoperative complications.
• Dr. Gold will alter his lifestyle to avoid conditions that cause venous stasis.

Implementation

NURSING BEHAVIORS	NURSING RATIONALES
Postoperative care	
1. Begin routine postoperative care.	**1.** See "Postoperative period," page 125, for specific nursing actions and rationales.
2. Apply firm, even pressure with elastic bandages over the entire leg. Do not remove bandages even for daily care.	**2.** This helps prevent bleeding and improve venous drainage.
3. Elevate the client's legs 15 degrees.	**3.** Leg elevation improves venous return from the legs.
4. Observe the incision sites for bleeding.	**4.** Vascular surgery can cause hemorrhage.

5. Check Dr. Gold's peripheral pulses and the color, movement, and temperature of his toes.

5. Inability to detect peripheral pulses indicates inadequate circulation. Leg constriction usually results from bandages wrapped too tightly. Temporary discoloration is expected.

6. Carry out the physician's orders for ambulation and pain medication. Encourage Dr. Gold to elevate his legs immediately after ambulation.

6. Ambulation, which usually begins the day of surgery, prevents circulatory stasis. Postoperative leg discomfort commonly lasts for several days, so the client will probably require pain medication, especially before ambulation. Elevating the legs after ambulation reduces discomfort.

7. Advise Dr. Gold not to dangle his legs over the edge of the bed.

7. Leg dangling impedes blood flow in the lower leg veins.

8. After removing pressure bandages, prepare Dr. Gold for discharge with these instructions:
• Wear elastic stockings for 3 to 4 weeks after surgery; thereafter, wear the stockings or support hose, donning them before getting out of bed.

8. The listed measures help prevent the recurrence of varicose veins. Elastic stockings and support hose compress the superficial veins, thus improving venous return. Leg crossing, prolonged standing or sitting, and constrictive clothing cause venous pooling.
• Avoid leg crossing and prolonged standing or sitting; elevate the legs periodically.
• Wear loose-fitting clothes.
• Prevent constipation by increasing fluid intake, eating a high-fiber diet, and exercising.
• Prevent or combat obesity by following a nutritious diet and exercising regularly. Constipation increases intra-abdominal pressure, which can contribute to venous pooling. Obesity increases venous pressure; muscle contraction from exercise promotes venous return and prevents pooling.

Evaluation

• Dr. Gold has no postoperative complications.
• Dr. Gold describes planned lifestyle changes that will prevent venous stasis.

Arteriosclerosis obliterans

Arteriosclerosis obliterans, a common arterial occlusive disorder, is a chronic progressive ischemia of the tissues, primarily in the legs (rarely affecting the arms), caused by progressive narrowing of the arteries from arteriosclerosis. The following clinical situation focuses on nursing care of a client learning to cope with peripheral vascular disease.

Clinical situation

George Franciscus is a 63-year-old postal worker whose job requires him to walk for several hours each day. When he walks, Mr. Franciscus experiences pain in the calf muscles; when he rests, the pain subsides. His medical diagnosis is arteriosclerosis obliterans.

Assessment

NURSING BEHAVIORS	NURSING RATIONALES
1. Assess for intermittent claudication (limb pain experienced as tiredness, aching, or constriction during exercise but relieved by rest).	**1.** Walking causes the muscles to contract, putting pressure on the blood vessels and further decreasing blood flow. Muscle contractions increase the need for oxygen, which can't be supplied because of the decreased blood flow that results from pressure and arteriosclerosis. Pain comes from ischemia and oxygen deficit in the muscles distal to the arterial obstruction.
2. Assess the client's pain site, and ask him to estimate how many minutes he can walk before experiencing calf pain.	**2.** Knowing the contributing factors of pain helps to determine its severity.
3. Ask Mr. Franciscus if he feels any pain at rest.	**3.** As arteriosclerosis progresses, the client may feel an intense, burning pain even when resting.
4. Assess skin color and temperature.	**4.** Pale, cool skin may indicate decreased capillary blood flow from arteriolar constriction. Reddish skin may indicate that peripheral vessels are damaged and remain dilated.
5. Check nail, hair, and skin texture.	**5.** Thick, hard nails, scant leg hair, and shiny, atrophic skin usually signal deficient blood flow to the tissues.
6. Observe for ulcers, cellulitis, and gangrene.	**6.** Ischemic tissues predispose the client to infection.
7. Note peripheral pulses (femoral, popliteal, posterior tibial, and dorsalis pedis) on both legs.	**7.** Assessment of peripheral pulses helps determine the client's heart rate and rhythm and vessel wall elasticity and may reveal a potential obstruction. Pulses are decreased or absent below the occlusion.
8. Check capillary refill time by compressing and then releasing the nail bed of the second or third toe. Note how long it takes the nail to turn pink.	**8.** Normally, the nail regains pink color in 2 to 4 seconds; a sluggish capillary refill time (5 seconds or more) is common with obstructive disease.

Diagnostic evaluation
- *Plethysmography:* assesses the degree of peripheral circulation
- *Angiography:* helps determine the extent of disease through visualization of arterial circulation
- *Exercise test for intermittent claudication:* measures the time that elapses between commencement of walking and onset of calf pain
- *Doppler ultrasonography:* determines the severity of ischemia

Nursing diagnoses
- Risk for infection related to peripheral ischemia
- Pain related to ischemic tissues
- Activity intolerance related to ischemic tissues
- Altered peripheral tissue perfusion related to arterial obstruction

Planning and goals

- Mr. Franciscus and his family will make lifestyle adjustments required to cope with a chronic health problem.
- Mr. Franciscus will understand how to prevent leg injury and infection.
- Mr. Franciscus will increase his activity without experiencing pain.

Implementation

NURSING BEHAVIORS

1. Administer medications, as ordered.

2. Help Mr. Franciscus perform Buerger-Allen exercises, if ordered: Elevate the legs for 2 to 3 minutes, then let the legs hang and exercise the feet and toes for 3 minutes, then place the legs flat for 5 minutes.

3. Encourage him to exercise regularly, as tolerated, alternating with frequent rest periods, and urge him to stop exercising at the first sign of pain.

4. Maintain complete bed rest if Mr. Franciscus has ulcers, cellulitis, or gangrene.

5. Provide Mr. Franciscus with the following basic health care instructions:

- Advise Mr. Franciscus to wear warm pants and socks during cold weather, to avoid constrictive clothing (such as garters or tight belts) at all times, and not to cross the legs when sitting.

- Don't place hot-water bottles, heating pads, or ice packs on the legs and feet.

- Periodically clean the legs and feet with a mild, nondrying soap; then apply oils or cream. Avoid strong antiseptic solutions, such as iodine, household disinfectants, and carbolic acid.

- Soak the feet in warm water before trimming toenails; trim straight across and not too close to the skin. Consult a podiatrist to trim corns and calluses.

- Advise Mr. Franciscus to wear properly fitted socks and never to go barefoot.

NURSING RATIONALES

1. Aspirin may be given to decrease aggregation of platelets. Pentoxifylline (Trental) may be given to make red blood cells more flexible and to decrease blood viscosity. Antilipemics may be ordered for elevated serum cholesterol.

2. Moderate exercise coupled with frequent rest periods helps increase circulation. Based on principles of gravity, the Buerger-Allen exercises promote increased blood flow.

3. Vascular rehabilitation via daily walking helps improve intermittent claudication.

4. Bed rest reduces the tissues' metabolic requirements for oxygen. (*Note:* If complications do not exist, activity should be encouraged.)

5. Health care teaching enables the nurse to review proper care procedures with the client and dispel any misconceptions he may have.

- Cold weather, constrictive clothing, and leg crossing can cause vasoconstriction and reduce circulation.

- Without a vigorous blood supply, peripheral nerves may be insensitive to heat or cold; if the client is unaware of extreme temperatures, tissue damage may result.

- Routine cleaning and moisturizing with mild soap and skin cream help prevent infection from organisms entering cracked skin tissue. Strong antiseptics may cause burns or other skin trauma.

- Soaking the feet in warm water softens the toenails, making trimming easier. The client should visit a podiatrist for removal of corns and calluses to prevent possible trauma from improper self-care.

- Foot protection prevents trauma and consequent infection.

ADULT NURSING

Surgical procedures for obstructed arterial vessels

Angioplasty. A small balloon-tipped catheter is inserted into an area of plaque in a coronary or peripheral artery. The balloon is inflated, flattening the plaque and increasing blood flow. The obstruction commonly recurs in 6 to 9 months, necessitating another angioplasty.

Bypass graft. A prosthetic graft is attached to the sides of an artery above and below an obstruction to bypass the obstruction.

Embolectomy. An embolus is removed from an artery.

Laser angioplasty. A laser-tipped catheter is threaded into the obstructed artery, and small-pulse laser beams are aimed at the plaque. The la-

ser heat vaporizes the plaque to reestablish circulation. The procedure requires cautious use of laser pulses to avoid burning through the artery or injuring the arterial wall (which could cause a clot to form at the site).

Prosthetic graft replacement. The diseased portion of an artery is removed and replaced with a synthetic prosthetic graft (the type commonly used to repair an abdominal aneurysm).

Thromboendarterectomy. A clot, plaque, and portions of the arterial intima are removed through an incision in the diseased artery. A temporary bypass is sutured into the artery above and below the operative site to detour the blood, preventing ischemia of tissues distal to the site.

• Notify the physician about redness, blisters, cuts, swelling, or pain in the legs or feet.

• Advise Mr. Franciscus to stop smoking.

• Advise Mr. Franciscus to maintain an average body weight to avoid obesity and to follow a diet low in saturated fats and cholesterol.

• An injury may become ulcerated and gangrenous, requiring prompt treatment.

• Nicotine causes vasospasm and vasoconstriction, thereby decreasing circulation more severely.

• Obesity places added stress on the leg muscles, increasing the need for arterial circulation.

Evaluation

• Mr. Franciscus increases his activity (1 mile of walking) without experiencing pain by resting 15 minutes between each 30 minutes of walking.
• Mr. Franciscus can explain how to prevent injuries to his legs and feet.

Clinical situation
(continued)

Initially, a client with arteriosclerosis obliterans receives medical treatment as previously described. If the disease progresses, the client may need surgery to correct an arterial obstruction (see *Surgical procedures for obstructed arterial vessels*). After such surgery, the nurse should closely monitor the neurovascular status at the surgical site and the tissue distal to the surgical repair. Other significant nursing behaviors are presented below.

Implementation
NURSING BEHAVIORS

NURSING RATIONALES

After any surgery to correct an arterial obstruction
1. Palpate or use ultrasound stethoscope to obtain peripheral pulses distal to the surgical site.

1. Palpation determines circulatory competence. All pulses should be palpable.

2. Compare the surgically repaired limb with its counterpart. Check color, temperature, motor and sensory functions, and capillary refill time. Determine the type and amount of pain and whether it is increasing or decreasing (increasing pain may signify reobstruction and anoxia). If surgery was performed on a carotid artery, compare by palpating both arteries and sides of the neck. Always perform neurologic checks if the carotid artery was surgically repaired.

2. Comparison helps determine circulatory adequacy.

3. If the obstruction hasn't been totally relieved, observe skin areas distal to it for signs of gangrene, such as edema, pain, red or darkening tissue, and cold skin.

3. Decreased or blocked circulation (stasis) impedes waste removal, allowing infection to begin early.

After a carotid endarterectomy
1. Elevate the head of the bed 20 to 30 degrees. Keep the head straight.

1. Head elevation aids venous return. Keeping the head straight maintains the airway and reduces incisional stress.

2. Apply an ice bag to the surgical site, if ordered. Avoid putting direct pressure on the incision. Observe for signs of bleeding.

2. Ice application helps decrease edema. Direct pressure on the incision could impede the client's circulation and lead to a stroke.

After a femoral-popliteal bypass graft
1. Instruct the client to remain supine for 24 to 48 hours.

1. This position allows the graft to have straight pathways without kinks or bends to interfere with blood flow.

2. After bed rest, allow the client to walk and stand but not to sit.

2. Sitting kinks the graft, decreasing blood flow to the tissues.

3. Instruct the client on proper care of the legs and feet, as described earlier.

3. Even after surgical repair, peripheral circulation may not be optimal. Therefore, infection and arterial constriction must be avoided.

4. Check for signs of airway obstruction, and have a tracheostomy set available.

4. Incisional bleeding and edema can cause airway occlusion.

Hypertension

Hypertension is chronically elevated blood pressure—a systolic blood pressure consistently above 140 mm Hg, a diastolic blood pressure consistently above 90 mm Hg, or both. Causes include fear, obesity, physical inactivity, severe pain, anxiety, and excessive sodium intake. The following clinical situation focuses on nursing care required to assist a client in reducing high blood pressure.

Clinical situation

Joan Winslow, a 46-year-old manager of a cosmetics company, is married with two teenage children. Currently 40 pounds (18 kg) overweight, Mrs. Winslow has been having headaches over the past 3 weeks and went to see the company nurse. After recording Mrs. Winslow's blood pressure as 160/100 mm Hg, the nurse provisionally assessed the condition as essential hypertension and referred Mrs. Winslow to her family physician for further evaluation.

Assessment

NURSING BEHAVIORS

1. Measure and record Mrs. Winslow's blood pressure in both arms on three separate occasions, with the client lying, sitting, and standing.

2. Assess stress factors in Mrs. Winslow's life, focusing on work and family relationships.

3. Ask Mrs. Winslow to describe her lifestyle; inquire about diet, exercise habits (amount and type), and social relationships.

NURSING RATIONALES

1. A temporary rise in blood pressure can occur with stress, pain, and such emotions as anger or fear. Taking several blood pressure readings provides an accurate assessment.

2. Stress, whether physical or psychological, can elevate blood pressure by stimulating the sympathetic nervous system.

3. With this assessment, the nurse begins to identify potential lifestyle changes necessitated by the client's hypertension.

Nursing diagnoses

• Altered health maintenance related to lack of knowledge about lifestyle changes and medication management
• Altered nutrition (more than body requirements) related to being 40 pounds overweight

Planning and goals

• Mrs. Winslow's blood pressure will be reduced.
• Mrs. Winslow and her family will understand and accept necessary lifestyle modifications.

Implementation

NURSING BEHAVIORS

1. Teach Mrs. Winslow the importance of following a low-sodium diet. Review the effects of excessive sodium intake, and identify high- and low-sodium foods. Advise her to read the ingredients on food and drug labels carefully.

2. Encourage Mrs. Winslow to reduce weight gradually and to decrease intake of dietary fat.

3. Instruct Mrs. Winslow on how to take prescribed medications and which side effects to report to the physician (see *Drug therapy for hypertension*).

NURSING RATIONALES

1. Reducing the client's sodium intake will decrease her fluid volume, thereby helping to reduce blood pressure. Many foods and some medications (especially nonprescription ones) contain high amounts of sodium.

2. Even moderate weight loss helps reduce blood pressure. Reducing fat intake will help to lower blood pressure and the serum cholesterol level.

3. The client is most likely to comply with drug therapy if she understands the administration method, dosage, purpose, side effects, and intended actions of prescribed drugs.

ADULT NURSING

Drug therapy for hypertension

The Fifth Report from the Joint National Committee on the Detection, Evaluation, and Treatment of High Blood Pressure recommended changes in the treatment of hypertension.

First, the committee reclassified hypertension. The new system considers systolic as well as diastolic pressures for the first time.

Certain terminology also has been changed. For example, the new system does not refer to "mild hypertension" because the term lulled people into thinking that treatment was optional.

Diuretics and beta blockers should be the first-choice agents because they are the only drugs that have been shown to reduce morbidity and mortality in long-term studies. Other drugs—namely calcium antagonists, angiotensin-converting enzyme (ACE) inhibitors, alpha-beta receptor antagonists (such as labetalol), or alpha$_1$-receptor blockers—can be considered as first-choice agents when treatment with beta blockers or diuretics is contraindicated, unacceptable, or conditions exist that demonstrate a preference for these drugs.

The treatment algorithm

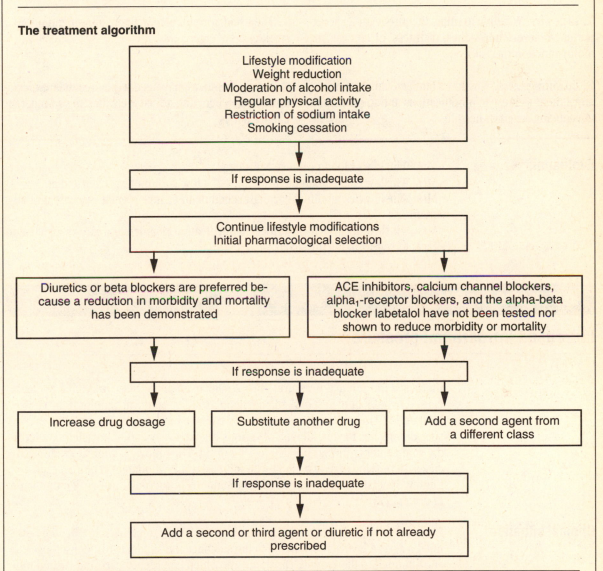

Lifestyle modification
Weight reduction
Moderation of alcohol intake
Regular physical activity
Restriction of sodium intake
Smoking cessation

↓

If response is inadequate

↓

Continue lifestyle modifications
Initial pharmacological selection

Diuretics or beta blockers are preferred because a reduction in morbidity and mortality has been demonstrated

ACE inhibitors, calcium channel blockers, alpha$_1$-receptor blockers, and the alpha-beta blocker labetalol have not been tested nor shown to reduce morbidity or mortality

If response is inadequate

Increase drug dosage | Substitute another drug | Add a second agent from a different class

If response is inadequate

↓

Add a second or third agent or diuretic if not already prescribed

Source: U.S. Department of Health and Human Services. National Institutes of Health, National Heart, Lung, and Blood Institute. *Fifth Report of the Joint National Committee on Detection, Evaluation, and Treatment of High Blood Pressure (JNC V)*. Washington, DC: Government Printing Office, Publication No. 93-1088, 1992.

ADULT NURSING

4. Help Mrs. Winslow design a regular exercise program appropriate to her needs. Suggest that she plan her daily schedule to include adequate rest and relaxation periods, and teach relaxation techniques, if desired.

4. Exercise reduces the effects of stress. Rest and relaxation lower blood pressure.

5. Teach Mrs. Winslow how to monitor her blood pressure.

5. The client should take her blood pressure regularly to monitor progress and to identify factors that exacerbate her condition.

6. Help Mrs. Winslow eliminate or reduce the stressors she has identified.

6. After stressors are identified, resources can be named to alleviate them. For instance, the client may need help at work or assistance with household chores.

7. Urge Mrs. Winslow to notify the physician if she experiences severe headaches, dizziness, or changes in motor function or vision.

7. The listed symptoms may signal an impending stroke.

8. Encourage Mrs. Winslow's family to support her adjustment to lifestyle modifications and to participate in reducing stress in her life.

8. Family members may need to change their expectations of the client and adjust their lifestyles to meet the client's needs.

Evaluation

• Mrs. Winslow's blood pressure is reduced.
• Mrs. Winslow can explain the principles of a low-sodium, low-calorie diet.
• Mrs. Winslow has modified her daily schedule to ensure regular exercise and adequate rest.
• Mrs. Winslow accurately describes the medication regimen and knows which side effects to report to the physician.

NEUROLOGIC SYSTEM

Increased intracranial pressure

Increased intracranial pressure (ICP) results from an increase in cranial contents caused by infection; cerebral edema; neoplasms; or epidural, subdural, or subarachnoid hemorrhage from trauma or a ruptured aneurysm. The building pressure diminishes the functioning of various cranial areas and, if unrelieved, affects the vital centers. Normal ICP is 0 to 15 mm Hg. The following clinical situation focuses on nursing care of a client with increased ICP who might require a craniotomy. Specialized care may include continuous intracranial pressure monitoring in critical care.

Clinical situation

Harry Spence, age 24, was playing touch football with some friends when he developed a severe headache. Walking to the sidelines, he suddenly lost consciousness and slumped to the ground. His friends provided emergency care and rushed him to the hospital.

Assessment

NURSING BEHAVIORS

NURSING RATIONALES

1. Perform a neurologic assessment as follows:

1. A neurologic assessment helps identify increased ICP as soon as possible.

• Determine the client's level of consciousness.

• A decreased level of consciousness is the most reliable indicator of increased ICP. Lethargy is a common early sign.

• Compare the client's pupils for size and reaction to light.

• The pupil on the side of increasing pressure dilates, reacts slowly to light, and eventually becomes fixed.

• Monitor the client's vital signs, noting changes in blood pressure, pulse rate, respiratory rate, and body temperature.

• Increased ICP results in a widening pulse pressure (from increasing systolic, but not diastolic, blood pressure), a slow pulse rate, and altered temperature regulation that eventually can lead to uncontrolled hyperthermia; respirations usually will be slowed if the respiratory center of the brain is affected.

• Observe for motor function changes: Check the client's hand grasp and leg extension bilaterally; observe facial expressions (hemiparesis or hemiplegia appears on the side opposite the affected area); check for Babinski's reflex on the side opposite the affected area; and assess for bowel and bladder incontinence.

• Increased ICP can impair motor function. The client's hand grasp, leg extension, and facial expressions may reveal deteriorating muscle strength in those areas. If hemiplegic, the client will have Babinski's reflex on the opposite side, which indicates damage to the corticospinal tract. The client may also lose bowel or bladder control, depending on the brain area affected.

• Assess bilaterally for sensory function changes, such as dull or sharp sensations and paresthesias.

• Numbness and tingling may occur on the side opposite the affected area.

2. Observe the client for other symptoms, such as blurred vision and diplopia; changes in behavior, judgment, and decision making; hearing deficit; ataxia and dizziness; aphasia; and seizures.

2. Increased ICP can affect the occipital lobe (blurred vision and diplopia), the frontal lobe (changes in behavior, judgment, and decision making), the temporal lobe (hearing deficit), the cerebellum (ataxia and dizziness), and the motor speech area (aphasia). A description of the seizure may help identify the cause and location of increased ICP.

3. Observe the client for decorticate posture (arms adducted and rigidly flexed, with the hands internally rotated and flexed) or decerebrate posture (all extremities rigidly extended, with hyperpronation of forearms and plantar extension of the feet; back arched; and toes pointed inward). (See *Pathologic postures,* page 458.)

3. The client's posture helps identify the brain area affected. The decorticate posture indicates corticospinal tract involvement, damage to the cerebral hemisphere, and depressed cerebral metabolic function. The decerebrate posture indicates midbrain or pons involvement; extensive involvement in these areas generally leads to a poor prognosis.

4. Assess the type and location of the client's headache, noting its frequency, duration, precipitating factors, and association with other neurologic symptoms.

4. Descriptions of the headache help identify its source. With increased ICP, a headache usually occurs suddenly, produces severe pain, and worsens with activity.

ADULT NURSING

Pathologic postures

Decorticate rigidity indicates corticospinal tract involvement.

Decerebrate rigidity indicates midbrain or pons involvement.

5. Document the frequency and characteristics of vomiting, if any.

5. Increased ICP may cause projectile vomiting.

6. Observe the client for nuchal rigidity, noting whether the neck is especially painful and stiff when the head is moved. Also assess for malaise, nausea and vomiting, increased body temperature, altered level of consciousness, and other signs of increased ICP.

6. Nuchal rigidity may signify either meningitis or encephalitis, which have similar symptoms. A decreased level of consciousness and other signs of increased ICP suggest encephalitis.

Diagnostic evaluation

- *Neurologic examination:* tests of cerebral, cranial nerve, motor, and sensory functioning; balance and coordination; and superficial and deep tendon reflexes to identify nervous system diseases
- *Computed tomography (CT) scan:* photographic series of the brain in 1-degree angles that precisely locates brain abnormalities
- *Arteriogram:* X-ray of an artery into which contrast medium has been injected to permit visualization of normal and abnormal arterial circulation and vessels
- *Brain scan:* scintillator-recorded photographs of radioactive accumulations in the brain (after oral or I.V. administration of a radioactive solution and medication to block radioactive uptake in the thyroid gland) that localize brain lesions, tumors, abnormal masses, and infarcts
- *Magnetic resonance imaging (MRI):* noninvasive brain scan without radiation or contrast media

| **Nursing diagnoses** | • Sensory or perceptual alterations (visual) related to cerebral ischemia
• Anxiety related to the perceived crisis |

Planning and goals • Mr. Spence will be physically and psychologically comfortable.
 • Mr. Spence will not experience preventable complications.
 • Mr. Spence's family and friends will support him.
 • Mr. Spence will not develop preventable increased ICP.

Implementation

NURSING BEHAVIORS

1. Elevate the head of the bed 30 degrees, and place the client in a side-lying position.

2. Maintain a calm atmosphere for the client; dim the room lights to prevent glare; and limit visitors, phone calls, and television time.

3. Maintain the client's complete physical and psychological rest, intervening, as follows, to prevent complications of immobility:

• Turn the client carefully.

• Perform passive range-of-motion exercises gently and slowly.

4. Closely monitor the client's respiratory status. Tell Mr. Spence to breathe deeply, but urge him to avoid coughing if he is hemorrhagic. Prepare for hyperventilation therapy. He may have to be intubated and placed on a ventilator. If suctioning is necessary, prepare to administer lidocaine, as ordered, via an endotracheal tube.

5. Urge the client to avoid emotional stress and such actions as bending, sneezing, coughing, lifting, vomiting, and straining for bowel movements.

6. If conscious, teach the client to avoid Valsalva's maneuver by breathing out through the mouth when turning.

7. Decrease the client's fluid intake, if ordered.

8. Monitor intake and output hourly until the client's condition stabilizes; also monitor fluid and electrolyte balance frequently.

NURSING RATIONALES

1. These measures improve venous drainage and help maintain an open airway. Preventing aspiration is particularly important if the client has a decreased level of consciousness.

2. These measures minimize stimulation, which can further increase ICP.

3. Stress increases ICP. Bed rest helps relieve stress but may cause problems related to immobility.

• Careful turning prevents rebleeding (if the client is hemorrhagic) and additional headache discomfort.

• This will prevent joint ankylosis and venous stasis from immobility.

4. Deep-breathing exercises help prevent pneumonia. Coughing may cause hemorrhage. Decreasing the client's PCO_2 to 27 to 33 mm Hg, makes him alkalotic, causes vasoconstriction, and reduces ICP.

5. All of these activities increase ICP.

6. Valsalva's maneuver further increases ICP.

7. Physicians commonly decrease the client's fluid intake to help reduce cerebral edema.

8. If the client doesn't eat and takes little fluid, fluid and electrolyte imbalance may result.

ADULT NURSING

Basics of I.V. therapy

I. Uses
A. To administer fluids, electrolytes, and other nutrients
B. To administer medications
C. To administer blood or blood products

II. Determining the flow rate
A. Check the physician's orders for the prescribed solution and either the duration of the infusion or the hourly infusion rate
B. Calculate the flow rate in drops per minute (gtt/minute) by using this formula:

$$\frac{\text{Volume of infusion (ml)}}{\text{time of infusion (minutes)}} \times \frac{\text{drop factor}}{\text{(drops/ml)}} = \text{drops/minute}$$

Example: The physician's order reads: *Administer 1,000 ml of D₅W in 8 hours.* The administration set delivers 10 gtt/ml. What is the flow rate in drops per minute?

$$\frac{1,000 \text{ ml}}{480 \text{ minutes}} \times 10 \text{ drops/ml} = 20 \text{ drops/minute}$$

Example: The physician's order reads: *Administer 1,000 ml of D₅W at 100 ml/hour.* The administration set delivers 20 gtt/ml. What is the flow rate in drops per minute?

$$\frac{100 \text{ ml} \times 20 \text{ drops/ml}}{60 \text{ minutes}} = 33 \text{ drops/minute}$$

Note: Standard I.V. administration sets deliver 10, 15, or 20 gtt/ml. Microdrip sets deliver 50 or 60 gtt/ml. This information, which appears on the box of the administration set, must be provided in any problem you are asked to solve in the NCLEX-RN.

III. Preventing complications
A. To prevent *clotting,* maintain a continuous flow rate or use a heparin lock
B. To prevent *infiltration,* use a plastic needle or catheter, and immobilize the infusion site
C. To prevent *too-rapid administration,* use an infusion pump, and frequently monitor the flow rate

---

9. Administer prescribed I.V. fluids slowly (see *Basics of I.V. therapy*). Dextrose 5% in half normal saline is commonly used.

10. Maintain seizure precautions: Keep the bed in the low position, and raise the side rails, padding them if necessary. Have suction equipment available.

11. Perform a neurologic assessment every 4 hours (hourly if the client has unstable signs).

12. Monitor the client frequently for leaking spinal fluid. To absorb the fluid, place a sterile cotton swab loosely in the ear or apply a nasal sling (gauze taped loosely under the nose to permit air passage); replace wet swabs and slings with dry ones, as needed.

13. Closely monitor the client's blood pressure.

9. Fluid overload from fast infusions can cause cerebral edema, which further increases ICP.

10. Seizures occur commonly with increased ICP. Anticonvulsants may be administered.

11. Frequent neurologic checks identify increased ICP.

12. Spinal fluid drainage is clear, with a yellow halo, and creates concentric circles on bed linen. The drainage will test positive for glucose. Changing saturated cotton swabs and nasal slings prevents infection.

13. If hemorrhage has caused increased ICP, the physician determines acceptable blood pressure limits. The blood pressure should be high enough for circulating blood to perfuse brain tissue but low enough to prevent rebleeding.

14. Provide continual emotional support to the client (even if he appears comatose) and to family and friends; encourage the client's loved ones to express their feelings.

14. Because hearing is the last sense to be lost, the client may benefit from the nurse's reassuring words. Family members and friends will surely need the nurse's understanding and support as they try to cope with the prognosis, which is usually uncertain for a client with increased ICP.

15. Explain treatments, realistic expectations for progress, and ways in which family and friends can help. Warn them not to discuss stress-inducing issues with the client.

15. Family and friends can provide valuable support to the client, particularly if they have adequate knowledge of his condition and guidance in coping with the situation. A major contribution is to avoid placing any stress on the client, which further increases ICP.

16. Administer a corticosteroid such as dexamethasone (Decadron) or a hypertonic diuretic such as mannitol (Osmitrol), as ordered. A loop diuretic such as furosemide (Lasix) may also be utilized. If a corticosteroid is prescribed, test the client's urine for glucose several times daily.

16. Corticosteroids are commonly prescribed to reduce cerebral edema, although they may elevate blood glucose levels. Hypertonic diuretics also reduce cerebral edema, raising osmotic pressure and pulling fluid from edematous cerebral cells.

17. Monitor the client's diet, and feed him as tolerated. Use a nasogastric tube or Dobhoff tube for feedings, as ordered, if the client has bowel sounds.

17. The client's level of consciousness, gag reflexes, and medical diagnosis determine dietary needs. Bowel sounds indicate peristalsis, which means the client can digest food.

18. Maintain aseptic technique during nursing care, and prohibit persons with infections from coming in contact with the client. Immediately notify the physician if the client has yellow sputum, a temperature above 100° F (37.8° C), or signs of infection at the I.V., indwelling catheter, or wound sites, and obtain tissue or discharge samples for culture.

18. The client with increased ICP is susceptible to infection. Aseptic technique and isolation help thwart infection; careful monitoring helps ensure early intervention if it develops.

19. Monitor the client for bleeding: Review hemoglobin and hematocrit values, obtain a hematest of stools three times weekly, inspect urine for blood, and monitor for abdominal tenderness and distention, hypotension, and sudden tachycardia. Administer antacids and histamine$_2$ antagonists (such as cimetidine or famotidine), as ordered.

19. A client on corticosteroid therapy may develop a stress ulcer. Antacids and cimetidine decrease the risk of GI bleeding.

Clinical situation
(continued)

Mr. Spence's ICP increased further. After his diagnostic test results were reviewed, he was prepared for a craniotomy, a surgical procedure that reduces ICP.

Implementation

NURSING BEHAVIORS

NURSING RATIONALES

Preoperative care
1. Obtain baseline information on the client's neurologic, respiratory, and cardiovascular status and fluid and electrolyte and acid-base balance.

1. Medical and nursing staff will use this baseline information for postoperative comparisons.

2. Assess the family's knowledge of the client's condition, resources, and stress level.

2. This information enables the nurse to plan care aimed at helping family members provide much-needed emotional support to the client.

3. Encourage family members to ask questions and voice concerns. Reassure them as much as possible while providing accurate information and realistic assessments. Explain that the client may have reduced intellectual functioning for a while.

3. The postcraniotomy prognosis remains uncertain; at best, the client faces a lengthy recovery period that can leave the entire family physically and emotionally drained.

4. Shave the client's head. If Mr. Spence is alert, assess his anxiety about the hair loss.

4. Hair must be removed before surgery. If the client is alert while being shaved, the nurse should expect to encounter anxiety arising from a potentially altered body image.

5. Explain postoperative nursing care, procedures, and equipment.

5. The client who understands these issues will be better prepared to participate in care.

6. Implement nursing care for increased ICP up to the time of surgery.

6. The client's condition warrants frequent monitoring.

7. Do not administer narcotics before surgery.

7. Narcotics can interfere with diagnosis, mask symptoms, and cause respiratory depression.

8. Administer a mild enema if the client had no bowel movement the day before surgery.

8. This will prevent fecal impaction and constipation.

Surgical intervention by craniotomy
The two major craniotomy types are supratentorial and infratentorial. The tentorium (a fold of the dura mater) separates the intracranial cavity into the supratentorial and infratentorial compartments. The supratentorial compartment includes the cerebral hemispheres and the diencephalon. The infratentorial compartment houses the pons, cerebellum, and medulla.

Supratentorial craniotomy
1. Elevate the client's head.

1. Elevating the head promotes venous drainage.

2. Don't position the client on the operative site.

2. This prevents pressure on the operative site.

3. Apply ice packs or pressure dressings over the client's eyes, if ordered.

3. Ice packs and pressure dressings reduce periocular edema, a possible consequence of supratentorial craniotomy.

Infratentorial craniotomy
Use the logroll maneuver to turn the client. Make sure he is flat in bed. Then, keeping his head aligned with his spine, turn him gingerly. *Do not flex his neck.*

Logrolling prevents tension on the surgical site and decreases client pain during turning.

Postoperative care
1. Implement nursing care for increased ICP.

1. The client's condition warrants frequent monitoring.

2. Position the client to maintain a patent airway and (if he has a Hemovac or other drainage apparatus) to prevent drainage tube tension or blockage. Support the client's head and neck when changing his position.

2. Maintaining a patent airway is critical, especially in light of the client's decreased level of consciousness, which can impede successful breathing. Preventing tube tension and blockage promotes the drainage needed for an uneventful recovery. Supporting the head and neck reduces pressure on the operative site and minimizes pain.

3. Perform neurologic assessments hourly.

3. These examinations provide data on nervous system functioning.

4. Reinforce dressings but do not change them unless ordered. Report signs of bleeding to the surgeon.

4. Neurosurgeons usually prefer to change dressings themselves.

5. Suction excess secretions as needed, but do not suction the nose if the frontal lobe was excised.

5. If the frontal lobe was excised, suctioning the nose may adversely affect the surgical site.

6. Monitor fluid intake and output hourly; notify the physician if the client has extreme thirst, excessive urine output, low specific gravity, urine retention, or low serum sodium levels.

6. If the client's condition has affected posterior pituitary function, he may develop either diabetes insipidus or syndrome of inappropriate antidiuretic hormone (SIADH). Diabetes insipidus, caused by a deficiency of ADH, is characterized by extreme thirst, excessive urine output, and low specific gravity of urine; the usual treatment is to administer pitressin (Vasopressin). SIADH, caused by excessive ADH secretion, leads to fluid retention and dilutional hyponatremia; treatment includes fluid restrictions.

7. Monitor the client for meningitis and encephalitis. If the client has meningitis, follow isolation precautions when disposing of discharge from the nose, mouth, throat, and wound.

7. Meningitis or encephalitis may result from inflammation caused by surgery or infection. Because meningitis is a communicable disease, precautions must be taken to prevent its spread.

8. Administer an analgesic for headache, as ordered.

8. The client will have pain in the incision site.

9. Administer an antipyretic, give the client a tepid sponge bath, or begin hypothermia therapy, as ordered.

9. These are standard fever-reducing measures. The fever's severity commonly dictates which therapy is chosen.

10. Assist with ambulation, as ordered, noting the client's out-of-bed behavior. Teach him to use safety restraints when sitting.

10. The client's physical strength may return before cognition and balance. Early ambulation is encouraged, and the client's activity level is progressively increased, with the goal of getting the client out of bed by the second to third postoperative day (possibly longer after infratentorial surgery).

11. Assess the client's neurologic deficits and strengths.

11. These data will determine rehabilitation potential.

12. Assess the family's resources, lifestyle, home setting, interpersonal relationships, and financial resources and limitations.

12. These data form a basis for developing an optimal rehabilitation plan.

ADULT NURSING

13. Develop a realistic plan for lifestyle changes and rehabilitation based on your assessment.

13. A plan that disregards the client's needs and the family's resources will probably cause frustration and squelch their desire to keep trying.

14. Encourage the client and family members to discuss their fears, frustrations, and anxieties. Promote their participation in assessment and planning.

14. The client needs as much support as possible, particularly from loved ones. The greater their knowledge and participation, the better equipped they will be to help.

15. Discuss realistic outcomes with the client and family, combining straightforward information with comforting reassurances.

15. The prognosis is uncertain and the extent of client function after rehabilitation is unpredictable; the client and family deserve accurate information from caring, supportive nursing staff.

Evaluation

- Mr. Spence and his family adjust to lifestyle changes required by his health.
- Mr. Spence's ICP is reduced.
- Mr. Spence experiences no preventable complications.

Cerebrovascular accident

A cerebrovascular accident (CVA), a severe disturbance in cerebral circulation, results from decreased perfusion in one or more brain areas. Predisposing factors include cerebral trauma, ruptured cerebral aneurysm, ruptured artery (such as from hypertension), spasm in a major cerebral artery, arteriosclerosis of cerebral vessels (for example, from diabetes mellitus or peripheral vascular disease), and obstruction of cerebral arteries by thrombi or emboli (see *Events that can cause a stroke*). The first three predisposing factors result in hemorrhage; the last three, in cerebral hypoxia. The following clinical situation focuses on nursing care of a client who has had a CVA (similar care would be provided to any unconscious client).

Clinical situation

Mary Avery, a 74-year-old retired schoolteacher, lives alone but has many friends nearby. She's been having transient ischemic attacks (TIAs) for the last few weeks, coupled with memory lapses and difficulty holding items in her left hand. Yesterday afternoon, after she failed to answer the telephone, some of her friends entered her house and found her on the floor, paralyzed on the left side. They gave her first aid and called an ambulance. Her medical diagnosis is CVA.

Emergency intervention

NURSING BEHAVIORS

NURSING RATIONALES

1. Establish and maintain an open airway.

1. An open airway is the initial emergency intervention consideration.

2. Check vital signs.

2. Absent pulse and respirations require immediate cardiopulmonary resuscitation.

3. Elevate the client's head slightly.

3. Head elevation may prevent increased intracranial pressure (ICP).

Events that can cause a stroke

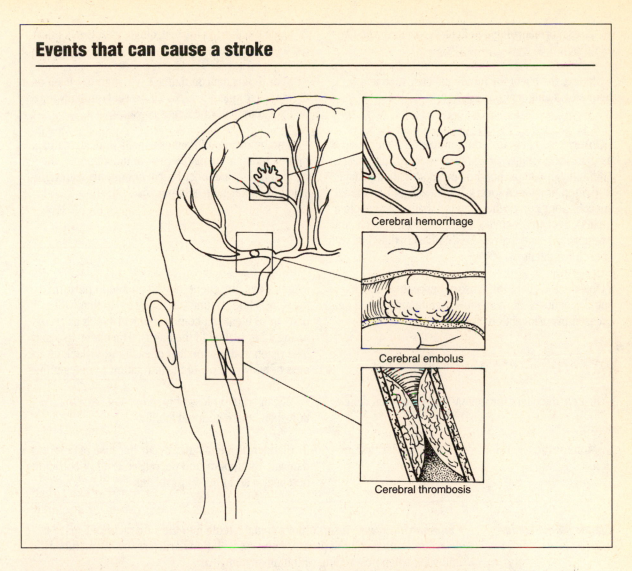

Cerebral hemorrhage

Cerebral embolus

Cerebral thrombosis

4. Loosen the client's clothing and remove potentially injurious items.

4. These are safety measures in case the client has seizures.

5. Observe the client's vital signs, level of consciousness, and skin color. Note the extent of paralysis, sensory loss, and seizures.

5. A decreased level of consciousness is the most reliable indicator of increased ICP. Weakening vital signs, pallor or cyanosis, paralysis, sensory loss, and seizures also may occur.

6. Give emotional support to the client, family, and friends.

6. Because the prognosis is uncertain at this point, the client and loved ones need encouragement.

Assessment
NURSING BEHAVIORS

NURSING RATIONALES

1. Assess as you would for increased ICP.

1. See "Increased intracranial pressure," pages 456 to 464, for specific nursing behaviors and rationales.

ADULT NURSING

2. Assess for neurologic deficits associated with CVA as follows:

2. Close monitoring for neurologic changes is essential to detect CVA.

• Observe the client for motor deficits, such as hemiplegia and hemiparesis.

• Upper motor neuron damage will manifest itself on the opposite side. Paralysis (if present) initially may be flaccid but later becomes spastic.

• Observe the client for communication deficits, such as dysarthria (poorly articulated speech), dysphasia (difficulty in comprehending or producing language in written or spoken form), global aphasia (minimal speech, poor comprehension for written and spoken forms), receptive aphasia (difficulty with speech comprehension), and expressive dysphasia (difficulty with speech production).

• Communication difficulties usually indicate damage to the dominant hemisphere—in most people, the left hemisphere—and occur most commonly with right-sided hemiplegia or hemiparesis.

• Observe the client for sensory-perceptual deficits, such as agnosia, homonymous hemianopsia, and decreased proprioception.

• After a CVA, the client may be unable to perform a previously known function (such as writing with a pen) or to identify a common object (such as recognizing a key placed in the hand). The client also may lose vision in the same half of each eye or lack awareness of body part positions in relation to one another.

• Observe the client for mental and emotional deficits.

• CVA can result in loss of memory, decreased attention span, and emotional lability.

3. Monitor the client for bowel and bladder dysfunction.

3. Bladder problems may occur because of cerebral damage. Immobility and decreased level of consciousness may lead to bowel problems.

Diagnostic evaluation

• *Lumbar puncture:* Insertion of a spinal needle into the subarachnoid space to determine spinal column pressure and spinal fluid characteristics. Remember the following when proceeding with lumbar puncture:
—Explain the procedure to the client. Then position the client on the side, with the legs flexed toward the abdomen and the chin bent toward the chest. This position separates the vertebrae, facilitating needle insertion into the subarachnoid space.
—Correctly label test tubes holding the collected spinal fluid: Clear fluid in the last tube obtained indicates cerebral thrombus, whereas bloody fluid indicates hemorrhage. Misnumbered, mislabeled tubes may cause misdiagnosis.
—After the test, keep the client flat in bed for 4 to 24 hours, as ordered; force fluids (unless contraindicated) because increased hydration promotes cerebrospinal fluid production to replace fluid removed; and observe for headache.
• *Computed tomography scan:* Also known as computerized axial tomography scan, this is the best diagnostic tool for identifying infarcted cerebral tissue. *Caution:* Monitor the client carefully for allergic reactions if a contrast medium is used.
• *Cerebral angiography:* Uses a radiopaque dye to visualize cerebral circulation. Monitor the client carefully for allergic reactions.

Nursing diagnoses
- Impaired verbal communication related to neurologic damage from CVA
- Feeding self-care deficit related to left-sided paralysis
- Bathing or hygiene self-care deficit related to left-sided paralysis
- Dressing or grooming self-care deficit related to left-sided paralysis
- Toileting self-care deficit related to left-sided paralysis

Planning and goals
- Ms. Avery will not experience preventable complications.
- Ms. Avery will be able to cope with the health problems associated with CVA.

Implementation

NURSING BEHAVIORS	NURSING RATIONALES
1. Implement the same measures as those used for a client with increased ICP.	**1.** See "Increased intracranial pressure," pages 456 to 464, for specific nursing behaviors and rationales.
2. If the client is unconscious, provide appropriate care.	**2.** See *Nursing interventions for the unconscious client*, page 468, for specific nursing behaviors and rationales.
3. Administer medications, as ordered.	**3.** Medications may include antihypertension agents and anticoagulants as well as platelet anti-aggregation therapy (aspirin or dipyridamole [Persantine]).
4. As ordered, administer heparin during the acute period and warfarin (Coumadin) in long-term care.	**4.** Anticoagulants help prevent further thrombi or emboli formation. Used for TIAs or thrombolytic strokes.
5. Position the client to maintain an open airway.	**5.** Paralysis and absent gag reflex compromise breathing.
6. Perform a neurologic assessment hourly, and report changes to the physician.	**6.** Neurologic checks identify changes in nervous system functioning (see "Increased intracranial pressure," pages 456 to 464).
7. Maintain the client on complete bed rest for 24 hours. Elevate the head of the bed 30 to 45 degrees. Maintain normal body alignment, and do not position the client on the affected side or place an unconscious client in the supine position. Reposition the client every 2 hours.	**7.** Bed rest is necessary until the diagnosis is confirmed because activity can increase cerebral hemorrhage. Elevating the head improves venous drainage. Correct positioning prevents deformities and maintains the client's airway (placing the client on the affected side reduces circulation to the affected muscles and increases stiffness; positioning an unconscious client on the back obstructs the airway). Frequent repositioning helps prevent complications of immobility associated with complete bed rest.
8. Administer tube feedings or I.V. infusions if the client has no gag or cough reflex.	**8.** Oral feedings should not be given to a client without a gag or cough reflex.
9. Initiate I.V. feedings (TPN, PPN) for the client without bowel sounds.	**9.** Bowel sounds indicate peristalsis in the GI tract. Without peristalsis, digestion cannot occur.

ADULT NURSING

Nursing interventions for the unconscious client

Unconsciousness is a state of depressed cerebral function. Loss of consciousness results in progressive inability to respond effectively to the environment. To assess the client's level of consciousness, observe for a loss of orientation—to time, place, and person. As level of consciousness decreases, the client initially responds to verbal stimuli, then only to painful stimuli, and finally to nothing. Observe for lost muscle, tendon, corneal, pupillary, swallowing, and cough reflexes, and perform a neurologic assessment.

Major goals include modifying the environment until the client can adapt to it and preventing complications. Nursing interventions for an unconscious client include the following:
1. Maintain an open airway.
2. Prevent complications of immobility.
3. Implement seizure precautions.
4. Use caution when applying heat or cold.
5. Perform neurologic checks hourly for a client with an unstable condition or increased intracranial pressure and every 4 hours for other clients.

6. If the client lacks a corneal reflex, patch both eyes to prevent corneal injury.
7. Instill artificial tears or ophthalmic ointment, as ordered, to prevent corneal injury.
8. Do not give food or fluid if the client cannot swallow. Begin tube feeding if bowel sounds exist; otherwise, feed the client intravenously.
9. In simple language, explain care that will be given to the client. (Hearing is the last sense to be lost.) Provide a calm environment, and continue giving emotional support.
10. If the client is delirious (a state of consciousness characterized by fears, hallucinations, irritability, and delusions), keep the lights on in the room to avoid shadows—which may increase hallucinations, adding to the client's fear. Instruct visitors not to whisper in the client's room because whispering increases hallucinations. Avoid restraints. They increase the client's fear.

---

10. Monitor the client's urine output and voiding pattern. Avoid using an indwelling catheter. If one is needed, however, use strict aseptic technique.

10. Monitoring urine output enables the nurse to detect inadequate renal function and fluid imbalances. Using an indwelling catheter increases the risk of urinary tract infection.

11. Establish a bowel retraining program for the client.

11. Bowel retraining may be needed if the client is incontinent.

12. Approach the client from the unaffected side, and place objects so the client can reach them from this side.

12. These measures help compensate for visual field deficits.

13. Speak slowly and clearly to the client, using simple sentences and gestures to promote communication.

13. These measures help compensate for aphasia, dysarthria, and dysphasia.

14. Provide emotional support to the client and loved ones while encouraging them to express concerns and feelings. Discuss ways in which friends can help the client now and after discharge.

14. Open expression of feelings commonly reduces anxiety for those involved. The uncertain prognosis and the potentially long rehabilitative period ensure the client's need for support from others.

Evaluation

• Ms. Avery experiences no preventable complications, such as pneumonia, skin breakdown, and urinary tract infection.
• Her friends assist Ms. Avery by visiting her in the hospital and by helping her make decisions about her future after discharge.

Spinal cord injury

Spinal cord injury can result from fracturing or dislocating one or more vertebrae and damaging the spinal cord or nerve roots or both. The following clinical situation focuses on nursing care of a client with a spinal cord injury.

Clinical situation

Henry House, an oil company executive who has a wife and eight children, was hospitalized after his private plane crashed. On admission to the emergency department, Mr. House complained of a severe headache along with numbness and weakness in his legs and arms.

Assessment

NURSING BEHAVIORS	NURSING RATIONALES
1. Assess motor and sensory function as you would for a client with increased intracranial pressure.	**1.** See "Increased intracranial pressure," pages 456 to 464, for specific nursing behaviors and rationales.
2. Assess for headache, inability to concentrate, and weak or labored breathing.	**2.** These symptoms suggest injured cervical vertebrae (C1 through C4) or head injury.
3. Assess for other injuries.	**3.** Violent physical trauma places all body systems at risk for injury.
4. Assess the client's relationships with family and friends.	**4.** The client's recovery time may be extensive, and he will need all available support systems.

Nursing diagnoses

• Impaired physical mobility related to motor deficit
• Ineffective airway clearance related to paralysis or weakness of respiratory muscles
• Feeding self-care deficit related to motor and sensory deficits
• Bathing or hygiene self-care deficit related to motor and sensory deficits
• Dressing or grooming self-care deficit related to motor and sensory deficits
• Toileting self-care deficit related to motor and sensory deficits
• Body image disturbance related to loss of use of the limbs
• Sexual dysfunction related to motor and sensory impairment
• Urine retention related to motor and sensory damage

Planning and goals

• Mr. House and his family will cope effectively with injury-related health problems.
• Mr. House will not develop preventable complications.

Implementation

NURSING BEHAVIORS	NURSING RATIONALES
1. Establish and maintain an open airway. Do not hyperextend the neck if the client has a cervical injury. Use the jaw thrust maneuver if cardiopulmonary resuscitation is necessary.	**1.** Spontaneous respiration may be impeded by impaired innervation of the intercostal muscles or the diaphragm or both. Using the jaw thrust maneuver to open the airway will prevent further cervical injury.

2. If the client's injury is in the high cervical spine, prepare for intubation or a tracheotomy and ventilatory support.

2. Intubation or a tracheotomy may be needed to maintain an open airway and to access obstructive secretions. Lesions above C4 require constant ventilatory support; those at or below C4 may require intermittent support.

3. Observe for weak or labored respirations, and arrange for mechanical ventilation, as ordered.

3. High cervical vertebral injuries can compromise the client's ability to breathe unassisted.

4. Encourage hourly deep breathing and coughing if the client can breathe effectively.

4. Deep breathing and coughing will prevent pneumonia.

5. Insert an I.V. infusion line, and keep the line open.

5. The client's precarious status requires that an open I.V. line be in place to administer medications and fluids if necessary.

6. Administer a steroid, such as dexamethasone (Decadron), or an osmotic diuretic, such as mannitol (Osmitrol), as ordered.

6. Anti-inflammatory drugs and diuretics reduce edema of the cerebrum and the spinal cord.

7. Administer prescribed fluids only.

7. Overhydration may cause spinal cord edema.

8. Monitor fluid and electrolyte levels hourly until the client's condition stabilizes.

8. Hourly monitoring enables medical and nursing staff to initiate prompt treatment of fluid and electrolyte imbalance.

9. Insert an indwelling urinary catheter, if needed; check frequently for kinks and obstructions.

9. A client who lacks motor and sensory function may be unable to initiate urination or perceive the need to urinate.

10. Observe the client for signs of spinal shock: lack of perspiration, urine and fecal retention, paralysis, and hypotension.

10. Manifested by loss of reflexes slightly above the lesion and in all areas below the lesion, spinal shock occurs 30 to 60 minutes after injury. Recovery usually occurs in 1 to 12 weeks.

11. Observe the client for signs of neurogenic shock: sudden hypotension, bradycardia, hypothermia, and syncope. Implement actions for neurogenic shock, as needed (see "Shock," pages 103 to 108).

11. An interruption of the sympathetic nervous system, neurogenic shock results from spinal cord injury. Any shock state can become irreversible and warrants immediate intervention.

12. Monitor bowel sounds every 8 hours.

12. Paralytic ileus, characterized by absent bowel sounds, may occur.

13. Immobilize the client by placing him on a Stryker frame or kinetic bed with Crutchfield tongs (if available). Maintain skeletal traction. Clean the tong sites (usually with hydrogen peroxide and saline solution) four times daily, using aseptic technique. Apply povidone-iodine ointment to the tong sites, as ordered.

13. Immobilization prevents further spinal cord damage. Skeletal traction maintains spinal column alignment. Aseptic technique helps prevent infection.

14. Use the logroll maneuver to turn a client without a Stryker frame or kinetic bed. Turn only if ordered by the physician.

14. Logrolling helps maintain spinal alignment; the maneuver requires three people, two to turn the body and one to support the head. Logrolling should not be performed without a physician's order because turning the client is dangerous until the fracture has been stabilized.

15. Assist the client with activities of daily living, as needed.

15. The client may be unable to perform activities of daily living independently.

16. Take steps to prevent thrombophlebitis and other complications of immobility (see "Immobility," pages 119 and 120, and interventions for thrombophlebitis in "Postoperative period," page 125).

16. Prolonged bed rest predisposes the client to thrombophlebitis and other complications of immobility.

17. Administer nothing by mouth until bowel sounds return.

17. Until bowel sounds return, the client is at risk for paralytic ileus.

18. Once oral feedings can begin, offer liquids with a high acid-ash content (such as cranberry juice) and restrict milk. Maintain the client on a high-fiber, vitamin-rich diet (especially the B-complex vitamins), and avoid foods that cause flatus.

18. Liquids with a high acid-ash content maintain acidic urine, thereby preventing renal calculi formation. High-fiber foods prevent constipation. The B-complex vitamins promote normal nerve function. Abdominal cramping from the client's inactivity will worsen with flatus.

19. Observe the client for symptoms of stress ulcer. Administer antacids every 2 hours or histamine$_2$ blockers, if ordered.

19. Stress ulcers commonly develop after major injuries.

20. Monitor for extreme hypertension, flushing, bradycardia, and headache. If the client has these symptoms, check for blockage or kinks in the indwelling urinary catheter (which may need replacement) and stop bowel stimulation (if stools are being digitally removed). If symptoms remain, raise the head of the bed, monitor vital signs, and call the physician. Be prepared to administer a vasodilator such as nitroprusside (Nipride).

20. These are symptoms of autonomic dysreflexia (reflex response to sympathetic nervous system stimulation), a life-threatening complication. Clients with lesions at T6 to T8 are most at risk. A full bowel or bladder is usually the cause, although autonomic dysreflexia can be triggered by any stimulus below the level of the injury. Eliminating the cause is a top priority.

21. Monitor the client's response to the room temperature, and take steps to prevent chilling or overheating.

21. Chilling can occur if the room temperature is too low. Overheating can occur if the room temperature is too warm and the client cannot perspire.

22. Handle paralyzed muscles gently. Eliminate stimuli that cause spasms.

22. During spastic paralysis, sudden or excessive jarring causes painful muscle spasms.

23. Ensure adequate urine output: For intermittent drainage, use Credé's maneuver (pressing on or tapping over the bladder) or intermittent catheterization; for continuous drainage, insert an indwelling urinary catheter. Maintain asepsis when providing care. Administer antibiotics and ascorbic acid, if ordered.

23. Maintaining adequate urine output helps prevent complications of urine retention. Catheterization may be needed because Credé's maneuver requires an intact reflex and bladder spasms, and these may be absent if the client's injury is below T12. Aseptic technique and antibiotic administration can help prevent urinary tract infection. Ascorbic acid acidifies urine.

ADULT NURSING

24. Begin bowel and bladder retraining, as needed, after the client's condition stabilizes. For bowel retraining, place the client on a bedpan or commode at regularly scheduled intervals and either provide a GI stimulus (caffeinated coffee works effectively) or administer a suppository. For bladder retraining, teach the client to use Credé's maneuver or intermittent catheterization, if possible.

24. Bowel retraining helps prevent constipation and incontinence. Without bladder retraining, damage to motor and sensory nerves can result.

25. Encourage Mr. House to express grief, stress, fears, and concerns related to his condition. Answer questions simply and honestly, correcting any misinformation he may have. Provide emotional support and positive reassurances without characterizing his condition unrealistically.

25. The client will experience loss and grieving because of his injury and its long-term consequences. His ability to cope with the current condition and future adjustments will be enhanced if the nurse focuses on positive aspects of his progress without raising false hopes.

26. Help Mr. House identify and use personal strengths to achieve his potential. Encourage his active participation in recovery by teaching him self-care and problem-solving techniques that use resources still available to him.

26. After the client begins to accept his situation, he needs to learn how to care for himself. Capitalizing on his strengths will help him adjust to physical limitations and lifestyle changes while promoting his independence.

27. Assess the family's emotional resources. Support family members as they learn to cope with the client's condition, and explain specific measures they can take to enhance the client's well-being.

27. Faced with profound lifestyle changes and a lengthy rehabilitation, the client will need tremendous support from loved ones, who will require similar support and encouragement from nursing staff.

28. Provide sexual counseling to Mr. and Mrs. House or refer them to a therapist.

28. The client's injury does not preclude sexual satisfaction, but the couple will need to develop new methods of sexual expression.

29. Implement rehabilitation strategies.

29. Paralyzed clients require long-term rehabilitation; the sooner it begins, the more successful it will be.

Evaluation

• Mr. House and his family understand and can explain the care he will require after discharge.
• Mr. House experiences no preventable complications.

Epilepsy

Epilepsy is a chronic condition characterized by seizures—excessive, uncontrolled discharges of impulses from cerebral neurons. Generalized seizures most commonly appear as tonic and clonic muscle contractions accompanied by loss of consciousness and respiratory cessation (see *International classification of seizures* for a more detailed discussion). The following clinical situation focuses on nursing care of a client with epilepsy.

Clinical situation

John Brady, a 38-year-old truck driver, had a generalized seizure while driving his truck. No one was injured, but he lost his job for safety reasons. His diagnosis is epilepsy with generalized seizures.

International classification of seizures

Partial (seizures begin locally)
Simple: No change in consciousness; motor activity; sensory response, such as hallucinations or tingling; autonomic nervous system response. Usually focal and may involve a personality change.
Complex: Impaired consciousness, confusion, impaired memory, bizarre behavioral changes, repetitive automatic activity. Progresses from partial to generalized convulsive activity.

Generalized (bilaterally asymmetrical)
Absence: Brief loss of consciousness (usually from a few seconds to a minute), staring or daydreaming, possibly eye blinking. Usually affects children. No convulsions present.
Tonic-clonic (includes tonic, clonic, myoclonic, atonic, infantile spasms, and unclassified seizures): Initially, all muscles in sustained contraction, with cessation of respiration; progresses to rapidly alternating periods of contraction and relaxation, with resumption of respirations.
Status epilepticus: Acute, prolonged seizures; no time for recovery between attacks. Includes those lasting at least 30 minutes without loss of consciousness.

Adapted from the Commission on Classification and Terminology of the International League Against Epilepsy, "Proposal for Revised Clinical and Electroencephalographic Classification of Epileptic Seizures," *Epilepsia* 22:489-501, 1981. Used with the permission of Raven Press, Ltd. New York.

Assessment

NURSING BEHAVIORS

1. Assess the client's lifestyle and occupation.

2. Identify the client's usual daily activities.

3. Assess the client's family relationships for evidence of tension and stress.

4. Obtain a description of seizures and their frequency.

NURSING RATIONALES

1. Because of seizures, a client with epilepsy may have to modify his lifestyle, alter job responsibilities, or change occupations.

2. The client may need to adjust some daily activities to prevent injury.

3. Stress increases seizure frequency.

4. Seizure descriptions help the physician classify the client's seizures.

Diagnostic evaluation
• *Electroencephalogram:* Records the brain's electrical activity patterns, which help identify seizure type. Similar to those in an electrocardiogram, the test electrodes are applied to the client's scalp to measure electrical impulses. Tell the client to wash his hair before the test for best results.
• *Serum chemistry:* Blood tests used to identify seizure causes, such as hypoglycemia, electrolyte imbalance, elevated blood urea nitrogen levels, or high blood alcohol levels
• *Computed tomography scan:* Identifies structural anomalies

Nursing diagnoses
• Risk for injury related to uncontrolled cerebral activity
• Social isolation related to the stigma sometimes associated with epilepsy
• Fear related to the unpredictable consequences of having a seizure

Planning and goals

• Mr. Brady will not be injured during a seizure.
  Mr. Brady and his family will cope effectively with the problems associated with a seizure disorder.

Implementation

NURSING BEHAVIORS	NURSING RATIONALES
1. Take the following seizure precautions: • Place the client in a flat, side-lying position. • Keep an artificial airway at the bedside. • Prevent the tongue from obstructing the airway. *Never use force or try to open a closed jaw.* • Have suction equipment available at the bedside. • Keep the bed in the low position, with the side rails up and padded.	**1.** The nurse implements seizure precautions to protect the client from serious injury.
2. Loosen clothing, but don't restrain the client. Remove potentially dangerous objects from the immediate vicinity.	**2.** These actions preserve client safety during a seizure.
3. Note the time, frequency, and duration of seizures, and describe their progression in sequential order:	**3.** These observations are vital aids in classifying the seizure and advancing the diagnosis:
• Aura (characterized by a high-pitched cry and abnormal sights, sounds, or odors)	• Produced as the client rapidly exhales air through the glottis, the high-pitched cry is the first indicator of seizure.
• Convulsive phase or ictal phase (consists of the tonic phase and the clonic phase) —Tonic phase (bilateral tonic contractions; legs extended, arms flexed, jaws clenched, eyes rolled upward; the client is unconscious and cyanotic)	—All muscles are in tonic contraction. The leg extensors have greater strength than the flexors, whereas the arm flexors have greater strength than the extensors. Respiration ceases (apnea). Incontinence may result. The tonic phase lasts less than 1 minute, with an average duration of 15 seconds.
—Clonic phase (clonic muscle contractions; shallow, irregular breathing; the client begins breathing again, but breathing isn't effective for maintaining oxygen level)	—Clonus consists of rapidly alternating muscle contractions and relaxation. Jerking movements decrease in frequency and strength over about 30 seconds.
• Postictal phase or relaxation phase (consciousness returns, and the client relaxes).	• The client needs to rest after a seizure.
4. When the client awakens, monitor vital signs and neurologic and respiratory status, and reorient him to the surroundings.	**4.** The client may be stuporous and limp and may feel confused and disoriented on awakening.
5. When the client is alert, explain the purpose, administration method, dosage, and side effects of prescribed medications. Warn him that he may have difficulty performing activities of daily living until he adjusts to the drug regimen, but urge him to continue taking medications as scheduled.	**5.** Drug therapy usually controls seizure disorders when the client strictly complies with the regimen. Effective teaching increases the client's knowledge, which will promote compliance and hasten seizure control.

ADULT NURSING

6. Encourage the client to establish and follow a daily schedule with minimal changes in the routine (for example, work the same shift and eat meals at the same time); urge him to incorporate a nutritious diet, adequate rest, and moderate exercise in the daily schedule.

6. Changes in daily habits can cause seizures. Adequate nutrition, rest, and exercise promote the client's health.

7. Teach the client, family, and friends about seizure disorders and their management.

7. This information enables the client and loved ones to plan preventive measures and to protect the client from injury if a seizure occurs.

8. Advise the client to wear an identification bracelet, such as a Medic Alert bracelet.

8. The client may be accused of drug or alcohol abuse if a seizure occurs in public. A medical identification tag will prevent embarrassment and promote assistance from others.

9. Help the client identify stressors that precipitate seizures.

9. High stress levels can precipitate seizures. Reducing stress, therefore, is a key preventive measure.

10. Advise the client to see the physician for regular checkups.

10. Certain medical problems can precipitate seizures. Regulating or correcting these problems helps control the client's condition.

11. Refer the client for counseling and vocational rehabilitation, if appropriate.

11. Safety-related job restrictions affect clients with seizure disorders. For example, in most states, only persons whose seizures are controlled for 1 year can qualify for a driver's license (which would affect Mr. Brady's career as a truck driver). Also, despite equal employment opportunity laws, some employers won't hire clients with seizure disorders. Counseling can prepare the client for a different career, if necessary, and can help the client and family cope with real or perceived social isolation (influenced by myths and ignorant of medical facts, many people still shun those with seizure disorders).

Evaluation

• Mr. Brady and his family are learning to cope effectively with epilepsy.
• Mr. Brady hasn't had any seizure-related injuries.

Multiple sclerosis

Multiple sclerosis (MS), a chronic disease caused by destruction of the myelin sheath of nerve fibers, results in motor and sensory dysfunction. The following clinical situation focuses on nursing care of a client with MS or spastic paralysis or both.

Clinical situation

Fred Johnson, a 32-year-old married construction worker, experienced fatigue, visual disturbances, and episodic paresthesias in various parts of his arms and legs. He later developed spastic paralysis of his legs. His physician says he has MS. Mr. Johnson has one child.

Assessment

NURSING BEHAVIORS	NURSING RATIONALES
1. Assess for blurred vision, nystagmus, and diplopia.	**1.** Optic neuritis is a common early sign.
2. Assess the client's sensory function by checking the arms, legs, and trunk for paresthesias.	**2.** Symptoms occur in areas supplied by peripheral nerves with demyelinated sheaths. Numbness and other paresthesias indicate the degree of nerve damage.
3. Assess the client's motor function.	**3.** Intention tremors and ataxic gait severely impair motor function.
4. Assess the client's bowel and bladder function and sexual function.	**4.** Nerve damage can cause urinary hesitancy, frequency, and retention; inability to move the bowels; and sexual impotence.
5. Determine how motor function changes affect the client's work performance and activities of daily living.	**5.** Knowing what the client can do enables the nurse to help the client use remaining abilities maximally.
6. Explore and identify the client's daily exercise habits.	**6.** Moderate exercise keeps unaffected muscles functioning and decreases pain in affected muscles. A physical therapist usually prescribes the exercise regimen.
7. Assess whether the client's emotional status affects family and work relationships.	**7.** Because of frontal lobe involvement, the client with MS may experience unrealistic mood swings (euphoria and depression), which can affect relationships.
8. Evaluate the client's relationships with family and friends to identify resources for emotional support.	**8.** As MS symptoms progress, the client will function less effectively, which, in turn, will strain relationships.
9. Assess the client's ability to do his current work.	**9.** The client may need to change jobs or quit working as his condition deteriorates.
10. Determine the family's financial resources.	**10.** Because MS requires costly treatment over an extended time, assistance from community resources may be required to meet the family's financial needs.

Diagnostic evaluation

- *Neurologic examination:* Tests all nervous system functions to identify dysfunctional sensory and motor areas
- *Computed tomography scan and magnetic resonance imaging:* Look for structural abnormalities
- *Serologic studies:* Identify high levels of marker antigens
- *Cerebral spinal fluid:* Analysis of fluid obtained by lumbar puncture commonly shows increased gamma globulin

Nursing diagnoses

- Impaired physical mobility related to paralysis of the lower limbs
- Feeding self-care deficit related to tremors, spasticity, and paralysis
- Bathing or hygiene self-care deficit related to tremors, spasticity, and paralysis

- Dressing or grooming self-care deficit related to tremors, spasticity, and paralysis
- Toileting self-care deficit related to tremors, spasticity, and paralysis
- Altered family processes related to the illness of the father and husband
- Body image disturbance related to decreased physical function
- Altered urinary elimination related to bladder spasms or retention

Planning and goals

- Mr. Johnson will have normal function of unaffected muscles.
- Mr. Johnson will have improved function in affected muscles.
- Mr. Johnson and his family will cope effectively with health problems associated with MS.
- Mr. Johnson will experience no complications.

Implementation

NURSING BEHAVIORS	NURSING RATIONALES
1. Provide the client with physical therapy (for example, stretching and strengthening exercises for muscles with paresis or spastic paralysis and active exercises for unaffected muscles). Caution the client not to become overfatigued.	**1.** Appropriate exercise decreases muscle spasticity and pain while maintaining function in unaffected muscles. Overfatigue increases muscle aches and spasms.
2. Gently handle muscles having spastic paralysis; don't bump the client's bed; identify movements and positions that initiate muscle spasms.	**2.** Rough handling causes painful muscle spasms. Positioning the client's body in normal alignment reduces the potential for spasms and pain.
3. Assist the client with activities of daily living, as needed, and teach self-care strategies.	**3.** Because MS is progressively debilitating, the nurse's objective is to help the client maintain independence for as long as possible.
4. Provide gait retraining for the ataxic (muscularly uncoordinated) client (who may also use a cane or walker), as necessary.	**4.** Because the client will be unsteady on his feet, safety precautions will prevent injury.
5. Provide bowel and bladder retraining if the client becomes incontinent.	**5.** If muscles facilitating defecation and urination are affected, retraining may be necessary.
• Administer propantheline (Pro-Banthine), if ordered.	• Anticholinergics are used to treat spastic bladder.
• Administer a cholinergic such as bethanechol (Urecholine).	• Cholinergics are used to treat bladder flaccidity, which causes urine retention.
6. Encourage fluid intake—up to 2,000 ml/day (about 2 quarts) for the constipated client, unless medically contraindicated.	**6.** Peristalsis slows with inactivity. Increasing fluid intake softens the stool. A high-fiber diet and stool softeners also may be recommended.
7. Assist the family and friends to understand the client's health problems; reinforce their support of the client.	**7.** Because of the many emotional problems accompanying MS, family members and friends may have difficulty being supportive. Divorce is common.
8. If ordered, administer cortisone or corticotropin.	**8.** These drugs weaken acute inflammation. Exacerbations may be treated with cyclophosphamide (Cytoxan) or interferon.

ADULT NURSING

Health teaching for clients with impaired physical mobility

Nursing behaviors	Nursing rationales
1. Plan a realistic daily schedule with the client.	1. Because of muscle dysfunction, the client requires additional time to perform activities of daily living.
2. Encourage moderate exercise—just enough to prevent progressive rigidity but not enough to cause fatigue.	2. Exercise maintains the tone and function of unaffected muscles and reduces disease effects on affected muscles. Fatigue increases muscle rigidity, precipitates muscle spasm, and lowers the client's resistance to infection.
3. Enforce adequate rest periods.	3. Rest contributes to optimal health while reducing muscle rigidity.
4. Reduce physical and emotional stresses.	4. Depression, emotional upsets, and anxiety increase muscle rigidity.
5. Teach the client to take safety precautions for walking, such as removing scatter rugs from the household and using a cane or walker.	5. A client with impaired physical mobility has a poor sense of balance.
6. Teach the client to use assistive devices when performing activities of daily living (for example, using clothing snaps instead of buttons and mesh fasteners instead of zippers).	6. Assistive devices enable the client to perform many self-care tasks independently.
7. Caution the client to avoid persons with infections and to follow a nutritious diet.	7. A disease progresses more slowly when the client is otherwise healthy.
8. Advise the client to wear medical identification, such as a Medic Alert bracelet.	8. The information enables others to provide appropriate care in an emergency.
9. Teach the client about medications and their side effects.	9. A client who complies with the medication regimen is most likely to benefit from it. Understanding drug actions and side effects usually enhances compliance.
10. Provide generous emotional support to the client and family.	10. The nurse's support and encouragement help the client and family cope with the many problems they will encounter.

9. Recommend psychological consultation if the client demonstrates emotional problems.

9. The problems of coping with and accepting the debilitating physical changes caused by MS are compounded by accompanying emotional changes. The client may require psychotherapy.

10. Suggest sexual counseling for the impotent client.

10. The client with MS needs to function sexually as normally as possible, which may mean learning alternative techniques.

11. Offer vocational counseling referral as appropriate.

11. The client's ability to work normally decreases as the disease progresses. Knowing about available and realistic work alternatives promotes a more positive outlook.

12. Suggest resources for financial assistance.

12. Treatment costs and family needs may exceed the client's and family's resources.

13. Teach the client to remain active and to avoid bed rest.

13. Bed rest and inactivity decrease motor function, worsening the client's condition.

14. Prevent complications of immobility.

14. During an exacerbation of MS or infection, the client may require bed rest. The complications of bed rest are pneumonia, urinary tract infection, and pressure ulcers.

15. Provide health teaching.

15. See *Health teaching for clients with impaired physical mobility,* for specific interventions and rationales.

16. Refer the client to the local chapter of the Multiple Sclerosis Society.

16. This organization can provide supportive services.

Evaluation

• Mr. Johnson and his family can cope effectively with MS-associated problems.
• Mr. Johnson has normal function in muscles unaffected by MS and improved function in affected muscles.

Myasthenia gravis

Myasthenia gravis is a chronic neuromuscular autoimmune disease characterized by rapid exhaustion of voluntary muscles during activity and profound muscular weakness after activity. The client's muscle strength improves with rest.

Nursing care of a client with myasthenia gravis includes monitoring for myasthenic or cholinergic crisis. Myasthenic crisis is caused by a sudden increase in motor symptoms, commonly from lack of medication; symptoms include ptosis, decreased blood pressure, absent cough reflex, and incontinence. Cholinergic crisis is caused by overmedication with anticholinesterase (cholinergic drugs); symptoms include nausea and vomiting, abdominal cramps, miosis, and blurred vision. Both conditions cause respiratory distress, weakness, and difficulty in swallowing and speaking. Tensilon may be given to determine which crisis the client is experiencing. In addition to treatments described below, plasmapheresis or thymectomy is used with some clients.

Clinical situation

Marjorie Hardy is a 35-year-old tightrope walker who began experiencing exhaustion of voluntary muscles during rehearsals and performances and severe muscular weakness afterward. On reviewing diagnostic test results, the physician has tentatively diagnosed her condition as myasthenia gravis.

Assessment

NURSING BEHAVIORS

NURSING RATIONALES

1. Assess the client's muscle weakness in the morning and evening.

1. Because muscles weaken with activity and regain strength with rest, the client with myasthenia gravis will have more severe muscle weakness in the evening.

2. Assess all voluntary muscles for weakness during activity and improvement with rest, including:

• muscles used in chewing and swallowing

• muscles used in breathing and laughing

• ocular muscles

• vocal weakness after talking.

2. The client will display a decreased response to nerve impulses, which decreases the strength of voluntary muscles because of an impaired conduction of nerve impulses at the myoneural junction.

• Nutrition may show impairment.

• Breathlessness is an early sign of respiratory involvement. If the intercostals or the diaphragm is affected, the client's condition can be life-threatening.

• Ptosis and diplopia commonly occur.

• Fatigue will weaken muscles needed for talking.

Diagnostic evaluation
• *Electromyography:* Assesses the functioning of affected muscles
• *Tensilon (edrophonium) test:* Confirms the diagnosis if the client's muscle strength increases after Tensilon administration; alternatively, neostigmine methylsulfate (Prostigmin) may be used
• *Computed tomography scan of the chest and chest X-ray:* Detect thymomas

Nursing diagnoses
• Feeding self-care deficit related to muscle weakness
• Bathing or hygiene self-care deficit related to muscle weakness
• Dressing or grooming self-care deficit related to muscle weakness
• Toileting self-care deficit related to muscle weakness
• Activity intolerance related to muscle weakness
• Impaired physical mobility related to muscle weakness
• Powerlessness related to lack of control over condition
• Ineffective airway clearance related to muscle weakness

Planning and goals
• Ms. Hardy will retain optimal functioning of unaffected muscles.
• Ms. Hardy and her family will learn to cope with the problems presented by this disease.
• Ms. Hardy will not experience complications of immobility.
• Ms. Hardy's muscular strength will improve.
• Ms. Hardy and her family will understand how they should manage myasthenia gravis.

Implementation
NURSING BEHAVIORS

1. Administer cholinergic medications, as ordered, such as pyridostigmine bromide (Mestinon) and neostigmine bromide (Prostigmin). Monitor the client for possible side effects, including abdominal cramping, diarrhea, muscle weakness (inadequate dose), nausea, vomiting, excessive salivation, and miosis.

2. Administer corticosteroids, as ordered. Clients are often maintained on alternate-day prednisone.

NURSING RATIONALES

1. These medications temporarily inhibit anticholinesterase at the neuromuscular junction, which enhances the action of acetylcholine. The response of muscles to nerve impulses increases. The physician should prescribe time-span tablets in a dosage high enough to provide maximum results without side effects. *Note:* Atropine sulfate is the antidote to cholinergic drugs.

2. Corticosteroids suppress the autoimmune response.

3. Schedule the client's daily activity and the action pattern of her medication to peak at the same time. Schedule realistic activity, balancing rest and exercise.

3. The client will receive maximum benefit from the drugs if their peak action occurs during her most active period. A realistic schedule will prevent excessive muscle weakness.

4. If the disorder affects the muscles of mastication, give soft, easily chewable food, and keep suction equipment in the client's room.

4. If chewing requires more energy than the client has, the client may aspirate unchewed food.

5. If the client's respiratory muscles are affected, make frequent assessments of breath sounds, respirations, and blood gases. If she has difficulty breathing, position her to maintain an adequate airway, and keep a ventilator and emergency drugs at her bedside.

5. Respiratory failure is a possible complication of myasthenia gravis.

6. If the client has many flaccid muscle groups, implement nursing care to prevent complications from immobility.

6. Myasthenia gravis can lead to complications of immobility (see "Immobility," pages 119 and 120).

7. As much as possible, prevent emotional upsets and unnecessary stress.

7. Emotional upsets can exacerbate myasthenia gravis.

8. Implement safety precautions related to affected muscles.

8. Suctioning, chest physiotherapy, oxygen administration, intubation, ambulation, and range-of-motion (ROM) exercises can prevent injury.

9. Provide physical therapy or passive or active ROM exercises.

9. Exercises within the client's ability will maintain functional muscles and improve the function of weakened muscles.

10. Provide speech therapy, as needed.

10. Speech therapy will enhance the client's ability to communicate.

11. Prevent constipation by promoting increased fluid intake and a high-fiber diet.

11. The client's inactivity may result in constipation.

12. Teach the client to follow a nutritious diet and to eat safely. Urge an overweight client to reduce caloric intake.

12. A nutritious diet will help prevent infection while providing adequate calories. The client should take small bites and chew thoroughly to avoid aspirating. Excessive weight increases the energy and strength needed to perform daily activities.

13. Teach the client how and when to take medications.

13. For drug therapy to be effective, the client must take all medications as ordered—on time, consistently, and without skipping doses.

14. Instruct the client to avoid alcohol, tobacco, and drugs that promote muscle relaxation; prolonged exposure to extreme heat or cold; and contact with persons who have upper respiratory infections.

14. Alcohol, tobacco, and muscle relaxants may increase muscle weakness. Exposure to extreme temperatures or to a person with an upper respiratory infection increases the client's susceptibility to infection, especially if the client is under stress.

ADULT NURSING

15. Have the client wear a medical identification tag.

15. In an emergency, caregivers should know the client has myasthenia gravis.

16. Teach the client symptoms to report to the physician.

16. The client will need rapid medical intervention to prevent further muscle weakness.

17. Refer the client and her family to the Myasthenia Gravis Foundation or a similar organization.

17. These agencies can provide emotional support and educational resources to help the client and her family cope with the disease.

18. Refer the client for vocational counseling as needed.

18. The client's condition may prevent her from resuming her previous occupation. Vocational counselors offer guidance and support in choosing and establishing a new career.

Evaluation

• Ms. Hardy has optimal functioning of unaffected muscles and increased muscular strength in affected muscles.
• Ms. Hardy and her family can explain the care she requires, medication dosages and side effects, her daily schedule of activities, and ways to maintain her independence.
• Ms. Hardy has not experienced complications of immobility during exacerbations.

Parkinson's disease

Parkinson's disease, a chronic, degenerative nervous system disease, affects the cells of the brain's basal ganglia. The following clinical situation focuses on nursing care of a client with tremors and muscle rigidity.

Clinical situation

Chad Faland, age 69, is a retired wood-carver who has tremors of the head and hands, especially when he rests. He has a masklike facial expression and muffled speech patterns. Mr. Faland's wife insisted that he see his physician, who has diagnosed Parkinson's disease.

Assessment

NURSING BEHAVIORS

NURSING RATIONALES

1. Assess for tremors.

1. Tremors are involuntary and occur when the client is at rest. The most common initial symptoms are pillrolling of the thumb and forefinger; up-and-down head tremors; and voice tremors.

2. Assess muscle rigidity, noting which muscles are affected and how severely.

2. The basal ganglia contribute to control of coordination associated with automatic and gross intentional muscle movements.

3. Determine how much difficulty the client has with changing positions and maintaining balance and posture.

3. As the cells in the basal ganglia degenerate, the client encounters progressive difficulty in maintaining posture and equilibrium and in changing position.

4. Assess the client's gait for festination.

4. Festination, or propulsive gait, commonly appears as the client, bent forward, takes a series of quick, short steps on his toes. Falls occur because of impaired equilibrium.

5. Evaluate motor function.

5. How well the client can perform activities of daily living determines nursing interventions.

6. Observe for emotional changes.

6. The cerebral cortex may be affected as the disease progresses.

7. Note the client's facial expression.

7. A client with Parkinson's disease typically has a masklike expression with a fixed stare.

8. Assess the client's relationships with his spouse, family, and friends.

8. A client with Parkinson's disease needs emotional support and understanding from loved ones. Stress and anxiety from strained relationships increase symptoms.

Diagnostic evaluation
- *Neurologic examination* (complete evaluation): Identifies dysfunctioning areas
- *Electromyography:* Determines muscle function

Nursing diagnoses
- Impaired physical mobility related to muscle rigidity and poor balance
- Feeding self-care deficit related to muscle tremors and deformity
- Bathing or hygiene self-care deficit related to muscle tremors and deformity
- Dressing or grooming self-care deficit related to muscle tremors and deformity
- Toileting self-care deficit related to muscle tremors and deformity
- Risk for injury related to poor balance

Planning and goals
- Mr. Faland will have normal functioning of unaffected muscles and improved functioning of affected muscles.
- Mr. and Mrs. Faland will cope effectively with the problems related to Parkinson's disease.
- Mr. Faland will experience no complications of immobility.

Implementation
NURSING BEHAVIORS

NURSING RATIONALES

1. Provide the client with physical therapy to reduce muscle rigidity and decrease deformities, and show him how to incorporate specific exercises into his daily schedule.

1. Daily exercise reduces muscle rigidity, minimizes deformity of affected muscles, and maintains normal functioning of the unaffected muscles. The nurse's encouragement, teaching, and guidance will help him accept a new routine.

2. As ordered, administer levodopa (Dopar) and carbidopa-levodopa (Sinemet) or an anticholinergic drug, such as benztropine mesylate (Cogentin) or trihexyphenidyl hydrochloride (Aparkane, Artane).

2. Antiparkinsonian agents help control Parkinson's disease. Levodopa relieves muscle rigidity and reduces tremors, and carbidopa-levodopa prevents levodopa's destruction. Anticholinergic drugs relieve muscle rigidity and tremors by decreasing the stimulating effects of acetylcholine.

ADULT NURSING

3. Monitor the client for side effects of antiparkinsonian agents. Teach the client preventive measures, such as slowly sitting and standing to prevent postural hypotension.

3. Side effects of levodopa (besides postural hypotension) include anorexia, vomiting, GI bleeding, cough, hoarseness, and jerky, involuntary movements. Side effects of anticholinergics include dry mouth, blurred vision, dizziness, urine retention, and glaucoma.

4. Take measures to prevent complications of immobility (see *Health teaching for clients with impaired physical mobility,* page 478).

4. When a client with Parkinson's disease is bedridden (from an exacerbation or an unrelated illness), complications of immobility commonly occur.

5. Provide emotional support for the client and family, and teach family members how they can support the client.

5. Parkinson's disease causes progressive functional loss, which is debilitating to the client and those close to him. Therapeutic support is vital.

6. Advise the client where and how to obtain financial assistance.

6. As the disease progresses, the client may be unable to meet health care costs independently.

7. Refer the client and family to the Parkinson's Disease Foundation.

7. Support groups can increase their understanding of the disease process and enhance their ability to learn new coping skills.

Evaluation

- Mr. Faland and his wife are coping effectively with Parkinson's disease.
- Mr. Faland has less muscle rigidity.

RESPIRATORY SYSTEM

Pulmonary tuberculosis

Caused by the acid-fast, gram-positive aerobic bacillus *Mycobacterium tuberculosis,* tuberculosis (TB) is considered preventable, although it continues to be a worldwide health problem. In the United States, its major incidence is in cities and in areas with high immigrant populations. TB occurs most commonly in the lower socioeconomic groups and is associated with overwork, poor nutrition, and overcrowding combined with poor ventilation. Individuals on steroid therapy and those positive for the human immunodeficiency virus have increased susceptibility to TB. After experiencing a decline, TB has steadily increased in the United States since 1986.

Inhaled bacilli, carried by droplet nuclei, usually settle in alveolar lung tissue, where they begin an inflammatory process. Leukocytes and macrophages phagocytize the invader but fail to kill it. Lymphocytes continue to surround the infecting organism for 10 to 20 days. The regional (hilar) lymph nodes become inflamed. A tubercle's center becomes necrotic, causing caseation (a process that changes dead tissue into a cheeselike substance). The organism may be walled off by the capsule and scar tissue. It may heal and produce no effects of illness, or it may progress to active disease. Sometimes the bacillus causes pneumonia-like symptoms. Most instances of active disease involve reactivation of the primary infection because the disease organisms remain dormant within the tubercle. Physical or emotional stress activates the organisms. (See *Guidelines for preventing tuberculosis.*)

Guidelines for preventing tuberculosis

The main purpose of preventive therapy is to keep latent infection from progressing to clinically active tuberculosis (TB). Therefore, persons with positive tuberculin skin test results who do not have clinically active disease should be evaluated for preventive therapy.

Preventive therapy for TB usually consists of treatment with isoniazid for 6 to 12 months. Treatment is recommended for:
• household members and others who have close contact with an infected individual
• newly infected individuals (positive tuberculin skin test conversion within the past 2 years)
• residents of long-term institutions (including correctional institutions and nursing homes) who have a positive tuberculin skin test result
• individuals with fibrotic infiltrates on chest X-ray that are thought to represent previously healed TB
• infected individuals (positive tuberculin skin test) with selected conditions (such as diabetes, silicosis, and acquired immunodeficiency syndrome) or circumstances (those who have tested positive for human immunodeficiency virus [HIV] or who are undergoing corticosteroid or immunosuppressive therapy)
• positive tuberculin skin test reactors under age 35
• I.V. drug users with a positive tuberculin skin test.

To ensure that persons in high-risk groups adhere to preventive therapy, health care workers are encouraged to use directly observed therapy (DOT). With DOT, a health care provider or designated person must directly observe a patient as he or she ingests anti-TB medications. The patient and provider should agree on a method that ensures the best possible DOT routine and that maintains the patient's confidentiality. Patients not receiving DOT who demonstrate noncompliant behaviors to preventive therapy (such as missed appointments) should be reported to the appropriate public health officials and be given DOT.

Source: U.S. Department of Health and Human Services. *TB Facts for Health Care Workers.* Centers for Disease Control and Prevention, Atlanta, Ga., 1993.

Clinical situation

Juan Lopez, age 40, works as a fruit picker in southern California. He entered the United States illegally and works long hours for meager wages to support his family. His fear of deportation initially caused him to conceal his symptoms (fatigue, anorexia, night sweats, weight loss, and productive cough). Eventually, he went to the clinic, where he was diagnosed as having pulmonary tuberculosis. His wife and four children have positive tuberculin skin-test reactions. Their chest X-rays reveal no lung changes, and they have no active TB symptoms. Hospitalized for 1 week, Mr. Lopez is discharged home for further treatment.

Assessment

NURSING BEHAVIORS	NURSING RATIONALES
1. Note early symptoms, including low-grade fever, fatigue, malaise, anorexia, weight loss, and night sweats.	**1.** Characteristic symptoms, including night sweats, result from inflammation. All are signs of generalized debility from untreated TB.
2. Observe for coughing that increases in frequency and productivity as the disease progresses; also observe for hemoptysis, dyspnea, and pleuritic pain.	**2.** This type of cough occurs if caseous material liquefies and erodes the bronchioles. Although frightening to most clients, bloody sputum, caused by erosion into the capillaries and blood vessels, rarely threatens life. Labored breathing shows extensive pulmonary involvement. Chest pain results from pleural effusion if the caseous material spreads into the pleural space.

ADULT NURSING

Diagnostic evaluation

• *Skin tests:* Evaluate the client's reaction to an intradermal injection of old tuberculin or purified protein derivative. The Mantoux test is considered the most accurate. Sensitized clients have a localized reaction in 24 to 72 hours. An induration, or welt, that measures more than 10 mm (about ¹/₂ inch) indicates a positive reaction; one that measures less than 4 mm (about ¹/₆ inch) indicates a negative reaction; those between 4 and 10 mm are inconclusive and require retesting.
• *Chest X-ray:* Shows lung changes consistent with TB.
• *Smear:* Detects disease organisms through acid-fast staining of secretion samples (sputum). Smear results can be obtained faster than culture results but may be diagnostically inconclusive.
• *Sputum culture:* The TB organism grows slowly. Sputum culture results take about 3 weeks to be determined positive and 6 weeks to be confirmed negative. The culture sample should be obtained first thing in the morning. Instruct the client not to use mouthwash, which may impair viability of the organism. Tell the client to cough deeply to produce about 1 teaspoon of sputum, and deposit it in a sterile container. Immediately send the sealed container to the bacteriology laboratory.

Nursing diagnoses

• Ineffective airway clearance related to increased respiratory secretions
• Altered health maintenance related to malaise
• Knowledge deficit related to medication management
• Altered nutrition (less than body requirements) related to anorexia and weight loss

Planning and goals

• Mr. Lopez will take prescribed medications as directed and will understand why he must do so.
• Mr. Lopez will explain ways to prevent organisms from spreading.
• Mr. Lopez's nutritional needs will be met.
• Mr. Lopez and his family will remain free of active pulmonary disease.

Implementation

NURSING BEHAVIORS	NURSING RATIONALES
1. Administer medications, as ordered, and teach the client the importance of following the prescribed regimen.	**1.** Initially, drug therapy with at least four primary drugs (used in combination to delay the disease organism's drug resistance) is the cornerstone of active disease treatment. Commonly, clients become discouraged by the long-term nature of TB treatment (6 to 24 months). However, the client who discontinues even one drug early may develop drug resistance, making the disease more difficult to treat.
2. Tell the client to cover his mouth when coughing, sneezing, or raising sputum.	**2.** Covering the mouth prevents organisms from spreading.
3. Have the client use disposable tissues and discard them according to institutional policy.	**3.** Tissues are infectious waste and should be treated as such.
4. Teach the client to wash his hands after handling handkerchiefs or other items that contact sputum.	**4.** Medical asepsis prevents the spread of disease.

Generalized guidelines for respiratory isolation

- Provide a private room for the client, and keep the door closed.
- Wash hands when entering and leaving the room.
- Use special handling procedures for sputum and secretions.
- Have the client wear a mask when being transported outside the room.
- Provide masks for people coming in direct contact with the client (depending on the organism, its mode of transmission, and the health care facility's infection control policy).

5. If the client's severe coughing bouts prevent sleep, administer a cough suppressant, such as codeine, hydrocodone bitartrate (Hycodan), or benzonatate (Tessalon), as ordered. Administer cough suppressants cautiously, however, and warn the client about side effects.

5. Although cough suppressants can minimize coughing spells that hinder sleep, they also can cause atelectasis and pneumonitis. Additionally, codeine may cause constipation and respiratory depression, and benzonatate may produce drowsiness, dizziness, nausea, and vomiting.

6. Expose the environment to ultraviolet light treatments, if ordered, and advise the client to let as much direct sunlight as possible into his home once he is discharged.

6. Sunlight kills bacteria in 1 to 2 hours.

7. Ensure that the client's environment is adequately ventilated.

7. Circulating air disperses airborne organisms to low levels, impeding potential contamination.

8. Tell the client he doesn't need to wear a mask for infection control if he can cover his mouth (see *Generalized guidelines for respiratory isolation*).

8. Droplet nuclei can pass through a mask, which provides less reliable protection than covering the mouth does.

9. Encourage the client to eat foods rich in protein, calcium, and vitamins C, D, and B complex.

9. These foods facilitate healing and improve overall nutritional status.

10. Review treatment measures for family members.

10. Adults take 300 mg of isoniazid daily for 1 year to prevent active disease. Children also receive isoniazid. Dosage follows body weight standards.

11. Refer the client for community health follow-up examinations.

11. The client's socioeconomic status may create complex problems affecting his ability to afford health care, purchase proper foods and adequate housing, and attain proper rest and relaxation.

Evaluation

- Mr. Lopez understands and follows the medication regimen.
- Mr. Lopez gains weight.
- The other Lopez family members comply with their medication regimen, and no one has active disease.
- Mr. Lopez can describe and demonstrate ways to prevent the spread of TB organisms.

Chronic airflow limitation

Chronic airflow limitation, commonly referred to as chronic obstructive pulmonary disease (COPD), encompasses a group of conditions that obstruct pulmonary air outflow, resulting in air being trapped in the alveoli.

Chronic obstructive bronchitis, a productive cough persisting for 3 months of the year for at least 2 consecutive years, causes inflamed airways that lead to increased mucus production and bronchospasms. Mucus plugs entrap air and result in alveolar hyperinflation. Clients with severe chronic bronchitis usually have severe hypoxemia and polycythemia, with hematocrit values from 50% to 55%.

Emphysema, characterized by enlargement of the alveoli distal to the terminal bronchioles, leads to alveolar wall destruction, obstructed expiratory airflow, and irreversible loss of lung elasticity. Emphysema causes less hypoxemia than chronic bronchitis does, and hematocrit values commonly are normal.

Asthma, marked by widespread airway narrowing in response to various stimuli, is considered a COPD only if airway obstruction becomes irreversible.

Clinical situation

Ronald Dawson works in a paper mill in the town where he has lived all his life. For 30 of his 50 years, he has been a smoker. His mill job exposes him to paper dust daily. Mr. Dawson's diagnosis is chronic bronchitis and emphysema.

Assessment

NURSING BEHAVIORS	NURSING RATIONALES
1. Investigate the prevalence of known COPD factors.	**1.** Smoking and air pollution are known factors contributing to COPD. White men, ages 50 to 70, are at greatest risk. In some people, a hereditary factor (genetic deficiency of antitrypsin) contributes to emphysema.
2. Observe for dyspnea.	**2.** Labored breathing, a common early subjective symptom, usually occurs on exertion in COPD's early stages. In later stages it also occurs at rest.
3. Watch for characteristic posturings, such as leaning forward and propping the arms on a table or chair.	**3.** This position compresses the abdomen, lifts the diaphragm, and increases intrathoracic pressure, permitting increased air expiration.
4. Evaluate the character and frequency of the client's cough and the time of day it occurs; if it is productive, note the sputum's color, consistency, and amount.	**4.** In chronic bronchitis, the sputum usually appears gray, sticky, and thick. In early stages, it is most abundant in the morning; later, it is produced throughout the day. In emphysema, sputum amounts are not so high. Yellow or green sputum may indicate infection, a common complication.
5. Listen for wheezing.	**5.** Wheezing results from air being expired against a collapsed airway.

6. Assess the physical appearance of the chest, and observe for decreased respiratory rate and the following:

6. Respirations are slower and deeper because of bronchial obstruction.

• prolonged expiratory time

• Pulmonary obstruction prolongs expiration times.

• barrel chest with increased anteroposterior diameter

• Hyperinflation causes diaphragm and rib fixation in inspiration.

• decreased chest excursion

• A fixed inspiratory position decreases chest movement.

• accessory muscle use

• The client uses the trapezius, pectorals, and sternocleidomastoid to help him breathe.

• hyperresonant lung sounds on percussion.

• Hyperresonance results from alveolar hyperinflation.

7. Assess the client's fatigue level.

7. The burden of increased breathing produces dyspnea, general fatigue, and tissue hypoxia.

8. Note signs of right ventricular failure.

8. With progressive COPD, pulmonary vascular resistance increases, which leads to pulmonary hypertension and, eventually, to cor pulmonale (right ventricular failure) secondary to lung disease.

9. Determine the effects of COPD on the client's lifestyle.

9. COPD may cause decreased activity tolerance, altered self-image, role changes that necessitate early retirement, and emotional changes that affect interpersonal and family relationships.

Diagnostic evaluation

• *Pulmonary function tests:* Spirometry is particularly valuable in screening lung function.
• *Chest X-ray:* This lung study provides baseline norms for each client with COPD. In late-stage disease, the client's diaphragm will appear flat on the X-ray film.
• *Arterial blood gas studies:* Elevated PCO_2 levels cause hypercapnia; decreased PO_2 levels result in hypoxemia. Bicarbonate levels may rise to compensate for chronic hypercapnia and the resultant respiratory acidosis.
• *Complete blood count (CBC):* In clients with COPD, the CBC shows elevated hemoglobin and hematocrit values.
• *Pulse oximetry:* Noninvasive monitoring of arterial oxygen saturation is performed at the bedside. Normal O_2 saturation is 95% to 98%; a falling O_2 saturation indicates impending hypoxia.

Nursing diagnoses

• Ineffective airway clearance related to thick secretions
• Impaired gas exchange related to loss of alveolar elasticity
• Self-esteem disturbance related to role changes

Planning and goals

• Mr. Dawson will maintain adequate gas exchange.
• Mr. Dawson will remain free of infection.
• Mr. Dawson will establish an effective breathing pattern.
• Mr. Dawson will have an adequately clear airway.
• Mr. Dawson will understand why he should avoid respiratory irritants.

Implementation

NURSING BEHAVIORS	NURSING RATIONALES
1. Teach the client how smoking and other respiratory irritants affect the lungs, and help him adopt a plan to give up smoking.	**1.** Smoking damages the ciliary clearing mechanism, thereby advancing inflammation. Because psychological addiction lasts for a minimum of several months, developing detailed strategies to quit smoking will increase the client's chances of success.
2. Teach the client pursed-lip breathing and abdominal breathing.	**2.** Breathing through pursed lips slows respiration and raises the intrabronchial pressure, which keeps the airway open longer, thereby decreasing alveolar air entrapment. Abdominal breathing increases respiratory excursion by elevating the diaphragm.
3. Teach the client effective deep-breathing and coughing techniques. Demonstrate how to sit, lean forward, take several deep breaths, and cough deeply several times without taking a breath in between coughs. Keep suction equipment on hand in case the client can't remove all secretions.	**3.** Effective deep-breathing and coughing techniques tense the abdominal muscles, putting more pressure on the diaphragm.
4. Use chest physiotherapy, as follows:	**4.** Chest physiotherapy helps remove secretions to improve breathing.
• Postural drainage: Position the client to drain all lung segments (include the head-down position to drain lower lobes, and modify positions according to the client's tolerance). Be sure to protect the client from falling and ensure his comfort. Gradually increase the position time to 20 minutes. Use a nebulizer first, and watch for such side effects as nausea and bronchospasm. Administer mucolytics, as ordered.	• Postural drainage uses gravity to remove retained secretions from the bronchial tree. Nebulization liquefies and loosens secretions. Mucolytics such as acetylcysteine decrease the sputum's viscosity.
• Percussion and vibration: Cup the hands and rhythmically strike the area to be drained. After percussion, use vibrations during expiration about five times.	• Percussion and vibration break up mucus plugs and move air into the alveoli, draining the lungs' deep periphery. The technique is contraindicated with hemorrhage or pain.
5. Provide adequate hydration, and watch for signs of fluid overload.	**5.** Fluid helps liquefy secretions to facilitate their removal. The client is at risk for fluid overload because of right-sided heart failure associated with COPD.
6. Teach the client to recognize signs of infection, such as fever and changes in the color and amount of sputum. Administer tetracycline, ampicillin, or another antibiotic, as prescribed.	**6.** Because infection frequently complicates COPD, antibiotic therapy (often used prophylactically) should start with the first infection sign.
7. Administer an expectorant, such as guaifenesin (Robitussin), or iodinated glycerol (Organidin), as ordered.	**7.** Expectorants are administered to liquefy secretions. Most expectorants have few side effects.

8. As ordered, administer a bronchodilator, such as epinephrine, metaproterenol (Alupent), albuterol (Ventolin), theophylline, or aminophylline. Explain appropriate administration routes, dosages, procedures to follow, and side effects to document or report.

8. Bronchodilators relieve bronchospasms, thereby increasing airway size. The drugs can be inhaled or given orally, subcutaneously, rectally, or (for acute bronchospasm) I.V. Inhalation therapy is commonly self-administered by metered-dose aerosol cartridge; the client should take bronchodilators as prescribed and keep an accurate administration record. Because bronchodilators interact with antihistamines, thyroid drugs, and other sympathomimetic drugs, they increase the potential for cardiac side effects, including tachycardia and palpitations. Other side effects include restlessness, nausea, and vomiting.

9. Administer corticosteroids, as ordered.

9. Corticosteroids decrease bronchospasms and bronchial inflammation. Current treatment includes increased use of inhaled corticosteroids.

10. Administer oxygen, as ordered, usually at 1 to 2 liters/minute in 24% to 28% concentrations (should not exceed 40%).

10. Because the client with COPD has chronically elevated PCO_2 levels and has lost the normal stimulus to breathe, he breathes from hypoxic drive; that is, chemoreceptors in the carotid and aortic arch, responding to the low PO_2 level, stimulate the respiratory center in the medulla. Breathing high oxygen concentrations can knock out the reflex hypoxic drive, decrease ventilation, raise PCO_2 values to toxic levels, and lead to carbon dioxide narcosis, confusion, coma, and death. Oxygen usually is administered only when the client shows signs of hypoxia and when PO_2 levels fall below 60 mm Hg.

11. Keep the client out of bed and walking.

11. Dyspneic clients, reluctant to move, are prone to complications of immobility.

12. Teach the client to maintain a normal weight by eating small, frequent meals; advise him to avoid gas-forming foods and to add fiber to the diet to prevent constipation.

12. Sensible eating will prevent increased pressure on the diaphragm and help decrease the work of breathing.

13. At discharge, make sure the client can describe healthful self-care and home-management routines, such as balancing frequent rest periods with activity each day. Explain the importance of avoiding people with respiratory infections and getting a yearly influenza vaccination. Also determine his need for support services and vocational or other counseling. Clients also should receive pneumococcal vaccine.

13. The client who understands why and how to implement a regimen to benefit him will be more likely to comply with treatment. Check history; if client has not received pneumococcal vaccine, he should discuss it with his physician.

14. As appropriate, refer the client for pulmonary rehabilitation and to a support group.

14. This increases the client's exercise tolerance and improves quality of life.

ADULT NURSING

Evaluation

• Mr. Dawson stops smoking and obtains a job with less exposure to respiratory irritants.
• Mr. Dawson remains free of respiratory infection.
• Mr. Dawson regularly practices breathing exercises, and his breathing efficiency increases.

Segmental resection of the lung

In a segmental resection, one or more lung segments are removed to retain as much functioning lung tissue as possible. An exacting surgical procedure, it may be used to treat bronchiectasis, lung abscess, metastatic cancer, or situations in which the client cannot tolerate a lobectomy or pneumonectomy. Chest tubes would be required postoperatively.

Any intrapleural pressure interruption requires the use of chest tubes. Normal intrapleural pressure is always negative, ranging from -2 to -4 cm during expiration and from -6 to -8 cm during inspiration. Atmospheric pressure replaces negative intrapleural pressure when the chest is opened during surgery or when it sustains a sucking injury, such as a gunshot wound. A sucking injury usually requires two chest tubes.

Chest tubes are used to remove blood and air, to reexpand the lung, and to restore negative pressure. The upper tube removes air; the lower tube removes fluid. The drainage system works by using a one-way valve system, or water seal. The water seal prevents air and blood from flowing back into the chest cavity. (See *Closed chest drainage system* for associated information, see *Points to remember in oxygen therapy,* page 494.)

Clinical situation

Diane Sharp, age 60, was admitted to the hospital with a cough and hemoptysis. She will undergo bronchoscopy and possible segmental resection of a coin-sized lesion in the lower lobe of her right lung. The lesion was detected by X-ray.

Assessment

NURSING BEHAVIORS

NURSING RATIONALES

Preoperative care
1. Prepare the client for bronchoscopy by explaining the procedure and providing emotional support.

1. Bronchoscopy is a diagnostic test that enables the examiner to visualize the bronchi and obtain a tissue sample for biopsy.

2. Give the client nothing by mouth for 8 hours before the test, and ask her to remove dentures, if she wears them.

2. These are precautions to prevent aspiration.

3. After bronchoscopy, give nothing by mouth until the gag reflex returns, discourage talking, and observe for signs of respiratory obstruction.

3. To prevent aspiration, the client should ingest nothing by mouth. Talking strains the vocal cords, thereby increasing the risk for laryngeal edema, a serious complication.

4. Carry out preoperative preparation for segmental lung resection. Explain the purpose of postoperative chest tubes, and help the client express concerns about the diagnosis.

4. As with any general surgical procedure, this information prepares the client for the operation and anticipates recovery.

Closed chest drainage system

Self-contained, disposable commercial closed-chest drainage systems are used exclusively today because they provide greater client mobility than the traditional closed-bottle systems previously used. Although many manufacturers make these systems, all models operate on the same principle: to maintain chest negative pressure. The unit below is a prototype.

PLEUR-EVAC

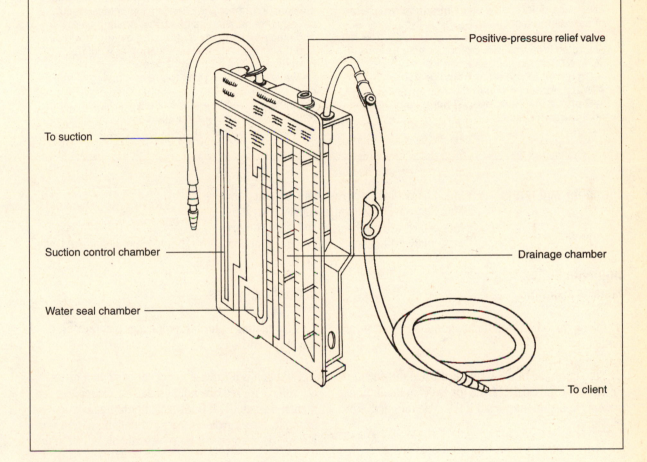

Positive-pressure relief valve

To suction

Suction control chamber

Water seal chamber

Drainage chamber

To client

Postoperative care

Perform all routine postoperative assessments, particularly those relating to possible chest surgery complications.

Review "Postoperative period," page 125.

Nursing diagnoses
• Anxiety related to the diagnosis and surgery
• Ineffective airway clearance related to anesthesia and postoperative discomfort
• Impaired gas exchange related to potential postoperative complications
• Pain related to the surgery

ADULT NURSING

Points to remember in oxygen therapy

Oxygen is administered to a client with hypoxia. Common signs and symptoms of hypoxia include tachycardia, restlessness, dyspnea, arrhythmias, headache, and cyanosis (a late sign).

Oxygen delivery (for an adult client)
• Nasal cannula: flow rates of 1 to 8 liters/minute; oxygen concentration of 24% to 40%
• Nasal catheters: now used infrequently because of associated discomfort
• Face mask: covers the nose and mouth; flow rate of 6 to 10 liters/minute; oxygen concentrations of 40% to 65%; may cause anxiety
—Do not let oxygen leak from the sides.
—Watch for facial skin irritation.
—Remove the mask every 2 hours, and wash and dry the client's face.

Note: The Venturi mask delivers precise oxygen concentrations (24%, 28%, 35%, or 40%); the flow rate varies with the concentration.
• Tracheal collar or mechanical ventilator
• Rebreathing mask

Safety considerations
• Because oxygen enhances combustion, prohibit smoking in or near the client's room, place electrical equipment (such as call bells, heating pads, and electric razors) away from the oxygen source, and do not use oil, grease, alcohol, or wool (all burn easily). Use a cotton blanket.
• Always humidify oxygen to prevent drying of mucous membranes.
• Monitor the client for signs of oxygen toxicity: sore throat, substernal pain, cough (caused by alveolar damage), inflammation, and hemorrhage.

Planning and goals

• Mrs. Sharp's lung will reexpand without difficulty.
• Mrs. Sharp will maintain an effective breathing pattern.
• Mrs. Sharp will not hemorrhage after surgery.
• Mrs. Sharp will maintain full range of motion of the shoulder on the affected side.

Implementation

NURSING BEHAVIORS	NURSING RATIONALES
1. Check for water level fluctuation in the water-seal bottle.	**1.** A fluctuating water level indicates that the chest tube is patent.
2. Note bubbling of the water seal when the client coughs or expires air. Check for leaks in the drainage system. Notify the physician if the system operates ineffectively.	**2.** Bubbling is normal if the client has had a procedure that exposes raw lung tissue (for example, a segmental resection). If unexpected bubbling occurs (for example, after cardiac surgery when lung parenchyma has not been entered), there is probably a leak in the system.
3. Check for bubbling in the suction bottle.	**3.** Bubbling must occur; otherwise, the suction is working improperly.
4. Always keep the drainage system below the client's chest level.	**4.** This maintains the water seal and prevents water and air reflux.
5. Keep tubing straight to avoid kinks.	**5.** Unkinked tubing ensures uninterrupted flow.
6. Reinforce all connections with tape.	**6.** Reinforcement prevents inadvertent disconnection.
7. Measure drainage at least hourly, marking the level with the date and time.	**7.** During the first 2 hours after surgery, drainage should be measured every time the nurse monitors vital signs. During the 1st hour, drainage may amount to 200 ml, depending on the surgery.

8. Support the client and help her deep-breathe hourly. Splint the chest as needed.

8. Support reduces discomfort; deep breathing prevents atelectasis and hypoventilation.

9. Reposition the client every 1 to 2 hours.

9. Repositioning supplies ventilation to all lung areas.

10. Help the client walk as soon as possible.

10. Walking increases ventilation and circulation and hastens recovery.

11. Have the client perform range-of-motion exercises for the affected shoulder.

11. Exercise helps prevent shoulder ankylosis.

12. Keep two clamps at the bedside in case the chest tubes disconnect. If the tube disconnects from the water seal, reconnect it if possible; if not, place the tube in any available water and summon the physician. Follow the same procedure if the water-seal bottle breaks. If the tube is pulled from the client's chest, cover the wound with petrolatum-coated gauze and call the physician.

12. Disruption of the water seal can cause atmospheric air to enter the chest cavity and collapse the lung. The best way to prevent this is to reestablish the water seal. *Note:* Traditionally, nurses have been taught to clamp the tube near the chest, but the literature overwhelmingly recommends caution. Clamping increases the danger of tension pneumothorax if an air leak exists and is therefore dangerous. It is left in this case study because some texts still say it may be needed.

13. Assess for tension pneumothorax; mediastinal shift, with signs of restlessness, dyspnea, tachypnea, and arrhythmias (especially tachycardia); and tracheal deviation.

13. Collapse of the lung under pressure can lead to mediastinal shift, a medical emergency that can lead to cardiac tamponade, heart failure, pulmonary edema, tracheal deviation, shock, and death.

14. Prepare the client for chest tube removal. (The physician will remove the chest tube when the lung fully reexpands and no air leaks.) Tell the client to take a deep breath and hold it or to perform Valsalva's maneuver (deep-breathe, blow air out, and bear down).

14. With the lung fully expanded, the tube is no longer needed. The physician will gently withdraw the tube and apply petrolatum-coated gauze and a pressure dressing to the wound. A sustained deep breath expands the lung and prevents entry of atmospheric air during tube removal. The dressing prevents entry of atmospheric air.

Evaluation

- Mrs. Sharp can breathe normally.
- Mrs. Sharp has no surgical complications.
- Mrs. Sharp's right shoulder has full range of motion.

MUSCULOSKELETAL SYSTEM

Injury to the vertebral column

Back injuries and low back pain are the two leading causes of lost work time. Trauma to the vertebral column may be to the vertebral body itself or to the disk, the inner part of the cartilage pads between two vertebrae. Usually, injury to the vertebral body results from a compression fracture. Both a ruptured disk (herniated nucleus pulposus) and a compression fracture cause pressure on the spinal nerves as they leave the spinal cord between the vertebrae. Conservative treatment

---

Surgeries for ruptured disk

Laminectomy or hemilaminectomy consists of removing the vertebral lamina (wing) to gain access to the disk area. The disk pieces are then removed from the annulus, the cartilage ring between the vertebrae. After a laminectomy, the client can get up (on the same day, if able) and move with minimal restriction. Recovery proceeds fairly steadily once the ruptured disk pieces are removed, relieving nerve pressure and pain. The client should be taught proper lifting techniques to prevent additional trauma and exercises to strengthen back and abdominal muscles after discharge.

Spinal fusion involves laminectomy to remove the ruptured disk pieces followed by placement of bone inserts (grafts), screws, or pins to fuse the vertebral segments solidly. After spinal fusion, the client may require bed rest for 1 to 3 days or more, depending on the fusion type. At times, a client may need a brace, which helps stabilize the fused parts for the lengthy healing time required (9 to 12 months for solid fusion). Postoperatively, the client must be positioned with the logrolling maneuver and will have limited ability to bend once the fusion heals.

Chemonucleolysis is the dissolution of ruptured disk pieces by injecting chymopapain, an enzyme from the papaya plant, into the affected disk. The enzyme dissolves the disk, which is replaced with scar tissue. Chymopapain can elicit severe anaphylactic responses and may result in death. Preoperative preparation includes obtaining a thorough allergy history and administering I.V. preoperative corticosteroids, antihistamines, and cimetidine to block histamine release.

Postoperatively, the client may have back muscle spasms of varying intensity and duration. Pain relief may be temporary, with pain returning 6 or more months later, possibly from scar tissue formation. The verdict on this controversial procedure's effectiveness and safety is out. Although initial enthusiasm for chemonucleolysis appears to be waning, the procedure is still being performed. For some clients, results have been good; other clients have resorted to laminectomy.

Microdiskectomy is similar to laminectomy but requires an incision measuring 1 to 3 inches (2.5 to 7.5 cm); only the disk fragments are removed, and recovery is faster. Sometimes, multiple operations are required because of retained disk fragments.

---

relies on analgesics and muscle relaxants, bed rest, and traction. Surgical options include laminectomy, spinal fusion, chemonucleolysis, and microdiskectomy (see *Surgeries for ruptured disk*). The following clinical situation focuses on nursing care of a client with a vertebral column injury.

Clinical situation

Clarence High, a 40-year-old construction worker, is hospitalized after falling from a scaffold. He complains of bilateral numbness of his fourth and fifth toes and pain that radiates down his buttocks and the back of his thighs. X-rays show that Mr. High has a compression fracture of the fourth lumbar vertebra (L4). He is admitted to the orthopedic unit for further evaluation and treatment.

Assessment

NURSING BEHAVIORS

1. Observe the client's general condition, assessing for altered level of consciousness, headache, blurred vision, respiratory irregularities, and other injuries, such as fractures, bruises, and open wounds.

2. Monitor and record the client's vital signs.

NURSING RATIONALES

1. Besides the vertebral injury and obvious bruises or wounds, the client may have sustained a serious head injury.

2. Vital sign measurements provide baseline data for future comparison.

3. Assess leg motor and sensory function, noting how well the client can move his legs, whether he can feel sharp and dull pressure, and whether he complains of numbness, tingling, or pins-and-needles sensations.

3. Because of pressure on spinal nerves as they exit the spinal cord areas, motor and sensory changes commonly accompany compression fractures.

4. Assess the intensity and character of the client's pain.

4. Pain usually results from muscle spasms and nerve pressure.

Diagnostic evaluation

• *X-ray studies of all musculoskeletal tissues:* Determines the extent of trauma and helps establish a medical diagnosis.

• *Hematologic studies and electrocardiography:* Determine the usual and current health status.

• *Myelography* (performed after the client's condition stabilizes): An X-ray study that uses radiopaque contrast medium to identify spine abnormalities. Used to determine whether the disk is intact, the myelographic contrast medium outlines any discontinuous areas and pressure on spinal nerves.

—Before myelography, explain the procedure and its purpose to the client.

—Allow the client only clear liquid nourishment on the morning of the examination; then give nothing by mouth. The client needs no other preparation.

—Follow orders accompanying the client's return from the examination. (Orders vary, depending on the contrast medium used.)

—Make sure the client remains flat in bed for 8 to 12 hours after the examination if oily-based iophendylate (Pantopaque) was used. Common side effects include headache and nerve root irritation.

—Allow the client to elevate the head and have bathroom privileges if watersoluble metrizamide (Amipaque) was used. Adverse reactions include headache, nausea, vomiting, and sometimes seizures.

—Force fluids to restore cerebrospinal fluid levels. If the client complains of a headache, relieve it by lowering the head of the bed.

• *Computed tomography or magnetic resonance imaging (MRI):* May be performed instead of or along with myelography. MRI clearly defines spinal tract tissues.

Nursing diagnoses

• Impaired physical mobility related to vertebral injury
• Feeding self-care deficit related to decreased mobility
• Bathing or hygiene self-care deficit related to decreased mobility
• Dressing or grooming self-care deficit related to decreased mobility
• Toileting self-care deficit related to decreased mobility

Planning and goals

• Mr. High will regain musculoskeletal and neurologic tissue function without complications.
• Mr. High will understand the implications of bone injury and healing and will participate in rehabilitation.

Implementation
NURSING BEHAVIORS

NURSING RATIONALES

---

1. Maintain bed rest, as ordered. The head of the bed usually is kept flat for 1 to 2 days.

1. Bed rest decreases inflammation and prevents further trauma.

ADULT NURSING

2. Perform neurovascular checks by assessing the client's color, temperature, capillary refill time, peripheral pulses, pain, motor and sensory functions, and edema. Compare findings bilaterally, and note regression or progression of symptoms.

2. Changes will reflect pressure on nerve endings as well as increasing (or decreasing) pain, numbness, tingling, and altered functions.

3. Continue to monitor the client's vital signs and level of consciousness.

3. Edema can cause sudden changes in these indicators.

4. Position the client comfortably, and use the logrolling maneuver to change positions (two nurses turn the client, who holds himself stiff as a log). Do not turn the client if the spine is unstable.

4. A side-lying position may be most comfortable. (When the client is on the side, place pillows between the legs to prevent back strain.) By keeping the spine straight, logrolling prevents additional injury to the client.

5. Observe the client's orientation and responses to care.

5. Trauma induces a stress-shock reaction.

6. Administer pain medication, as ordered and needed.

6. Pain may be localized in the client's back. Pain medication rarely relieves numbness, whereas relieving pressure on the nerve does.

7. If ordered, administer a skeletal muscle relaxant, such as baclofen (Lioresal), carisoprodol (Soma), cyclobenzaprine (Flexeril), diazepam (Valium), methocarbamol (Robaxin), or orphenadrine citrate (Norflex). Observe for side effects.

7. These drugs aid in relaxing muscle spasms associated with vertebral column injuries. Side effects include dizziness, weakness, drowsiness, blurred vision, fatigue, headache, nausea, vomiting, and constipation. Long-term use may cause bone marrow depression. The client may develop dependence on diazepam.

8. Assess whether the client's injury has affected the GI, genitourinary, respiratory, and other body systems.

8. Trauma imposes stress on the entire body. Signs may not be readily apparent and can occur over time. Bed rest affects all body systems.

9. Evaluate the client's psychological state.

9. Each client has a prolonged or shortened stress response. How stress manifests and to what degree depends on the client's perception of the threat.

Clinical situation
(continued)

After bed rest and diagnostic tests, Mr. High was found to have no additional injuries. His treatment plan included wearing a body cast for 2 weeks, after which he would wear a back brace. He was discharged when the body cast dried. (*Note:* Clients with nondisplaced fractures may be mobilized with a brace or corset. Be sure it is applied before the client gets out of bed.)

Implementation
NURSING BEHAVIORS

NURSING RATIONALES

1. Before applying the body cast, carefully observe and clean the client's skin.

1. Once the cast is applied, no skin care can be provided from the nipple line to the hips; open skin areas inside the cast can become infected.

2. Explain the body cast procedure and what the client can expect afterward.

2. Preparing the client helps relieve apprehension.

3. Handle the damp cast with the palms, not the fingertips. After cast application, have the client lie on a firm mattress with a rolled blanket or small pillow supporting his back curvature. Leave the casted areas uncovered to dry (except the genital area, for privacy). Use a fan (not a heat lamp) to speed drying.

3. Handling a damp cast with the fingertips would place too much pressure on skin tissues inside the cast. The cast must stay uncovered for full drying to occur (1 to 2 days). Fanned air may be used to aid drying, but a heat lamp concentrates energy on too small a tissue area, predisposing it to burns inside the cast.

4. Turn the client to the sides and abdomen every 2 to 4 hours.

4. Turning exposes the cast's damp areas to air, which hastens drying. Turning also maintains the client's mobility and aids body functions.

5. Observe the client's reaction to the body cast, and encourage him to express his feelings about it. Monitor vital signs, appetite, urine output, and bowel movements, and note any passing of flatus or expressions of discomfort. Notify the physician of adverse reactions.

5. The immobile client will undoubtedly feel some frustration from his confinement and may experience other adverse reactions, including claustrophobia and cast syndrome (increased anxiety, vital sign changes, nausea, and vomiting) from abnormal kinking of the superior mesenteric artery. This is caused by the body's in-cast position and by abdominal distention, which can lead to small-bowel obstruction requiring surgical correction. The cast's sides may need to be cut (bivalved) to ease adverse reactions.

6. Before discharge, teach the client proper cast and skin care, and caution him to put nothing in the cast. Show him how to turn, prop himself, and get into and out of bed safely. Discuss elements of a sound diet that will prevent weight gain, minimize flatus, and help meet fluid, nutritional, and elimination needs. Review appropriate exercises he can perform, and suggest ways to decrease boredom from imposed inactivity.

6. Proper instruction helps the client prevent complications of immobility and promotes safety and comfort. The cast can get too tight if the client gains weight or has flatus. Lack of exercise may increase intestinal gas. Increased fluid intake helps maintain normal urinary functions.

7. Schedule appointments for follow-up care, as needed.

7. This ensures continuity of care. The cast will be removed in the physician's office, and the back brace will be fitted by a brace specialist.

Evaluation

• Mr. High will regain full leg motor and sensory functions as healing continues.
• Mr. High understands how to maintain a strong cast and why he must increase fluid intake during inactivity.
• Mr. High will regain limited mobility while in the cast or brace and, later, full mobility when out of the brace.

ADULT NURSING

Hip fracture

Older adults are particularly prone to fractures of the hip. Two fracture types commonly occur: intracapsular fractures, involving the femoral head and neck, and extracapsular fractures, most commonly involving the trochanters (intertrochanteric). Intracapsular fractures predispose the client to avascular necrosis of the femoral head because the injury can disrupt blood supply to it. As with osteoporosis, women are especially vulnerable to intracapsular fractures. The following clinical situation focuses on nursing care of a client with a fractured hip.

Clinical situation

Roberta Joseph, a 73-year-old widow, is admitted to the hospital for treatment of an intracapsular fracture of the left femur. She has been placed in Buck's extension traction with a 7-lb (3.2-kg) weight. Because of marked osteoporosis revealed by X-rays, Mrs. Joseph will undergo prosthetic replacement of the femoral head. Expected length of stay is 7 days.

Assessment

NURSING BEHAVIORS

1. Orient the client to time, place, and person.

2. Check the client's vital signs and level of consciousness.

3. Assess the traction for proper functioning, and observe the client's skin surfaces for tolerance to traction. (Traction can be removed for nursing care according to institutional policies.) Turn the client to the side away from the leg in traction. (See *Types of skin traction*.)

4. Assess the client's pain level, and identify pain patterns; administer a narcotic or analgesic, as ordered.

5. Assess the client's muscle strength.

NURSING RATIONALES

1. Aging predisposes the client to confusion; trauma leads to displacement from familiar areas, adding to the confusion.

2. A fracture can result in hemorrhage, with the client losing up to 1,000 ml (about 2 pints) of blood into the hip joint area. The elderly client may have established circulatory disorders and, with the fracture, a subnormal temperature, hypotension from trauma or bleeding, confusion from displacement, and hypovolemia.

3. Traction prevents additional trauma and overcomes muscle spasm before surgery. If the skin cannot tolerate the prescribed weight, the physician may decrease it. The usual weight for Buck's extension traction is 5 to 7 lb (2.3 to 3.2 kg).

4. Pain usually is minimal with traction but may intensify on moving or turning. (The client can be turned for care if she cannot raise herself with the help of a trapeze.) Because the elderly client may have an increased tolerance for pain, medication may be administered less frequently and in lower doses.

5. Inactivity can quickly reduce an elderly client's muscle strength and increase mobilization of calcium from the bone.

ADULT NURSING

Types of skin traction

TRACTION TYPE	APPLICATION SITE	WEIGHT	CARE FACTORS
Buck's extension	Arm or leg (one or both)	5 to 7 lb per extremity	• Clean and dry the skin. Be sure the client has no open cuts or wounds. • Make sure equipment (tape, bandages, traction straps, or boot) is new (when appropriate) and functioning properly. • Remove the traction apparatus to care for and observe tissues. • Keep the client recumbent to obtain the most effective traction. • Teach the client how to use traction at home.
Russell's extension	Leg only (one or both)	5 to 10 lb per leg	• Arrange pulleys and ropes, and determine the weight by the principle "for every force in one direction, there's an equal force in the opposite direction." • Loosen the knee sling for care and observation. • Keep the client recumbent. • Remove the traction to care for the client (always check with the physician before removing).
Bryant's extension	One or both legs (usually both)	Varies— enough weight to raise the buttocks off the bed	• Use for children under 35 lb. • Position both legs at right angles to the buttocks. • Position the child's buttocks slightly off the bed to ensure correct amount of pull. • Supervise the child closely to maintain the recumbent position. • Remove the traction to provide care, according to the physician's orders or institutional policy (requires two people, with one gently maintaining manual traction). • Teach the child and parents or guardians how to use this traction at home.
Pelvic belt	Around abdomen and pelvis, like a girdle	20 to 35 lb	• Use for conservative low-back pain and possible ruptured disk. • Use traction intermittently and never at night. • Keep the client recumbent, with knees and hips flexed at 45-degree angles. • Teach the client how to use traction at home.
Pelvic sling	Under the pelvis like a hammock	20 to 35 lb	• Use for pelvic bone fractures. • Advise the client to stay in the sling except when it is removed for care. • Wean the client from the sling to prevent dependency. • Keep the sling clean and dry to prevent pressure areas. • Position the client's buttocks slightly off the bed to ensure correct use of the sling. • One person can remove the client from the sling, but two are needed to reapply it to center the client properly.
Head halter	Under the chin and around the skull base	5 to 15 lb (8 to 10 lb most common)	• Use for neck muscle disorders, degenerative cervical conditions, and (rarely) cervical vertebral fractures. • Explain that the pull comes mostly from the occipital area of the halter, not from the chin. • Tell the client that pressure exerted on the chin reverts to the temporomandibular joint, causing pain and soreness when chewing. • Remove the client from the traction for care before inserting skull tongs (if the client has a fractured cervical vertebra, only the physician removes the traction). • Show the client (especially one with arthritis) how to use traction at home. • Avoid pressure exerted over the facial nerve by a halter that is too small or incorrectly applied.

ADULT NURSING

Types of skin traction (continued)

TRACTION TYPE	APPLICATION SITE	WEIGHT	CARE FACTORS
90°-90° (ninety-ninety)	Lower legs and thighs	5 to 15 lb	• Relieves lumbosacral muscle spasms by applying principle of 90-degree angle of knees and hips. • Keep the client flat in bed while in this traction. • Use traction intermittently, and usually not at night.
Dunlop's	Humerus	8 to 15 lb	• Use for humeral fractures to decrease muscle spasms and align bone fragments. • Hold the client's forearm in Buck's extension vertically, with the elbow at a right angle to the arm for most effective traction. • Keep the client recumbent for effective traction.
Cotrel's	Head halter to the head and a pelvic belt to the pelvis	15 to 30 lb for pelvic belt; 8 to 15 lb for head halter	• Use to assist straightening scoliotic curvature (commonly used before brace application or surgical correction). • Maintain the client flat in bed so that the spine is pulled lengthwise in opposite directions by the head halter and pelvic belt. • Use intermittently, but not at night unless curvature and muscle spasms are severe.

6. Assess serum calcium levels.

6. Osteoporosis (indicated by elevated serum calcium levels) may predispose the client to renal calculi. Increased serum calcium levels result from mobilization of calcium from the bone.

7. Assess urine output, and inspect the urine for calculi.

7. Small calculi may be excreted in urine.

8. Assess the client's appetite, dietary preferences, and food intake, especially calcium and vitamin D intake (estimate the client's exposure to sunlight).

8. Elderly clients who live alone commonly do not eat enough quality foods to meet all of their nutritional requirements. Many of them have a vitamin D deficiency, resulting in reduced absorption and use of calcium and phosphorus.

Diagnostic evaluation
• *Admission studies:* Assess hematologic, urinary, and fluid and electrolyte status to determine the client's blood loss and tolerance for surgery
• *Electrocardiography and chest X-ray:* Determine cardiac and circulatory status
• *X-rays and bone scan:* Identify fracture and skeletal status (osteoporosis) and determine whether the femur can tolerate a prosthesis

Nursing diagnoses
• Impaired physical mobility related to hip fracture and traction
• Fluid volume deficit related to hemorrhage
• Risk for injury related to brittle bones and immobility
• Pain related to fracture and muscle spasms
• Impaired home maintenance management related to decreased mobility

Planning and goals
• Mrs. Joseph will withstand surgery without complications.
• Mrs. Joseph will use a walker with limited weight bearing.
• Mrs. Joseph will return home when she is ambulatory and the incision has healed.

Implementation

NURSING BEHAVIORS	**NURSING RATIONALES**

Preoperative care

1. Provide routine preoperative care.

1. Preparation enhances the client's physical and mental status for tolerating surgery.

2. Assess the client's skin turgor, appetite and food intake (if not fasting for surgery), and elimination patterns.

2. These indicate fluid and electrolyte status.

3. Before surgery, inform the client of anticipated postoperative activities, including deep breathing and use of a walker for mobility and limited weight bearing.

3. Instruction helps reduce the client's anxiety and prepares her for postoperative rehabilitation.

4. Determine the client's vital capacity.

4. The vital capacity indicates the client's respiratory status, which, from age or inactivity, may be abnormal. Vital capacity is based on age, sex, and body size. Normal vital capacity is 4,000 to 5,000 cc.

5. Consult with social service personnel.

5. Expected length of stay is 7 days. Social services can help the client to plan care after discharge and to obtain a home health aide.

Clinical situation
(continued)

Mrs. Joseph successfully undergoes Austin-Moore prosthetic replacement of the femoral head. An abduction pillow (foam, A-shaped) placed between her legs helps maintain the desired postoperative abduction position, which keeps the prosthesis within the acetabulum. The physician's orders include walking with limited weight bearing on the affected leg.

Implementation

NURSING BEHAVIORS	**NURSING RATIONALES**

Postoperative care

1. Provide routine postoperative care. Help the client sit on the edge of the bed, and assess her vital signs.

1. Monitoring the client's vital signs determines circulatory adequacy, oxygenation, and ability to stand without becoming hypotensive or weak.

2. Demonstrate how to use a walker without bearing weight on the affected leg. Before the client uses the walker, have her repeat explanations and steps, and consult with a physical therapist.

2. If the client accurately repeats explanations and steps, she probably understands how to use the walker correctly. The physical therapist evaluates the client's musculoskeletal strength and ability to begin rehabilitation.

3. Assist the client to a standing position, and help her take several steps. Then allow her to sit in a chair with her legs uncrossed and her feet on the floor; avoid extreme hip flexion. Closely monitor the amount of weight placed on the affected leg. Increase weight bearing, as ordered, after X-rays confirm that the hip joint and incision are healing.

3. Bearing more than the allowable weight on her leg may dislodge the prosthesis. Adduction also can dislodge the prosthesis during the early postoperative period; therefore, abduction remains the required position. Flexion and internal rotation also can cause the prosthesis to dislodge.

ADULT NURSING

4. Monitor the wound area as needed; inspect and measure drainage from the Hemovac catheter.

4. The client may have moderate edema, discoloration, and pain in the incision area. Within 48 hours, drainage usually is minimal and the Hemovac catheter is removed.

5. Intervene to prevent common postoperative complications, such as deep vein thrombosis and pressure ulcers.

5. Anticoagulants, antiembolic stockings, and pneumatic compression devices may be used. Proper skin care and use of eggcrate mattresses and heel rolls aid in preventing ischemia.

6. Assist the client with deep breathing, coughing, and using respiratory aids every 2 hours.

6. Elderly clients require vigorous pulmonary care because they are prone to postoperative atelectasis (collapsed or partially expanded lung) and pneumonia.

7. Note positioning instructions when the client is in bed.

7. Do not turn the client to the affected side without orders from the physician. The internal rotation can cause dislodgement of the prosthesis.

8. Monitor urinary and bowel elimination patterns.

8. The client may dribble or be incontinent with sphincter tone loss. Trauma and inadequate fluid intake can cause constipation.

9. Update social service personnel on the client's progress.

9. The client will probably need home care assistance for general hygiene, proper nourishment, mobility, and other activities of daily living. Full weight bearing may not be permitted for 3 months or longer. Furthermore, osteoporosis may prevent the client from regaining her former strength and mobility, and the hip may never heal completely.

10. Provide the client with appropriate discharge instructions:
• Do not flex the hip greater than 90 degrees.
• Do not cross the legs.
• Have help putting on shoes and socks,
• Report sudden, sharp pain to the physician.

10. The first three discharge instructions are designed to help the client avoid dislodging the prosthesis. Sudden, sharp pain may indicate dislodgement, which would require the physician's attention. Ongoing postdischarge rehabilitation is necessary to return the client to a prefracture level of functioning.

Evaluation

• Mrs. Joseph underwent prosthetic replacement of the femoral head without complications.
• Mrs. Joseph can use a walker, bearing only limited weight on her affected leg.
• Mrs. Joseph was discharged to an extended care facility for full recuperation; since returning home, she has been assisted by a home health care aide.

Displaced comminuted fracture of the femur

Motorcycle accidents and injuries are a major cause of illness and disability in adolescents and young adults, predominantly male, age 15 to 30. Multiple injuries are common and affect more than the musculoskeletal system. A fractured femur usually requires traction and surgery followed by a long recovery period. The following clinical situation focuses on nursing care of a client with a comminuted fracture of the femur. (For more information, see *Common conditions affecting musculoskeletal tissues,* page 506.)

Clinical situation

James Wyman, age 20, was hospitalized after a motorcycle accident left him with a displaced comminuted midshaft fracture of the right femur. On admission, he was hypotensive and confused, at times screaming in pain. His urine output showed oliguria and hematuria. He was placed in balanced-suspension skeletal traction with a 35-lb (16-kg) weight.

Assessment

NURSING BEHAVIORS

NURSING RATIONALES

1. Assess the client's response to sudden trauma necessitating hospitalization.

1. Displacement from usual activities results in stress. The threat to the self causes alarm.

2. Monitor the client's vital signs.

2. Femoral shaft fractures may cause hemorrhage, with 1,000 to 1,500 ml (about 3 pints) of blood lost, leading to hypovolemic shock.

3. Evaluate the client's orientation to time, place, and person.

3. The client may have a head injury. Displacement and anoxia, resulting from hypovolemia, may account for disorientation and confusion.

4. Identify the type, location, and amount of pain.

4. Displaced fractures place pressure on nerve endings, which causes pain. Hemorrhage also causes pressure pain—sharp, continuous, and localized in the fracture area. Young men (ages 20 to 26) metabolize drugs faster than women; therefore, they need higher doses of narcotics for effective pain relief.

5. Assess the skeletal traction for proper functioning.

5. Treating a displaced fracture requires continuous and sufficiently weighted skeletal traction to relieve muscle spasm that results from trauma and to aid bone fragment realignment. Traction must be maintained continuously until surgery is performed.

6. Monitor the client's urine output, and inspect the urine for blood.

6. Because of shock, hemorrhage, and stress, urine output will be less than normal. Trauma to the muscles and kidneys can cause hematuria, which may lead to acute renal failure from shock, hemorrhage, or trauma.

Common conditions affecting musculoskeletal tissues

I. Osteomyelitis

A. Definition—infection of bones and surrounding tissues

B. Etiology—most commonly from staphylococci, streptococci, or tubercle bacilli. In children, osteomyelitis commonly develops secondary to strep throat, the infection being spread by the bloodstream. Open wounds also allow bacterial invasion and development of osteomyelitis.

C. Symptoms—heat, redness, pain, and edema at the infection site; inability to use body part normally; malaise, headache, and moderately high (102° to 103° F [38.9° to 39.4° C]) systemic fever. If diagnosis is not made early in the disease, purulent drainage may flow through sinus tracts from the site to the skin. Common osteomyelitis sites include the distal femur, upper tibia, and upper humerus, although no bone is immune.

D. Treatment—initially, I.V. antibiotic administration at high doses after completing culture and sensitivity studies. Follow I.V. antibiotic therapy (lasting a minimum of 6 weeks) with oral antibiotic therapy. When cultures indicate the infection site is "sterile," the surgeon opens the site, scrapes out dead bone, and may apply bone grafts. If necessary, drains are inserted to irrigate wounds as well as to permit drainage. Administer I.V. antibiotics postoperatively to prevent reinfection or chronic osteomyelitis. If chronic osteomyelitis does develop, the site is drained repeatedly, dead bone is scraped away, and the site is irrigated with antibiotics. If the infection progresses, the affected arm or leg may be amputated. Fortunately, because of vigorous and prolonged initial therapies, amputation occurs infrequently.

II. Osteoporosis

A. Definition—bodywide decrease in bone mass

B. Etiology—several possible causes, including bone resorption from disuse (as with paralysis or immobility), postmenopausal hormonal shifts, and calcium and vitamin D deficiencies

C. Signs and symptoms—vague low-back pain, bone weakness or soreness, height loss caused by changes in vertebral height or shape, bone fractures, X-ray evidence of decreased bone mass, pathologic fractures (especially of the hip) with minor trauma

D. Treatment—exercise (muscle activity) to retain calcium in bones; increased calcium, phosphorus, and vitamin intake (either from foods or tablets); estrogen-progesterone medication to delay or treat osteoporosis; splint or brace for weakened bones; analgesics for pain relief

III. Bone tumors

A. Definition—growth in or around bone tissues

B. Types—benign, such as bone cysts and osteoma, and malignant, such as osteogenic sarcoma and Ewing's sarcoma (malignant bone tumors most commonly affect persons aged 5 to 30); primary or secondary (spreading to bone from another site)

C. Symptoms—soreness and persistent dull ache in the tumor area (malignant bone tumors occur most frequently around the knee in the distal femur or upper tibia); night pain; X-ray evidence of mass; swelling or mass at the site

D. Treatment—varies according to tumor type and stage (local or systemic spread) and may include wide excision of tumor, bone, muscle, and contiguous tissues; removal of the affected bone and replacement with bone from a cadaver donor or a bone bank; administration of preoperative and postoperative radiation or chemotherapy or both; amputation of the affected limb; or removal of the affected bone and muscles and replacement with metallic prostheses.

E. Prognosis—depends on tumor type, whether the tumor has metastasized, and therapeutic vigor. Bone metastasis occurs commonly with primary and secondary tumors. Advances in drug therapies and adequate surgical excision are improving overall life expectancy, although with metastasis, life expectancy remains limited. Fortunately, of all malignant tumors, bone tumors make up only 1% to 2%.

Diagnostic evaluation	• *Laboratory tests* (complete blood count, hematocrit, hemoglobin, blood urea nitrogen, creatinine, electrolytes, CO_2 content, urinalysis): Determine the client's general health status on admission and may be performed daily to evaluate blood loss and renal function • *X-ray studies:* Help define the type and extent of trauma
Nursing diagnoses	• Impaired physical mobility related to the fracture and traction • Pain related to the fracture • Fluid volume deficit related to hemorrhage • Risk for infection related to skeletal traction • Posttrauma response related to the overwhelming experience of the accident
Planning and goals	• Mr. Wyman's fractured bone fragments will realign and unite. • Mr. Wyman's fracture will heal without complications. • Mr. Wyman will regain mobility over time. • Mr. Wyman's fluid and electrolyte balance will be restored. • Mr. Wyman will learn to walk with crutches without bearing weight on the affected leg.

Implementation

NURSING BEHAVIORS	**NURSING RATIONALES**
1. Monitor vital signs every 2 to 4 hours.	**1.** The client may have hypovolemia for 12 to 24 hours, until fluid volume is replaced and bleeding stops.
2. Perform neurovascular circulation checks, as follows:	**2.** The listed nursing behaviors help determine the client's neurovascular status.
• Compare the affected leg with the unaffected one, monitoring color and temperature, peripheral pulses, and capillary refill time (gently compress the middle toenail and release it quickly).	• The injured leg will be slightly paler and slightly cooler than the opposite leg. Popliteal, posterior tibialis, and dorsalis pedis pulses should be palpable. The toenail should pink up in 2 to 4 seconds (4 to 6 seconds is sluggish and requires close monitoring).
• Determine the amount and type of the client's pain.	• With a fractured femur, pain usually is sharp, continuous, and localized to the thigh.
• Determine the client's ability to move the toes and ankle of the affected leg and to perform quadriceps-setting exercises. If the client cannot actively move muscles, perform passive movements and assess for increased pain (passive movements stretch muscles, increasing pain with muscle anoxia or ischemia). Check muscle compartment pressure with a tissue pressure manometer.	• The client should be able to move his muscles and joints. Compartment syndrome, indicated by an inability to perform active movements and by increasing pain with passive movements, results from compromised arterial and venous circulation caused by hemorrhage into the muscle mass. The resultant edema increases venous pressure. Arterial circulation decreases, leading to anoxia and cell death in 6 to 8 hours if the pressure is not reduced. Treatment (fasciotomy) involves cutting the fascia over affected muscles to permit muscle expansion. About 7 to 10 days later, when the swelling subsides, the muscle fascia can be closed secondarily or covered with a skin graft if the fascial opening is large.

ADULT NURSING

• Monitor sensory functions, and assess the client for paresthesias (numbness, tingling, or pins-and-needles sensations).

3. Monitor fluid intake and output, I.V. fluids, and the I.V. site hourly.

4. Initially, check the client's overall condition and orientation to time, place, and person every 1 to 2 hours.

5. Monitor respiratory functions and breathing. Observe for sudden tachypnea, tachycardia, shortness of breath, feeling of danger, chest pain, and petechial rash on the chest and neck and in conjunctiva. Immediately report these signs and symptoms to the physician.

6. Assist the client with deep breathing, coughing, and using respiratory aids every 4 hours.

7. Monitor the client for pain; administer a narcotic every 3 to 4 hours or as ordered.

8. Assist the client with eating when oral intake is permitted. Provide a high-protein, high-calorie diet and increased fluids, as ordered.

9. Provide thorough skin care, especially to the back and buttocks. Inspect all bony prominences. Supply skin protectors and pads as needed.

10. Monitor the skeletal pin entrance and exit sites daily, following institutional policies for pin-site care.

11. Assess bowel functions, noting abdominal girth, distention, bowel sounds, and constipation; check the amount, color, and consistency of bowel movements.

• The client should be able to feel and sense body parts touched. Increasing numbness and tingling indicate increasing anoxia and ischemia.

3. The client will receive I.V. fluids and nothing by mouth until he is fully conscious and his condition stabilizes.

4. Shock and hypovolemia predispose the client to anoxia, accounting for confusion and disorientation.

5. These signs and symptoms suggest fat emboli syndrome, which can develop 1 to 3 days after a long-bone fracture. Treatment includes oxygen administration, I.V. therapy, antibiotic and steroid administration, and I.V. dextrose infusion. Because the mortality connected with fat emboli ranges from 30% to 50%, these symptoms must be anticipated, recognized, and treated early to prevent death.

6. Bed rest restricts pulmonary functions associated with impaired gas exchange.

7. Around-the-clock narcotics administration maintains therapeutic blood levels. A nonnarcotic analgesic, such as aspirin or acetaminophen, may be given between narcotic doses after bleeding stops. Aspirin, an anti-inflammatory medication, enhances narcotic action but also impedes blood coagulation. Pain decreases dramatically when muscle spasms diminish.

8. A client in skeletal traction and on bed rest loses $1/4$ to $1/2$ lb/day. Proteins promote cell growth and bone union. Increased fluids aid renal elimination. The client's appetite will return gradually.

9. Bed rest decreases circulation. Pressure over bony prominences contributes to skin breakdown and pressure ulcers. Padding provides support to alleviate pressure and irritation.

10. Some institutions advise applying dry sterile dressings to the pin sites, changing them every 3 days. Some physicians order cleaning of the sites with hydrogen peroxide, if drainage occurs, to lower the risk of infection.

11. Shock may cause abdominal distention and paralytic ileus because blood is shunted from the GI tract to vital organs. Constipation is a side effect of bed rest, decreased fluid intake, and narcotic administration.

12. Monitor urine output, and note signs of urinary tract infection.

12. Bed rest, decreased fluid intake, and shock decrease urine output. Signs of urinary tract infection include fever, chills, back pain, elevated white blood cell count, and urinary urgency, frequency, burning, and clouding.

13. Check the traction setup and functioning every shift. Show the client how to use the trapeze to adjust body position.

13. For traction to be effective, weights must hang freely, ropes must be on pulleys, the client must be lying on his back and away from the foot of the bed, and splints must be properly positioned on the leg and thigh.

14. Assist the client with range-of-motion exercises; perform quadriceps-setting and triceps-strengthening exercises four times daily.

14. Exercises maintain muscle mass and prepare the client for walking with crutches. The increased circulation resulting from exercise hastens resolution of inflammation.

15. Explore the client's interests; suggest diversionary activities as needed.

15. An active client with a positive outlook recovers more quickly than a passive, bored client.

16. Explain what the client can expect if the treatment plan calls for surgically inserting a compression plate with screws or placing an intramedullary rod. Instruct the client on walking with crutches.

16. Surgical repair hastens the client's recovery by immobilizing the fracture fragments compactly. The client may be up on crutches without weight bearing on the right leg. Three-point gait may be used with crutches.

Clinical situation
(continued)

After 5 to 7 days in skeletal traction to align the fractured bone fragments and after achieving hematologic stability, James Wyman underwent open insertion of a compression plate with screws to hold the multiple (comminuted) fracture pieces. His postoperative recovery was uneventful. By discharge, he was walking on crutches, with instructions not to bear weight on his right leg for 1 week.

Evaluation

• Mr. Wyman recovers from the surgery without such complications as infection, bleeding, phlebitis, or pneumonia.
• Mr. Wyman walks with crutches (with no weight bearing on his right leg) and navigates stairs safely.
• Mr. Wyman is discharged home for recuperation and bone healing.
• Mr. Wyman experiences no fat emboli or neurovascular compromise.

Rheumatoid arthritis

Rheumatoid arthritis, a systemic disease with signs of inflammation in many body tissues, appears locally in joints as well as systemically with pain, fever, soreness, weakness, and malaise. Subcutaneous nodules appear near joints. (For associated information, see *Gout,* page 510, and *Differences between rheumatoid arthritis and osteoarthritis,* page 511.) The following clinical situation focuses on nursing care of a client with rheumatoid arthritis.

ADULT NURSING

Gout

Gout, a genetic defect of purine metabolism, results in overproduction or decreased excretion of uric acid. Urate crystals precipitate out of the serum and urine and are deposited in and around joints (tophi) and in the kidney.

Gout attacks usually affect the great toe, finger joints, and wrists. Symptoms result from an inflammatory reaction to the urate crystals. Daily ingestion of anti-uric acid medication prevents attacks. Other preventive measures include avoiding foods high in purines, such as organ meats (liver, brains, kidneys), sardines, and anchovies.

For acute attacks, colchicine is commonly prescribed. Drugs used for long-term and maintenance therapy include allopurinol (Zyloprim) and probenecid (Benemid).

Clinical situation

Betty Marks, a 53-year-old librarian, is admitted for synovectomy (surgical removal of the synovial sheath) to correct finger deformities caused by rheumatoid arthritis. The deformities prevent her from performing her responsibilities as a librarian. She is being prepared for synovectomy later in the week.

Assessment

NURSING BEHAVIORS	NURSING RATIONALES
1. Observe the client's posture and the functional capacities of musculoskeletal tissue: skin turgor, color, temperature, edema, pain location, deformity, and joint movement limitations.	1. Rheumatoid arthritis, a systemic inflammatory disease, affects multiple organ systems, including integumentary, renal, circulatory, respiratory, and musculoskeletal. The disease diminishes capacities in all involved tissues.
2. Assess vital signs, peripheral pulses, and respiratory patterns.	2. This baseline information helps identify changes from the norm.
3. Evaluate the client's appetite, nutritional intake, and GI functioning.	3. Treatment medications can cause GI irritation (nausea, vomiting, ulcer formation, and bleeding).
4. Determine the client's energy level and rest and activity patterns.	4. Chronic debilitating illness saps energy; insomnia, anemia, and depression may add to the client's problems. In rheumatoid arthritis, optimal exercise will keep the joints functioning. Medications can cause blood dyscrasias (abnormalities) and anemia.
5. Find out how well the client understands the disease and its management (for example, the reasons for and effects of various treatments).	5. Knowing the rationale for treatment is vital for safe and therapeutic results. Initially, new techniques may be insufficiently learned (see *Rheumatoid arthritis treatments,* page 512).
6. Assess the client's readiness for surgery, both psychologically and physiologically.	6. Rheumatoid arthritis affects the synovial linings of joints, affecting smaller joints symmetrically and laterally. Synovectomy removes the irritated lining but doesn't halt the disease's systemic effects. Other joints also may eventually require surgical repair.

Differences between rheumatoid arthritis and osteoarthritis

RHEUMATOID ARTHRITIS	OSTEOARTHRITIS
• Systemic disease: affects multiple body systems	• Local disease of joints only
• Affects synovial membranes initially, then other joint structures	• Affects cartilage initially, then other joint structures
• Affects symmetrical joints bilaterally; affects proximal joints and smaller joints most frequently	• Asymmetrical joint involvement; distal joints and larger weight-bearing joints most likely to be involved
• Multiple subcutaneous nodules under skin surfaces, not in joints	• Bony enlargements of distal joints common (Heberden's nodes)
• Dislocations, subluxations (partial dislocations), and deformities common (swan neck and boutonnière deformities of joints)	• Dislocation and subluxation uncommon; deformity from bony outgrowths
• Signs of inflammation: heat, fever, swelling, malaise, elevated erythrocyte sedimentation rate	• No systemic signs of inflammation; joints may be swollen but rarely hot
• Affects women three times as often as men; affects those between ages 30 and 55	• Not gender-specific; affects those ages 45 and older

7. Consult social service personnel.

7. This preliminary consultation enables the nurse to identify social services that can help the client with rheumatoid arthritis, if needed.

Diagnostic evaluation

• *Musculoskeletal tissue X-rays* (throughout the body as needed): Determine the status and progression of the disease
• *Hematologic studies* (rheumatoid factor, C-reactive protein, erythrocyte sedimentation rate [ESR], complete blood count, and immunologic assay): Accurately establish the diagnosis and current disease activity. Negative results may occur in rheumatoid factor and C-reactive protein even with active disease. In inflammatory rheumatic diseases, the ESR usually is elevated. Anemia commonly accompanies chronic and rheumatic diseases. Immunologic studies help confirm the diagnosis of rheumatoid arthritis, an autoimmune disease.
• *Other diagnostic tests* (electrocardiography, chest X-ray, blood urea nitrogen, and creatinine): Identify how rheumatoid arthritis affects various systems and whether the client can tolerate anesthesia and surgery
• *GI series:* Determines whether GI involvement results from rheumatoid arthritis or side effects of medications

Nursing diagnoses

• Impaired physical mobility related to joint stiffness and deformity
• Activity intolerance related to joint stiffness
• Risk for infection related to disruption of skin integrity
• Feeding self-care deficit related to joint stiffness and surgery
• Bathing or hygiene self-care deficit related to joint stiffness and surgery
• Dressing or grooming self-care deficit related to joint stiffness and surgery
• Toileting self-care deficit related to joint stiffness and surgery

ADULT NURSING

Rheumatoid arthritis treatments

Step 1
• Client and family education about rheumatoid arthritis
• Heat applications
• Exercise programs
• Rest for joints and body
• Salicylate medications

Step 2
• Physical and occupational therapy
• Splints and other orthotic devices
• Nonsteroidal anti-inflammatory drugs
• Analgesic drugs

Step 3
• Gold therapy
• Low-dose glucocorticoids
• Hydroxychloroquine
• Intra-articular glucocorticoids

Step 4
• High-dose glucocorticoids
• Hospitalization
• Reconstructive surgery

Step 5
• Immunosuppressive drugs
• Antineoplastic drugs
• Penicillamine

Planning and goals

• Mrs. Marks will undergo synovectomy without complication.
• Mrs. Marks will continue other required treatments, such as medications, splints, heat and cold applications, and adequate rest.
• Mrs. Marks will perform postoperative exercises, when ordered, to regain joint function and mobility.

Implementation

NURSING BEHAVIORS	NURSING RATIONALES
Medical therapy	
1. Administer medications, as ordered.	1. Drug administration maintains a serum drug level sufficient to produce therapeutic effects.
2. Encourage the client to perform exercises specifically designed for joint problems and conditioning exercises for unaffected joints.	2. These exercises strengthen muscles that support joints and increase endurance.
3. Encourage the client to wear the splints, as ordered.	3. Splinting decreases synovitis and reduces pain, stiffness, and swelling, thereby enhancing joint functioning.
4. Encourage physical therapy such as paraffin soaks.	4. Heat reduces muscle spasms and after-rest stiffness. Many clients take a warm shower in the morning to relieve stiffness after sleeping.
5. Apply ice packs, as ordered, for acute inflammation.	5. Cold relieves edema and pain and helps restore joint function.
6. Promote 30- to 60-minute rest periods (at least one daily) and 8 to 9 hours of sleep at night.	6. Fatigue increases inflammation and discomfort.
Preoperative care	
1. Provide routine preoperative care.	1. See "Preoperative period," pages 123 and 124, for specific nursing behaviors and rationales.

2. Check the client's vital signs and skin condition; then, if ordered, do skin scrubs and teach the client to do them (in some institutions, scrubs may be done only in the operating room before surgery).

2. Preparations for surgery reduce infection risks by decreasing microorganisms on the skin.

Postoperative care

1. Provide routine postoperative care.

1. See "Postoperative period," page 125, for specific nursing behaviors and rationales.

2. Elevate the client's hands, as ordered; use slings if they will help.

2. Elevation promotes circulation by decreasing edema.

3. Perform neurovascular checks.

3. Neurovascular checks enable the nurse to detect untoward conditions quickly.

4. Administer medication every 3 to 4 hours, as ordered, to relieve the dull, throbbing pain that commonly occurs after surgery.

4. Throbbing pain may also indicate that too-tight bandages are impeding arterial circulation.

5. Provide food and fluids, as ordered, and assist the client who had bilateral repairs.

5. Food and fluids help maintain fluid and electrolyte balance. If surgery affected both hands, the client will need help with eating.

6. Apply ice bags, if ordered, to operative sites.

6. Ice reduces swelling.

7. Administer medications for rheumatoid arthritis, as ordered, and review the medication regimen with the client.

7. Compliance with the drug regimen (including administration of the correct dose) maintains the therapeutic serum drug levels necessary to control the disease.

8. When ordered, teach the client exercises to regain mobility and strength of muscle and joints (or have a physical therapist do this).

8. Initially, exercises will be passive, then active-assisted and repetitive (see "Rehabilitation," pages 69 to 72). The joint is usually kept at rest for 3 to 5 days.

9. Observe the degree to which the client can perform activities of daily living; assist as needed.

9. This helps determine the client's ability to regain independence or the need for assistance or retraining.

10. Update social service personnel on the client's progress.

10. This information enables the social worker to identify how much assistance, if any, the client needs.

11. Inspect the client's wound.

11. The wound's appearance can be a clue to healing or infection.

Evaluation

• Mrs. Marks recovers from surgery with improved joint movements.
• Mrs. Marks performs required exercises and can perform activities of daily living independently.
• Mrs. Marks states she will continue to take her arthritis medications and will use hot and cold applications.
• Mrs. Marks returns to her librarian job after convalescing for 6 weeks.

ADULT NURSING

Leg amputation

Complete or partial leg (or arm) amputation may be required after trauma, neoplasms, infections, and peripheral vascular conditions, such as frostbite and gangrene. Amputations and the areas involved include the following:
- Lower leg: below-the-knee (BK) amputation
- Thigh: above-the-knee (AK) amputation
- Ankle, foot, toe: forepart of the foot removed at metatarsal joints
- Fingers: partial or complete amputation
- Arm: the forearm or above the elbow
- Hip: disarticulated at the hip, including all surrounding tissues; referred to as a hemipelvectomy or hindquarter amputation
- Shoulder: disarticulated at the shoulder, including the arm, forearm, and hand; called a forequarter amputation.

Lower limb amputations of parts of the toes, foot and leg, or thigh may be necessary after such complications of diabetes as gangrene. The following clinical situation focuses on nursing care of a diabetic client with a leg amputation.

Clinical situation

Richard Card, age 53, has had diabetes since childhood. Now, three toes of his right foot have gangrene, with surrounding cellulitis and inflammation of the entire foot. He is scheduled for a BK amputation tomorrow.

Assessment

NURSING BEHAVIORS

1. Identify the client's overall health status.

2. Assess for diabetic neuropathy (numbness, tingling, and other circulatory changes), retinopathy (decreased vision or blindness), and renal function indicators, such as fluid intake and output, edema, and blood volume.

3. Monitor the client's vital signs.

4. Assess the client's neurovascular status, checking circulation bilaterally. Monitor peripheral pulses, tissue color, skin temperature, and pain level, if any. Also note the following:

- skin changes, including atrophy, shiny skin, and hair loss; wet or dry skin; edema; and capillary refill status

NURSING RATIONALES

1. The client's overall health status indicates his ability to tolerate general anesthesia, surgery, and recovery processes.

2. In long-standing diabetes, small arteries sustain disease and damage. These assessments help the nurse determine the degree of damage.

3. Pulse, respiration, and temperature provide clues to possible systemic infection.

4. Neurovascular checks help detect compromised peripheral circulation.

- Moist skin may signify venous stasis; dry skin, arterial obstruction. With pressure, capillaries should blanch and turn pink in 2 to 4 seconds after pressure release.

• intermittent claudication, if the client is ambulatory

• Intermittent claudication results from peripheral neuropathy and tissue anoxia (oxygen deprivation). Rest relieves pain if the client has intermittent claudication only. With additional conditions (such as gangrene and obstruction), pain will persist despite rest.

• open lesions or ulcerations (compare diseased tissues with counterparts) and the extent and progression of gangrene, if any.

• Ulcerations and gangrene indicate poor tissue perfusion.

5. Evaluate the client's psychological outlook and feelings about proposed surgery.

5. Positive adjustment requires that the client accept an altered body image.

Diagnostic evaluation

• *Hematologic studies* (complete blood count, blood urea nitrogen, creatinine, and fasting blood glucose levels): Reveal the client's general health and diabetic control
• *Angiography* (femoropopliteal arteriogram): Shows condition of arterial circulation (for wound healing) and identifies the correct amputation level
• *Urinalysis:* Determines kidney function, which may be altered with diabetes

Nursing diagnoses

• Altered peripheral tissue perfusion related to atherosclerotic vessels
• Risk for infection related to impaired wound healing
• Body image disturbance related to loss of the limb
• Pain related to postamputation status

Planning and goals

• Mr. Card will undergo amputation without complications.
• Mr. Card will control diabetes during postoperative recovery and thereafter.
• Mr. Card will regain mobility with ambulatory aids and a prosthesis.
• Mr. Card will adjust to an altered body image after amputation.

Implementation

NURSING BEHAVIORS

NURSING RATIONALES

Preoperative care

1. Explain the procedure to the client, repeating the physician's explanations, as needed.

1. Anxiety prevents many clients from fully understanding explanations in one session.

2. Give the client opportunities to voice feelings and concerns.

2. Voicing concerns may reduce the client's anxiety and provide some measure of comfort.

3. Administer medications to relieve pain, as ordered.

3. The client may have severe burning and constant throbbing in affected tissues; pain results from tissue anoxia and infection.

4. Clean the skin with antiseptics, as ordered.

4. Cleaning with antiseptics commonly begins several days before surgery to reduce pathogens and prevent infection.

5. If time and the client's condition permit, arrange a visit from a healthy, rehabilitated amputee (of the client's sex and age, when possible).

5. In many cases, visits from persons who have successfully adjusted to amputation encourage the client to share feelings and may help diminish loneliness and helplessness.

ADULT NURSING

6. Carry out ordered and routine preoperative care.

6. Preoperative care enhances the client's ability to tolerate surgery and recover.

Postoperative care

1. Monitor the client's vital signs and level of consciousness.

1. Such monitoring helps determine fluid balance (blood loss) and the degree of recovery from anesthesia.

2. Perform reagent strip analysis or blood glucose determinations and urine testing, as ordered.

2. Test results determine the degree to which diabetes is being controlled.

3. Administer I.V. therapy and insulin as necessary.

3. Increased gluconeogenesis from the stress of surgery elevates blood glucose levels. Insulin helps restore normal levels to aid healing and recovery.

4. Check the stump dressing, if any.

4. Two amputation types are common: *closed* (skin is closed over the wound) and *open*, or *guillotine* (tissues are cut straight across and remain open). The client returns to surgery for wound closing after the wound is cleaned, irrigated, and infection free. Usually, the surgeon applies skin traction to open amputations to prevent skin retraction.

5. Use strict aseptic technique to change the dressing and irrigate the wound as required.

5. Dressings usually remain intact for 24 hours, then are changed as needed. Aseptic technique prevents additional infection.

6. Observe the color and condition of the stump; monitor for edema, drainage, pain, and signs of infection.

6. Observations indicate healing or continuing gangrene.

7. Elevate the stump on a pillow for 24 hours; then place the limb flat on the bed.

7. Elevating the stump decreases edema; subsequent lowering prevents contractures.

8. As the client's condition permits, turn the client to the abdomen four times daily for 30 minutes, with both knees extended.

8. Turning the client prevents flexion contractures of the knee. For AK amputation, turning is especially important to prevent hip flexion contractures.

9. Keep a tourniquet at the bedside if the client has an open wound. Should hemorrhage occur, apply the tourniquet 3″ to 4″ above the stump, and notify the physician immediately. Loosen the tourniquet every 20 minutes.

9. Sudden hemorrhage commonly occurs after open amputations (rarely after closed amputations). Using a tourniquet may cause vasospasm in arteries near the stump; loosening it permits arterial perfusion. A bleeding artery requires closing on the unit or in surgery.

10. Have the client perform deep-breathing and coughing exercises every 2 hours.

10. Breathing exercises help prevent pulmonary complications.

11. Provide food and fluids as ordered.

11. When the client's condition permits oral intake, the physician will prescribe a diet to help the client regain and maintain diabetic control.

12. Administer pain medications every 3 or 4 hours, as ordered.

12. The client's pain usually is confined to the incision site for 3 to 4 days after surgery.

13. Observe for indications of phantom pain, such as complaints of cramping in the toes or foot.

13. Phantom pain varies but should diminish over time. It may develop from nerve trauma related to surgery, tissue anoxia, or preoperative infection. Long-standing phantom pain may be caused by neuromas.

14. If the client is able, have him walk with a walker or crutches. Watch for dizziness and weakness.

14. A client with a leg amputation usually walks on the night of surgery or the next day. Walking will be delayed if the client's diabetes produces orthostatic changes from diseased arteries.

15. Assist the client with exercises—flexion, extension, adduction, and abduction—or arrange for a physical therapist to do it.

15. Exercise helps the client regain or maintain strength in the biceps, triceps, quadriceps, and hamstrings.

16. Using strict aseptic technique, clean the wound as needed and apply sterile bandages to the stump. (When healing permits, begin using elastic bandages.) Wrap the stump to look like a cone. Teach the client or a family member proper wound and stump care.

16. Suture line care requires strict asepsis, especially for a diabetic client, who develops infection more readily than others. A conical shape allows the stump to fit snugly into a prosthesis. Proper wrapping promotes venous return and reduces edema.

17. Arrange for stump measurements for a prosthesis (performed by an orthotist, a specialist in prosthetic fitting).

17. The orthotist will help the client learn to apply the prosthesis and walk effectively with it.

18. Assess the client's adjustment to amputation, and encourage him to express feelings and concerns.

18. The client may go through the stages of grief—denial, depression, anger, and withdrawal—before accepting the situation. Voicing feelings indicates progress.

19. Monitor food and fluid intake, noting the client's appetite for and tolerance of a diabetic diet.

19. While recovering from surgery, the client may have to follow a modified diet that does not include many preferences.

20. Monitor the client's insulin administration and blood and urine testing.

20. The insulin dosage may need adjustment until the client regains balance. Stress commonly disrupts diabetic control.

21. To preserve tissues in the remaining leg, teach the client proper foot care and provide these instructions:
• Do not wear tight garters or stockings.
• Alternately elevate and lower the leg every 4 hours for 20 minutes each.
• Wash the skin daily, dry carefully between the toes, and apply a moisturizer.
• Wear a new shoe or slipper only for brief periods to break it in slowly.
• Do not walk barefoot (to avoid cuts and bruises).
• Check the condition of the toes and foot daily.
• Test bath water with an elbow before immersing the foot (to prevent scalding).

21. Following these instructions will help maintain sound circulation in the remaining limb and promptly alert the client to changes.

ADULT NURSING

Postamputation discharge instructions

To prevent infection and other complications of amputation (which are especially problematic for the diabetic client), the nurse must teach the client about self-care. Be sure to cover the following points:
• Examine the stump daily for signs of redness and skin breakdown.
• If the stump looks irritated, stop using the prosthesis and notify the physician.
• Clean the stump daily with mild soap and water.
• Do not apply alcohol or other substances to the stump.
• Wear only a clean, approved stump sock that is free from holes or tears.
• To prevent edema, apply the stump sock immediately on arising in the morning.

---

22. Include family members in exercises, stump care, and diabetic teaching. (See *Postamputation discharge instructions.*)

22. The client's anxiety may diminish if he knows that the family supports him and can participate in his care.

Evaluation

• Mr. Card's wound is healing satisfactorily, and the stump is becoming cone-shaped without signs of infection or contractures.
• Mr. Card has regained diabetic control.
• Mr. Card walks with crutches (eventually, with a prosthesis).
• Mr. Card states acceptance of his altered body image.

INTEGUMENTARY SYSTEM

Burns

When a person is burned, all body functions undergo dramatic changes. The results include an inability to maintain a constant temperature, shock from fluid shifts and losses, increased susceptibility to life-threatening infections, altered sensory impulses causing mild to severe pain, and altered vitamin D production. These problems are accompanied by psychological and physiologic reactions to scarring, repeated skin grafts, and a long restorative process.

Burn types include thermal (from fire, steam, hot metal, and grease splatters), chemical (from acids and lye), and electrical (from live wires and lightning). (See *Principles of emergency burn care.*) The following clinical situation focuses on nursing care of a burn victim during the emergency, long-term, and skin-graft stages.

Clinical situation

Mark Raymond, a 29-year-old factory worker, was burned during a flash fire of chemicals he mixed incorrectly. After sustaining burns over his face, neck, chest, arms, and hands, he was rushed to the emergency department by the emergency medical team.

Principles of emergency burn care

Nursing behaviors

1. Stop the burning process.
• *Chemical burn:* Remove clothes if splattered; flush burned areas with cool, clean water for 10 to 15 minutes. Wear double gloves.
• *Thermal burn:* Remove objects that retain heat (such as rings and medals). Remove the client's clothes, if dirty, and cover the client with clean cloths or dressings, moistening them for easy removal.
• *Electrical burn:* Monitor vital functions of the brain, heart, and lungs. The human body is electrolytic (it conducts electricity). Be sure the current is off.

2. Prevent infection.

3. Determine the extent and degree of tissue burned.

Nursing rationales

• Flushing the area dilutes the chemicals and washes them away. Wearing double gloves aids in avoiding contact with the chemical.

• Electricity that passes through the body (the body will have an entrance and exit site) affects all body systems.

• Because skin is the body's first line of defense against infecting organisms, its disruption by burning predisposes the client to infection—the major cause of death among burn victims. When caring for a burned client, always use aseptic techniques and equipment. Cover the burn area to keep it soil-free, prevent heat loss, and protect exposed nerve endings, thereby decreasing pain.

• The Rule of Nines, a formula used to estimate body surface area burned, assigns 9% to the head and each arm, twice 9% to each leg and to the posterior and anterior trunk, and 1% to the perineum. The physician adds the percentages to arrive at the percent of total body surface area burned. Although for children the estimate considers age and size, for adults it does not, making it a valid guideline only in an emergency.

Depth of burns

• *Partial thickness:* superficial; epidermis only. Example: sunburn—marked reddening from dilated dermal blood vessels.
• *Deep:* between dermis and epidermis; dilated vessels begin to leak plasma and blisters of plasma fluid form between the skin layers.
• *Full thickness:* complete damage of epidermis, dermis, and skin appendages (sweat glands, sebaceous glands, and hair follicles). Burned areas appear black, brownish, and leathery and fail to heal (reepithelialize) without grafting.

Rule of Nines

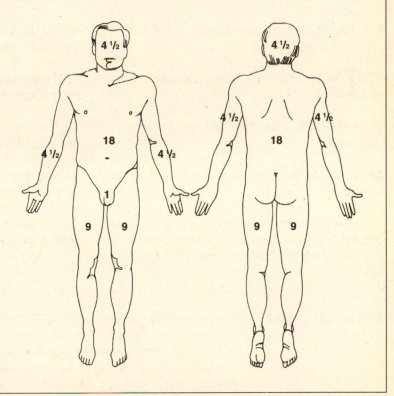

Assessment

NURSING BEHAVIORS	NURSING RATIONALES
1. Record the client's respiratory rate and evaluate the airway, noting shortness of breath, wheezing, splinting, sputum containing debris, smoky breath odor, hoarseness, accessory muscle use, and singed nostrils or nasal hairs. Prepare for possible endotracheal intubation.	**1.** These observations enable the nurse to assess laryngeal or pulmonary damage, swelling, or both. Smoke inhalation increases the likelihood of airway obstruction. A client with burns of the face, head, or neck may need intubation to aid breathing.
2. Look for blisters, edema, and charring.	**2.** Blisters indicate that plasma is being lost from the blood, which leads to hypovolemia and shock.
3. Choose appropriate veins (cephalic, jugular, subclavian) for I.V. access.	**3.** To replace fluid loss, central and peripheral I.V. lines must be established (see *Physiologic responses to burns*).
4. Monitor for nausea and vomiting; check emesis for occult blood.	**4.** Burns predispose the client to formation of stress ulcers, which may bleed.
5. Evaluate renal function and urine output.	**5.** A consequence of severe burns, renal shutdown arises from hypovolemia and shock.
6. Look for foreign matter, dirt, and other contaminants on the skin.	**6.** Wherever the skin barrier breaks, infectious agents can enter.
7. Identify the client's allergies and tetanus immunization history.	**7.** Allergy and vaccine data establish bases for selecting antibiotic and other drug therapies.
8. Collect health history and laboratory test data.	**8.** The client's general health history and laboratory test results serve as a treatment baseline.
9. Monitor the client's vital signs; maintain a warm environment.	**9.** These measures help prevent shock and ensure prompt intervention if shock occurs.
10. Assess the location, type, and severity of the client's pain.	**10.** Common in partial-thickness burns, pain is minimal with full-thickness burns.
11. Administer pain medication every 3 to 4 hours or as ordered.	**11.** Relieving the client's pain conserves energy for recovery efforts.
12. Assess the client's psychological status (fear, anger, and other emotions), sensory status, level of consciousness, and orientation to time, place, and person.	**12.** Being burned poses great psychological as well as physiologic threats.

Nursing diagnoses

- Impaired tissue integrity related to full-thickness burns
- Impaired skin integrity related to burns
- Ineffective thermoregulation related to loss of skin surfaces
- Risk for infection related to disrupted skin integrity
- Body image disturbance related to burns and scarring

ADULT NURSING

Physiologic responses to burns

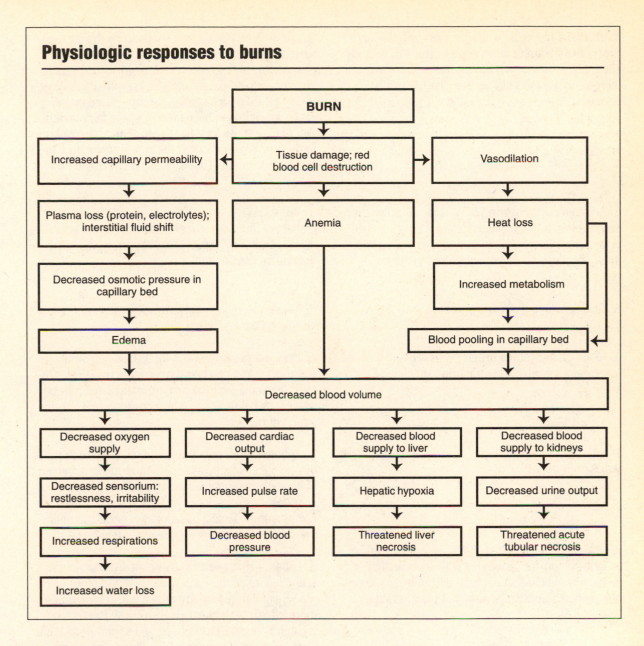

Planning and goals
- Mr. Raymond's burns will heal without infection or contractures.
- Mr. Raymond's fluid, electrolyte, and cellular balances will be restored.
- Mr. Raymond's self-concept will be restored without lasting deficits.

Implementation

NURSING BEHAVIORS

1. Maintain a patent airway by suctioning or by preparing for endotracheal intubation; administer oxygen therapy, as ordered.

2. Assist with the client's physical examination to identify the extent and degree of his burns.

NURSING RATIONALES

1. Smoke inhalation and fumes from burning materials predispose the client to pulmonary edema that compromises the airway. Intubation is preferred to tracheostomy because the latter poses a greater risk of infection.

2. The physical examination establishes baseline data, permitting definitive short- and long-term care.

3. Establish (or assist with) I.V. therapy following a prescribed formula: water and electrolytes, colloids (blood, plasma), and sugar (dextrose). Follow I.V. therapy orders carefully, and use an I.V. pump (Imed).

3. Hypovolemia is the primary concern during the first 48 to 72 hours after a burn (the hypovolemic phase). The client's recovery depends on adequate and accurate fluid replacement. The physician determines the fluid replacement formula based on rules set by specialists in burn therapy (for example, infuse half of the client's total fluid requirement for 24 hours in the first 8 hours; supply the rest over the next 16 hours). I.V. pumps (Imed) maintain accurate flow rates.

4. Administer tetanus prophylaxis (tetanus hyperimmune globulin, plus tetanus toxoid if the client had no prior prophylaxis). Administer tetanus toxoid booster if the client has not been immunized in the last 5 years.

4. Prophylaxis prevents tetanus by assisting passive and active immunity. Hyperimmune serum confers passive immunity. Tetanus toxoid permits the client to build active immunity.

5. Give the client nothing by mouth.

5. Nausea, vomiting, and paralytic ileus commonly occur in response to burns.

6. Insert an indwelling urinary catheter, and monitor urine output hourly. Obtain a urine specimen for analysis.

6. Urine output determines fluid replacement needs. Renal shutdown can result from tubular necrosis related to shock, hypovolemia, or toxins from burned tissues. The diuretic stage may begin 48 to 72 hours after a burn.

7. Administer I.V. antibiotics as ordered (usually every 6 to 8 hours).

7. Antibiotics are commonly administered to burn victims to fight gram-positive and gram-negative bacteria. The most common infections stem from *Staphylococcus aureus, Escherichia coli,* and *Pseudomonas* microorganisms. Fungal infections secondary to antibiotic administration are increasing in incidence.

8. Draw blood specimens for laboratory analysis of hematocrit, hemoglobin, blood urea nitrogen, creatinine, blood glucose, and arterial blood gas values.

8. Laboratory test values enable medical and nursing staff to compute fluid and colloid (blood plasma) replacement. Specimens are drawn daily (sometimes more often). With burns, as with crush injuries, potassium is released from cells, and serum potassium levels can rise dangerously high during the hypovolemic phase. Hypokalemia may occur during the diuretic phase.

9. Assist with radiologic studies, as needed.

9. Smoke inhalation warrants a chest X-ray to check for pulmonary edema and inhaled particles.

10. Attach electrocardiogram (ECG) leads for cardiac monitoring.

10. An ECG records the heart's response to increased potassium levels and other cardiac data. Monitoring is mandatory for electrical burns, which affect the cardiovascular system.

11. Monitor the client's vital signs every 30 minutes; check central venous pressure (CVP), and weigh the client, if possible.

11. Decreases in vital signs, CVP, and weight suggest shock, commonly resulting from burn trauma or hypovolemia (see "Shock," pages 103 to 108).

12. Use strict aseptic technique to assist with cleaning and dressing burns (may be done in the emergency department, the operating room, or burn rooms). Assist with hydrotherapy, if prescribed. Handle the client gently to prevent further trauma. Apply mafenide acetate ointment (Sulfamylon) to burned areas before applying a loose dressing. Administer an analgesic before debriding burned areas.

12. Wound sepsis is the leading cause of death among clients with burns. Aseptic technique and mafenide acetate ointment guard against infection. Mafenide acetate penetrates eschar but can be painful when applied. Silver sulfadiazine is also used; although less painful than mafenide acetate, it is also less likely to penetrate eschar. Rarely used today, liquid silver nitrate 0.5% may be applied if the client is allergic to sulfa drugs. Fingers and toes should be wrapped separately to prevent skin surfaces from adhering. Circumferential dressings (around the trunk, arms, and legs) must be loose to allow for edema.

13. Insert a rectal temperature probe to monitor body temperature.

13. The client may be cool from loss of skin surfaces, which function as a heat regulator.

14. Monitor the client's sensorium as well as sensory and pain levels. As ordered, administer I.V. narcotics and analgesics cautiously to prevent respiratory or neurologic depression.

14. The client may be confused or disoriented, especially if he was burned electrically. Intramuscular administration of narcotics into edematous tissue is contraindicated because the drug may not be absorbed. Initially, narcotics are given I.V.

15. Position the client to prevent contractures and further trauma to affected skin areas.

15. Usually, the client is placed in a special bed (CircOlectric) if the trunk and back are burned.

16. Inform the client and family about the short- and long-term care he requires; encourage them to express their feelings and concerns.

16. Fear and anxiety are typical responses to shock or trauma. Because outcomes are uncertain for most burn victims, the client and family need support and understanding from the nursing staff.

Clinical situation
(continued)

Long-term care of the client with burns

After treatment in the emergency department, clients with burns usually are cared for in specially equipped and staffed burn units, where they receive specialized long-term therapy vital to improved health. Ultimate recovery (if it occurs) usually is prolonged, marked by gains and setbacks. The following nursing care of Mark Raymond is common.

Assessment
NURSING BEHAVIORS

NURSING RATIONALES

1. Assess for anorexia, paralytic ileus, loss of appetite, nausea, vomiting, indigestion, headache, constipation, and diarrhea.

1. Anorexia and paralytic ileus commonly affect clients with burns. Appetite returns slowly after the client resumes eating. Nausea, vomiting, indigestion, headache, constipation, and diarrhea are common side effects of narcotics and antibiotics.

2. Check the range of motion of muscles and joints.

2. Stiffness and contracture are common.

3. Observe burn wounds for signs of healing or infection.

3. Infection commonly occurs, characterized by increased drainage, purulent discharge, redness, and edema.

4. Assess the client's mood over several weeks and months, noting any mood swings. Consult a mental health counselor, if appropriate.

4. The client typically experiences anger, hostility, and depression, and the feeling "Why me?" predominates. Mental health counseling can assist the client in successfully adapting to his condition.

Nursing diagnoses

- Altered nutrition (less than body requirements) related to anorexia and paralytic ileus
- Risk for infection related to loss of protective skin barrier
- Self-esteem disturbance related to role changes and scarring
- Chronic pain related to joint stiffness and contractures
- Powerlessness related to an inability to control the current situation

Planning and goals

- Mr. Raymond will retain nutritional intake and regain lost weight.
- Mr. Raymond will experience minimal drug side effects.
- Mr. Raymond will regain satisfactory muscle and joint functions.

Implementation

NURSING BEHAVIORS

NURSING RATIONALES

1. Provide foods rich in calories, proteins, vitamins, and minerals; force fluids; and weigh the client daily.

1. The client requires optimum intake of all nutrients to regain lost weight and nutritional balance and to achieve full recovery.

2. Administer oral antibiotics, multivitamins, analgesics, and other medications, as ordered, and give antacids every 2 hours. Monitor for occult blood, a sign of Curling's (stress) ulcer.

2. Antibiotics are administered orally rather than intravenously once the client resumes eating. Curling's ulcer, a duodenal ulcer, may develop in clients with severe body-surface burns.

3. Help the client perform range-of-motion exercises.

3. Exercise prevents contractures and maintains joint movements.

4. Clean the client's wounds in a Hubbard tank or shower. Assist in debriding wounds, if feasible. (Eschar, leatherlike encrustation, may require surgical removal.) Apply solutions or creams two or three times daily.

4. Cleaning wounds, debriding dead skin, and applying ointments help granulation tissue develop, providing a healthy base for skin grafts.

5. Promote ambulation, occupational therapy, and physical therapy.

5. Walking and other forms of exercise (with the assistance of the nurse and therapists) enhance physiologic recovery.

6. Teach family members and friends to participate in the client's care.

6. Through their participation, loved ones help keep the lines of communication open, promote ongoing relationships, and provide support and security to the client.

ADULT NURSING

7. Encourage the client to express his feelings about disfigurement and scarring. Consider a psychiatric consultation, if applicable.

7. Disfigurement and scarring alter the client's body image and self-concept; his adjustment to body image changes may be reflected in periods of anger, depression, withdrawal—even suicidal feelings. Expressing these feelings is an early step toward resolving them. When such feelings persist despite the nurse's efforts, psychiatric therapy may be warranted.

8. Prepare the client for skin grafts, if necessary; use pigskin (porcine) or similar material to cover the flesh temporarily before grafting.

8. The client may require several grafting sessions. Temporary coverings decrease fluid loss and help prevent infection.

Clinical situation
(continued)

Skin grafts, applied to healthy granulating tissues, close the open skin areas produced by burns. The grafts conserve fluids and electrolytes and cosmetically restore the skin's appearance. Skin grafts also are used to cover chronic draining lesions, such as stasis ulcers. (See *Skin graft types,* page 526.)

Mark Raymond's emergency and long-term burn care is behind him. Now he is preparing to have split-thickness skin grafts applied to his chest and shoulders, which sustained third-degree burns.

Assessment

NURSING BEHAVIORS

1. Before skin grafting, continue to assess the client's overall health and his recovery from burn trauma.

2. Assess burned areas for appearance of granulating tissues.

3. Review laboratory test results.

4. Observe burn areas for contractures.

5. Teach the client about skin grafts.

NURSING RATIONALES

1. Ongoing assessments determine the client's readiness for skin grafting.

2. Healthy granulating tissue looks pink and moist without purulent drainage. Wet-to-dry dressings aid drainage removal and development of healthy granulating tissue.

3. This review gives medical and nursing staff the information necessary to correct deficiencies before the procedure.

4. Scar tissues contract as they heal. Scars across joints may pull the joint into contractures. Contracted scars may need surgical corrrection (such as a Z-plasty) or removal of the contracted scar graft.

5. Knowledge will relieve some of the client's anxiety.

Nursing diagnoses

• Impaired skin integrity related to skin grafting
• Body image disturbance related to scarring and skin grafts
• Pain related to the surgical procedure

Planning and goals

• Mr. Raymond will regain skin integrity, with healed grafts and no contractures.
• Mr. Raymond will resume social roles and relationships, having accepted his altered body image.

ADULT NURSING

Skin graft types

Split-thickness skin grafts
Using a dermatome, the surgeon slices layers of skin from a donor site and applies the material to a prepared recipient site. Layers can be sliced in desired thicknesses by adjusting the instrument's gauge. They are called split- or partial-thickness grafts.

Full-thickness skin grafts
These grafts contain dermis, epidermis, and skin appendages acquired from the client's unaffected skin areas. Because it will not heal spontaneously, the donor site must be covered by a split-thickness graft (or its edges sutured shut). Full-thickness grafts are called free grafts when they come from a distant site and flap grafts (or pedicle grafts) when they are slid over to the burned area from an adjacent site. One end of the flap graft remains attached to the donor site, which ensures a continuous blood supply. Again, the donor site must be grafted or closed.

Tube pedicle grafts
Full-thickness skin grafts loosened from underlying tissues by parallel vertical incisions, tube pedicle grafts are skin pieces with edges sewn together to form a cylinder-like tube (hence the name). After 2 to 3 weeks, one end of the tube is cut off and reattached closer to its eventual home site. Gradually (every 3 weeks), the tube is "walked" to the desired site by cutting the distal end while the proximal end remains attached to the blood supply. Pedicle grafts are rare because of advanced microsurgical techniques that permit moving and reattaching full thicknesses of skin easily.

Implementation

NURSING BEHAVIORS

1. After skin grafting, maintain the client in a supine position in bed.

2. Check the graft sites and dressings, noting drainage, numbness or tightness, and the color of surrounding tissue.

3. Administer analgesics as ordered.

4. If ordered, roll cotton-tipped applicators over the graft, applying steady, gentle pressure from the center of the graft to the edges. Roll the entire site, taking care not to push the graft ahead of the applicator, which could loosen the graft.

5. Protect graft sites from bumping and stretching.

NURSING RATIONALES

1. With the client in this position, gravity helps grafts adhere to underlying tissues.

2. Dressings should be snug but not too tight. Drainage is usually serosanguineous. Skin surrounding the graft should be pink and warm and may appear slightly edematous. The skin graft, if visible, should be pink and warm; a bluish or cool edematous site may indicate venous stasis, which may impair graft adherence.

3. The donor site has exposed nerve ends, causing much pain for most clients with split-thickness grafts. A pressure dressing that initially covers the site usually is removed in 24 to 48 hours. The site is then covered with a thin, transparent dressing or with petrolatum-coated gauze. In 7 to 10 days, new skin forms over the donor site, relieving pain. Usually, the recipient site is only minimally painful.

4. Rolling mobilizes fluid, which promotes graft adherence.

5. New blood vessels growing into the graft can break easily with slight trauma. These blood vessels remain delicate for several weeks after the procedure.

ADULT NURSING

6. Encourage the client to perform range-of-motion (ROM) exercises when ordered. Elevate the head of the bed and assist with ambulation as needed.

6. ROM exercises maintain muscle and joint functions and help prevent new contractures. Split-thickness skin grafts contract as they heal; full-thickness grafts do not contract.

7. Encourage the client to discuss how he feels about himself and his situation.

7. Even at later stages of burn care, the client may still harbor anger, hostility, or depression. Psychiatric counseling may be helpful.

8. Encourage the client to perform or assist with self-care.

8. Self-care enhances the client's independence while furthering rehabilitation. A client who is fearful, reluctant, or anxious about self-care may require gentle prodding.

9. Allow the client time to discuss fears or anxieties about returning home.

9. Because of disfigurement or scarring, the client may have fear or anxiety about returning to family and societal roles.

Evaluation

- Mr. Raymond regains skin integrity of the donor site.
- Mr. Raymond's graft sites heal without infection or undue contracture.
- Mr. Raymond returns to societal roles and accepts his altered body image.

EYE, EAR, NOSE, AND THROAT

Detached retina

The retina transmits impulses from its nerve cells to the optic nerve. A *detached retina* occurs when the neural retina (the layer of rods and cones) is separated from the pigmented epithelium. Retinal tears and holes can result from aging, trauma, and disease. When such tears occur, vitreous humor or other substances from the eye's interior seep behind the neural retina, causing the detachment. The following clinical situation focuses on nursing care of a client with a detached retina.

Clinical situation

Theresa Carmello, age 55, visits her physician after experiencing sudden flashes of light and floating spots in her left eye. She is scheduled for surgery when ophthalmologic examination confirms the physician's diagnosis of retinal detachment in the upper part of the left eye. (Surgery may be done on an outpatient basis or may require an overnight stay, depending on the client's condition.)

Assessment
NURSING BEHAVIORS

NURSING RATIONALES

1. Assess floating spots in the client's left eye.

1. When the retina tears, blood cells ooze into the vitreous humor, causing the floating spots.

2. Assess the frequency of light flashes.

2. The vitreous humor pulls on the retina, causing the light flashes.

3. Assess for vision loss in the upper part of the left eye.

3. Retinal detachment that develops slowly (such as from aging) will result in gradual loss of the visual field.

4. Ask the client if she has blurred vision.

4. Blurred vision will increase as detachment continues.

Diagnostic evaluation

• *Full ophthalmoscopic examination:* Reveals a retinal tear draping into the vitreous humor

Nursing diagnoses

• Sensory or perceptual alterations (visual) related to a detached retina
• Anxiety related to sudden vision loss
• Risk for injury related to further detachment

Planning and goals

• Mrs. Carmello will remain free of injury.
• Mrs. Carmello will understand treatment options.
• Mrs. Carmello will be free of permanent visual impairment.

Implementation

NURSING BEHAVIORS

NURSING RATIONALES

1. Help the client into a comfortable position, with the retinal tear in the lowest part of the eye. Keep her eyes covered.

1. These measures will help prevent further detachment. A client with upper left detachment should lie on the left side, with the head of the bed flat. Activity restrictions may be necessary, although bathroom privileges are usually allowed.

2. Implement nursing interventions for blind clients, as needed.

2. See "Cataract extraction," pages 529 to 531, for specific nursing behaviors and rationales.

3. Prepare the client for surgery by explaining possible surgical interventions and techniques.

3. Preparation may alleviate some of the client's anxiety. Surgical interventions include the following:
• Cryotherapy uses a probe to freeze the borders of the retinal tear, leading to inflammation, scarring, and retinal reattachment.
• Photocoagulation uses heat from a bright light to coagulate the retina with underlying tissues.
• Diathermy applies heat directly to the sclera, causing the retinal tear to adhere to it.
• Scleral buckling splints the choroid to the retina, thus sealing the retinal tear.

4. Postoperatively, position the client as ordered.

4. The surgeon determines the position based on the procedure and the area of detachment. If an air bubble is injected, the client will have to lie in a position that causes the air bubble to rise and place pressure on the area of detachment for at least 24 hours.

5. Instruct the client to avoid activities that may increase intraocular pressure.

5. See "Cataract extraction," pages 529 to 531, for examples.

6. Notify the physician if the client complains of floating spots, flashes of light, or blurred vision.

6. These symptoms suggest a recurrence of the detachment.

7. Before discharge, provide the following health teaching instructions:
• Care for the eye properly, and use aseptic technique when administering eye medications.
• Avoid rapid eye movements and head jarring.
• Follow a diet and exercise program that prevents constipation.
• Vary the activity level only according to the physician's orders. Discourage driving or engaging in strenuous activity until cleared by the physician.

7. Health teaching reinforces the client's knowledge of her condition and prepares her for self-care at home. Proper eye care and aseptic technique help prevent infection and promote healing. The other measures help prevent increased intraocular pressure.

Evaluation

• Mrs. Carmello remains free of injury.
• Mrs. Carmello understands her discharge restrictions.
• Mrs. Carmello's vision is restored.

Cataract extraction

A cataract, an opacification of the eye's lens, causes vision loss. Cataracts usually develop in both eyes, but vision does not decrease at the same rate in both eyes. Cataracts are removed surgically by intracapsular or extracapsular extraction, and vision can be restored by intraocular lens implantation. The following clinical situation focuses on nursing care of a client with limited vision who will undergo surgery for cataract removal.

Clinical situation

Over the past 6 months, Rita Henry, age 69, has been losing her vision. She is blind in the left eye and perceives only light and dark with the right eye. She lives with her sister. Mrs. Henry was admitted to the same-day surgery unit for an extracapsular cataract extraction with intracapsular lens implant.

Assessment

NURSING BEHAVIORS

Determine how well the client sees and how well she moves about in her environment without assistance.

NURSING RATIONALES

This assessment clarifies the type and degree of assistance the client will need in the surgery center.

Diagnostic evaluation (before admission)

• *Vision screening* (for clients who have some vision in one or both eyes): Identifies the amount of vision in each eye and the total visual effectiveness of both eyes. Common ophthalmologic abbreviations used in vision screening tests include O.D. (right eye), O.S. (left eye), and O.U. (both eyes).
• *Ophthalmoscopic examination:* Identifies abnormalities in the fundus of each eye.

Nursing diagnoses

• Sensory or perceptual alterations (visual) related to lens opacity
• Risk for infection related to impending surgery
• Risk for injury related to decreased vision
• Knowledge deficit related to postoperative management

Planning and goals
- Mrs. Henry will perform needed postoperative self-care.
- Mrs. Henry will take steps to prevent infection and reduce intraocular pressure.

Implementation

NURSING BEHAVIORS	NURSING RATIONALES
Preoperative care **1.** A few days before surgery, contact the client to verify that she has received and understands the physician's preadmission instructions: Remind her to take a laxative the day before surgery if she hasn't had a bowel movement in the past 2 days; tell her to shampoo her hair; and be sure someone will drive her to and from the same-day surgery unit and stay with her at home for several days afterward.	**1.** Well in advance of surgery, the physician provides the client with preadmission instructions; the nurse's verification serves as a reminder to ensure compliance. A laxative may be needed to prevent constipation and resultant straining at stool, which increases intraocular pressure. Such activities as shampooing and shaving are not permitted soon after surgery to prevent head jarring. The client should not drive or remain alone until vision has sufficiently improved to ensure safety.
2. Caution the client not to bend, strain, or lift and to avoid coughing, sneezing, and squeezing the eyes shut. Remind her to lean her head backward (not forward) when washing the hair. Repeat these instructions during postoperative teaching.	**2.** The restricted activities can increase intraocular pressure, possibly causing hemorrhage and vision loss.
3. Perform routine preoperative procedures when the client enters the same-day surgery unit.	**3.** Although the client won't stay overnight in the surgical unit, routine preoperative care remains the same (see "Preoperative period," pages 123 and 124, for specifc nursing behaviors and rationales).
4. Advise the client to keep both eyes closed during eye patch application.	**4.** This prevents trauma, which may occur if the patch scratches the cornea.
Postoperative care **1.** Review postoperative care instructions with the client after she recovers from anesthesia. Make sure she has a copy of the instructions.	**1.** By following postoperative care instructions, the client can prevent complications. Written instructions help ensure compliance.
2. Tell the client to wear eyeglasses during the day and a metal shield over the affected eye at night for several weeks.	**2.** The covering protects the eye and prevents injury to the incision.
3. Caution the client not to rub her eyes.	**3.** Rubbing the eyes increases the potential for infection.
4. Advise the client to lie on her back or on the side opposite the surgical site when resting or sleeping.	**4.** These positions help prevent injury to the incision.
5. Teach the client to clean the affected eye from the inner to the outer canthus, using sterile cotton balls. Also advise her to apply a warm, moist cloth twice daily.	**5.** Proper eye care helps prevent infection. The warm, moist cloth soothes the eye and reduces inflammation.

6. Review instructions for administration of eye medications:
- Always wash hands first.
- Use sterile equipment only.
- Do not touch the eyeball with the eyedropper.

6. The client must understand how to administer eye medications to protect the cornea from trauma and infection.

7. Tell the client to walk only in familiar surroundings.

7. Because of limited vision, the client may fall or bump into an unfamiliar object and injure the affected eye.

8. Teach family and friends to increase the client's stimulation, especially if she is elderly or has mental clouding or confusion.

8. Decreased sensory stimulation from vision loss can cause disorientation.

9. Encourage the client to increase her intake of fiber and fluids, to walk regularly, and to take psyllium (Metamucil) and a stool softener, if prescribed.

9. These measures help prevent constipation and resultant straining, which increases intraocular pressure.

10. Urge the client to notify the physician of distorted, blurred, or clouded vision (if a lens was implanted); nausea, vomiting, halos around lights, and pain unrelieved by medication; a temperature over 100° F (37.8° C) and foul-smelling yellow drainage on the eye patch; and sudden sharp pain in the affected eye.

10. Visual complaints may stem from a dislocated lens. Nausea, vomiting, halos around lights, and pain unrelieved by medication all signal increased intraocular pressure. A temperature over 100° F or foul-smelling yellow drainage indicates infection. Acute pain in the affected eye may result from intraocular hemorrhage.

11. Reinforce teaching to prevent increased intraocular pressure: Caution the client to avoid bending, straining, lifting, coughing, sneezing, squeezing the eyes shut, and leaning forward.

11. Increased intraocular pressure can cause hemorrhage and vision loss. (*Note:* If the client's cataract was removed by phacoemulsification, restrictions concerning intraocular pressure are less rigid.)

12. Help the client adjust to cataract glasses. Advise her to remain seated while wearing them the first time and to avoid using the stairs.

12. Until the other cataract is removed, the glasses will make objects appear about one-third closer than they are, distorting the client's vision.

Evaluation

- Mrs. Henry can perform required eye care.
- Mrs. Henry knows how to prevent infection and increased intraocular pressure.
- Mrs. Henry states the signs she must report to the physician.

Glaucoma

Glaucoma, a disease that encompasses various conditions associated with increased intraocular pressure, occurs when an obstruction limits aqueous humor outflow from the eye's anterior chamber. Although usually managed medically, the disease sometimes requires surgery, such as *trabeculoplasty* and *trabeculectomy*. With trabeculoplasty, a laser beam is passed through the trabecular meshwork. Scarring that occurs from the burn changes the fibers, thus increasing the outflow of aqueous humor. Trabeculectomy is a filtering procedure that creates a new opening, bypassing the obstructed outflow. Other procedures such as peripheral iridectomy may be used with acute glaucoma to prevent the iris from obstructing the anterior chamber.

Narrow-angle glaucoma has a sudden onset and is characterized by acute pain, nausea, vomiting, diaphoresis, fixed and dilated pupils, and dramatically elevated intraocular pressure (50 to 60 mm Hg). This medical emergency requires immediate surgery. The preoperative objective is to decrease intraocular pressure by administering pilocarpine (every 5 minutes for up to 1 hour); an osmotic diuretic such as mannitol (to decrease eye fluid); and acetazolamide (Diamox) I.V. (to reduce formation of aqueous humor). The following clinical situation focuses on nursing care of a client having surgery for glaucoma.

Clinical situation

Vera Smith, age 55, sees halos around lights and has had mild pain in both eyes for several weeks. She works as a bookkeeper and lives alone. She has been diagnosed with primary open-angle glaucoma. She arrives at the ambulatory surgical unit on the morning she is scheduled for a laser trabeculoplasty. She will be discharged the same day.

Assessment

NURSING BEHAVIORS	NURSING RATIONALES
1. Assess the client's understanding of surgery and presence of support persons.	**1.** After surgery, the client will need a ride home.
2. Review the client's symptoms, such as red eye (also called steamy cornea), a pupil that is moderately dilated and unresponsive to light, head and eye pain from pressure on the sensory distribution of the trigeminal nerve, and decreased visual acuity.	**2.** These are common symptoms of glaucoma.

Diagnostic evaluation

• *Tonometry:* Measures intraocular pressure (normal value: less than 20 mm Hg). Before administering the test, instill eyedrops to anesthetize the cornea, prevent injury, and promote accurate measurement. Instruct the client not to blink during the test and to hold her head still.

Nursing diagnoses

• Sensory or perceptual alterations (visual) related to increased intraocular pressure
• Pain related to increased pressure
• Knowledge deficit related to medication management
• Risk for injury related to possible further damage

Planning and goals

• Mrs. Smith's vision will improve and pain will decrease.
• Mrs. Smith will be able to perform needed postoperative self-care.
• Mrs. Smith will take steps to prevent infection and reduce intraocular pressure.

Implementation

NURSING BEHAVIORS	NURSING RATIONALES
Preoperative care	
1. Explain the procedure to the client, and provide routine preoperative care.	**1.** Clear explanations teach the client what to expect and usually help lessen the client's anxiety (see "Preoperative period," pages 123 and 124, for specific nursing behaviors and rationales).

2. Provide analgesics to reduce the client's pain.

2. As intraocular pressure increases, eye pain becomes more severe.

Postoperative care

1. Evaluate the client's intraocular pressure 1 hour after surgery and before discharge.

1. Laser procedures may increase intraocular pressure.

2. Instruct the client not to lie on the operative site.

2. Increased pressure on the operative site must be avoided.

3. Advise the client to wear eyeglasses or an eye shield.

3. This provides necessary eye protection.

4. Caution the client to avoid bending, sneezing, straining, lifting, coughing, squeezing eyes shut, and leaning forward. Recommend that she add fiber and fluids to her diet.

4. The client should avoid activities that can increase intraocular pressure. Added fiber and fluids will help prevent constipation.

5. Be sure the client understands discharge instructions, especially those related to eye medications.

5. Ocular steroids (such as prednisolone acetate) decrease inflammation. Miotics (such as pilocarpine or carbachol) constrict the pupil. Beta blockers (such as timolol) and carbonic anhydrase inhibitors (such as acetazolamide) decrease production of aqueous humor.

6. Instruct the client to report eye pain that is unrelieved by analgesics, occurring over the eyebrow, or accompanied by nausea or decreased vision.

6. These are signs of increased intraocular pressure.

Evaluation
- Mrs. Smith accurately explains the medication regimen.
- Mrs. Smith plans to modify her lifestyle to cope effectively with glaucoma.
- Mrs. Smith's vision is improved.

Rhinoplasty

A rhinoplasty is a reconstruction of the external nose to repair structural defects that impair nasal breathing. The surgery is also performed for cosmetic reasons. The following clinical situation focuses on nursing care after nasal surgery.

Clinical situation

Ron Holmes, a 24-year-old professional baseball player, was hit in the nose during a fracas at a baseball game. After receiving first aid for his nosebleed, he was admitted to the hospital for a rhinoplasty (frequently a same-day surgical procedure). His medical diagnosis is a fractured nose.

Assessment

NURSING BEHAVIORS

1. Determine the amount of airway obstruction sustained by the client.

NURSING RATIONALES

1. A patent airway is the immediate consideration in all first aid. Heavy bleeding can obstruct the client's airway.

2. Determine the amount and cause of nasal bleeding, and check the client's vital signs.

2. Nasal injuries can cause severe hemorrhage, creating the potential for fluid volume loss.

3. Determine the severity of the client's pain.

3. Most injuries cause pain. Identifying the severity of the pain enables the nurse to determine appropriate comfort measures.

Nursing diagnoses
- Ineffective airway clearance related to posttraumatic bleeding
- Risk for infection related to the client's postoperative status
- Pain related to trauma and surgery

Planning and goals
- Mr. Holmes will be physically and emotionally prepared for surgery.
- Mr. Holmes will not experience preventable complications.

Implementation

NURSING BEHAVIORS

NURSING RATIONALES

Preoperative care

1. Provide routine preoperative care.

1. See "Preoperative period," pages 123 and 124, for specific nursing behaviors and rationales.

2. Instruct the client to practice mouth breathing.

2. Nasal packing after surgery will force the client to breathe through his mouth.

3. Keep scissors readily available in the client's room.

3. Should the client's airway become obstructed, the strip holding the nasal packing can be cut and the obstructive packing removed.

Postoperative care

1. Elevate the head of the bed about 45 degrees.

1. Head elevation promotes drainage, enhances breathing, and prevents airway obstruction.

2. Monitor the client's vital signs, and check for bleeding and frequent swallowing. Change nasal slings (the compress under the nose) when saturated with blood. Instruct the client not to remove nasal packing.

2. Nasal hemorrhage is a common complication of rhinoplasty. Frequent swallowing is a clue to possible hemorrhage. The client usually has nasal packing for 1 to 2 days and wears a splint for about 1 week.

3. Administer pain medication as needed (usually, acetaminophen, codeine, or both).

3. The client will have moderate discomfort for 2 to 3 days. Aspirin is not given because of the risk of bleeding.

4. Use ice compresses on the client's nose for 24 hours as needed.

4. Cold compresses reduce edema and bruising.

5. Humidify the client's room air with cool mist and provide mouth care four times daily and as needed.

5. Mouth breathing causes secretions to dry.

6. Allow the client food as tolerated.

6. The client will probably tolerate liquids better on the day of surgery but proceed to his usual diet thereafter. A soft diet may be better tolerated for several days.

7. Caution the client not to blow his nose for 48 hours after packing is removed.

7. The client's nose will feel full from edema and packing. Blowing the nose could dislodge the packing and precipitate further hemorrhage.

8. Observe the client frequently for signs of airway obstruction. If the airway is obstructed, cut the nasal plug's posterior string and remove the packing.

8. The nasal packing can slip, blocking the airway.

9. Give the client a timetable for postoperative healing.

9. Swelling and discoloration will remain around the eyes and nose for several weeks. The final cosmetic results won't be known for 3 months to 1 year.

10. Instruct the client to notify his physician of nasal bleeding, increased pain and swelling, redness, tenderness, foul-smelling drainage, and fever.

10. Signs and symptoms of inflammation and infection warrant medical attention. Hemorrhage can occur up to 1 week after surgery.

11. Caution the client not to bump his nose when playing baseball or engaging in other vigorous activities. Suggest that he wear a nose guard.

11. These precautions protect the client's nose from injury.

Evaluation

• Mr. Holmes can breathe effectively through the nose.
• Mr. Holmes accurately describes the signs and symptoms he should report to his physician.

Laryngectomy

A laryngectomy is performed for cancer of the larynx. It may be partial (surgical removal of a portion of one vocal cord) or total (complete removal of the larynx), with an incision made in the thyroid cartilage.

With a partial laryngectomy, the client's voice is preserved; aspiration is a risk because the epiglottis has been removed. With a total laryngectomy, aspiration is not a risk because the trachea and esophagus are completely separated; the client loses sense of smell (no air passes through the nose) and speech and requires a permanent stoma. Apart from these differences, nursing care is the same for both procedures.

The following clinical situation focuses on nursing care of a client undergoing a laryngectomy and facing speech loss.

Clinical situation

Stephan Conly, age 62, is a car salesman who has been hoarse since recovering from the flu 6 weeks ago. After examining Mr. Conly, the physician admits him to the hospital for diagnostic tests to determine the source of his chronic hoarseness. Test results confirm the need for laryngectomy.

Assessment

NURSING BEHAVIORS

NURSING RATIONALES

1. Determine whether the client has symptoms besides hoarseness, such as difficulty swallowing (or a lump in the throat), a burning sensation in the throat when drinking hot beverages, and a persistent sore throat.

1. Feeling a lump in the throat may indicate a tumor. A burning sensation and a sore throat are signs of inflammation, which is present in laryngeal cancer.

2. Assess the client's relationships with family, friends, and coworkers, and identify his job responsibilities.

2. The client's diagnosis and impending speech loss may damage personal relationships and alter his job performance.

Diagnostic evaluation

• *Laryngoscopy:* Permits visualization of tumors and other laryngeal masses

Nursing diagnoses

• Impaired verbal communication related to removal of the larynx
• Risk for infection related to the client's postoperative status
• Body image disturbance related to speech loss
• Ineffective airway clearance related to increased respiratory secretions
• Impaired social interaction related to speech loss

Planning and goals

• Mr. Conly's family and friends will provide emotional support.
• Mr. Conly's fluid and electrolyte levels will remain within normal limits.
• Mr. Conly's nutrition will be adequate to meet his needs.
• Mr. Conly will:
—have an unobstructed airway
—experience no preventable complications
—adjust to and care for his stoma
—communicate effectively with others
—be physically and emotionally prepared for surgery.

Implementation
NURSING BEHAVIORS

NURSING RATIONALES

Preoperative care
1. Provide routine preoperative care. Explain the procedure, the nursing care the client will receive after surgery, and his postoperative appearance (tracheostomy, neck drains, nasogastric [NG] tube).

1. Uninformed clients become frightened when they wake up after anesthesia and notice their appearance, replete with drains and many tubes.

2. Encourage frequent deep breathing and coughing.

2. Deep breathing and coughing clear the lungs and promote optimal respiratory system functioning.

3. Encourage the client to express concerns related to the stoma, loss of oronasal breathing, disfigurement, and speech loss.

3. Frankly addressing the client's concerns preoperatively prepares the course for postoperative adjustment.

4. Have the client practice the communication method he will use after surgery.

4. The client will have to communicate nonverbally after surgery, usually by writing.

Postoperative care
1. Provide routine postoperative care. Elevate the client's head, and keep it slightly flexed to ease tension on the incision.

1. Breathing is easier and edema is decreased when the head is elevated.

2. Give the client constant attention until he adjusts to stomal breathing.

2. The nurse's attention helps lessen any anxiety the client may have about choking.

Suncioning guidelines

- Use aseptic technique throughout the suctioning procedure to prevent infection.
- Insert a catheter when suction is turned off to prevent injury to the respiratory tract.
- Do not use suction more than 15 seconds at a time (hypoxia may result).
- Hyperventilate the client before and after suctioning to prevent hypoxia.
- Maintain suction pressure between −80 and −120 mm Hg. Limit the diameter of the catheter to half the diameter of the airway.

---

3. Keep laryngectomy tubes and the stoma free of obstructions, including bedclothes. Encourage the client to cough and deep-breathe hourly or as needed, staging the coughing from shallow to progressively deeper coughs. Suction the client every 2 hours (more frequently if needed) for the first 24 hours (see *Suctioning guidelines*).

3. An obstructed stoma compromises the client's airway. Frequent coughing and deep breathing prevent atelectasis. Copious secretions in the first 24 hours must be removed to maintain an open airway.

4. Support the client's head when repositioning him.

4. Supporting the client's head minimizes pain and promotes comfort.

5. Assist the client with deep-breathing and coughing exercises after administering analgesics and before walking or a position change.

5. These strategies promote comfort, reduce pain, and prevent complications.

6. Administer prescribed narcotics with caution, observe the client's respirations, and notify the physician of problems.

6. Narcotics decrease the respiratory rate and inhibit coughing. The pain medication should be changed if the client's respiratory rate falls below 12 breaths/minute.

7. Humidify the client's room air, and provide an oxygen mist as needed.

7. The physiologic mechanisms that normally moisten inspired air are bypassed after a laryngectomy. Oxygen supplements help maintain normal arterial oxygen levels in the client's blood.

8. Maintain I.V. therapy until tube feeding begins, and frequently monitor fluid and electrolyte levels.

8. I.V. therapy decreases the potential for fluid and electrolyte imbalance from blood loss and wound drainage.

9. Provide frequent oral hygiene.

9. Oral hygiene helps prevent infection and provides comfort.

10. Attach an NG tube to low suction for 24 to 48 hours or until bowel sounds return. Be alert for abdominal distention when first clamping the tube.

10. NG suctioning prevents abdominal distention, an early sign of paralytic ileus.

11. Check the Hemovac to ensure that it is removing neck drainage.

11. After surgery, the drainage system removes fluid from potential dead space and prevents suture line tension.

12. Adopt the most effective method of communicating with the client (for example, paper and pencil, toy slate, picture cards, gestures, and sign language). Resist the urge to shout and to complete the client's sentences. Consult a speech therapist as needed.

12. The best communication method will depend on the client's coping skills and his capacity to communicate. Regardless of which method is used, the nurse should not shout or finish the client's sentences. Shouting increases the client's anxiety (and is unnecessary if the client does not have a hearing problem). Finishing the client's sentences diminishes his feeling of self-worth. Speech therapy will assist the client in speech retraining or learning new communication methods.

13. Observe for hemorrhage—check the color of secretions, wound drainage, and Hemovac drainage.

13. Hemorrhage is a common complication of laryngectomy.

14. Notify the physician of temperature elevation or changes in the amount, color, and odor of secretions.

14. Fever and changes in secretions signal infection.

15. Teach the client to use aseptic technique when cleaning laryngectomy tubes and the stoma.

15. Until the incision heals, aseptic technique is used to prevent infection.

16. If the client has a laryngectomy tube, show him how to insert another one correctly.

16. This prepares the client for self-care at home.

17. Feed the client by mouth or by tube, as appropriate. Consult a dietitian if needed.

17. Some clients require tube feeding, whereas others can take food by mouth.

18. Review activity and recreation limitations with the client; for example, caution him about stoma care related to showering and swimming, and tell him to avoid using inhalant irritants and pollutants (paint, hair spray, and other aerosol products) near the stoma.

18. Water, aerosols, and sprays can cause severe inflammation of the tracheobronchial tree.

19. Inform the client that gustatory changes may be permanent.

19. Absence of taste may be temporary (when using an NG or gastrostomy tube) or permanent (if the tongue and taste buds were removed during surgery).

20. Provide referrals to the local Visiting Nurse Association or community health nursing agency; to a speech therapist; and to the Lost Chord Club, New Voice, or a similar support group.

20. A visiting nurse or community health nurse can provide home nursing care related to nursing diagnoses and implementations developed by hospital staff nurses. A speech therapist can help with speech retraining or suggest new ways to communicate (such as esophageal speech, mechanical aids, and surgical voice restoration using a prosthesis). Support groups serve members who have had laryngectomies.

21. Advise the client to wear a medical identification tag.

21. In an emergency, the medical identification tag informs caregivers that the client has a stoma and that resuscitation efforts should be mouth to stoma.

ADULT NURSING

22. Encourage the client to express his feelings about his appearance and voice loss, and the rehabilitation and lifestyle changes awaiting him. Urge family and friends to support the client, and offer your support and understanding to all of them.

22. The client will grieve over his appearance and voice loss, and will probably react negatively at first to rehabilitation demands and lifestyle changes, although expressing these feelings will strengthen his self-concept. Because the client's condition also affects the lives of family and friends, they all need encouragement from the nursing staff.

23. Support the client's efforts to cope with career-related problems.

23. A client who must communicate verbally may be unable to return to his job. (Mr. Conly, a car salesman, will certainly have difficulty.) Counseling or job retraining may be needed.

24. Teach the client's family how to suction the stoma.

24. Family members or friends should learn how to maintain a patent airway in case the client cannot do it.

25. As the client relearns communication skills, allow time for him to respond. Maintain a calm environment.

25. Patience and understanding alleviate the client's anxiety and boost his self-confidence and motivation to continue with rehabilitation.

Evaluation

- Mr. Conly underwent surgery successfully and experienced no preventable complications.
- Mr. Conly can demonstrate how to care for his stoma.
- Mr. Conly's nutrition is adequate to meet his needs.
- Mr. Conly's family and friends are providing emotional support.
- Mr. Conly is beginning to communicate effectively with others.

Stapedectomy

A stapedectomy is surgery to remove the stapes bone in the ear and replace it with a prosthesis. The following clinical situation focuses on nursing care of a client undergoing ear surgery to treat a hearing loss.

Clinical situation

Over the past few years, Harry Thornby, a 45-year-old auto mechanic, has had gradual hearing loss. After administering an audiometric examination, Mr. Thornby's physician told him he had otosclerosis, which was causing conductive deafness, and that stapedectomy could correct it. The nurse scheduled Mr. Thornby for same-day surgery.

Giving Mr. Thornby a copy of instructions, she reviewed what he should do to prepare for the procedure. For instance, because ear surgery would affect his equilibrium, he should arrange for someone to transport him to and from the surgical unit and stay with him at home for a few days after surgery. The nurse also explained that Mr. Thornby could expect diminished hearing for a day or so after surgery because of inflammation and swelling and that it would take about 3 months to determine the operation's success—measured by how well the prosthesis (or graft) attaches and whether adhesions result. Mr. Thornby agreed to bring the copy of these instructions with him on the day of stapedectomy.

ADULT NURSING

Assessment

NURSING BEHAVIORS	**NURSING RATIONALES**
1. Determine the degree of the client's hearing impairment.	**1.** Conductive deafness is impaired air conduction of sound waves reaching the inner ear. Sometimes hearing aids help, but many clients must learn alternative communication methods.
2. Assess the client's speech, vision, ability to write, and facility at lipreading.	**2.** This assessment enables the nurse to plan effective and comfortable client communication.
3. Find out whether the client wears a hearing aid.	**3.** The client's hearing aid (if he uses one) must be removed before surgery.

Nursing diagnoses

• Sensory or perceptual alterations (auditory) related to poor bone conduction
• Knowledge deficit related to postsurgical care
• Risk for infection related to the client's postoperative status

Planning and goals

• Mr. Thornby will communicate effectively with others.
• Mr. Thornby will experience no preventable complications.
• Mr. Thornby will be physically and emotionally prepared for surgery.

Implementation

NURSING BEHAVIORS	**NURSING RATIONALES**
For all clients with hearing loss	
1. Get the client's attention by approaching so that he can see you coming.	**1.** Approaching the client from behind may startle or frighten him.
2. If the client can lip-read: • Face the client directly; don't shout or exaggerate lip movements.	• Straightforward, natural speech will help the client read lips.
• Don't talk with anything in or covering the mouth.	• An object in or over the mouth makes lip movements unintelligible.
• Speak to the client with a light source shining on your face.	• Direct lighting makes lip movements easier to see.
3. If the client wears a hearing aid: • Don't shout. • Speak slowly and clearly. • Make sure the client turns on the hearing aid before you speak.	**3.** Hearing aids amplify sound. People who have hearing aids are sensitive to loud noises.

4. If the client has speech limitations or can't understand you:
• Speak slowly, using simple words.
• Use gestures.
• Allow time for the client's response.
• Repeat words, more than once if necessary.
• Don't shout.
• Remain calm and avoid distractions.

4. These techniques facilitate the client's understanding of spoken words. Giving the client time to respond decreases his anxiety. Shouting will not improve the client's hearing.

5. Provide writing instruments for the client who can't hear or speak.

5. Writing is an effective form of communication.

Preoperative care

1. Perform routine preoperative preparations.

1. Preoperative preparations for same-day surgery are the same as those for hospitalized clients.

2. Allow the client to wear his hearing aid into the operating room, if applicable.

2. The client needs to maintain communication until he's anesthetized.

3. Warn the client not to make quick, jerky movements or turn his head when he recovers from anesthesia.

3. Rapid movement can dislodge the prosthesis.

Postoperative care

1. Review postoperative instructions with the client after he recovers from anesthesia. Supply a copy of instructions for him to take home.

1. Written instructions prompt the client's memory, especially if anesthesia or anxiety impairs his comprehension during the initial review.

2. Tell the client to lie in bed on his unaffected side for 24 hours.

2. This position prevents trauma to the surgical site.

3. Change the client's ear cotton as prescribed.

3. This is usually done to maintain an infection-free environment.

4. Be alert to fluctuations in the client's hearing.

4. Fluctuations may result from closure of the oval window.

5. Observe for tinnitus, vertigo, and nystagmus.

5. These symptoms indicate developing labyrinthitis.

6. Observe the client's ability to frown, wrinkle the forehead, and grimace.

6. If the client cannot make facial expressions, he may have edema or a facial nerve injury.

7. Review activity restrictions ordered by the client's physician.

7. Usually, no physical activity is allowed for 1 week and no exercise and sports for 3 weeks. Heavy lifting should be avoided.

8. Advise the client to sneeze or cough with the mouth open and to blow his nose gently one side at a time for 1 week after surgery. Also tell him to avoid airplane flights for 1 week.

8. These precautions help prevent buildup of pressure inside the ear.

ADULT NURSING

9. Caution the client not to get water in the ear (no shampooing, showering, or swimming) for 6 weeks and to avoid people with upper respiratory tract infections.

9. These precautions guard against infections.

10. Teach the client to change ear cotton aseptically.

10. Aseptic technique prevents infection.

11. Explain that the client's hearing will return slowly.

11. The client's hearing will return when edema decreases and the prosthesis is firmly attached.

12. Instruct the client to move slowly until the ear heals.

12. Slow movements help avoid vertigo (dizziness). Falling may dislodge the prosthesis.

13. Tell the client to notify the physician of dizziness, ear pain, and sudden hearing loss.

13. These symptoms indicate that the prosthesis may have separated from the surgical site.

14. Caution the client not to return to work until his ear heals.

14. The client should allow appropriate healing time (usually 1 week; 3 weeks if the work is strenuous).

Evaluation

- Mr. Thornby underwent surgery successfully and experienced no preventable complications.
- Mr. Thornby can explain how to care for his ear at home.
- Mr. Thornby accurately describes measures to prevent infection.

ENDOCRINE SYSTEM

Diabetes mellitus

Diabetes mellitus is a chronic disturbance in the production, action, or rate of use of insulin, resulting in disturbed metabolism of carbohydrates, protein, and fats. A client may develop either insulin-dependent (Type I) or non-insulin-dependent (Type II) diabetes.

The hormone insulin, produced in the islets of Langerhans in the pancreas, performs three major functions: it helps glucose enter body cells, inhibits protein and fat breakdown, and assists in the liver's storage of glycogen.

Factors that increase the blood glucose level include glucocorticoids, epinephrine, glucagon, somatotropin, emotional stress, pregnancy with multiple births, surgery or trauma, and obesity (overeating). Factors that lower the blood glucose level include insulin, exercise, and decreased food intake. (See *Major complications of diabetes mellitus*, for additional information.)

The following clinical situation focuses on nursing care of an adult client with diabetes mellitus.

Clinical situation

Shauna Holmes, a 53-year-old married homemaker and the parent of one child, has had frequent skin infections recently. When she went to the physician for a routine checkup, she learned that her blood glucose level was 225 mg/dl (normal: 80 to 120 mg/dl). The physician arranged for her to enter the hospital for diagnostic tests, which resulted in a provisional diagnosis of non-insulin-dependent (Type II) diabetes mellitus.

Major complications of diabetes mellitus

ARTERIOSCLEROSIS

Assess for ulcers on legs, lack of sensation in legs and feet, angina pectoris, pyelonephritis and reduced renal function, and retinopathy (observe for visual impairment). Note that the client should undergo an annual vision check by an ophthalmologist. The diabetic client is susceptible to peripheral vascular disease, neuropathy, and early coronary artery disease. Glomerulosclerosis is a common complication. Retinopathy is the major cause of acquired blindness in diabetic adults. With severely impaired vision, the client may require modifications in self-care management.

METABOLIC ACIDOSIS

Diabetic ketoacidosis, more common in Type I diabetes, has a slow onset. It results from acute insulin deficiency, causing acidosis from metabolism of fats (ketone bodies). Assess for dehydration caused by polyuria and hypovolemia as well as acid-base imbalance and electrolyte changes caused by acidosis and ketone excretion. Determine the client's blood glucose level, and assess the client's history for recent infection, severe stress, and noncompliance with insulin therapy. Depending on the severity of the acidosis, the client may need I.V. insulin, plasma expanders to prevent shock, and electrolyte replacement. Monitor the client's blood glucose level frequently to assess progress. Teach the client how to avoid recurrence by adhering to the planned diet, exercise, and medication program.

HYPEROSMOLAR HYPERGLYCEMIC NONKETOTIC SYNDROME (HHNK)

The client with Type II diabetes is at risk for this life-threatening complication, which occurs when elevated blood glucose leads to severe dehydration and electrolyte imbalance. Treatment resembles that for ketoacidosis; however, correcting dehydration is even more important.

HYPOGLYCEMIA (INSULIN REACTION)

Assess the client for hunger, anxiety, blurred vision, sweating, and tremors. Unconsciousness can occur if the blood glucose level falls below 50 mg/dl. Provide a source of rapidly absorbed carbohydrate (for example, 4 oz of orange juice, regular soda pop, or 5 Life Savers). If the client cannot swallow, administer 25 ml of 50% glucose by I.V. bolus, as ordered. (Glucagon, which converts glycogen stored in the liver to glucose, can also be administered to a client who cannot swallow; for example, a family member can administer glucagon intramuscularly to an unconscious client. Once the client regains consciousness, the family member should provide small, frequent meals.) Monitor the blood glucose level to prevent relapse. Teach the client to avoid hypoglycemia by regulating diet, exercise, and insulin or oral hypoglycemic drugs.

Assessment

NURSING BEHAVIORS	NURSING RATIONALES
1. Determine the client's age.	1. Clients over age 40 show a high incidence of Type II diabetes mellitus.
2. Check the family history for diabetes mellitus.	2. A family history of diabetes mellitus predisposes the client to the disease.
3. Assess the client's weight.	3. Obesity is a predisposing factor.
4. Identify the client's medications.	4. The client's medications may contain substances that elevate the blood glucose level.
5. Ask the client to describe her food intake for a typical day.	5. Medical and nursing staff use this essential baseline information to plan the client's meal pattern.

ADULT NURSING

6. Ask the client if she is experiencing urinary frequency (polyuria), hunger (polyphagia), or thirst (polydipsia).

6. Excess glucose acts as an osmotic diuretic thereby pulling fluid from the cells and causing polyuria. Excess fluid loss causes thirst; insufficient cellular nourishment causes hunger.

7. Observe for weakness.

7. Generalized weakness results from fat and protein breakdown for energy.

8. Observe for pruritus vulvae.

8. Pruritus indicates excretion of glucose and ketones in the urine.

9. Check for infections.

9. Infections indicate an impaired ability to form antibodies and a disturbed protein metabolism. Blood glucose presents a good culture medium.

10. Assess the client's and family's lifestyle.

10. This information helps determine lifestyle modifications necessitated by diabetes mellitus.

Diagnostic evaluation

• *Fasting blood glucose test:* The client should not eat for 6 hours before the test; a fasting blood glucose evaluation prevents the error of measuring normal increases in the blood glucose level that occur after eating.
• *Postprandial blood test:* Draw blood from a fasting client, have the client eat a high-carbohydrate meal or drink 100 mg/dl glucose in solution, then draw blood 2 hours after the client eats. An elevated blood glucose level 2 hours after a meal indicates diabetes mellitus.
• *Glucose tolerance test:* Draw blood from a fasting client, have the client drink 100 mg/dl glucose in solution, then collect blood (and urine) specimens, as ordered, for testing. In a client without diabetes, the blood glucose level initially will range from about 140 to 150 mg/dl but will return to normal (80 to 120 mg/dl) within 2 hours. In a client with diabetes mellitus, the blood glucose level initially will be higher than 150 mg/dl and will remain elevated for a longer time before returning to its previous level.
• *Glycosylated hemoglobin level:* A level above 7% indicates poor glucose control over the past 3 months.
• *Urinalysis:* Obtain a urine specimen to test for glycosuria and ketonuria. When the blood glucose level is higher than the renal threshold, the excess spills into the urine, causing glycosuria. Ineffective carbohydrate metabolism causes mobilization of fat to supply energy; excess ketones (organic acids) spill into the urine, causing ketonuria.

Nursing diagnoses

• Risk for infection related to the effects of the disease
• Knowledge deficit related to self-care and disease management
• Fluid volume deficit related to polyuria
• Altered nutrition: Less than body requirements, related to the inability to use glucose

Planning and goals

• Mrs. Holmes and her family will be able to cope with lifestyle changes caused by diabetes mellitus and associated therapy.
• Mrs. Holmes will not experience complications resulting from ignorance of diabetes mellitus or appropriate therapy.
• Mrs. Holmes's blood glucose level and body weight will approach normal limits as much as is physiologically possible.

Implementation

NURSING BEHAVIORS

1. Monitor the client's meal pattern, using the American Diabetic Association's food-exchange system (see *Planning a meal pattern using the food-exchange system,* page 546).

2. Teach the client who requires insulin to regulate dietary intake, as needed, to accommodate changes in activity level or medication dosage. (Some clients with Type II diabetes and all clients with Type I diabetes require insulin.)

3. For the client receiving insulin, explain insulin administration, as follows:

• Tell the client to administer insulin daily, in amounts consistent with diet, exercise, and health status.

• Advise the client that infection, surgery, emotional stress, and acidosis increase the amount of insulin required.

• Explain how to manage periods of increased exercise (for example, by eating an extra snack of whole wheat crackers and cheese).

• Urge the client to be aware of the insulin's expiration date and whether the insulin is bovine, porcine, or human.

• Show the client how to draw up and administer insulin using sterile technique and subcutaneous injection; demonstrate preferred locations and proper rotation of injection sites.

4. Administer an oral hypoglycemic agent, as ordered, and monitor the client for side effects. If necessary, administer treatment for hypoglycemia (treatment may be continued longer than for insulin-caused hypoglycemia). If the physician prescribes a long-acting drug, increase the client's food supplement at bedtime.

NURSING RATIONALES

1. The amount and type of foods depend on the client's age, desirable weight, and usual activity level. The plan is developed in collaboration with the client, based on her usual meal pattern. Dietary management may be sufficient to control blood glucose in the client with Type II diabetes.

2. The client must learn to balance changes in activity level or insulin dosage with appropriate dietary modifications. For example, if the client wants to exercise more often or more vigorously and the insulin dosage remains the same, the client must eat enough to offset the increased exercise; on a reduced insulin regimen, the client must eat less.

3. See *Common insulins and their action,* page 547.

• Insulin requirements vary according to diet, exercise, and health.

• These health problems cause the liver to release glucose, which increases the blood glucose level.

• As exercise increases and insulin is used more effectively, the client must increase complex carbohydrate and protein consumption.

• Human insulin, made by the recombinant DNA technique, does not cause the sensitivity problems associated with animal insulin.

• U-100 insulin, the standard concentration used today, is compatible with the decimal system and reduces confusion and dosage errors. Rotating the site prevents tissue damage.

4. Hypoglycemic agents, administered to lower the blood glucose level in some Type II diabetic clients, offer a long duration of action (see *Common oral antidiabetic drugs,* page 548). Side effects include hypoglycemic reaction, GI disturbances, nausea, vomiting, diarrhea, headache, paresthesias, allergic reactions (for example, skin rash), and pruritus. Some of the drugs produce a hypoglycemic reaction in the middle of the night.

ADULT NURSING

Planning a meal pattern using the food-exchange system

Foods in the six exchange lists contain about the same amount of carbohydrate, protein, fat, and calories; that is, in the given amounts, all choices on each list are equal, and any food on a list can be exchanged or traded for any other food on the same list. Using the exchange lists provides variety in food choices and a means of balancing the distribution of nutrients throughout the day.

Milk exchange list
One exchange of milk contains about 12 g of carbohydrate and 8 g of protein. The amount of fat and the number of calories vary, depending on the kind of milk chosen. One cup of skim milk, 1% milk, or nonfat yogurt equals one exchange.

Vegetable exchange list
One exchange of vegetables contains about 5 g of carbohydrate, 2 g of protein, and 25 calories. Vegetables contain 2 to 3 g of dietary fiber. One half cup of a cooked vegetable or vegetable juice equals one exchange.

Fruit exchange list
One exchange of fruit contains about 15 g of carbohydrate and 60 calories. A typical serving of fruit is $1/2$ cup of fresh fruit or fruit juice or $1/4$ cup of dried fruit.

Starch and bread exchange list
One exchange of bread or starch contains about 15 g of carbohydrate, 3 g of protein, and 80 calories. Whole-grain products contribute about 2 g of fiber per exchange. One slice of bread or $1/2$ cup of

cereal, grain, pasta, or starchy vegetable (potato, corn) equals one exchange.

Meat exchange list
One exchange of meat contains about 7 g of protein. The amount of fat and the number of calories vary with the kind of meat chosen. One ounce of meat equals one exchange. Cheese, eggs, and legumes are included in this exchange.

Fat exchange list
One exchange of fat contains about 5 g of fat and 45 calories. One teaspoon of margarine or butter, one tablespoon of mayonnaise or salad dressing, one slice of bacon, or varying amounts of nuts equals one exchange.

SAMPLE MENU USING EXCHANGE LIST
(assuming IDDM, requiring three meals and three snacks daily)
This is a sample of using the exchange list, not a sample diet plan, and does not include the amount of calories, carbohydrates, protein, and fats.

DAILY EXCHANGE PATTERN	SAMPLE FOODS FOR 1 DAY	DAILY EXCHANGE PATTERN	SAMPLE FOODS FOR 1 DAY
Breakfast		**Snack**	
1 fruit	$1/2$ grapefruit	1 bread	3 graham crackers
2 bread	$1/2$ cup shredded wheat $1/2$ English muffin	$1/2$ milk	$1/2$ cup 1% milk
$1/2$ milk	$1/2$ cup 1% milk	**Dinner**	
1 fat	1 tsp. margarine coffee/tea (free)	3 meat	$1/2$ cup ground beef, cooked 1 oz. shredded cheese
Snack		1 bread	2 taco shells lettuce, tomato, onion in taco (free)
1 meat	1 tbs. peanut butter	2 vegetables	$1/2$ cup cooked zucchini $1/2$ cup cooked wax beans
1 bread	6 saltine crackers	1 fat	1 tsp. margarine
Lunch		1 fruit	2 plums coffee/tea (free)
2 bread	2 slices whole-wheat bread		
1 meat	$1/4$ cup tuna fish	**Snack**	
1 fat	1 tbs. mayonnaise lettuce (free)	$1/2$ milk	$1/2$ cup plain yogurt
1 milk	1 cup 1% milk	1 fruit	$1/2$ cup canned peaches
1 vegetable	1 cup carrot sticks	1 bread	6 Ritz crackers
1 fruit	1 medium apple	1 fat	

Adapted with permission from *Exchange Lists for Meal Planning*, American Diabetes Association, Inc., Alexandria, Va. ©1995 American Diabetes Association, Inc., and the American Dietetic Association.

Common insulins and their action

TYPE	ONSET (HOURS)	PEAK ACTION (HOURS)	DURATION OF ACTION (HOURS)
Rapid-acting insulins			
Insulin Injection, Regular	$1/2$ to 1	Varies	6 to 8
Prompt Insulin Zinc Suspension (Semilente)	1 to $1^1/_2$	5 to 10	12 to 16
Intermediate-acting insulins			
Isophane Insulin Suspension (NPH)	1 to $1^1/_2$	4 to 12	24
Insulin Zinc Suspension (Lente)	1 to $2^1/_2$	7 to 15	24
Isophane (NPH) 70% and regular insulin 30%	$1/2$ to 1	4 to 12	18 to 24
Long-acting insulins			
Protamine Zinc Insulin Suspension (PZL)	4 to 8	14 to 24	36
Extended Insulin Zinc Suspension (Ultralente)	4 to 8	10 to 30	>36

5. Show the client how to use glucose strips and the blood glucose monitor for self-testing. If the client is taking insulin, teach the importance of regular use.

5. This test determines the client's blood glucose level. It offers the most reliable means to monitor diabetes control and is recommended for clients taking insulin.

6. Obtain a urine specimen to determine the ketone level. Have the client empty the bladder, and obtain another specimen for testing in 30 minutes.

6. This test determines the ketone level in the urine. Testing the second specimen yields more accurate results.

7. Review the physician's instructions on what the client should do if self-test results fall outside the range established by the physician. Be sure the client understands the instructions.

7. If urine contains ketones, the physician may increase the insulin dosage. The blood glucose level may be normal. If it isn't, the client will be instructed to administer regular insulin according to an individualized schedule.

8. Teach the client proper skin care.

8. The client will be susceptible to peripheral vascular disease and will have decreased circulation and neuropathy (see the implementation section of "Arteriosclerosis obliterans," pages 449 to 453, for specific nursing behaviors and rationales).

9. Encourage the client to wear a medical alert bracelet.

9. Signs of hypoglycemia mimic signs of alcohol intoxication. The bracelet identifies the client's medical condition so that police officers, health care personnel, and others can respond appropriately to ensure prompt treatment.

Evaluation

On discharge, Mrs. Holmes can explain how to:
• prevent hypoglycemic reaction and metabolic acidosis
• administer insulin
• modify the family menu so that she can follow her prescribed diet.

ADULT NURSING

Common oral antidiabetic drugs

DRUG	DURATION OF ACTION	SIDE EFFECTS
Sulfonylureas glipizide (Glucotrol)	10 to 24 hours	Hypoglycemia, nausea, heartburn, rash, flushed face
glyburide (DiaBeta)	18 to 24 hours	Same as above
tolazamide (Tolinase)	12 to 24 hours	Same as above
tolbutamide (Orinase)	6 to 12 hours	Same as above
Biguanides metformin (Glucophage)	8 to 12 hours	Nausea, vomiting, diarrhea, generalized abdominal distress
Oligosaccharides acarbose (Precose)	1 to 5 hours	Abdominal discomfort, diarrhea, flatulence

Cushing's syndrome

Cushing's syndrome (hypercortisolism) is associated with excessive production of hydrocortisone resulting from malfunction of the adrenal or pituitary glands. Causes include increased production of adrenocorticotropic hormone (ACTH) by the pituitary, a tumor of the adrenal cortex that increases the production of glucocorticoids, and excess intake of glucocorticoids.

Located above the kidneys, the two adrenal glands are major endocrine organs. They make a vital contribution to maintaining body systems. The adrenal glands consist of the cortex and the medulla. The cortex produces glucocorticoids (cortisol), mineralocorticoids (aldosterone), and sex hormones. The medulla produces catecholamines, epinephrine, and norepinephrine. Adrenal cortex dysfunction produces marked changes in metabolism, fluid and electrolyte balance, response to stress, and an anti-inflammatory response.

Clinical situation

Danielle Dawson, age 58, has been taking hydrocortisone orally to treat rheumatoid arthritis. During a recent examination, her physician noted that Mrs. Dawson was developing signs of Cushing's syndrome.

Assessment

NURSING BEHAVIORS	NURSING RATIONALES
1. Observe the client for a swollen, puffy appearance.	1. Increased secretion of aldosterone, which leads to sodium and water retention, causes the swelling and puffiness.
2. Observe the client for hypertension.	2. Increased fluid retention causes hypertension.
3. Check laboratory data for the client's serum potassium level.	3. Increased aldosterone secretion results in sodium retention and potassium excretion.

4. Observe the client for increased fat deposits in the face and abdomen.	**4.** The characteristic moon face and buffalo hump result from an increased secretion of cortisol.
5. Observe the client for weakness and muscle wasting.	**5.** The catabolic effects of glucocorticoids are weakness and muscle wasting.
6. Assess the client for easy bruising.	**6.** Decreased collagen support around the blood vessels produces bruising.
7. Observe for striae.	**7.** Striae develop from skin stretching caused by fluid retention.
8. Assess for hyperglycemia.	**8.** In impaired glucose use, gluconeogenesis increases.
9. Observe for osteoporosis.	**9.** This results from mobilization of calcium from the bones.
10. Observe the client for emotional lability and suppressed inflammatory and stress response.	**10.** Glucocorticoids produce all these effects.
11. Assess for hirsutism and decreased menses.	**11.** Increased androgen secretion causes these symptoms.

Diagnostic evaluation
- *Urine cortisol:* The level will be elevated with Cushing's syndrome.
- *Blood cortisol:* The level will be elevated, especially at night.
- *Urine 17-hydroxycorticosteroid and 17-hydroxyketosteroid:* Adrenal gland hyperfunction may increase both of these levels.
- *Dexamethasone suppression:* Cushing's syndrome alters pituitary-adrenal feedback. A low dose of dexamethasone does not cause the pituitary's expected suppression of ACTH.
- *Serum sodium:* The level will increase.
- *Serum potassium:* The level will decrease.

Nursing diagnoses
- Risk for injury related to muscle weakness
- Fluid volume excess related to sodium and water retention
- Body image disturbance related to swollen, puffy appearance

Planning and goals
- Mrs. Dawson will have adequate metabolic function and normal fluid and electrolyte balance.
- Mrs. Dawson will be free from injury and complications.
- Mrs. Dawson will regain emotional stability.

Implementation

NURSING BEHAVIORS	**NURSING RATIONALES**
1. Develop rapport with the client by providing emotional support.	**1.** The client will have an altered body image because of the changes in her physical appearance. Understanding and support help the nurse develop a therapeutic relationship with the client.

ADULT NURSING

2. Protect the client from injury.

2. Protein catabolism, muscle weakness, and osteoporosis leave the client at risk for injury.

3. Apply prolonged pressure at the site of intrusive procedures such as venipuncture.

3. Vessel weakness places the client at increased risk for bleeding.

4. Check carefully for signs of infection.

4. Signs of infection may be masked. A small temperature elevation assumes increased significance.

5. Teach the client and family about the effects of glucocorticoid therapy.

5. The client and family must understand the risks of glucocorticoid therapy. Side effects include edema, hypertension, moonface, weakness, muscle wasting, hyperglycemia, emotional lability, steroid-induced psychosis, osteoporosis, suppressed inflammatory response, and gastric ulceration.

6. Replace potassium as needed.

6. Cushing's syndrome decreases serum potassium levels.

7. Explain the rationale behind treatments, and encourage the client to comply with the medical regimen.

7. The physician may gradually decrease the drug dosage to allow the client's adrenal glands to resume functioning. If a tumor caused Cushing's syndrome, the appropriate treatment may be surgical removal of the gland.

Evaluation
- Mrs. Dawson's electrolyte levels have returned to normal.
- Mrs. Dawson's blood glucose level remains within normal limits.
- Mrs. Dawson is coping with an altered body image.
- Mrs. Dawson remains free of infection and trauma.

Addison's disease

Decreased pituitary function, rapid cessation of steroid treatment, or adrenalectomy can cause Addison's disease (also called adrenocortical insufficiency), a condition that results from a lack of adrenocorticotropic hormone (ACTH). Addison's disease may occur in a person of any age; incidence among men and women is virtually the same.

Clinical situation

Sam Valdez, age 36, enters the hospital with symptoms of Addison's disease. He relates that he was taking cortisone pills for his severe contact dermatitis, but they bothered his stomach so he quit taking them.

Assessment

NURSING BEHAVIORS

NURSING RATIONALES

1. Observe the client for hypoglycemia.

1. Altered glucose metabolism and decreased gluconeogenesis render the client incapable of maintaining an adequate blood glucose level.

2. Observe the client for elevated serum potassium and decreased serum sodium levels.

2. Decreased aldosterone secretion produces these effects.

3. Assess the client for hypotension and a decreased ability to cope with stress.

3. Cortisol deficiency causes low blood pressure, and reduced adrenal output contributes to lowered ability to cope with stress.

4. Observe the client for dehydration and weight loss.

4. Decreased aldosterone leads to loss of sodium and water.

5. Observe the client for increased pigmentation.

5. If the pituitary compensates by increasing ACTH, melanin production and skin pigmentation will increase.

6. Assess the client for anorexia, nausea, vomiting, and diarrhea.

6. The decreased cortisol level causes a decrease in gastric enzymes.

Diagnostic evaluation

- *ACTH stimulation test:* The plasma cortisol level will not increase after administration of corticotropin.
- *Urine 17-hydroxycorticosteroid and 17-hydroxyketosteroid:* Levels will drop with Addison's disease.
- *Serum cortisol:* The level will drop.
- *Serum potassium:* The level will rise.
- *Serum sodium:* The level will drop.
- *Fasting blood glucose:* The level will drop.

Nursing diagnoses

- Risk for injury related to hypotension and hypoglycemia
- Altered nutrition: Less than body requirements, related to electrolyte depletion and hypoglycemia
- Decreased cardiac output related to hypovolemia

Planning and goals

- Mr. Valdez will have normal serum cortisol and blood glucose levels.
- Mr. Valdez will understand how to take medications.
- Mr. Valdez's blood pressure will be controlled.
- Mr. Valdez will be free from injury.
- Mr. Valdez will have normal GI functioning.

Implementation
NURSING BEHAVIORS

NURSING RATIONALES

1. As needed, provide hormone replacement with hydrocortisone or another steroid. Give the medication with milk or antacids, and administer a larger dose in the morning than in the afternoon.

1. Milk or an antacid will reduce gastric irritation. The larger morning dose coincides with the diurnal peak of the body's cortisone production.

2. Teach the client self-injection, and urge him to carry a syringe containing a prescribed dose of cortisone.

2. The client (and a family member or friend, if possible) should learn how to inject the medication intramuscularly to prepare for a crisis.

Clinical situation
(continued)

Adrenocortical tumors commonly receive surgical treatment. The following implementations apply to the client whose symptoms of adrenocortical insufficiency result from adrenalectomy.

ADULT NURSING

Implementation

NURSING BEHAVIORS	NURSING RATIONALES
1. Monitor bowel sounds.	**1.** Nausea, vomiting, and paralytic ileus present particular problems after an adrenalectomy.
2. Monitor for hemorrhage.	**2.** A possible complication after any surgery, hemorrhage is common after an adrenalectomy.
3. Monitor for Addison's crisis, checking the client's vital signs, central venous pressure (CVP), and urine output hourly.	**3.** Addison's crisis is characterized by profound adrenocortical insufficiency with manifestations of dehydration, restlessness, tachycardia, decreased CVP, and increased urine output.
4. As needed, treat the client for shock.	**4.** In Addison's crisis, the client can quickly go into profound shock.
5. Administer cortisone, as ordered, parenterally at first and then orally as the client's condition improves. Teach the client and family the importance of continuing cortisone therapy at home, and caution them about possible side effects.	**5.** The client must take cortisone until the remaining adrenal gland can take over functioning from the removed adrenal gland. Lifetime replacement follows a bilateral adrenalectomy. Cortisone produces side effects similar to those of Cushing's syndrome.
6. Instruct the client to wear a medical identification bracelet.	**6.** The bracelet alerts police officers, medical personnel, and others to the client's medical condition in the event of a crisis that requires prompt treatment.

Evaluation

- Mr. Valdez recovers from surgery without complications.
- Mr. Valdez takes replacement hormone as directed.

Hyperthyroidism

The thyroid produces two hormones—triiodothyronine (T_3) and thyroxine (T_4)—known together as the thyroid hormone. Thyroid hormone is produced when the hypothalamus secretes a hormone that causes the pituitary to release thyrotropin.

The thyroid hormone regulates metabolic activities in various ways. Besides affecting cholesterol metabolism, it increases oxygen consumption, food metabolism, protein catabolism, growth rate, and heart rate. Any change in the amount of thyroid hormone affects all these activities. Excess production causes hyperthyroidism, known as Graves' disease or exophthalmic goiter.

Treatment for hyperthyroidism varies with the client's age and childbearing status and the cause and severity of illness. Options include drug therapy, administration of radioactive iodine (^{131}I), and surgery. A common choice is treatment with ^{131}I. Symptoms begin to subside within several weeks of treatment, although normal thyroid functioning usually takes 6 months to occur. Almost all clients treated in this manner ultimately become hypothyroid and require close monitoring for associated symptoms.

Depending on dosage, precautions may be needed after ingestion of ^{131}I. The low dose typically given makes precautions unnecessary. If needed, the client should: flush the toilet several times after each use; refrain from kissing, sexual intercourse, and other sustained physical contact; and use separate dishes, glasses, silverware, bed linens, towels, and washcloths. The goal is to protect others from coming in contact with the client's secretions (such as urine, sweat, feces, and saliva), which eliminate ^{131}I.

Clinical situation

Jane Wilson, a 34-year-old businesswoman, is admitted to the hospital after complaining of heart palpitations and weight loss and feeling very edgy. With a tentative medical diagnosis of hyperthyroidism, Ms. Wilson will receive drug therapy followed by a thyroidectomy.

Assessment

NURSING BEHAVIORS	NURSING RATIONALES
1. Observe the client for heat intolerance, rapid speech, tachycardia and palpitations, exophthalmos, diaphoresis, weakness, and menstrual changes.	**1.** These signs and symptoms follow the profoundly increased production of the thyroid hormone and its effect on body metabolism.
2. Observe the client for hoarseness.	**2.** Hoarseness results when the goiter puts pressure on the recurrent laryngeal nerve.
3. Note increased food intake and weight loss.	**3.** The basal metabolic rate (BMR) drastically increases with hyperthyroidism.
4. Assess the client for nervousness and excitability.	**4.** Increased sensitivity to catecholamines causes these symptoms.

Diagnostic evaluation

• *Serum T$_3$, serum T$_4$, and radioactive iodine uptake tests:* All levels will be elevated with hyperthyroidism. Medications that contain iodine and tests that use contrast media can affect test accuracy. Obtain a thorough history.

Nursing diagnoses

• Risk for injury related to exophthalmos and excitability
• Altered nutrition: Less than body requirements, related to increased metabolism
• Ineffective individual coping related to nervousness and excitability

Planning and goals

Ms. Wilson will:
• be free of toxic effects of thyroid hormone
• feel rested and comfortable
• maintain adequate nutrition
• have an uncomplicated postoperative course
• understand how to take medications.

Implementation

NURSING BEHAVIORS	NURSING RATIONALES
Preoperative care	
1. Maintain a calm, quiet environment and a cool room temperature.	**1.** Calm and quiet reduce external stimulation that can unduly excite the client. A cool room is most comfortable for a client with heat intolerance.
2. Protect the client's eyes, if necessary, by taping them shut for sleep or by having the client wear sunglasses. Offer eye drops.	**2.** The client may require protection if exophthalmos is severe. Methylcellulose eye drops prevent drying.

3. Provide a diet high in calories, nutrients, and fluids.

3. The client's increased BMR may necessitate daily consumption of 4,000 to 5,000 calories, mostly in protein and carbohydrates. Up to 4 qt (4,000 ml) of fluid may be needed daily to replace fluid loss from perspiration.

4. Prohibit all stimulants, such as caffeine and tobacco.

4. The client must avoid excessive stimulation.

5. Provide prescribed drug treatments, as follows:

5. Drug therapy helps control hyperthyroidism.

• Administer radioactive ^{131}I, and observe the client for symptoms of hypothyroidism, such as fatigue, changed facial appearance, alopecia, brittle hair and nails, increased serum cholesterol, and cold intolerance.

• ^{131}I limits thyroid hormone secretion by destroying thyroid tissue. The drug is sometimes used to treat older clients. Because a high incidence of hypothyroidism follows treatment, the client should be observed for relevant symptoms.

• Administer an antithyroid drug, such as propylthiouracil (Propyl-Thyracil) or methimazole (Tapazole). Observe the client for side effects, including dermatitis, GI disturbances, liver damage, and blood dyscrasias.

• Antithyroid drugs inhibit thyroid hormone synthesis, thereby decreasing the amount of hormone circulating in the body and preventing thyroid storm. The listed side effects all require medical attention.

• Administer an iodine preparation, such as potassium iodide or a saturated solution of potassium iodide. Observe the client for hypersensitivity reactions, including dermatitis, ulceration of the mucous membrane, GI upset, and metallic taste (iodism).

• Iodine preparations are administered before surgery to decrease the thyroid gland's functioning, friability, and vascularity. Many clients are sensitive or allergic to iodine and require close monitoring for symptoms.

• Administer a beta blocker such as propranolol.

• These drugs block catecholamine synthesis and help control sweating, palpitations, and nervous tremors.

6. Provide preoperative care and teaching (for example, how to prevent strain on the neck incision).

6. After surgery, the client will have an incision at the collar line and will need to support the neck when she moves.

Postoperative care

1. Keep the client in semi-Fowler's position.

1. This position facilitates drainage from the surgical wound.

2. Support the client's neck.

2. This prevents strain on the suture line.

3. Limit the client's talking.

3. This decreases irritation of the vocal cords.

4. Observe the client for complications, as follows:

4. Complications from thyroid surgery require immediate attention.

• Check for signs of hemorrhage; be sure to inspect drainage behind the client's neck.

• Hemorrhage can occur 12 to 24 hours after surgery. The client's position may obscure drainage behind the neck.

• Observe for signs of airway obstruction, such as stridor and crowing respirations. Keep a tracheostomy set at the bedside.

• Any blood or fluids collecting under the suture line can lead to tracheal compression, which must be relieved.

NURSING BEHAVIORS	NURSING RATIONALES
• Listen for hoarseness.	• Hoarseness may indicate a damaged laryngeal nerve.
• Monitor for signs of tetany, such as twitching and positive Chvostek's or Trousseau's signs. Have calcium gluconate readily available.	• Tetany, leading to laryngospasm from severe hypocalcemia, can be life-threatening. Calcium gluconate combats hypocalcemia.
• Observe the client for increased pulse and respiratory rates, signs of possible thyroid storm. Be prepared to administer oxygen and I.V. drugs and to control the client's body temperature.	• Glandular manipulation during surgery causes increased thyroid hormone release, resulting in hormonal instability. Mortality from thyroid storm is about 20%.

Evaluation
- Ms. Wilson recovers from surgery without complications.
- Ms. Wilson's weight and pulse and respiratory rates are within normal limits.
- Ms. Wilson takes drugs as prescribed without adverse effects.

Hypothyroidism

Hypothyroidism results from a decreased secretion of thyroid hormone. A common disorder, it affects men and women of all ages. Symptoms vary according to the degree of hormone deficiency.

Clinical situation

Rick Foster, age 65, recently retired after 50 years as a butcher. He has gradually become lethargic and frequently sits idly all day. His physician has diagnosed his condition as hypothyroidism.

Assessment

NURSING BEHAVIORS	NURSING RATIONALES
1. Evaluate the client for mild, vague complaints of aches, pains, and fatigue.	**1.** A decreased secretion of thyroid hormone causes signs and symptoms (listed in 1 through 3 at left) known collectively as myxedema.
2. Assess the client for an enlarged, swollen tongue; alopecia; dry, brittle hair and nails; elevated serum cholesterol level; constipation; cold intolerance; poor concentration; and (in female clients) menstrual changes.	**2.** All are signs of hypothyroidism.
3. Assess for lethargy and slowness, increased weight, and decreased appetite.	**3.** Inactivity and a decreased basal metabolic rate cause weight gain despite decreased appetite.

Diagnostic evaluation
- *Serum T_3, serum T_4, and radioactive iodine uptake tests:* All levels will be decreased with hypothyroidism. Medications that contain iodine and tests that use contrast media can affect test accuracy. Obtain a thorough history.

Nursing diagnoses
- Constipation related to decreased peristalsis
- Risk for injury related to the client's response to drug therapy
- Altered nutrition: More than body requirements, related to decreased metabolism

- Activity intolerance related to lethargy
- Knowledge deficit related to medication management

Planning and goals

Mr. Foster will:
- resume a normal activity level
- be free of cardiac complications
- understand how to take medications.

Implementations

NURSING BEHAVIORS	NURSING RATIONALES
1. Treat the hormone deficiency with prescribed drugs, such as levothyroxine sodium (Synthroid) or liothyronine sodium (Cytomel).	**1.** These drugs decrease fatigue and edema, reduce weight, and minimize cold intolerance. Side effects may include symptoms of hyperthyroidism.
2. Replace thyroid hormone gradually.	**2.** The client is especially susceptible to cardiac problems such as angina because of the increased metabolic demand and the vessel changes produced by elevated cholesterol levels.
3. Prepare the client for self-care at home by teaching him to monitor his pulse rate; tell him to notify the physician if the rate exceeds 100 beats/minute.	**3.** A rapid pulse rate may indicate drug toxicity.
4. Inform the client and family that thyroid hormone therapy must continue for the rest of the client's life. Remain available to answer their questions and listen to their concerns.	**4.** The client may be discouraged by the prospect of facing lifelong treatment. Health teaching that combines clear explanations with generous emotional support usually alleviates the client's anxiety and shows other family members how they can help.

Evaluation

- Mr. Foster is taking thyroid hormone replacements as prescribed.
- Mr. Foster maintains a pulse rate below 100 beats/minute.
- Mr. Foster does not experience chest pain.
- Mr. Foster resumes his previous activity level.

REPRODUCTIVE SYSTEM

Cervical cancer and hysterectomy

Cervical cancer is a common cancer in women. When detected and treated early (in situ), it is virtually 100% curable. To promote early detection of cervical cancer, some authorities recommend an annual Papanicolaou (Pap) smear test for all women age 18 or over and for sexually active girls. After three consecutive normal examinations, the client may undergo the test less frequently, as determined by her physician. The client's age, health history, and current health help determine the recommended frequency for a Pap test. Treatment methods for cervical cancer include radiation, surgery, or a combination of the two, depending on the woman's age, general health status, cancer stage, and complications.

The following clinical situation focuses on a client undergoing an abdominal hysterectomy for cervical cancer.

Clinical situation   Clara Cannon, age 38, enters the hospital for a total hysterectomy for microinvasive cervical carcinoma. She has had a Pap test highly suggestive of cancer and a positive cervical biopsy. Mrs. Cannon has two teenage children and teaches English at a local high school. Her husband owns a gymnastics school, and both enjoy gymnastics as a favorite activity.

Assessment

NURSING BEHAVIORS	NURSING RATIONALES
1. Assess the client's general health status.	**1.** General health assessment consists of a complete health history and a physical examination, including a pelvic examination. This client shows no symptoms of early cancer of the cervix other than vaginal discharge and spotting. Any other medical problems (such as diabetes mellitus and anemia) should receive appropriate treatment before major surgery.
2. Assess the client's instructional and psychological needs.	**2.** The client must acquire a basic understanding of the planned surgery. Clients display a wide range of emotional responses to a cancer diagnosis and to impending surgery. This client may be deeply concerned over the potential change in her body image and the loss of her reproductive function. Some women associate their reproductive capacity with femininity or harbor a strong fear of death during surgery or from cancer.
3. Assess the results of such diagnostic tests as the Pap test and cervical biopsy.	**3.** The Pap test has a high accuracy rate for detecting early cancer of the cervix. The client should not douche for 24 to 48 hours before the examination and should be midcycle (not having a menstrual period). The results are reported as normal or describe the cellular changes in detail. A cervical biopsy involves removing a small portion of cervical tissue for microscopic examination. The results can confirm or establish a diagnosis.

Nursing diagnoses
- Impaired skin integrity related to the surgical incision
- Pain related to incisional discomfort and flatus
- Body image disturbance related to surgical removal of the uterus

Planning and goals   Mrs. Cannon will:
- be physically and emotionally prepared for surgery
- state the effect of the hysterectomy on her reproductive capacity
- maintain a positive body image and positive self-concept
- receive, together with her husband, adequate information and support in coping with potential and perceived threats to their sexual relationship
- recover from surgery without complications.

Implementation

NURSING BEHAVIORS

NURSING RATIONALES

Preoperative care

1. Validate the client's physical preparation, including routine preoperative care, vaginal douche with Betadine or insertion of a tampon soaked with Betadine, and enema or laxative at home the day before surgery.

1. Preparation includes such routine preoperative screening as the client's history, physical examination, and evaluation of pulmonary, cardiac, and renal status. The objective is to determine the client's state of health and ability to withstand surgery. The douche and enema serve as cleaning measures that help prevent postoperative infection. Preoperative teaching is completed in the preadmission testing unit.

2. Prepare the client for the postoperative period with instructions about turning, coughing, and deep breathing; tubes and dressings; pain management; walking; and other activity.

2. Turning, coughing, and deep breathing help restore normal respiratory function after surgery. An indwelling catheter may be inserted to facilitate bladder emptying until spontaneous voiding is adequate. The client will have an abdominal dressing. She may have a choice of pain medications for incisional pain and discomfort from gas. Patient-controlled analgesia may be used. Early walking helps improve GI functioning and relieve gas pain.

3. Administer preoperative medication.

3. The preoperative medication may include a narcotic for sedation and an anticholinergic to decrease secretions.

4. Complete the client's procedural and charting requirements.

4. Specific procedural and charting requirements (such as consents, laboratory results, and identification bracelet) will be completed the day of surgery.

5. Review psychological preparation with the client by explaining the expected outcome and effects of a total hysterectomy.

5. A total hysterectomy involves removal of the cervix and uterus, resulting in the cessation of menstruation and of the ability to bear children. It will *not* cause menopausal symptoms, such as hot flashes and hormonal disturbances, because the ovaries will remain intact.

6. Allow the client to express her fears and ask questions.

6. Although the grief response is inevitable, stressing the positive outcome (a high cure rate) associated with early diagnosis and treatment helps many clients cope with the loss of the uterus. Hysterectomy does not cause obesity or mental illness or make a woman less feminine. The client should expect some grieflike responses (crying, depression) during the postoperative period. Supportive care from her family (especially the spouse) and from the nurse can help the client regain composure and her feminine perspective.

Postoperative care

1. Check abdominal and perineal dressings for excessive bleeding every 15 minutes for 2 hours, then every 4 hours for at least 8 hours. A moderate amount of sanguineous drainage on the perineal pad is normal.

1. The risk of hemorrhage after an abdominal hysterectomy is greatest during the first 24 hours because of the abundant blood supply to the pelvis.

2. Maintain urine output by inserting an indwelling urinary catheter or by encouraging the client to void.

2. The bladder may temporarily be atonic; if a urinary catheter is necessary, it usually remains in place for 24 hours postoperatively. If the client does not have a catheter, she must void within 8 hours. If the client cannot void or incompletely empties her bladder, she may need catheterization for residual urine.

3. Prevent abdominal distention, as follows:
• Allow no food or fluids for 24 to 48 hours, as ordered, until peristalsis returns and bowel sounds are normal. When the client is able to eat, allow no gas-forming foods because flatus causes intense discomfort.
• Administer an enema on the 2nd or 3rd postoperative day, as ordered.
• Insert a rectal tube for flatulence, as ordered.
• Encourage ambulation.

3. Abdominal distention commonly results from nerve damage and handling of the viscera during surgery. A full lower bowel places stress on the abdominal incision. Normal GI functioning will be impaired by the deep levels of anesthesia required for surgery. A rectal tube helps relieve discomfort from gas and promotes peristalsis. Ambulation promotes peristalsis.

4. Promote circulation through ambulation and leg exercises. Have the client walk the day after surgery, if ordered. Avoid high Fowler's position, which may result in pelvic congestion. Do not use the knee gatch on the bed. Use antiembolic stockings and pneumatic compression stockings as appropriate.

4. The client is susceptible to thrombophlebitis after pelvic surgery from venous stasis in the pelvis and lower extremities. Early, frequent walking (starting the evening of surgery or the next day) is usually ordered. Leg exercises promote circulation and help prevent postoperative thrombophlebitis. Stockings help prevent venous pooling.

5. Provide comfort measures, including position changes, back rubs, and analgesic medication, as ordered.

5. Pain and discomfort after abdominal hysterectomy may come from many sources, such as incision, shoulder and back pain from the position on the operating table, and postoperative gas pain.

6. Provide the following discharge instructions:

6. The client should understand that a hysterectomy is a major operation, from which she will need adequate time to recover.

• Avoid sexual intercourse and douching until instructed otherwise by the physician.

• Early resumption of sexual activity and douching may interfere with healing and introduce infection.

• Avoid heavy lifting and other strenuous activities for about 2 months, as instructed by the physician.

• Mrs. Cannon should not participate in gymnastics until her physician says it is safe to do so. For several months, she should avoid activities such as dancing and horseback riding, which increase pelvic congestion. Swimming, which promotes physical and mental well-being, would be an appropriate nonstrenuous activity after a few weeks, if the physician allows it. The client should have a regular program of abdominal strengthening exercises.

• Notify the physician of bleeding or abnormal vaginal discharge.

• Late hemorrhage (10 to 14 days after surgery) is a possible complication. An abnormal (other than nonodorous liquid or whitish) vaginal discharge may signal an infection.

ADULT NURSING

• Schedule follow-up care.

• The importance of continued follow-up care demands emphatic repetition. Follow-up at frequent intervals also allows for an assessment of the client's psychological adjustment. While most clients successfully resolve their feelings of loss and fear associated with hysterectomy and a diagnosis of cancer, some will have unusual difficulty coping and may need referral for psychological counseling.

Evaluation

• Mrs. Cannon recovers from surgery without complications.
• Mrs. Cannon can state the expected results of her surgery and its effects on her reproductive capacity.
• Mrs. Cannon expresses positive feelings about herself as a woman and her ability to cope successfully with a diagnosis of cancer.
• Mrs. Cannon can state the specific requirements for self-care after discharge and follow-up care by the physician.

GASTROINTESTINAL SYSTEM

Peptic ulcer disease

Peptic ulcer disease is a major cause of illness. Duodenal ulcers are more common than gastric ulcers. Medical therapy is the first line of treatment, but ulcers that resist medical control, perforate, or hemorrhage may necessitate surgery. Surgical repairs include laser cauterization, gastric resection, and, more rarely now, gastroduodenostomy or gastrojejunostomy. The following clinical situation describes the medical, surgical, and nursing care of a client with a GI ulcer.

Clinical situation

Carl Unter, a 35-year-old bank manager, enters the hospital for a diagnostic workup and treatment of his duodenal ulcer. He has been having increasing episodes of upper epigastric pain that medications and diet cannot relieve. On occasion, he has noticed dark-colored stools. He finds it difficult to perform his bank duties because of his preoccupation with his condition.

Assessment

NURSING BEHAVIORS

1. Determine the client's pain patterns: type, location, severity, and means of relief.

2. Assess the client's dietary intake.

3. Assess the client's bowel movement patterns: type, color, and pain, if any.

NURSING RATIONALES

1. The recurring pain of duodenal ulcers may be sharp or dull, localized or spread throughout the epigastrium, more severe in the fall and spring seasons, and temporarily relieved by antacids.

2. Current research supports allowing a diet as tolerated while avoiding gastric stimulants, such as nicotine, caffeine, alcohol, and pepper.

3. Alteration in bowel elimination commonly accompanies ulcers. The client may have diarrhea or constipation, depending on the type and amount of antacid used. Dark-colored stools may indicate bleeding or may result from antacids or foods.

4. Check vital signs and assess the client's history for dizziness, fainting, abnormal weight patterns, and anemia.

4. The client's history may indicate more extensive bleeding, leading to orthostatic hypotension or hypovolemia from blood volume deficit.

5. Determine any medications ingested for concurrent conditions.

5. Many medications taken for other conditions can cause or exacerbate ulcers—for example, aspirin, steroids, and anti-inflammatory drugs used for arthritis.

6. Assess stressors: work, relationships at work, and interaction with family, friends, and associates.

6. Stress can predispose a person to ulcers from ineffective coping behaviors.

Diagnostic evaluation

- *GI series, gastroscopy, gastric analysis, esophagoscopy, duodenoscopy:* These studies determine the site of ulceration, localize bleeding points, and assess acid production.
- *Chest X-ray, electrocardiogram:* The client is under stress. Other organs may have function changes.
- *Hematologic studies, guaiac tests of stools:* Hematologic studies detect other conditions. The red blood cell count and hematocrit will be low with bleeding. These studies also detect bleeding into the GI tract. *Note:* Perform studies serially to detect bleeding at different times.
- *Acid-base studies:* Overuse of antacids may cause metabolic alkalosis.
- *Gastric sampling:* This is done to detect presence of *Helicobacter pylori.*

Nursing diagnoses

- Pain related to gastric distress
- Fluid volume deficit related to risk of GI bleeding
- Ineffective individual coping related to stressors

Planning and goals

Mr. Unter will:
- experience pain relief through healing
- have few adverse reactions to medications
- acquire positive outlets for stress and learn stress management techniques.

Implementation

NURSING BEHAVIORS

NURSING RATIONALES

Medical therapy

1. Administer antacids as ordered—aluminum hydroxide (Amphojel), calcium carbonate suspension, aluminum hydroxide and magnesium hydroxide (Maalox).

1. Antacids neutralize gastric acid and help decrease pain. They are usually taken 1 to 3 hours after meals and before sleep. They should not be given within 1 hour of a histamine-2 (H_2) antagonist because they will impair its absorption.

2. Observe the client for side effects, such as constipation, diarrhea, and altered urine output.

2. Aluminum hydroxide and calcium carbonate can cause constipation, and aluminum hydroxide or magnesium hydroxide can cause diarrhea. Aluminum hydroxide contains sodium and must be used cautiously with low-sodium diets. If taking magnesium hydroxide, a client with poor renal function may retain magnesium.

Administering tube feedings

Tube feedings can be administered to a client through one of three tubes: A *nasogastric tube* passes from the nose to the stomach, a *gastrostomy tube* passes through the surgical incision into the stomach, and a *transpyloric tube* passes through the pylorus into the duodenum or jejunum. The following list highlights important nursing considerations when administering tube feedings:

- Start with half-strength formula and gradually increase the strength according to the client's tolerance.
- Provide adequate fluids to prevent dehydration (a common complication of tube feedings).
- Assess the client for diarrhea (the most common complication of tube feedings).
- Refrigerate noncommercial preparations to prevent bacterial overgrowth.
- Warm the preparation to room temperature because the procedure bypasses the usual ingestion processes.

- Verify the tube's location and the absorption of the previous feeding. Aspirate contents; if more than 100 ml is returned, do not feed.
- Return aspirated contents to the client to prevent electrolyte imbalance.
- Position the client in semi-Fowler's position to facilitate passage of the feeding through the pylorus and to decrease the risk of vomiting and aspiration.
- Clear the tube with water before and after feeding to provide fluids and to prevent tube clogging.
- Keep in mind that many clients better tolerate a feeding by continuous drip, using either gravity or a feeding pump.
- If using a transpyloric tube, monitor the client for dumping syndrome and hypovolemic shock, complications that can result from bypassing the stomach.

---

3. Teach the client how to administer cimetidine (Tagamet), ranitidine (Zantac), famotidine (Pepcid), or nizatidine (Axid). Caution him about drug interactions with cimetidine.

3. These H_2 blocking agents inhibit gastric acid secretion.

4. Observe for adverse reactions of the H_2 blockers: mild, transient diarrhea; muscle or joint pain; dizziness and rash; headache; and lowered sperm counts.

4. H_2 blockers potentiate the action of certain anticoagulants. Cimetidine demonstrably lowers sperm count and impairs metabolism of many drugs. The other H_2 antagonists do not have this problem.

5. If ordered, administer sucralfate (Carafate).

5. Sucralfate is thought to coat the ulcer and protect it from acid, pepsin, and bile salts.

6. Review negative stress response behaviors with the client. Encourage him to practice relaxation techniques, as desired, to decrease his stress response; encourage behaviors to lessen the negative responses.

6. Stress causes increased secretion of gastric acid, which produces a predisposition to recurring ulcerations. If the client perceives the therapeutic behaviors as beneficial to him, he will have increased interest and he will practice the behaviors over time.

Evaluation

Mr. Unter does not have any adverse reactions to his medications.

Clinical situation
(continued)

After medical treatment and diagnostic tests, Mr. Unter received a diagnosis of multiple bleeding ulcerated areas too large to cauterize with laser therapy. He subsequently underwent a gastric resection and duodenostomy. He returned from surgery with a nasogastric (NG) tube to be connected to suction (see *Administering tube feedings,* above, and *Gastrointestinal tubes,* at right).

Gastrointestinal tubes

NAME	SITE	PURPOSE	IRRIGATION	SOLUTION	NURSING CONSIDERATIONS
Salem sump	Nasogastric	Suctioning or feeding	Yes	Normal saline solution; 20 to 30 ml	Blue tubing must be free of secretions; clamp tube for ambulation and to note tolerance; use for feeding.
Levin tube	Nasogastric	Suctioning or feeding	Yes	Normal saline solution; 20 to 30 ml	Must be connected to low suction to prevent gastric irritation; use for feeding.
Nutriflex	Nasogastric	Feeding	Yes	Water; 20 ml	Use 50-ml syringe with 20 ml water to irrigate (small syringe may cause tube to rupture from excessive pressure); use infusion pump, which can exert only up to 40 psi (tube bursting pressure is 80 psi).
Gastrostomy	Stomach	Suctioning or feeding	Yes	Normal saline solution; 20 to 30 ml	Uses gravity drainage; as required, clamp and open for residuals; use for feedings to supplement oral intake.
Sengstaken-Blakemore	Esophagus and stomach	Compressing esophageal varices	No	See Nursing considerations.	Use esophageal balloon inflated with air (*never irrigated*) and a tube into the stomach that can be irrigated with 20 to 30 ml normal saline solution as required.
Jejunostomy	Jejunum	Feeding	Yes	Normal saline solution; 10 to 20 ml	Feedings may be intermittent or continuous with an infusion pump.
Dobhoff	Jejunum	Feeding	Yes	Water; 20 to 30 ml	Has mercury tip for X-ray visualization and to assist passage; has same cautions as Nutriflex tube.
Cantor	Small to large intestine	Suctioning	Yes	Normal saline solution; 20 to 30 ml	Mercury is inserted into balloon before insertion to aid passage; connect to suction.
Miller-Abbott	Small to large intestine	Suctioning	Yes	Normal saline solution; 20 to 30 ml	Mercury is instilled into properly marked opening after tube reaches stomach, to aid passage.

Nursing diagnoses
- Impaired tissue integrity related to the surgical incision
- Pain related to the surgical incision
- Risk for fluid volume deficit related to nasogastric drainage and risk of postoperative hemorrhage

Planning and goals
Mr. Unter will:
- have ulcerated areas relieved through surgery
- continue to learn stress management techniques
- not have dumping syndrome
- not experience postoperative complications.

ADULT NURSING

Assessment

NURSING BEHAVIORS	NURSING RATIONALES
Preoperative care Review routine preoperative care and explain what the client can expect postoperatively (NG tube, no nourishment by mouth for a time; turning, deep breathing, coughing; and measures to control pain).	Explaining postoperative routines lessens the client's anticipatory anxiety and promotes postoperative comfort.
Postoperative care **1.** Monitor NG tube drainage; irrigate with 20 ml of normal saline solution; measure output. *Caution:* Do not reposition the NG tube if it is not draining. Notify the physician if irrigation does not restore patency.	**1.** NG tube drainage initially will be sanguineous and gradually will become brown and then serous. Drainage may be copious from intestinal secretions. The physician (not the nurse) should reposition the tube because the tube is in the surgical site.
2. Maintain I.V. fluids, with nothing by mouth; record the client's intake and output, weight, and abdominal girth.	**2.** The client will receive nothing but I.V. fluids for 2 to 5 days, so weight loss is common.
3. Inspect the client's stools; administer a suppository, as needed and ordered.	**3.** Melena (black stools) indicates upper GI bleeding. Because straining at stool increases intra-abdominal pressure, a suppository softens stool to lessen straining, which may exert undue pressure on the suture line.
4. Have the client turn, deep-breathe, and cough every 2 hours and use a respiratory aid every 2 hours. Help the client walk, increasing to four times daily.	**4.** The client may be reluctant to breathe deeply because of the incision's location near the chest. A high abdominal incision places the client at increased risk of respiratory complications. Ambulation aids peristalsis to stimulate bowel function.
5. Administer pain medication and antacids as ordered and needed.	**5.** Pain decreases by the 2nd or 3rd postoperative day. Antacids decrease irritation while the client has nothing by mouth.
6. Offer a small amount of clear liquids after the physician has discontinued food restrictions; advance to small, frequent meals of soft, high-protein, moderate-fat, low-carbohydrate foods. Avoid simple sugars. Give fluids between meals, not with meals.	**6.** This prevents dumping syndrome.
7. Discuss dumping syndrome with the client, and review steps to prevent or minimize its effects. Dumping syndrome has 2 phases:	**7.** The client needs to know how to minimize the effects of dumping syndrome.
• *Phase 1*. Rapid pouring of fluids and hypertonic foods or solutions causes a vasomotor response in the small intestine, causing more fluids to be drawn into the gut lumen. The client experiences tachycardia, pallor or flushing, and hypotension, which produces syncopal symptoms.	• Shifts in blood fluid volume cause the symptoms.

• *Phase 2*. Rapid glucose absorption causes increased insulin secretion, which eventually leads to hypoglycemia, causing weakness, pallor, hypotension, and sweating.

8. Discuss with the client positive outlets and strategies to modify negative stress responses.

• The syndrome can be avoided by maintaining the client on small, dry, frequent meals that are low in carbohydrates and high in fat. The client should lie down after eating to reduce vasomotor responses by permitting blood flow to the intestine.

8. Stress produces increased secretions of gastric acid and can cause ulcers to recur.

Evaluation

• Mr. Unter recovers from surgery without infection, obstruction, or wound disruption.
• Mr. Unter resumes eating, following recommended dietary principles, by increasing his intake to six small meals per day, with low-carbohydrate foods and fluids between meals.
• Mr. Unter experiences no symptoms of dumping syndrome by the time of discharge.
• Mr. Unter learns new coping strategies to modify his stress response behaviors.
• Mr. Unter can verbalize stress management techniques.

Cholelithiasis

Cholelithiasis—the formation of gallstones—commonly occurs in adults ages 30 to 50 and affects women more frequently than men. Stones can remain in the gallbladder or move into the common bile duct (choledocholithiasis); in the latter condition, an obstruction can cause bile to back up into the liver, which predisposes the client to stasis and liver inflammation.

Clinical situation

Mae Green, a 45-year-old homemaker, is hospitalized after experiencing jaundice for 3 days. She has a history of nausea, intolerance to fatty foods, and pain in her right upper abdomen. Diagnostic studies include hematologic, radiologic, and ultrasound examinations. Results show an enlarged, edematous gallbladder with multiple stones, radiolucent masses in the common bile duct, and a slight liver enlargement that suggests stasis. The client also has an elevated bilirubin level.

Assessment
NURSING BEHAVIORS

1. Assess the severity of jaundice by checking the color of skin, urine, stools, and conjunctiva.

2. Assess the client's appetite, food intake, likes, dislikes, and tolerances.

NURSING RATIONALES

1. Jaundice (yellowish skin coloration) results from elevated bile pigmentation in the serum. Obstruction of bile flow through the common bile duct into the small intestine leads to a backup of bile, which is then absorbed into the serum, with bile pigments deposited in the tissues. Serum also shows increased bilirubin levels.

2. Loss of appetite usually results from inadequate digestion of nutrients, slowed absorption, and nausea from inadequate fat emulsification (metabolism requires the emulsification of fats by bile).

ADULT NURSING

3. Determine pain patterns and sites of radiating pain.

3. Pressure and obstruction in the common bile duct cause pain, which may be constant and gradually increasing in intensity, especially during digestion and metabolism of fats. Pain in the right upper quadrant may radiate to the right shoulder area (Kehr's sign); it may be sharp and stabbing at times from peristaltic waves in the duct (biliary colic).

4. Assess the types (and dosages) of medications that the client is taking.

4. Severe pain usually requires narcotics and antispasmodics for relief.

5. Weigh the client daily.

5. Weight loss may result from inadequate food intake.

6. Check vital signs and temperature patterns.

6. Chills and fever commonly occur. Inflammation in the common bile duct or the gallbladder may cause an elevated temperature.

Diagnostic evaluation

• *Hematologic studies* (complete blood count, serum bilirubin levels, aspartate aminotransferase, alanine aminotransferase, alkaline phosphatase, serum amylase): Enzyme levels will be elevated if the liver has stasis or cell destruction. Bilirubin levels will be elevated (as will alkaline phosphatase) from obstructed bile flow through the common bile duct. Elevated serum amylase levels may indicate concurrent pancreatitis.
• *Radiologic studies* (GI series, ultrasound, chest X-ray, cholecystogram [rare], and endoscopic retrograde cholangiopancreatography): These studies help determine any abnormalities, the extent of disease, and the client's ability to tolerate the proposed surgery.
• *Color of urine and stools:* Bilirubin darkens the urine (cola-colored). Normally, stools contain excreted bilirubin; without bilirubin they have a clay color. With obstruction, bilirubin is excreted in urine.

Implementation
NURSING BEHAVIORS

NURSING RATIONALES

Diagnostic period

1. Prepare Mrs. Green for an upper GI series, explaining procedures and rationales. Administer a laxative the afternoon preceding the examination, if possible. Provide clear liquids for dinner and nothing by mouth after midnight. After the upper GI series, administer a laxative to clear barium from the GI tract.

1. An upper GI series is performed to pinpoint the medical diagnosis. Explanations help relieve the client's anxiety.

2. Prepare Mrs. Green for the cholecystogram, as follows:

2. If an ultrasound examination indicates choledocholithiasis, this step is not necessary.

• Explain the procedure and its rationale to the client.

• Explanations help relieve fear and anxiety.

• Provide a clear-liquid dinner the evening before the cholecystogram.

• Clear liquid helps reduce contents in the GI tract.

• Administer dye tablets, as ordered (usually, Telepaque, Tablets VI, one every 5 minutes beginning at 6 p.m.); provide a full glass of water with each tablet.

• Telepaque is a dye that collects in the gallbladder to outline it on the X-ray. Ultrasound examinations substitute for or accompany the cholecystogram.

• Administer enemas, as ordered.

• One or two enemas may be needed to clean the colon.

• Provide nothing by mouth after midnight.

• This keeps the colon free of contents.

• After the client returns from the examination, resume the client's diet and fluids, as ordered.

• Resuming food and fluids promotes return to a normal bowel pattern.

3. Use the guaiac test to detect occult blood in stools.

3. Guaiac testing detects occult bleeding caused by decreased prothrombin synthesis if the liver is inflamed.

4. Weigh the client daily.

4. Weight loss can occur from decreased food intake.

5. Monitor the client's appetite, food intake, and food tolerance; assess the client for pain after eating, abdominal distention, nausea, and vomiting.

5. These measures help determine the client's nutritional status and can detect passage of stones from the duct or increasing obstruction.

Nursing diagnoses	• Altered nutrition: Less than body requirements, related to pain and nausea • Pain related to obstruction • Risk for infection related to wound incision
Planning and goals	Mrs. Green will: • regain pain-free digestion and relief of jaundice • retain liver functions • undergo surgical removal of gallstones without complications.
Clinical situation *(continued)*	After reviewing the results of diagnostic studies, the physician concludes that Mrs. Green can safely undergo surgical removal of the stones in the bile duct and removal of her inflamed gallbladder, via traditional cholecystectomy. (Some clients do not undergo surgical removal of gallstones; see *Alternative treatments for gallstones,* page 569, for more information.) Also, clients who require gallbladder removal increasingly are undergoing laparoscopic cholecystectomy. In this ambulatory surgery procedure, the surgeon makes four small incisions into the abdomen. Pain is minimal; the client is discharged the same day or on the first postoperative day and can resume activities after a few days. In contrast, with traditional cholecystectomy, the client typically is discharged in about 5 days. Postoperatively, the client has a T tube in place (see *T-tube placement,* page 568).

Implementation

NURSING BEHAVIORS

NURSING RATIONALES

Preoperative care

Perform usual preoperative preparations, including an explanation of the T tube the client will have after surgery.

A client undergoing common bile duct surgery usually has a T tube in the common bile duct to promote drainage.

ADULT NURSING

T-tube placement

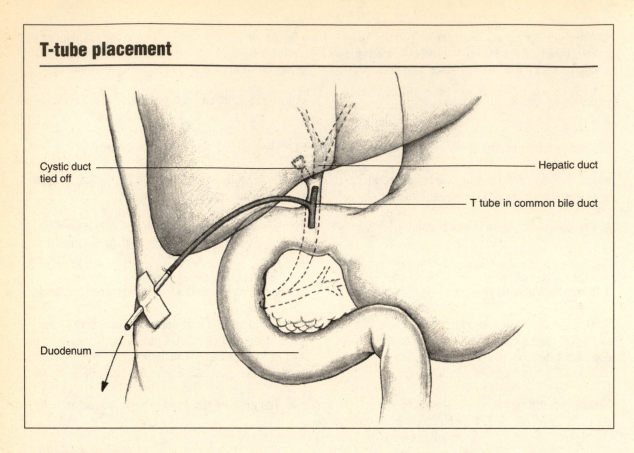

Cystic duct tied off

Hepatic duct

T tube in common bile duct

Duodenum

Postoperative care

1. Provide routine postoperative care. Check the client's vital signs, fluid and electrolyte levels, hemoglobin level, white blood cell count, and PCO_2 level.

1. These will help determine the client's postoperative status.

2. Check the client's skin for relief of jaundice and edema.

2. Jaundice should gradually fade. Edema should not be present postoperatively.

3. Have the client turn, deep-breathe, cough, and use a respiratory aid every 2 hours; increase walking, as tolerated; administer pain medications, as needed.

3. An incision in the right upper quadrant causes pain with breathing. Although possibly reluctant to take deep breaths, the client must persist and needs encouragement for her efforts. Atelectasis commonly occurs after this type of surgery.

4. Observe drainage in the T-tube bile collection container, and keep the container below the incisional level; maintain the client on I.V. fluids only, as ordered.

4. Because of trauma to the common bile duct, the T tube is inserted to allow bile to drain; the drainage system uses gravity. I.V. fluids nourish the client until GI functions return; then food intake provides nourishment.

5. Clamp the T tube when ordered; prepare for a possible T-tube cholangiogram about 1 week after surgery. If the client is discharged with a T tube in place, provide instructions for home care. Maintain gravity drainage until surgeon decides healing has occurred. The tube will then be clamped. Instruct the client to take a daily shower to keep insertion site clean.

5. If the client experiences no pain, nausea, or vomiting after eating, the physician removes the T tube. A cholangiogram confirms the absence of stones before the T tube is removed.

Alternative treatments for gallstones

Extracorporeal shock wave lithotripsy: This procedure is designed for a client with a small number of stones and mild to moderate symptoms. The client sits in a tank of water or holds a water-filled cushion against the appropriate place on the abdomen. Shock waves are sent through the water until the stones disintegrate (1 to 2 hours). The client is on a cardiac monitor throughout the procedure because shock waves must be coordinated with cardiac rhythm to prevent arrhythmias. After the procedure, observe the client for hematuria, hematoma, nausea, and biliary colic.

Endoscopic sphincterotomy: This procedure uses an endoscope to remove stones from the common bile duct. After the procedure, monitor the client for bleeding, pain, and fever. Promote bed rest for 6 to 8 hours, and give the client nothing by mouth until the gag reflex returns.

Cholesterol dissolvent: Monoctanoin is administered through a nasal biliary catheter to dissolve stones left in the bile duct after cholecystectomy. Dissolution may take 1 to 3 weeks. Observe the client for anorexia, nausea, vomiting, and abdominal pain.

Oral bile acids: Chenodiol (Chenix) and ursodiol (Actigall) are administered to dissolve small stones. Side effects include diarrhea (especially with chenodiol), elevation of hepatic enzymes, gastritis, and gastric ulcers. Dissolution takes between 6 months and 2 years, and the success rate is only about 30%.

---

6. Check the wound site every 4 hours for 24 to 48 hours. Change the dressing as needed and perform wound care, using aseptic technique.

7. Measure the client's abdominal girth, check stool color, and monitor for flatus. Begin a clear liquid diet, when ordered, after bowel sounds return and the client can pass flatus; advance to a regular diet as tolerated.

8. Prepare the client for discharge by reviewing home care instructions and activity restrictions.

6. The wound may bleed after surgery. Aseptic technique helps prevent infection (the liver's ability to overcome infection is decreased).

7. The GI tract begins to regain function after the 2nd postoperative day. Passage of flatus represents significant progress. The client's appetite slowly increases. Abdominal girth measurement will detect the development of ileus.

8. Wound care includes washing the area while the client is bathing, noting untoward signs (drainage, warmth, tenderness), and keeping the area free of dressings and pressure from clothing. The client may not lift or carry heavy items for 6 weeks but can perform light household activities and cooking, as desired. The client should return to the physician if pain or food intolerance recurs.

Evaluation

Mrs. Green:
• gains relief from jaundice, gallstones, and pain after surgery
• has no postoperative complications
• performs self-care activities and increases nutritional intake to restore nutritional balance.

ADULT NURSING

Cirrhosis of the liver

Cirrhosis of the liver is a severe, life-threatening condition. Fibrotic, scarred tissues and fatty deposits within the cells gradually replace functioning liver cells. Although about 50% of cirrhosis results from alcoholism, other causes include hepatitis, chemical destruction (from drugs, such as vinyl chloride), and bacterial liver infections. The cirrhotic liver shows patchy areas of regenerated cells that give the liver capsule a hobnailed, irregular appearance.

The pathophysiologic changes of cirrhosis arise from portal vein hypertension, leading to hypoalbuminemia and excessive venous pressures causing esophageal varices and hemorrhoids, ascites, hyperaldosteronism, and hepatic encephalopathy. (See *Pathophysiologic changes caused by cirrhosis of the liver*.)

Clinical situation

Vaughn Zimmer, a 54-year-old manufacturer of plastic ornaments, enters the hospital with a tentative medical diagnosis of cirrhosis of the liver. Mr. Zimmer has been ill at home for the past 6 weeks after developing viral hepatitis B. For 25 years he has been working in a plastics factory, handling liquid materials. Mr. Zimmer appears pale, weak, and fatigued.

Assessment

NURSING BEHAVIORS

1. Check the client's overall health: weight, skin turgor, and vital signs.

2. Assess the client's appetite, food intake, likes, and dislikes.

3. Assess for edema, jaundice, pallor, petechiae, and spider nevi (dilated arterioles with branches like spider legs).

4. Measure the client's abdominal girth, assess for abdominal pain, and percuss for fluid levels in the abdomen; weigh the client daily.

5. Assess for gynecomastia and testicular atrophy.

NURSING RATIONALES

1. These data establish baseline patterns. Weight loss and emaciation commonly occur in cirrhosis. Fever may be present.

2. Extended illness or the liver's inability to metabolize foods may result in poor appetite.

3. Edema commonly occurs from hypoalbuminemia, hyperaldosteronism, and pressure from ascites. Jaundice occurs from the enlarged liver and obstructed bile ducts. Pallor indicates anemia. Petechiae result from hypoprothrombinemia. Ascites results from malnutrition, GI blood loss, and red blood cell destruction by the enlarged spleen.

4. The abdomen is usually enlarged, with skin that is shiny and thin from ascites. Ascites results from portal hypertension, hypoalbuminemia, and hyperaldosteronism. Pain results from edema and pressure on body organs.

5. Abnormal hormone metabolism results in estrogen excess, breast enlargement, and testicular atrophy.

Pathophysiologic changes caused by cirrhosis of the liver

CHANGES	DEFINITION
Portal vein hypertension	The portal vein empties into the liver. Scarring or obstruction in the liver causes backup in the portal vein, producing portal vein hypertension.
Hypoalbuminemia	The contents of the portal vein and blood serum contain albumin and globulin, two serum proteins. Albumin leaks out of the portal vein into the peritoneal cavity because the portal vein is distended by portal vein hypertension. Hypoalbuminemia is loss of albumin from the blood serum.
Esophageal varices	Portal vein hypertension leads to increased pressures in veins, causing esophageal varices and hemorrhoids.
Ascites	Albumin draws fluids with it into the abdominal cavity, causing a fluid accumulation called ascites.
Hyperaldosteronism	Only the liver metabolizes aldosterone. A cirrhotic liver cannot perform its normal functions. Therefore, aldosterone builds up (hyperaldosteronism), leading to fluid retention and edema.
Portal-systemic (hepatic) encephalopathy	Buildup of nitrogenous and biliary products in the blood causes a pathologic brain cell condition (encephalopathy). The wastes accumulate because the dysfunctional liver cannot metabolize and excrete them.

Diagnostic evaluation

• *Hematologic studies* (complete blood count, electrolyte levels, aspartate aminotransferase, alanine aminotransferase, lactate dehydrogenase, total protein, albumin-globulin [A/G] ratio, prothrombin time): All tests will show altered results, with anemia common, enzymes elevated, total protein and albumin decreased, and globulin increased (the A/G ratio will be reversed from the usual 2:1 ratio). Prothrombin time will be prolonged.
• *Radiologic studies* (chest X-ray, liver biopsy, electroencephalogram [EEG]): Chest X-ray determines pulmonary condition; liver biopsy confirms the diagnosis. An EEG determines cerebral functioning.

Nursing diagnoses

• Feeding self-care deficit related to altered metabolic state
• Bathing/hygiene self-care deficit related to altered metabolic state
• Dressing/grooming self-care deficit related to altered metabolic state
• Toileting self-care deficit related to altered metabolic state
• Risk for impaired skin integrity related to pruritus
• Altered nutrition: Less than body requirements, related to anorexia and decreased albumin

Planning and goals

Mr. Zimmer will:
• retain maximum liver functioning
• not experience uncontrolled bleeding episodes
• not suffer severe infections
• retain mental capacity and functions.

Implementation

NURSING BEHAVIORS	NURSING RATIONALES

Preoperative care

1. Check vital signs every 4 hours, or as ordered.

1. Changes can indicate bleeding or infection.

2. Perform a guaiac test of stools. Check the color and consistency of stools, and monitor for straining with a bowel movement.

2. GI bleeding commonly occurs with cirrhosis. Hemorrhoids frequently develop from increased venous congestion. Straining increases the risk of bleeding.

3. Observe the client's food intake and tolerance; monitor for fluid and electrolyte imbalance, nausea, and vomiting.

3. Foods should be soft and low in roughage to prevent bleeding of esophageal varices. Because the client's serum sodium level will increase and may lead to edema, foods should be low in sodium.

4. Provide extended rest periods.

4. Anemia and malnutrition lead to decreased oxygenation.

5. Observe the skin for breakdown and edema.

5. Because of decreased albumin, the client's skin is extremely susceptible to breakdown from edema.

6. Observe for pruritus.

6. This results from irritation caused by elevated serum bilirubin deposited in skin tissue.

7. Prepare the client for liver biopsy, as follows:
• Explain the procedure and its rationale.
• Give nothing by mouth after midnight, if ordered.
• Instruct the client to breathe deeply four to five times and then hold his breath during the biopsy (this procedure generally takes 1 minute); have him practice beforehand.
• Clean the biopsy site (in the right upper quadrant) with an antiseptic solution. Explain that a local anesthetic will be injected.
• Check vital signs immediately before the biopsy.

7. A liver biopsy is performed to confirm the diagnosis. Explanations and rehearsals prepare the client for what to expect, help relieve anxiety, and promote safety.

Postoperative care

1. Apply a snug dressing over the biopsy site. Have the client lie on his right side to assist in splinting the site for 1 to 4 hours, as ordered. Take vital signs every 15 minutes for 1 hour, then every 30 minutes for 1 hour, then every hour for the first 8 to 12 hours. After 8 to 12 hours, begin ambulation, if ordered. If bleeding occurs, notify the physician, who may prescribe vitamin K to control it.

1. A snug dressing and a right side-lying position help prevent hemorrhage (the liver is highly vascular). Postoperative care ensures the client's safety.

2. Check the results of the liver biopsy.

2. Biopsy tissues should indicate the extent of cirrhosis.

3. Monitor Mr. Zimmer for nausea and vomiting. If vomitus contains blood, prepare for treatment of esophageal varices. Treatment can vary as follows: Minor bleeding may warrant nasogastric tube insertion and antacid administration; major bleeding may require I.V. administration of vasopressin to cause splanchnic vasoconstriction, and uncontrolled bleeding may necessitate a Sengstaken-Blakemore (S-B) tube. (See *Sengstaken-Blakemore tube*.) Deflate and reinflate the esophageal balloon, as ordered.

3. The S-B tube has a triple lumen to the esophageal balloon, gastric balloon, and gastric suction. Periodically, the esophageal balloon must be deflated and reinflated to prevent compression trauma to the esophageal venous circulation. The physician may order ice-water saline lavages to decrease the client's bleeding.

Sengstaken-Blakemore tube

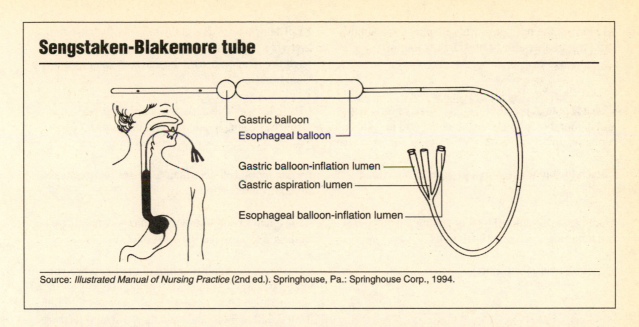

Gastric balloon

Esophageal balloon

Gastric balloon-inflation lumen

Gastric aspiration lumen

Esophageal balloon-inflation lumen

Source: *Illustrated Manual of Nursing Practice* (2nd ed.). Springhouse, Pa.: Springhouse Corp., 1994.

---

4. Administer vitamin K, neomycin, and lactulose, as ordered.

4. Vitamin K improves blood clotting. Neomycin destroys normal flora that can increase the risk of portal-systemic (hepatic) encephalopathy by breaking down blood protein in the GI tract. Lactulose decreases the serum ammonia level and, by causing diarrhea, helps eliminate blood protein in the GI tract.

5. Observe Mr. Zimmer for dyspnea.

5. Dyspnea may occur if the S-B tube becomes dislodged from the stomach.

6. Provide thorough oral hygiene as long as the client can take nothing by mouth.

6. The client cannot swallow secretions. His breath may have a fetid odor from high serum ammonia levels.

7. After the physician removes the S-B tube, observe the client for renewed bleeding and laryngospasm.

7. Removing pressure causes the veins to refill. Vein injury or excessive hydrostatic pressure can produce rebleeding. Laryngospasm can occur from edema or trauma from the S-B tube.

8. Observe the client for confusion, disorientation, and restlessness.

8. Hepatic encephalopathy can occur from increased ammonia levels in the circulation because the liver is not detoxifying amino acids properly.

9. Administer cleaning enemas, as ordered.

9. Medical orders may include frequent enemas to rid the bowel of putrefying foodstuffs, which contain high protein and ammonia levels that the cirrhotic liver cannot detoxify.

10. Administer diuretics, such as furosemide and spironolactone, as ordered.

10. Furosemide, a potent diuretic, inhibits sodium reabsorption. Spironolactone inhibits aldosterone, causing sodium loss while sparing potassium. Hypokalemia may require potassium supplementation.

11. Review the prognosis with the client and family, and prepare them for home care, as follows:

11. The prognosis is usually negative because the liver cells will eventually cease to regenerate. Thorough preparation before discharge helps promote optimal home care.

• Review potential complications, such as esophageal and hemorrhoidal bleeding, anemia, and hepatic encephalopathy.

• The enlarged spleen destroys red blood cells and platelets, leading to anemia and hemorrhage.

• Teach the client measures to prevent infection.

• White blood cell destruction causes increased susceptibility to infection.

• Emphasize the importance of getting adequate rest and adhering to activity restrictions.

• The client's condition necessitates extended rest periods and avoiding of strenuous activity.

• Review dietary instructions.

• The client must follow a diet of modified protein (70 to 100 g daily), carbohydrate intake to spare protein, and modified fat as desired; total intake should range from 2,000 to 3,000 calories daily. Dietary needs result from the liver's inability to use nutrients properly.

• Explain other medical treatments for cirrhosis of the liver.

• Other medical treatments may include the LeVeen shunt (to lessen and drain peritoneal ascitic fluids into the superior vena cava) or a surgical shunt. The most commonly performed surgical shunt is the *portacaval*, which detours (shunts) the portal vein into the vena cava to lessen its pressure. Other shunts (splenorenal and mesocaval) also decrease portal vein pressure. After a shunt, the client eliminates proteins and wastes through the renal system, which can precipitate renal failure.

Evaluation

• Mr. Zimmer retains optimum liver functioning despite cirrhosis.
• Mr. Zimmer's bleeding is under control.
• Mr. Zimmer has no severe infections.
• Mr. Zimmer retains his mental capacity and functions.

Ulcerative colitis

A major health problem and a potentially debilitating disease, ulcerative colitis, a type of inflammatory bowel disease, produces lesions primarily confined to the large bowel, with ulcerations of the large bowel's mucosa and submucosa. Healing of lesions causes scarring and strictures, leading to bowel obstruction, and ulcers may perforate, causing hemorrhage and peritonitis. Ulcerative colitis usually develops in those between ages 18 and 35 and occurs more frequently in women than in men. The following clinical situation focuses on nursing care of a client undergoing treatment for ulcerative colitis.

ADULT NURSING

Clinical situation   Kathleen Jones, a 22-year-old college senior, is admitted to the hospital. The medical diagnosis is ulcerative colitis. Her history reveals severe abdominal cramping and diarrhea containing blood and mucus.

Assessment

NURSING BEHAVIORS	NURSING RATIONALES
1. Assess the client's weight (noting recent loss or gain), vital signs (noting recent fever), skin turgor, and nutritional and dietary patterns.	**1.** These data establish baseline patterns and help determine the extent of the disease.
2. Assess the characteristics of the diarrhea.	**2.** Frequent, bloody diarrhea and abdominal cramping are common in ulcerative colitis.
3. Monitor the client's intake and output and fluid and electrolyte status.	**3.** This establishes baseline patterns for future comparison.
4. Assess the client's understanding of her disease and of past treatments.	**4.** This information enables the nurse to plan appropriate health teaching.
5. Assess the client's stresses and relationships with family, friends, and associates.	**5.** Researchers believe ulcerative colitis to be of autoimmune origin and to be worsened by individual stress-response behaviors.

Diagnostic evaluation

• *Lower GI series* (barium enema): This test is administered to detect bowel obstruction and help confirm the diagnosis.
—Explain the procedure and its rationale to the client.
—Administer a laxative, if ordered, on the afternoon before the procedure. *Caution:* Check for bowel sounds before administering the laxative, and measure the client's abdominal girth.
—Provide a clear liquid diet up to the night before surgery (after midnight, the client usually is given nothing by mouth).
—Administer enemas until return is clear on the evening before and the morning of the procedure.
—After the procedure, administer a cleaning enema (to rid the bowel of barium) or a laxative, as ordered.
• *Intestinal cell biopsy:* Intestinal cell biopsy offers one means of differentiating ulcerative colitis from regional enteritis (see *Comparing ulcerative colitis and regional enteritis,* page 576, for more information).
—Explain the procedure and its rationale to the client.
—Give the client nothing by mouth.
—Administer an enema to clear the bowel, if necessary.

Nursing diagnoses

• Diarrhea related to colon irritation
• Fluid volume deficit related to fluid loss from diarrhea
• Altered nutrition: Less than body requirements, related to electrolyte loss
• Impaired skin integrity related to anal excoriation

Planning and goals

• Ms. Jones will understand the possible complications of ulcerative colitis.
• Ms. Jones will follow her treatment regimen.

Comparing ulcerative colitis and regional enteritis

The following chart compares and contrasts ulcerative colitis and regional enteritis. Clinical symptoms usually do not aid differentiation.

	ULCERATIVE COLITIS	REGIONAL ENTERITIS (CROHN'S DISEASE)
Site of inflammation	Colon and rectum	Small intestine (primarily terminal ileum), although the disease may occur in any part of the small or large intestine
Type of lesion	Continuous ulcerated lesions involving mucosal and submucosal layers; may create abscesses	Skip lesions (inflamed areas skip around in the tract); lesions involve all intestinal layers (mucosa, submucosa, muscle, and serous layers); may abscess or perforate, scar, or form fistulas
Common patterns	Frequent diarrhea (30 to 40 bowel movements per day)—profuse, mucus-filled, watery, bloody, and debilitating; dehydration and weight loss; electrolyte imbalances are common; fever is common in acute attacks	Watery, mucus-filled diarrhea, less bloody than in ulcerative colitis; cramping, distention, and low-grade fever
Treatments	*Medical:* a diet high in protein, calories, and vitamins; anticholinergic drugs and anti-inflammatory, antibacterial, or antibiotic drugs; emotional support	*Medical:* same as for ulcerative colitis
	Surgical: ileostomy, with colectomy and removal of the rectum	*Surgical:* bowel resection; the client may need repeated resections

Implementation

NURSING BEHAVIORS

1. Administer steroids and antibacterial medications, such as corticosteroids and sulfasalazine (Azulfidine), as ordered. Administer antidiarrheals, such as diphenoxylate (Lomotil), loperamide (Imodium), kaolin and pectin mixtures (Kaopectate), and bismuth subcarbonate, as ordered.

2. Observe the client for side effects.

3. Monitor the client's food and fluid intake. During periods of extreme inflammation, provide tube feedings or total parenteral nutrition (TPN), if ordered (see *Total parenteral nutrition*). During acute exacerbations, provide plenty of fluids and electrolytes and a low-residue, high-nutrient diet (see *Low-residue diet,* page 578).

NURSING RATIONALES

1. Ulcerative colitis follows a pattern of alternating remission and exacerbations; medications help maintain control. Corticosteroids may decrease the immune response. Antibacterials may combine antimicrobial (sulfonamide) with anti-inflammatory (aspirin) actions. Anti-diarrheals help decrease gastric motility and water in the stool.

2. The drugs may cause constipation and abdominal pain and distention. Lomotil also may cause dependence.

3. Dietary modifications reduce bowel irritation. TPN permits total rest for the GI tract. Tube feedings provide predigested nutrients, minimizing digestive function.

ADULT NURSING

Total parenteral nutrition

PURPOSE
To meet a client's total nutritional needs when oral feedings, tube feedings, and standard I.V. feedings are contraindicated; used for clients with various gastrointestinal problems and in other situations necessitating nutritional support (for example, with the oncology client)

PRINCIPLES
- In most cases, administer total parenteral nutrition (TPN) via a central vein, such as the subclavian. The fluid is highly concentrated to provide rapid dilution and thus decrease the risks of peripheral inflammation and thrombosis.
- Administer fluid at a constant rate, using an infusion pump. The fluid's high concentration means that rapid administration can lead to circulatory overload, potassium depletion, and cellular dehydration.
- Do not abruptly discontinue the infusion. Administer dextrose 10% in water if you must stop the infusion. During TPN, the pancreas secretes increased insulin, and abrupt cessation can lead to hypoglycemia.
- Maintain *strict* asepsis. Use an occlusive dressing and change the dressing, tubing, and filter every 48 hours. Note that glucose and protein make effective bacterial media.
- Monitor blood glucose levels or check urine for glucose every 6 hours. Note that the client might need insulin.
- Observe the client for headache, nausea, vomiting, and fever. These indicate an allergy to the protein.
- Closely monitor intake and output.
- Weigh the client daily. Expect a weight gain of ¼ lb per day.
- Never use a filter with fat emulsions. Monitor for nausea and fever, common adverse reactions.

---

4. Assist the client with sitz baths several times daily, and apply ointment to the perianal area after each bowel movement.

4. These measures reduce discomfort from anal excoriation.

Evaluation	Ms. Jones can explain her treatment regimen and possible complications.
Clinical situation *(continued)*	Because the medical treatment proved ineffective in controlling Ms. Jones's ulcerative colitis, she is scheduled for an ileostomy.
Assessment	See the nursing behaviors and rationales previously listed for ulcerative colitis.
Nursing diagnoses	• Altered health maintenance related to lack of knowledge about the disease and ileostomy care • Body image disturbance related to frequent diarrhea • Impaired skin integrity related to anal excoriation
Planning and goals	Ms. Jones will: • understand and eventually participate in self-care after the ileostomy • regain skin integrity after incisions heal • learn long-term care techniques.

Implementation

NURSING BEHAVIORS

NURSING RATIONALES

Preoperative care
1. Provide routine preoperative care.

1. See "Preoperative period," pages 123 to 125, for specific nursing behaviors and rationales.

Low-residue diet

A low-residue diet is prescribed to avoid irritation of the mucosal lining. A regular diet containing normal amounts of protein and gradually incorporating fiber should be instituted when the client can tolerate it.

FOODS	ALLOWED	NOT ALLOWED
Breads and cereals	Refined breads without seeds	High-fiber cereals (All Bran, Grape Nuts); whole-grain breads
Fruit	Canned fruits without skins or seeds; ripe banana; strained fruit juice	Raw fruits
Fats	All	None
Meats, fish, poultry	Roasted, baked or broiled	Fried or highly spiced
Dairy	Milk, eggs, cheese	Fried eggs
Soups	Bouillon, broth, strained cream soups	All others
Vegetables	Canned or cooked strained vegetables; tomato juice	Raw or whole cooked vegetables
Miscellaneous	Salt, gravy, jelly, syrups, chocolate, puddings, and plain cakes	Nuts, olives, pickles, jam, alcohol, rich pastries

2. Instruct the client in measures to clear the bowel, as follows:
• Clear liquid diet for 1 to 2 days before surgery.
• Enemas the evening before and the morning of surgery.
• Laxative, such as bisacodyl or magnesium citrate, if ordered (usually not done if the client has diarrhea and ulceration).
• Oral antibacterial (usually sulfonamide) or antibiotic (usually neomycin sulfate) medication, as ordered (usually every 4 hours in large doses, beginning 48 hours before surgery).
• Administer vitamin K, if ordered, to increase prothrombin synthesis.

2. Before major surgery on the small or large bowel, the bowel must be cleared of fecal material to reduce the risk of contaminating the abdomen. Antibacterials decrease bacterial growth and functions in the intestine, predisposing the client to bleeding from decreased synthesis of vitamin K.

3. Prepare Ms. Jones for the ileostomy by providing appropriate teaching and consultation with enterostomal therapist.

3. An ileostomy, a curative treatment for ulcerative colitis, involves removal of the colon and rectum (see *Comparing ileostomy and colostomy* for more information). Long-standing ulcerative colitis (of more than 10 years' duration) predisposes the client to colon cancer, which an ileostomy will prevent.

4. Provide emotional support to the client and family.

4. The prognosis is uncertain before surgery.

Postoperative care
1. Provide routine postoperative care.

1. See "Postoperative period," page 125, for specific nursing behaviors and rationales.

Comparing ileostomy and colostomy

TYPE OF SURGERY	OPERATIVE SITE AND TISSUES REMOVED	PURPOSE OF SURGERY	NURSING CONSIDERATIONS
Ileostomy	Terminal ileum; colon removed	Curative for ulcerative colitis	Has one stoma at the terminal ileum; it drains gastric juices that are destructive if they contact the skin. Change the stoma appliance if a leak develops. Protect the client's skin with karaya powder. Use an adhesive spray to keep the appliance attached to the skin.
Colostomy Double barrel (loop colostomy)	Transverse colon; usually temporary. Stomas may be side by side or separated. The distal loop is called a mucus fistula, as it allows mucus to be expelled from the colon.	Relieves obstruction distal to colostomy site	Has two openings (proximal and distal stomas); may have a rod under openings to hold the colon on the abdomen. The proximal loop may be irrigated before closure; the distal loop may be irrigated as needed or before surgery to reconnect the bowel. Drainage from the proximal stoma is proteolytic (use same cautions as with ileostomy).
Single barrel (end colostomy)	Sigmoid or descending colon; rectum may be removed	Curative for colon or rectal cancer	One small stoma, usually on the lower left abdominal area; the client may be taught to irrigate colostomy to help regulate fecal discharge, which is nonirritating. The client may wear only a small cover over stoma. Teach the client to avoid or limit gas-forming foods, high-residue foods (to lessen fecal mass), and nuts and skins, which increase elimination frequency.

2. Monitor the client's vital signs, fluid intake and output, and daily weight.

2. Monitoring helps detect fluid and electrolyte imbalances and inflammation.

3. Maintain the patency of the nasogastric (NG) tube by low intermittent suction and irrigation with normal saline solution; maintain nothing-by-mouth status.

3. Maintaining tube patency decreases the risk that the client will develop paralytic ileus after surgery. The client must have nothing by mouth until GI tract functioning returns. Irrigating the NG tube with normal saline solution helps prevent metabolic alkalosis.

4. Inspect the stoma site for color, edema, and drainage.

4. The stoma site should be pink, with a small amount of edema. Initially, drainage may be scant and sanguineous, gradually becoming mucoserous, with flatus in the bag in 2 to 3 days. After bowel functions return, drainage increases markedly and becomes semiliquid, with unformed stools from the loss of the colon and the ileocecal sphincter.

5. Periodically inspect the stoma and the surrounding skin to detect irritation and to ensure adherence of the stoma appliance to the skin. Change the appliance regularly, usually every 5 to 7 days (change it immediately if leaking occurs), and empty it every 4 to 6 hours: Gently wash the client's skin with soap and water, dry it, protect it with a skin barrier, and carefully fit the new appliance around the stoma (the appliance opening should be approximately 1/8″ larger than the stoma to prevent constriction). Place deodorant tablets or drops in the appliance before closing the stoma. Apply adhesive sprays or tape to hold the appliance in place, and leave it open at the bottom for easy emptying. Measure output to determine fluid and electrolyte status.

6. Have the client turn, deep-breathe, and cough, and show her how to use a respiratory aid, if ordered; gradually increase ambulation as strength returns; administer antibiotics as ordered; and have the client move her legs and change her position frequently.

7. Change rectal and abdominal wound dressings as necessary. If ordered, perform rectal wound irrigations (when the drain is out) after a sitz bath three times daily. Keep the abdominal wound clear of ileostomy drainage, and change dressings before applying the ileostomy appliance.

8. After the nasogastric tube is removed, provide a clear liquid diet, advancing to a regular diet as tolerated. Explain the importance of increased fluid and electrolyte intake, and describe signs of fluid and electrolyte imbalance.

9. Teach the client self-care of the ileostomy, with help from an enterostomal therapist. Be certain the client understands dietary needs and stoma and wound care.

10. Prepare the client for discharge by reviewing sitz bath and wound care techniques, appliance care, symptoms to report to the physician, and the medication regimen (if any). Caution the client to avoid heavy carrying and lifting for 6 weeks, and tell her that she can resume sexual relations as healing permits. Finally, refer the client to an ostomy association.

5. An ileostomy drains from the small intestine. The juices contain proteolytic enzymes that can be destructive if they contact unprotected skin. Commercially prepared skin care sprays, powders, disks of karaya, and double-backed adhesive disks are available. Stoma appliances may be reusable according to the manufacturer's specifications.

6. Recovery from surgery that involves removal of the rectum usually is lengthy, predisposing the client to respiratory, circulatory, and GI complications. Ambulation decreases the risk of developing atelectasis, emboli, ileus, and infection.

7. The rectal wound may have suture closure except for a 1″ opening for one or two drains. Drainage initially appears sanguineous and may be profuse, requiring frequent dressing changes. Rectal wounds must heal from the inside out to prevent abscesses; irrigations and sitz baths bring more blood to the rectal area to aid healing. Keeping the abdominal wound clear of drainage prevents contamination.

8. The client can follow a regular diet with increased fluid and electrolyte intake, especially sodium. The client should understand the need for increased fluid and electrolytes: output is liquid, and the body does not reabsorb water sufficiently. The client must learn signs of fluid and electrolyte imbalances to ensure early detection and prompt treatment.

9. An enterostomal therapist can supply invaluable information on appliance care (including proper fitting and adherence) and resources (such as an ostomy association) for obtaining equipment, supplies, and psychological support.

10. The client should be able to perform (or assist with) appliance and stoma care and know how to recognize signs of inadequate healing, fluid and electrolyte imbalances, and bowel obstruction. The client no longer needs medication for ulcerative colitis, although she may need analgesics and sedatives temporarily while healing. Activity restrictions usually are temporary; having an ileostomy does not preclude childbearing, swimming, and most other activities (although the client must learn how to ensure adherence of the appliance during strenuous activities). An ostomy association can provide emotional support and educational guidance. (*Note:* Some clients undergo a Koch ileostomy, which creates a pouch of ileum with a one-way valve, making the ileostomy continent—that is, no spillage occurs except when a catheter enters the pouch for drainage. Clients usually catheterize every 4 hours, including nighttime. The small stoma has only a dry dressing, or it may be left uncovered.)

Evaluation

- Ms. Jones recovers from surgery without infection.
- Ms. Jones's abdominal and rectal wounds are healing.
- Ms. Jones can care for her ileostomy.

Bowel obstruction

Bowel obstruction, which can become life-threatening, occurs most frequently in people over age 40; usually, surgical treatment yields satisfactory results. Common causes of bowel obstruction include adhesions, which frequently develop after previous surgery, and cancer.

Clinical situation

Fred Martin, a 59-year-old garage mechanic, enters the hospital with a diagnosis of large-bowel obstruction. Three years ago, Mr. Martin underwent surgery to remove his inflamed gallbladder, and his physician suspects he now suffers from abdominal adhesions. Mr. Martin appears acutely ill; his condition must be stabilized before he can have surgery to remove the obstruction. His Salem sump nasogastric (NG) tube is connected to suction. Mr. Martin's temperature is 101° F (38.3° C); pulse rate, 92 beats/minute; respiratory rate, 24 breaths/minute; and blood pressure, 140/90 mm Hg.

Assessment

NURSING BEHAVIORS

1. Assess the client's general health, including vital signs, skin turgor, weight, appetite, and abdominal girth. Inquire about nausea and vomiting.

2. Assess the client's knowledge of his condition and of the need for diagnostic tests and surgery.

NURSING RATIONALES

1. These data constitute a baseline for future comparison. Bowel obstruction usually produces nausea, vomiting, constipation or obstipation, weight loss, distention, and prostration. The overdistended bowel can rupture, perforate, or become gangrenous (predisposing the client to peritonitis).

2. This assessment enables the nurse to plan appropriate teaching.

ADULT NURSING

Diagnostic evaluation

• *Hematologic studies* (complete blood count, clotting studies, blood urea nitrogen levels, creatinine study, and urinalysis): Test results provide data about the client's health and his ability to tolerate surgery.
• *Radiologic studies* (abdominal and chest X-rays and a GI series, when the client can tolerate these): These will determine the cause and site of obstruction.
• *Electrocardiogram:* This will help determine the client's circulatory status.

Nursing diagnosis

• Risk for infection related to the risk of peritonitis
• Risk for fluid volume deficit related to risk for bowel perforation

Planning and goals

• Mr. Martin will undergo bowel resection without complications.
• Mr. Martin's bowel function will return.
• Mr. Martin will be able to return to work.

Implementation

NURSING BEHAVIORS	NURSING RATIONALES
Preoperative care	
1. Administer enemas, as ordered (usually in a 500-ml solution). Do not administer a laxative.	**1.** Enemas help clear the bowel before surgery. A laxative is not administered for bowel obstruction.
2. Explain the procedure and its rationale to the client.	**2.** Explanations help the client anticipate probable events, which may alleviate some of his anxiety.
3. Provide emotional support to the client and family.	**3.** Any surgical procedure carries certain risks, and the prognosis for this acute illness is uncertain.
4. Measure the client's abdominal girth, intake and output, and weight; monitor I.V. fluids; administer antibiotics, as ordered; maintain the client on nothing-by-mouth status.	**4.** Weight loss will occur without oral intake. Abdominal distention should lessen after the bowel obstruction is relieved. Antibiotics help prevent peritonitis.

Clinical situation
(continued)

Measurement of Mr. Martin's vital signs reveals these increases: temperature (rectal), 102° F (38.9° C); pulse rate, 104 beats/minute; respiratory rate, 32 breaths/minute; and blood pressure, 150/90 mm Hg. His abdominal girth has increased 2″ (5 cm) over his admission finding. The NG tube is draining clear fluid. The physician decides to remove the NG tube and insert an intestinal (Miller-Abbott) tube. The nurse assists with the insertion and connects the tube to suction.

Implementation

NURSING BEHAVIORS	NURSING RATIONALES
1. Turn Mr. Martin on his right side for 2 hours, then on his back for 2 hours, then on his left side for 2 hours (or as ordered).	**1.** Turning the client sequentially facilitates passage of the tube through the intestinal tract and through the sphincters.
2. Inspect the drainage in the suction container.	**2.** The drainage may become bile-colored or brownish and profuse as the tube reaches the obstructed area.

3. Continue to measure the client's abdominal girth, record vital signs, and administer I.V. fluids.

3. As the intestinal tube reaches the obstruction and removes drainage, the abdominal girth should decrease. Temperature elevation may indicate peritonitis. I.V. fluids prevent hypovolemia and dehydration.

4. Provide thorough skin care.

4. If his temperature drops, the client may perspire.

Clinical situation
(continued)

Eight hours later Mr. Martin's condition appears improved, with the following vital signs: temperature (rectal), 101° F (38.3° C); pulse rate, 100 beats/minute; respiratory rate, 28 breaths/minute; and blood pressure, 146/90 mm Hg. The abdominal X-ray showed a loop of dilated bowel, confirming the diagnosis. Mr. Martin receives an intramuscular injection of vitamin K and his skin is cleaned with antiseptic solutions in preparation for surgery. His schedule calls for lysis (cutting) of adhesions. He enters surgery with I.V. antibiotics and the intestinal tube in place; later, in the recovery room, the intestinal tube is replaced with an NG tube.

Implementation

NURSING BEHAVIORS

NURSING RATIONALES

Postoperative care

1. Besides providing routine postoperative care, continually monitor the client's vital signs, bowel sounds, and abdominal girth.

1. The client needs continual observation to detect peritonitis or paralytic ileus.

2. Change the client's position hourly; have him turn, deep-breathe, cough, and use a respiratory aid; and assist with ambulation and leg exercises, as ordered.

2. These measures are taken to minimize the potential for respiratory complications associated with the surgical incision and acute illness.

3. Check the amount and type of drainage from the Salem sump tube; irrigate the tube with normal saline solution, if needed.

3. Drainage should be yellow-green and may contain mucus and blood. No more fecal material should appear in the suction drainage.

4. Change dressings as necessary, using aseptic technique, and monitor wound healing.

4. Aseptic technique helps prevent contamination and infection.

5. After the NG tube is removed and the client resumes a regular diet, monitor his appetite, intake, and ability to digest food. Note distention, passing of flatus, and bowel movements (especially stool size and shape).

5. This information enables medical and nursing staff to evaluate the client's health and the effectiveness of surgery.

6. Review the specifics of home care, including self-care measures, activity precautions, and the importance of rest and ambulation.

6. Mr. Martin should not resume sexual activity or drive a car for 3 weeks and should not return to garage mechanic work for 6 weeks. He also must acknowledge the possibility of recurrent obstruction.

Evaluation

- Mr. Martin recovers from surgery without complications.
- Mr. Martin's appetite and digestion return.
- Mr. Martin's bowel movements are normal, with soft, formed stools.

ADULT NURSING

GENITOURINARY SYSTEM

Benign prostatic hyperplasia

Benign prostatic hyperplasia affects about half of all men over age 50. Medical management to shrink the size of the prostrate includes administration of finasteride (Proscar), which blocks the production of dihydrotestosterone, and alpha-adrenergic blockers, such as prazosin (Minipress) and phenoxybenzamine (Dibenzyline), which relax muscles and improve urination. Clients taking these drugs should be cautioned about orthostatic hypotension. If hyperplasia becomes severe and causes obstruction, infection, or impaired renal function, surgical intervention becomes necessary. Surgeons most commonly use transurethral resection, the subject of the following clinical situation.

Clinical situation

Ellis Stern, age 60, is an active businessman who recently married a 48-year-old woman. Having experienced acute urine retention for the past several days, Mr. Stern is admitted to the hospital after the physician diagnoses his condition as benign prostatic hyperplasia. Mr. Stern has an indwelling urinary catheter and is now awaiting surgery for a transurethral resection. He seems quiet and withdrawn. Finally, he confides to the nurse that he is concerned about how his "inability to perform" may affect his new marriage.

Assessment

NURSING BEHAVIORS	NURSING RATIONALES
1. Assess for decreased urine stream and difficulty in starting the stream if a catheter is not in place.	**1.** Partial obstruction of the urethra by the enlarged prostate gland causes this.
2. Observe the client for urinary frequency and urgency, burning on urination, and nocturia if a catheter is not in place.	**2.** These are symptoms of cystitis, which occurs because of residual urine. If the obstruction continues, signs of hydroureter, hydronephrosis, and calculi may appear.

Diagnostic evaluation

• *Blood urea nitrogen* (normal: 8 to 20 mg/dl): An elevated level indicates dehydration or renal damage.
• *Creatinine* (normal: 0.8 to 1.5 mg/dl): An elevated level indicates renal damage.
• *I.V. pyelogram:* This is an X-ray of the kidney and pelvis using a contrast material injected intravenously. A check for hypersensitivity to the dye may be necessary.
• *Cystoscopy:* This permits visualization of the bladder and the urethra through a lighted tube.

Before cystoscopy

1. Force fluids for several hours.	**1.** This will maintain a constant flow of urine and prevent bacterial stasis.
2. Provide sedation 1 hour before the cystoscopy with either diazepam (Valium) or meperidine, as ordered.	**2.** The procedure usually produces a great deal of stress and anxiety in the client.

After cystoscopy

1. Check the client's voiding.	**1.** Urine may be pink-tinged from the trauma of cystoscopy.
2. Check for complaints of pain, spasms, and urinary frequency.	**2.** Warm sitz baths may provide relief. The client also may need analgesics or antispasmodics.
3. Force fluids.	**3.** This will keep the urinary tract flushed and provide internal irrigation.
4. Observe the client for complications.	**4.** An elevated temperature, chills, flushing, and hypotension may signal hemorrhage or infection.

Nursing diagnoses
- Pain related to the obstruction
- Urinary retention related to the obstruction
- Altered urinary elimination related to the indwelling catheter

Planning and goals

Mr. Stern will:
- have normal urine output and unobstructed flow
- be free of postoperative complications
- discuss concerns related to temporary sexual dysfunction.

Implementation

NURSING BEHAVIORS

NURSING RATIONALES

Preoperative care

1. Relieve the obstruction by gradually draining urine through a urethral catheter.	**1.** With severe obstruction, the bladder may contain more than 1,000 ml of urine; gradual decompression is necessary to prevent shock and hemorrhage.
2. Prepare the client for the transurethral resection. Tell him to expect a catheter in the bladder. Explain that he will feel like voiding and that urine will drain through the tube.	**2.** The client should not attempt to void around the tube. That would strain the bladder and contribute to spasms.
3. Reassure the client that he will probably be able to resume sexual activity once he is healed.	**3.** This information helps alleviate the client's fears about sexual dysfunctioning. Impotence rarely occurs except after a radical prostatectomy for prostate cancer.

Postoperative care

1. Inspect the client's urine, and observe the client for signs of shock.	**1.** Dark red blood in the urine is normal for the first few days after surgery; bright red blood and clots indicate an active hemorrhage. Tissue sloughing and straining can cause delayed hemorrhaging 6 to 10 days postoperatively.
2. Maintain catheter patency. Keep accurate intake and output records, and account for irrigating fluid. Assess the client for water intoxication. Force fluids.	**2.** The client is likely to have a three-way urinary catheter in place with continuous irrigation for the first 24 hours. The catheter maintains flow and prevents and eliminates clots. The venous sinusoids of the bladder may absorb the irrigating fluid. Forcing fluids keeps the urine dilute.

ADULT NURSING

3. Reduce the discomfort of bladder spasms. Remind the client not to void around the catheter, and irrigate as needed.

3. This will decrease strain. Irrigation removes clots. The catheter has a 30-ml balloon, and applied traction prevents bleeding. Both the large balloon and traction contribute to spasms, which usually decrease within 24 to 48 hours.

4. Administer anticholinergic drugs (for example, belladonna and opium suppositories), as ordered.

4. Anticholinergic drugs decrease bladder spasms.

5. Remove the catheter 2 to 3 days after surgery.

5. The catheter typically is removed by the time the client is discharged, usually 3 days after surgery. The nurse should periodically check for voiding, however, because the client may have occasional dribbling.

6. Teach perineal (Kegel) exercises, with the client tightly squeezing the perineal muscles 5 to 10 times each hour.

6. Perineal exercises increase sphincter tone. Full bladder capacity may not return for 2 months.

7. Help the client walk.

7. This prevents a thromboembolism and reduces bladder spasms.

8. Before discharge, provide these instructions:
• Do not strain at stool.
• Use a stool softener.
• Do not drive a car for 3 weeks.
• Do no heavy lifting for 6 weeks.
• Resume sexual activity when healing is complete.

8. These measures protect the client from injury and hemorrhage, which can occur if the client sustains trauma before healing is complete. Without complications, the client is usually discharged on day 4.

Evaluation

• Mr. Stern shows no evidence of hemorrhage or infection.
• Mr. Stern has an unobstructed urine flow.
• Follow-up care reveals that Mr. Stern is not experiencing sexual dysfunction.

Cystitis

Cystitis, an inflammation of the urinary bladder, usually results from pathologic microorganisms. The following clinical situation focuses on nursing care of a client with cystitis.

Clinical situation

Helen Davis is a 25-year-old college student who has urinary urgency and frequency, with a burning sensation during urination. Her physician diagnoses her condition as cystitis.

Assessment

NURSING BEHAVIORS

NURSING RATIONALES

1. Assess the client for urinary burning, frequency, and urgency and for suprapubic tenderness.

1. These constitute signs of inflammation and infection of the urinary bladder.

2. Check her urine for pyuria (pus) and hematuria (blood).

2. Pyuria and hematuria will be present with advanced infection.

3. Obtain a history of the client's voiding frequency and daily fluid intake.

3. The history provides baseline data for future evaluations of the client's response to treatment.

4. Assess for predisposing factors: urinary stasis; presence of calculi or an indwelling catheter; lowered body resistance; disease, such as diabetes mellitus or hypertension; and trauma.

4. Identifying factors that contributed to the current condition enables caregivers to correct them and prevent recurrence.

Nursing diagnoses	• Altered urinary elimination related to urinary tract infection • Risk for infection related to urinary stasis
Planning and goals	Ms. Davis will: • be free of cystitis • understand how to prevent cystitis.

Implementation

NURSING BEHAVIORS

NURSING RATIONALES

1. Administer prescribed antibiotics.

1. Antibiotic therapy is initiated to combat infection.

2. Encourage high fluid intake (up to 3 qt [3,000 ml] /day).

2. Fluids will decrease discomfort and flush microorganisms out of the bladder.

3. Encourage the client to void every 2 to 3 hours, emptying the bladder completely.

3. This enhances bacteria removal and reduces urinary stasis.

4. Encourage bed rest during the acute phase.

4. Rest decreases the client's metabolic rate and promotes comfort.

5. Provide sitz baths, analgesics, and warmth to the perineum.

5. These interventions decrease discomfort.

6. Teach the client proper perineal hygiene, and emphasize the need for follow-up urine studies.

6. Proper hygiene helps prevent reinfection, and follow-up examinations ensure prompt detection and treatment if cystitis recurs.

Evaluation	Ms. Davis: • remains free of cystitis • can explain how to prevent recurrence.

Renal calculi

Renal calculi result from the precipitation of salts in the urine. These salts include phosphate, oxalate, carbonate, uric acid, urate, and cystine. Conditions that may lead to calculi formation include urinary stasis, infection, altered urine pH, certain diseases (such as leukemia and hyperparathyroidism), dehydration, and immobilization. The following clinical situation focuses on nursing care of a client with renal calculi.

ADULT NURSING

Clinical situation   Harold Downs, age 42, has urinary frequency, flank tenderness, and spasms of acute back pain. His physician diagnoses renal calculi.

Assessment

NURSING BEHAVIORS	NURSING RATIONALES
1. Obtain the client's health history.	**1.** This will identify any conditions contributing to calculi formation.
2. Determine the client's dietary pattern.	**2.** Diet can alter urine pH to increase the potential for calculi formation.
3. Assess the client for increased temperature, chills, and dysuria.	**3.** These symptoms may indicate urinary or renal infection.
4. Obtain a urine specimen to determine urine pH and specific gravity values and to detect hematuria.	**4.** The client's urine pH may enhance calculi formation. A urine culture can identify the organisms causing the infection, which enables the physician to determine the appropriate antibiotic therapy.
5. Assess the client for an allergy to iodine, and administer a laxative, as ordered, to prepare the client for a pyelogram. Then check the X-ray of the client's urinary tract.	**5.** A pyelogram, which uses a radiopaque contrast medium to permit visualization of the urinary tract, can identify abnormalities. Many renal calculi are radiopaque. (In an I.V. pyelogram, a radiopaque medium is infused intravenously; in a retrograde pyelogram, the medium is injected through ureteral catheters, as is done during a cystoscopy. In both cases, the contrast medium contains iodine.) Laxatives help eliminate intestinal gas and fecal material that can impair visualization of the urinary tract.
6. Check the client's blood studies—serum concentrations of calcium, phosphorus, oxalate, and uric acid.	**6.** These studies can identify the type of calculi, which will dictate the appropriate diet.
7. Frequently assess the client to determine if he has any discomfort along the course of the ureter, with sudden, sharp pain radiating down the ureter.	**7.** This indicates that the calculi are moving or trying to move down the urinary tract. Ureteral colic is acute spasmodic pain caused by calculi lodging in the ureter.

Nursing diagnoses   • Altered urinary elimination related to urinary tract obstruction
• Pain related to calculi lodged in the ureter

Planning and goals   Mr. Downs will:
• eliminate calculi
• experience pain relief
• not experience complications
• understand how to prevent calculi.

Diet considerations for clients with renal calculi

A. Foods to acidify urine

Fish (halibut)	Roast Beef
Bacon	Pork
Veal	Cranberries
Lamb	Prunes
Chicken	Plums

B. Foods to alkalinize urine

Dried apricots	Dandelion greens
Dried figs	Navy beans
Molasses	Milk
Beet greens	Milk products
Green olives	Citrus fruit and juices

C. Foods to avoid with calcium calculi

Cheddar cheese	Whole milk
Cheese food	Evaporated milk
Cheese spread	Skim milk
	Powdered dry skim milk

D. Foods to avoid with oxalate calculi

Rhubarb	Chocolate
Asparagus	Cocoa
Dandelion greens	Okra
Spinach	Potatoes
Cranberries	Tomatoes
Beets and beet greens	Corn
Cashew nuts	Swiss chard

Implementation

NURSING BEHAVIORS	NURSING RATIONALES
1. Force fluids (3 to 4 qt [3,000 to 4,000 ml] daily).	**1.** Increasing fluid intake will reduce the concentration of crystals in the urine (dilute the urine) and help flush the urinary tract.
2. Strain all urine for calculi.	**2.** Straining retrieves any calculi, which must go to the laboratory for analysis.
3. Administer prescribed anticholinergics, such as atropine sulfate, methantheline bromide (Banthine), and propantheline bromide (Pro-Banthine).	**3.** Anticholinergic agents relax the ureteral and bladder muscles.
4. Administer analgesics and I.V. morphine, as ordered.	**4.** Analgesics reduce acute pain. Morphine, which may be required for ureteral colic, depresses the central nervous system and alters pain perception and response.
5. Administer medications and offer foods to acidify or alkalinize the urine (as ordered, depending on the type of calculi). (See *Diet considerations for clients with renal calculi*.)	**5.** Changing the urine pH prevents calculi formation.

ADULT NURSING

Surgeries for renal calculi

When calculi are too large to pass through the urinary tract, the surgeon may choose among the following types of surgery:

Cystoscopy
After the instrument has been inserted into the bladder, ultrasound crushes the calculi.

Ureterolithotomy
Using an abdominal incision, the surgeon makes an opening into the ureter to remove calculi. Postoperatively, a ureteral stent (tube) is inserted to maintain patency until healing occurs.

Pyelolithotomy
Using a flank incision, the surgeon opens the kidney pelvis to remove calculi.

Nephrolithotomy
Using a flank incision, the surgeon opens the kidney to remove calculi.

Percutaneous lithotripsy
An endoscope is passed in the region around the kidney. Either a snare basket is used to get the calculi, or the surgeon delivers ultrasound waves through a probe placed on the stone, fragmenting it.

Extracorporeal shock wave lithotripsy
The client is placed in water, and the surgeon sends shock waves through the water to break up calculi, which are passed within a few days. Complications include hematoma and hemorrhage.

• Choice A: Administer ammonium chloride, ascorbic acid, and an acid-ash diet to acidify the client's urine.

• Some calculi form in an alkaline medium.

• Choice B: Administer potassium citrate or acetate, sodium bicarbonate, and an alkaline-ash diet to alkalinize the client's urine.

• Uric acid calculi form in an acid medium.

• Choice C: Decrease dietary calcium. Thiazide diuretics may be used.

• Increased dietary calcium results in calcium calculi. Thiazide diuretics decrease urinary calcium.

• Choice D: Decrease dietary oxalate. Allopurinol may be administered.

• Increased dietary oxalate results in oxalate calculi. Allopurinol inhibits synthesis of uric acid.

6. Administer antibiotics, as ordered.

6. Antibiotics are administered to treat or prevent infection.

7. Observe the client for abdominal distention and absent bowel sounds. If bowel sounds are absent, do not give the client anything by mouth.

7. Paralytic ileus commonly complicates kidney surgery. Some types of renal calculi, such as staghorn calculi, may require nephrectomy (see *Surgeries for renal calculi*).

8. Encourage a client who has undergone a nephrectomy to deep-breathe and cough every hour; monitor the client's hourly urine output, and obtain a specimen to determine urine pH and specific gravity values.

8. Deep breathing and coughing help prevent atelectasis and pneumonia; because the high incision near the diaphragm will cause pain on breathing, a surgical client may be reluctant to do the required exercises. Urine monitoring and testing will measure how effectively the remaining kidney is functioning.

9. Discuss the causes of renal calculi and ways to prevent recurrence.

9. Enhancing the client's knowledge of his condition will probably promote compliance with treatment.

10. Stress the importance of fluids (3 to 4 qt [3,000 to 4,000 ml] /day) and a diet appropriate for the client's type of calculi.

10. Fluids help reduce urinary stasis, thereby impeding the formation of calculi. A diet specifically designed for the client can promote a urine pH level that hinders calculi development.

11. Review the medication regimen and adverse reactions (if any).

11. Drugs maintain proper urine pH.

12. Advise a surgical client to avoid heavy lifting for 6 weeks.

12. Complete healing of a surgical incision requires 6 weeks.

Evaluation

• Mr. Downs excreted calculi without complications.
• Mr. Downs can explain how to prevent renal calculi.

Acute renal failure

Renal failure is a marked decrease in function by the nephrons of the kidneys, resulting in electrolyte imbalance and retention of nitrogenous substances. A major cause of renal failure is a reduction in blood supply to the kidneys because of congestive heart failure, hemorrhage, shock, dehydration, or obstruction of the renal arteries by thrombi and emboli. Other causes of renal failure include infections (such as pyelonephritis or septicemia) and hypersensitivity reactions from poisons, allergens, mismatched blood transfusions, and drug toxicity. Regardless of the cause, the result is destruction of the renal tubules.

Acute renal failure has four phases: onset, oliguric-anuric, diuretic, and convalescent. The convalescent period can last up to 12 months. The following clinical situation focuses on nursing care of a client with acute renal failure.

Clinical situation

Mary Harrigan, age 56, a single woman who works as a bookkeeper for a lumber company, was spraying insecticide on her roses when she became ill and had to be rushed to the hospital. She has an anaphylactic reaction to the insecticide, leading to shock and renal failure. This was the precipitating event or onset phase.

Oliguric-anuric phase

During this period, the client's urine output falls below 400 ml/day, with resultant electrolyte imbalance, metabolic acidosis, and retention of nitrogenous wastes from nonfunctioning nephrons. This phase may last up to 14 days.

Assessment

NURSING BEHAVIORS

NURSING RATIONALES

1. Observe the client for signs and symptoms related to the cause of the dysfunction.

1. Besides treating acute renal failure, medical and nursing staff must also treat its cause.

2. Assess fluid and electrolyte balance by checking intake and output and urine specific gravity.

2. The kidneys play a major role in regulating the body's fluid and electrolytes.

3. Assess the client's and family's knowledge of renal failure.

3. These data form a necessary baseline for teaching.

4. Assess the emotional status of the client and family.

4. The client is facing a life-threatening illness, and she needs her family's emotional support.

Diagnostic evaluation	Draw blood samples to determine blood pH, bicarbonate levels, and urea nitrogen levels. The normal values are as follows: • *Blood pH*—7.35 to 7.45: The blood pH indicates the presence or absence of uncompensated metabolic acidosis. If the mechanisms to maintain the acid-base balance prove effective, the blood pH remains within normal limits. • *Blood urea nitrogen (BUN) levels*—10 to 15 mg/dl: Elevated BUN levels indicate urea retention, which shows the kidneys are not functioning effectively. • *Creatinine level*—0.7 to 1.5 mg/dl: Elevation indicates renal damage.

Nursing diagnoses

• Altered renal tissue perfusion related to decreased arterial circulation
• Fluid volume excess related to impaired renal function (oliguric phase)
• Risk for infection related to acute metabolic disruption
• Fluid volume deficit related to fluid loss (polyuric phases)

Planning and goals

Ms. Harrigan will:
• have normal fluid and electrolyte levels
• experience no preventable complications
• understand the means by which she and her family will implement health teaching after her discharge.

Implementation

NURSING BEHAVIORS

NURSING RATIONALES

1. Maintain the client on complete bed rest; organize her care to provide long rest periods.

1. Activity increases the rate of metabolism, which increases production of nitrogenous waste products.

2. Implement interventions to prevent infection and the complications of immobility.

2. Because she is on bed rest, the client becomes susceptible to the hazards of immobility. Infection is a serious risk and the leading cause of death in clients with acute renal failure.

3. Observe the client for metabolic acidosis.

3. Retention of acids causes metabolic acidosis—one of the complications of renal failure.

4. Observe fluid and electrolyte balance. Insert an indwelling urinary catheter, and measure output and specific gravity hourly.

4. The kidneys have the major role in regulating fluid and electrolyte balance. High potassium levels can occur.

5. Provide only enough fluid intake to replace urine output.

5. Excessive fluid intake produces edema.

6. Monitor the client's diet to provide high carbohydrates, adequate fats, and low protein. (Protein should be of high biologic value, or complete protein, such as from beef, eggs, milk, and chicken. See *Low-protein diet*.) Offer carbohydrate supplements (hard candy, jelly beans, Kool-Aid, tapioca, honey, and jelly).

6. If the client receives adequate calories from fat and carbohydrate metabolism, the body does not break down protein for energy. Protein is thus available for growth and repair. There is an accompanying decrease in nonprotein waste products, which result from protein metabolism.

Low-protein diet

In acute and chronic renal failure, as the client can excrete fewer nitrogenous waste products, medical and nursing staff must reduce the client's protein intake while continuing to maintain nitrogen balance. A major part of the client's diet protein should be of high biologic value, or complete protein, to ensure meeting needs for essential amino acids (examples of foods containing protein of high biologic value include eggs, meat, fish, poultry, milk, and cheese). Use endogenous nitrogen to synthesize nonessential amino acids, thus reducing the amount of urea formed. Supply adequate calories to spare protein for tissue-protein synthesis. Include protein-free or low-protein foods to provide calories. As necessary, control sodium and potassium intake. Protein-free or low-protein foods include the following:
• Butter ball (composed of butter and sugar)
• Controlyte (made by Doyle)
• Polycase (made by Ross)
• Calpower (made by General Mills)
• Hycal (made by Beecham)
• Low-protein flour, pasta, bread, muffins, and cereals.

---

7. Reduce the client's potassium intake.

7. Protein catabolism causes potassium release from cells into the serum.

8. Observe for arrhythmias and cardiac arrest.

8. High serum potassium can cause arrhythmias.

9. Provide frequent oral hygiene by gently cleaning the client's mouth and administering antacids.

9. Urea and other acid waste products excreted through the skin and mucous membranes cause tissue irritation and sometimes ulcer formation.

10. Provide the client with hard candy and chewing gum.

10. These substances will stimulate saliva flow and decrease thirst.

11. Maintain skin care with cool water.

11. This will relieve pruritus and remove uremic frost (white crystals formed on the skin from excretion of urea).

12. Administer stool softeners.

12. These medications prevent colon irritation from high levels of urea and organic acids.

13. Provide emotional reassurance to the client and her family.

13. The client has an acute illness with an unknown prognosis.

14. As necessary, explain treatments and progress to the client.

14. This information may help reduce anxiety.

15. Provide hemodialysis or peritoneal dialysis.

15. Dialysis reduces nonprotein nitrogen waste levels in the blood and improves the fluid and electrolyte balance until the kidneys regain function.

Early diuretic phase   During this period, which lasts about 10 days, the client excretes a large volume (usually over 3,000 ml/day) of very dilute urine; the glomeruli are beginning to function effectively, but the tubules are not, and the client still experiences electrolyte imbalance, retention of nitrogenous waste products, and metabolic acidosis.

ADULT NURSING

Assessment

NURSING BEHAVIORS	NURSING RATIONALES
1. Assess fluid and electrolyte balance.	**1.** When the renal tubules are not functioning, fluid and electrolyte imbalance continues.
2. Assess the client's and family's emotional status.	**2.** Facing a prognosis that is still uncertain, the client and family need support.
3. Continue interventions used during the oliguric-anuric phase, *except:* • Increase fluid intake dramatically to keep up with output. • Administer potassium or other electrolyte replacements, if needed.	**3.** During the polyuric phase the client may experience dehydration. Electrolytes and fluid may be lost.

Late diuretic phase   The client is still excreting more fluid than normal; urine specific gravity is increasing because the tubules are beginning to function effectively; fluid, electrolyte, and acid-base balances are returning to normal.

Implementation

NURSING BEHAVIORS	NURSING RATIONALES
1. Continue implementations of the early diuretic phase. Allow the client to engage in nonstrenuous activity for brief periods, and increase the activity level gradually; do not let her become fatigued.	**1.** Too much activity may increase the rate of metabolism and overwork the kidneys.
2. Teach the client to prevent infection and to avoid the factors that caused renal failure.	**2.** This information may prevent a recurrence.

Evaluation   • Ms. Harrigan regains fluid and electrolyte balance.
• Ms. Harrigan understands the rationale behind activity restrictions.

Chronic renal failure

Chronic renal failure involves a chronic, progressive deterioration of renal function. Its major causes are diabetic nephropathy, hypertension, and glomerulonephritis.

Clinical situation   Amos Harvey, a 67-year-old retired steelworker, has had several urinary tract infections. Recently, he has been experiencing muscle weakness, and he tires more easily than usual. After the physician examines him, Mr. Harvey receives a medical diagnosis of chronic renal failure.

Assessment

NURSING BEHAVIORS	NURSING RATIONALES
1. Assess the client's fatigue and muscle weakness.	**1.** Anemia, resulting from decreased formation of red blood cells and hemolysis, causes the client to tire easily and to develop muscle weakness and spasms.
2. Observe the client for delayed wound healing and susceptibility to infection.	**2.** General physical deterioration from chronic kidney disease delays healing and weakens the immune system.
3. Assess for anorexia, nausea, and vomiting.	**3.** They result from an electrolyte imbalance or high urea levels.
4. Assess the client for pruritus, uremic frost, and ulcerations in the mouth (stomatitis) and GI tract.	**4.** The skin and mucous membranes excrete urea and other salts, causing irritation.
5. Observe the client for irritability (early metabolic acidosis) and for apathy, drowsiness, and coma (late metabolic acidosis).	**5.** A high serum urea level affects the central nervous system and also causes metabolic acidosis, which produces these symptoms.
6. Assess the client for other symptoms of the cause of the renal failure (for example, hypertension can cause decreased vision).	**6.** Another condition can produce its own set of symptoms as well as cause renal failure.
7. Check for fluid and electrolyte imbalance.	**7.** The client has many nonfunctional glomeruli and tubules.

Nursing diagnoses
- Altered tissue perfusion related to decreased renal circulation
- Fluid volume excess related to impaired excretory function
- Impaired physical mobility related to fatigue and anemia
- Powerlessness related to dependence on dialysis

Planning and goals
- Mr. Harvey will understand how dialysis works and why he needs it.
- Mr. Harvey and his family will be able to cope with lifelong dialysis and the accompanying prognosis.

Implementation

NURSING BEHAVIORS	NURSING RATIONALES
1. Allow the client to select foods from the diet prescribed by the physician.	**1.** This will encourage the client to eat. The client may be on a high-carbohydrate, protein-limited diet.
2. Administer epoetin alfa (Epogen), as ordered.	**2.** This drug replaces natural erythropoietin, which is destroyed in chronic renal failure. It also stimulates red blood cell production and corrects anemia.
3. Provide frequent mouth care (gentle cleaning), especially before meals.	**3.** The client's breath will have an ammonia odor, resembling that of urine, which will limit his ability to eat. His gums may bleed, and stomatitis or ulcers may form.

4. Gently bathe the client, using lukewarm water with soap only on body areas that require cleaning.

4. Pruritus and uremic frost result from the skin's excreting urea and other acid waste products.

5. Avoid medications that the kidney must excrete.

5. Because of impaired kidney function, medications cannot be excreted effectively.

6. Observe the client for side effects of medications.

6. He will be sensitive to all medications.

7. Assist the client with activities of daily living, as needed. Encourage him to do as much as possible without becoming fatigued.

7. Chronic renal failure follows a progressive course. The client's dependency will gradually increase.

8. Maintain a diet based on the client's serum electrolyte and blood urea nitrogen (BUN) levels; continue to offer foods the client will eat.

8. The nurse can assist in maintaining fluid and electrolyte balance by not increasing the client's intake of already elevated electrolytes. Protein intake may have to be adjusted according to the BUN level.

9. Provide hemodialysis or peritoneal dialysis several times each week.

9. This lowers the client's blood pressure, improves fluid and electrolyte balance, and reduces symptoms.

10. Teach the client and family the required care techniques and which symptoms to report to the physician.

10. This disease follows a chronic, progressive course. Correct teaching will enable the client to remain at home as long as possible.

11. Record the client's weight daily.

11. Recording the daily weight helps monitor the body's fluid balance (one pint of fluid weighs one pound).

12. Maintain the client's daily fluid intake, as ordered.

12. The client will retain excess amounts of fluid, which elevates the blood pressure and causes edema. The client on dialysis will have fewer restrictions on food and liquids than the diet-controlled client.

13. Encourage low-protein intake (protein of high biological value) to reduce risk of infection (see *Low-protein diet,* page 593).

13. Reducing protein intake decreases BUN. Protein of high biological value helps maintain nitrogen balance.

14. Provide emotional support to the client and family.

14. The client and family may become depressed by the problems of continuing therapy and the poor prognosis.

15. Teach ways to avoid infection.

15. The client will be susceptible to infection.

Dialysis

Dialysis is the process of diffusion, osmosis, and ultrafiltration used to reestablish fluid and electrolyte balance and to remove toxic substances and metabolic wastes. *Diffusion* is the passage of ions from an area of high concentration across a semipermeable membrane to an area of lower concentration. *Osmosis* is the passage of water molecules across a semipermeable membrane from a less concentrated solution to a more concentrated one. *Ultrafiltration* uses positive pressure to cause fluid to pass across a semipermeable membrane from an area of lesser concentration to one of greater concentration. It is faster than osmosis.

ADULT NURSING

There are two types of dialysis, *peritoneal dialysis* and *hemodialysis.* In peritoneal dialysis, a commercially prepared sterile dialysate, an electrolyte solution, flows by gravity through a catheter inserted through the abdominal wall into the peritoneal cavity. The peritoneum acts as a semipermeable membrane for osmosis and diffusion. After the solution has remained in the peritoneal cavity for the prescribed time, the dialysate is removed. The physician will order this process repeated until the client's fluid and electrolyte levels fall within acceptable limits.

In hemodialysis, the client's blood is passed through a dialyzer where, via the processes of diffusion and ultrafiltration, body fluids and electrolytes are exchanged with the dialysate. In this way excess fluid, electrolytes, and nitrogenous wastes are removed from the body. Access to the client's bloodstream is essential in hemodialysis. This is achieved via external arteriovenous shunt (for acute situations), subclavian or femoral catheters (for acute situations), or internal arteriovenous fistula or graft (used for chronic dialysis).

Continuous ambulatory peritoneal dialysis (CAPD) is a recent variation of peritoneal dialysis. CAPD involves infusing 500 to 1,000 ml of a personalized dialysate through a peritoneal catheter, clamping the catheter with the empty bag still attached, rolling the bag up, and placing it in a waistband, with the client then going about his usual activities. Every 4 hours the client drains the fluid from his peritoneal cavity into the empty bag, removes the bag and drainage from the catheter, aseptically attaches a new bag of dialysate, and repeats the infusion. CAPD proves much less confining to those who can assume the responsibility of maintaining the proper techniques. Major complications of CAPD include peritonitis, fluid and electrolyte imbalances, dehydration, catheter sepsis, abdominal pain and tenderness, organ trauma, and hemorrhage.

Continuous cyclic peritoneal dialysis (CCPD) uses a machine to deliver and drain the peritoneal fluid. Since cycling time lasts from 6 to 8 hours, the client can usually be dialyzed while sleeping at night. The machine has an alarm to protect the client from malfunction.

Implementation

NURSING BEHAVIORS

NURSING RATIONALES

Before dialysis

1. Explain the procedure to the client (see *Nursing measures in peritoneal dialysis and hemodialysis*, page 598.).

1. Explanations help reduce the client's anxiety.

2. Weigh the client, using a bed scale, and measure the client's vital signs.

2. This information establishes a baseline for future comparison.

3. Place the client in a comfortable supine or semireclining position.

3. The client must remain in one position for 6 to 8 hours.

During dialysis

1. Provide emotional reassurance to the client and family throughout the procedure.

1. This will assist in decreasing their anxiety.

2. During peritoneal dialysis, carefully provide passive range-of-motion exercises to all the limbs of a client, and during hemodialysis, to every limb except the arm or leg with the shunt.

2. This will prevent muscle stiffness and soreness. With hemodialysis, the arm or leg with the shunt is left unexercised to avoid dislodging the catheter.

ADULT NURSING

Nursing measures in peritoneal dialysis and hemodialysis

Peritoneal dialysis
• Ask the client to urinate before you insert the catheter into the peritoneum, to prevent bladder puncture.
• Warm the bottles of dialysate in warm water.
• Permit 2 liters of dialysate to flow unrestricted into the peritoneal cavity (this should take about 10 minutes).
• Allow fluid to remain in the cavity for the time ordered by the physician (about 20 to 30 minutes).
• Reverse the bottles; allow fluid to drain from the peritoneal cavity unrestricted (about 20 to 30 minutes). Facilitate drainage by changing the client's position or massaging the abdomen.
• Keep accurate intake and output records related to the amount of dialysis fluid entering the peritoneal cavity and the amount in the drainage. *Important:* Remove all the dialysis fluid.

Hemodialysis
• Observe carefully for breaks or kinks in membranes to prevent hemorrhage.
• Monitor the chemical composition of the dialysate solution, the fluid rate and pressure, and blood clotting time (anticoagulants are administered throughout hemodialysis).
• Provide shunt care:
—Keep the area clean, dry, and sterile.
—Observe the internal fistula for patency. If it is working, you can feel a thrill on palpation or hear a bruit with a stethoscope; if the shunt is discolored, patency is questionable.
—Immediately report clotting to the physician.
—Avoid trauma to the extremity with the shunt (no blood pressure measurement, intramuscular or intravenous medications, or blood drawn).
—Have clamps available to prevent exsanguination if the external shunt disconnects.
• Provide comfort measures for the client.

---

3. Maintain aseptic technique in peritoneal dialysis, with care of the peritoneal catheter and the area around it, and in hemodialysis, with all tubing connections and at the shunt site.

3. Aseptic technique helps prevent infection, a potentially serious complication.

4. Monitor the client's vital signs every 15 minutes (blood pressure will go down as the body loses fluid).

4. Monitoring vital signs helps determine whether the client is losing fluid too rapidly; early detection can prevent complications, such as infection, arrhythmias, and shock.

After dialysis

1. Monitor the client's pulse rate and blood pressure every 15 minutes until the client becomes stable, then every 4 hours.

1. Arrhythmias pose a threat. A client who loses fluid too rapidly will go into hypovolemic shock.

2. Monitor the client's weight daily.

2. This identifies when the client will need dialysis again.

3. Monitor the client's temperature every 4 hours.

3. Infection poses a possible complication.

Evaluation

• Mr. Harvey can explain the principles of dialysis and his participation in the procedure.
• Mr. Harvey and his family are learning to cope with their situation.

COMMUNICABLE DISEASES

Hepatitis B

Viral hepatitis occurs in five major types: hepatitis A, hepatitis B, hepatitis C, hepatitis D, and hepatitis E. A separate virus causes each type of the disease. Each virus destroys liver cells. Viral hepatitis causes the parenchymal or Kupffer's cells of the liver to become severely inflamed, enlarged, and necrotic, leading to stasis of bile outflow. Clients vary somewhat in the severity of the inflammation, which can be mild, moderate, or severe enough to cause death. Bacteria, drugs, chemical agents (such as halothane anesthetic and vinyl chloride), and unknown agents can also cause hepatitis. (See *Comparing types of hepatitis,* page 600.)

The following clinical situation focuses on hepatitis B, the most severe type of hepatitis.

Clinical situation

John Waterman, age 26, enters the hospital with possible viral hepatitis B. A heavy cigarette smoker and a known user of intravenous drugs, he shares an apartment with several persons who also have drug habits. Mr. Waterman has lost weight and appears jaundiced.

Assessment

NURSING BEHAVIORS	NURSING RATIONALES
1. Assess the client's overall health and lifestyle habits.	**1.** Viral hepatitis B can affect people of any age. It spreads by means of blood and blood products, communal use of intravenous needles, sexual intercourse, and human carriers of the virus.
2. Assess the client's vital signs and weight.	**2.** A client with viral hepatitis B may have weight loss, a moderately elevated temperature, hypotension, tachycardia, and tachypnea.
3. Assess the client's food intake, likes, and dislikes.	**3.** A client with viral hepatitis B will have anorexia, nausea, vomiting, and diarrhea or constipation.
4. Assess the color of the client's skin, urine, and stool. Ask him if he has itching (pruritus).	**4.** The client may have jaundice (noted in yellowish conjunctiva and skin tones); urine will be dark from bile content; stools will be clay-colored. Bile pigments irritate nerve endings in skin, causing itching.
5. Assess the location and severity of pain, muscle aches, soreness, and fatigue.	**5.** The client will have headache, malaise, and fatigue and complain of fullness and tenderness in the right upper abdomen. The liver will be markedly enlarged and tender.

Comparing types of hepatitis

Types of hepatitis viruses are named alphabetically in their order of discovery. Knowing the type of virus that has infected a person aids in planning treatment and anticipating outcomes.

	Type A	Type B	Type C	Type D	Type E
Transmission route	Fecal/oral; water-borne, contaminated shellfish or food	Blood or blood products; sexual intercourse; contaminated needles	Transfusion of blood and blood products	Same as C; I.V. drug use	Fecal/oral
Average incubation period	30 days	70 to 80 days	50 days	35 days	42 days
Symptoms	May be absent; headache and other flulike symptoms. Extreme malaise and fatigue, dark urine, jaundice, tender upper right quadrant	Same as A; rash, easy bruising, joint pain	Same as B	Same as B	Same as A; pregnancy increases severity
Treatment	Bed rest, high caloric/protein diet, forced fluids	Same as A; interferon may help if disease course is prolonged	Same as B	Same as B	Same as B
Outcomes	Good. Low mortality (<1.0%), no carrier state	Major cause of cirrhosis. Mortality as high as 10%. Carrier and chronic hepatitis state.	Chronic carrier state. High risk of liver cancer.	Same as B	Same as A; prolonged in pregnancy

6. Assess the client's intake and output.

6. Intake and output will be less than normal body requirements.

Diagnostic evaluation

• *Hematologic and liver function tests* (complete blood count, hematocrit, hemoglobin level, prothrombin time, aspartate aminotransferase, alanine aminotransferase, lactate dehydrogenase, alkaline phosphatase, total protein, albumin-globulin levels, fasting blood glucose, and bilirubin levels): Anemia commonly results from decreased red blood cell life. Prothrombin times may be prolonged because of liver dysfunction. Enzymes will show elevation 4 to 10 times normal because of liver cell necrosis. Protein and serum A/G levels will be abnormally low; serum bilirubin levels will be elevated. (Appendix 1 shows normal liver function levels).

• *Urinalysis:* This will show elevated bilirubin levels. Proteinuria and hematuria may be present.

• *Chest X-ray and electrocardiogram:* These determine the condition of respiratory and cardiac tissues.

• *Liver biopsy:* This may show local or diffuse, widespread necrosis.

• *Serum studies for hepatitis B surface antigen:* This confirms the diagnosis if the antigen is present.

Nursing diagnoses
- Altered nutrition: Less than body requirements, related to anorexia
- Fluid volume deficit related to nausea, vomiting, and diarrhea
- Impaired physical mobility related to bed rest
- Risk for impaired skin integrity related to pruritus
- Social isolation related to bed rest and separation from peers

Planning and goals

Mr. Waterman will:
- recover from hepatitis B without life-threatening sequelae
- regain adequate nutritional and fluid intake
- learn how to prevent reinfection.

Implementation

NURSING BEHAVIORS	NURSING RATIONALES
1. Assist the client with activities of daily living, as needed.	**1.** Hepatitis B commonly causes fatigue and malaise. The client needs frequent rest periods, with activity as tolerated.
2. Monitor vital signs and weight, as ordered.	**2.** The client's temperature may fluctuate and his weight may continue to decrease during the acute stage of the disease.
3. Maintain universal precautions to prevent the spread of hepatitis. Use only disposable equipment. Safely dispose of used materials by bagging and destroying items according to institutional policies.	**3.** Maximum precautions help prevent infecting others with the client's equipment and utensils.
4. Promote gradual intake of high-biologic-value protein with vitamins and minerals; encourage fluid intake; measure intake and output levels.	**4.** Although anorexia may be pronounced, the client's appetite will slowly improve as he recovers. High-biologic-value protein contains all the essential amino acids.
5. Refrain from administering medications, if possible.	**5.** A dysfunctioning liver can't metabolize medications; thus, the client could develop toxicity.
6. Assist the client with range-of-motion exercises, as needed.	**6.** Bed rest and fatigue may prevent the client from maintaining satisfactory muscle mass or function. Hepatitis B has a 6-month recovery period.
7. Teach the client about the disease, methods of transmission, and preventive measures.	**7.** Knowledge deficit is an associated nursing diagnosis. (See *Comparing types of hepatitis* for details.)
8. As the client's condition permits, provide activities to induce a positive mood and self-concept.	**8.** Fatigue and depression may hinder the client in investing full interest or participation.
9. Prepare for home care.	**9.** The client with hepatitis B is discharged when his condition improves sufficiently for him to continue recovery at home.

10. Contact community nursing service personnel.

10. Follow-up care at home is vital to the health and safety of the client and of those in contact with him. Epidemiologic studies and actions help prevent additional transmission.

Evaluation

Mr. Waterman:
• follows a progressive course toward recovery by the time of discharge
• has no apparent sequelae (sequelae include chronic hepatitis, cirrhosis, and hepatoma)
• regains a healthy appetite and fluid intake
• can state ways to prevent transmission to others.

Acquired immunodeficiency syndrome (AIDS)

Researchers first recognized AIDS in 1981. A severe immune deficiency that leaves the individual susceptible to life-threatening, opportunistic illness characterizes this disorder, which arises from the human immunodeficiency virus (HIV). The virus enters the T lymphocytes and reproduces, damaging the lymphocytes.

Modes of transmission include sexual contact, exposure to infected blood or blood products, and pregnancy (mother to neonate). Current epidemiologic evidence shows blood, semen, vaginal secretions, and breast milk to be sources of transmission. AIDS can occur in sexual partners (male and female) of infected individuals, injection drug users who share equipment, clients who received contaminated blood transfusions (particularly before routine blood screening), and babies of infected mothers.

HIV infection runs a continuum from HIV-positive but without symptoms, to mild symptoms, to full-blown clinical disease. Present knowledge indicates that 6 to 11 years can pass between the asymptomatic phase and the active phase. Current research indicates that zidovudine, or AZT, an antiviral agent, is effective in delaying the onset of clinical disease. The availability of HIV protease inhibitors (such as ritonavir) has increased therapeutic options. Ongoing research continues to change recommendations regarding drug therapies. Clinical disease is present when the client develops life-threatening infections or cancer.

As with all communicable diseases, nursing considerations for a client with HIV include strict attention to the universal body fluid precautions, including those listed here:
• Promote barrier protection by all health care workers.
• Wash hands thoroughly, using aseptic technique, before and after contacting the client.
• Wear gloves, masks, goggles, a face shield, and a gown, as necessary, to prevent direct contact with blood and body fluids.
• Immediately discard used needles and syringes in puncture-proof containers. Do not recap the needle or attempt to remove it from the syringe.

The following clinical situation focuses on nursing care of an injection drug user infected with HIV.

Clinical situation   LaMont Williams, age 30, has a history of I.V. drug abuse. He arrives at the medical clinic complaining of shortness of breath, hacking cough, and loss of appetite. He has lost 20 lb over the past several months. Diagnostic testing reveals that he has *Pneumocystis carinii* pneumonia and HIV. His CD4 lymphocyte count has decreased from 220 to 160/mm^3.

Assessment

NURSING BEHAVIORS	NURSING RATIONALES
1. Assess the client for fatigue, lethargy, weakness, anorexia, weight loss, enlarged lymph glands, diarrhea, night sweats, pallor, and fever.	**1.** These are all nonspecific signs of decreasing immunocompetence seen in people with AIDS.
2. Note signs of increasing dyspnea, cyanosis, and pain on respiration.	**2.** Extensive infection with *P. carinii* causes shortness of breath and extreme air hunger.
3. Examine the skin for dark purplish-blue lesions that may be ulcerated.	**3.** These are signs of Kaposi's sarcoma, an otherwise rare cancer that commonly occurs in those with AIDS. It affects the endothelial lining of the heart, vascular system, lymph tissue, and serous membranes.
4. Assess for herpesvirus.	**4.** All types of herpes are common in AIDS.
5. Examine the client's mouth for white plaques and hairy leukoplakia.	**5.** Candidiasis is a common opportunistic infection. Infection with Epstein-Barr virus is common in clients whose first manifestation of AIDS is *P. carinii* pneumonia.
6. Observe for signs of cytomegalovirus (CMV), which can affect many organs and cause retinitis, pneumonitis, and colitis.	**6.** CMV is a common opportunistic infection.
7. Thoroughly assess the neurologic system for flulike symptoms (fever, headache, sweats), aseptic meningitis (headache, stiff neck), AIDS dementia complex (headache, inability to concentrate, forgetfulness), spinal cord degeneration (myelopathy), and peripheral neuropathy.	**7.** These symptoms can result when HIV directly invades the brain cells. Neurologic infections from *Toxoplasmosis* and *Cryptococcus neoformans* can also occur.
8. Continually monitor the client's vital signs, and immediately report significant changes to the physician.	**8.** Ongoing assessment of the client's condition is vital—immunosuppression can make almost any organ system vulnerable to breakdown.

Diagnostic evaluation   • *Screening:* The enzyme-linked immunoassay (ELISA) test will detect HIV antibodies, indicating exposure (false-positive results are possible, however). If this test yields a positive result, test with the Western blot assay, which is more specific and thus acts as a follow-up test for antibodies if ELISA proves seropositive.

   Important: Antibodies require 6 to 8 weeks to develop after the client's exposure to HIV. Some authorities believe antibody development occurs for as long as 1 year, which would produce many false-negative results.

• *Chest X-ray:* Identifies pulmonary pathologic conditions.

ADULT NURSING

• *Bronchoscopy:* Confirms *P. carinii.*
• *Stool culture:* Detects such organisms as *Cryptosporidium muris,* a common cause of diarrhea in those with AIDS.
• *Viral titers:* Confirm presence of certain viral infections
• *Serum blood tests:* Identify decreased white blood cell and lymphocyte counts.
• *Tissue biopsy:* Tests for Kaposi's sarcoma, if suspected.

Nursing diagnoses

• Impaired gas exchange related to respiratory infection
• Altered nutrition: Less than body requirements, related to anorexia, weight loss, and possible GI manifestations
• Risk for infection related to impaired immunocompetence
• Diarrhea related to GI infection
• Activity intolerance related to weakness and air hunger
• Body image disturbance related to weight loss
• Impaired home maintenance management related to debilitation
• Social isolation related to possible rejection by peers
• Fear related to the disease's life-threatening consequences
• Sensory or perceptual (visual) alterations related to neurologic complications

Planning and goals

Mr. Williams will:
• make lifestyle adjustments required to cope with AIDS
• maintain adequate oxygenation
• engage in behaviors that prevent the spread of HIV
• remain free of complications for as long as possible.

Clinical situation
(continued)

Nursing implementations for Mr. Williams will not necessarily apply to all clients with pneumonia and HIV. Interventions vary according to each client's unique problems. For instance, if the client is receiving chemotherapy for Kaposi's sarcoma or another cancer, implementations on pages 609 to 615 in "Chemotherapy" also apply.

Implementation

NURSING BEHAVIORS

1. Encourage the client to enter a drug treatment program. If the client refuses, teach safe handling of equipment. The client must *never* share equipment with anyone.

2. Instruct the client on sexual practices that reduce the risk of transmission, such as using a latex condom, spermicide, and water-based lubricant (such as K-Y jelly) for vaginal or anal intercourse.

NURSING RATIONALES

1. A drug treatment program may help the client reduce or eliminate his dependency on drugs. A client's refusal to participate in such a program should not prevent the nurse from teaching safe handling of equipment, which not only will benefit the client but also will reduce the risk of his spreading HIV via contaminated equipment.

2. Abstinence is the only sure way to prevent the spread of HIV through sexual contact. When this is not realistic, so-called safer sexual practices reduce the risk of transmission. A condom provides a barrier for semen. Nonoxynol 9, contained in spermicide, may give added protection but should be used with a condom. Water-based lubricants help prevent the condom from breaking; oil-based lubricants such as petrolatum (Vaseline) weaken latex and may cause the condom to break.

ADULT NURSING

3. Relieve respiratory distress, as follows:

• Administer oxygen.

• Institute chest physiotherapy.

• Teach the client diaphragmatic and pursed-lip breathing, and tell him to avoid smoking.

• Administer antibiotics, such as trimethoprim sulfamethoxazole (TMP-SMZ) and pentamidine (an antiprotozoal agent), as ordered, and monitor the client for side effects. Preventive treatment is recommended for a client whose CD4 lymphocyte count drops below 200/mm^3.

4. Take steps to increase the client's appetite: Administer an antiemetic 30 minutes before meals; provide small, frequent meals; and encourage frequent oral hygiene. (See *Nutrition and AIDS,* page 606.)

5. Administer antidiarrheals and prevent perianal skin breakdown.

6. Prevent complications from immobility by turning and repositioning the client frequently and by promoting ambulation.

7. Thoroughly wash the client's skin, pat dry (do not rub), and apply lotion.

8. Provide oral care. Have the client use a soft toothbrush or cotton swab, and tell him to brush after each meal. Moisturize the lips if needed.

9. Teach the client to balance activity with rest.

10. Protect the client from injury; for example, have him use a nonskid bath mat, and caution him not to use throw rugs.

11. Support all medical therapies.

3. Respiratory distress warrants immediate relief.

• Oxygen administration relieves hypoxemia present with extensive *Pneumocystis* infection.

• This mobilizes secretions from the chest and helps maintain a patent airway.

• Breathing exercises enhance respirations. Smoking (and other forms of smoke) should be avoided to prevent further lung damage.

• *P. carinii* pneumonia (PCP) is treated with TMP-SMZ; side effects include rash, decreased white blood cell count, and fever. For those who can tolerate it, TMP-SMZ is used to prevent PCP. Pentamidine is used to treat and prevent PCP; side effects include leukopenia, sterile abscesses, and renal damage.

4. Antiemetic medications help control nausea. Small, frequent meals are more appealing to and better tolerated by an anorectic client than the standard three meals a day. Frequent oral hygiene refreshes the mouth and may help improve appetite.

5. Diarrhea is a common complication of GI infection and chemotherapy.

6. As the client gets weaker, the risk of complications from immobility becomes greater.

7. Proper skin care helps prevent irritation and drying.

8. Oral care prevents trauma, reduces the risk of infection, and refreshes the mouth. Moisturizing the lips prevents drying and cracking.

9. This helps avoid fatigue, which becomes a more challenging task as the client's condition weakens.

10. The client's weakened immune system renders him highly susceptible to injury.

11. Various treatments may be used to delay progression of the client's disease and to prevent replication of HIV. Treatment may include chemotherapy as well as administration of antifungal agents, acyclovir (for herpes), and antiviral agents such as azidothymidine (zidovudine; Retrovir).

ADULT NURSING

Nutrition and AIDS

Clinical manifestations that alter nutritional status
• Weight loss
—Progressive and unexplained loss (wasting syndrome)
—Massive loss (20 to 40 lbs) with severe diarrhea
—Reduced appetite secondary to malaise, depression, or drug therapy
—Early satiety related to massive hepatomegaly or splenomegaly
• Diarrhea (can be severe, as much as 1 liter/day)
• Other GI symptoms
—Dysphagia
—Steatorrhea
—Lactose intolerance
—Nausea and vomiting
—Abdominal pain
—Taste alterations
—Malabsorption
—Alterations in metabolism of nutrients

Nutrition support
• For outpatient clients (those infected with HIV) to supplement calories and protein:
—Whole milk and cream
—Liberal use of butter, margarine, and mayonnaise

—Sauces and gravies
—Toppings (nuts, whipped cream, sour cream, frostings)
—Nonfat dry milk added to home-baked goods, hot cereals, soups, and desserts
• For inpatient clients (those with AIDS or AIDS-related complex) who have a good appetite, minimal malabsorption, moderate diarrhea, and semi-solid stool:
—High calories
—High protein
—Low fat (about 3% of total calorie intake)
—Lactose-free dairy foods
—Oral food supplement (such as Vivonex TEN or Resource)
• For inpatient clients with severe diarrhea:
—Short-term use of the BRAT diet: Bananas, Rice, Apples, and Tea or Toast
—Oral food supplement (such as Vivonex TEN or Resource)

Note: Vivonex TEN is best accepted in chilled water, soft drink, or juice when taken orally. Enteral feeding may be accomplished with Vivonex TEN or Compleat Modified Formula. Parenteral nutrition for AIDS clients remains controversial because of the increased risk of infection at the catheter site.

---

12. Provide generous emotional support to the client and loved ones. Encourage the client to voice concerns and grieve for losses. Refer him to professional and lay support services for additional guidance and comfort.

12. A multidisciplinary, holistic approach best serves the client, who is striving to cope with grieving, social isolation, job loss, financial devastation, physical and emotional depletion, and the fear of suffering and death.

13. Continually monitor the client for opportunistic infections.

13. *Mycobacterium avium complex* (MAC) occurs later in the disease when the CD4 level drops below 100/mm^3. The client may be placed on prophylactic therapy with the antitubercular rifabutin.

Evaluation

• Mr. Williams has entered a drug treatment program.
• Mr. Williams reports that he now uses a condom when having intercourse.
• Mr. Williams is currently free of respiratory distress.
• Mr. Williams is receiving support services through his community's AIDS Project.

ONCOLOGY NURSING

Introduction

Cancer is a malignant neoplasm, or tumor, characterized by uncontrolled cell growth that can metastasize (spread). Characteristically, malignant neoplasms are poorly differentiated, immature cells lacking resemblance to the parent cell. These cells grow rapidly, are not encapsulated, frequently recur after removal, and infiltrate surrounding tissues. Metastasis proceeds in three ways: by local extension, by movement through the blood or the lymphatic system, or by seeding in the serous membrane of the peritoneum or pleura. Common sites for metastasis include the long bones, brain, lungs, heart, liver, and skin. Some form of cancer develops in one of four Americans, making it the second leading cause of death in the United States.

Cancer screening and assessment

I. **Risk factors**
    A. Heredity
        1. Retinoblastoma and Wilms' tumor are examples of genetic neoplasms
        2. Cancer incidence increases with genetic disorders, such as Down syndrome
    B. Family history
    C. Acquired disorders (for example, pernicious anemia, ulcerative colitis, cirrhosis, hepatitis, and obesity)
    D. Environmental hazards
        1. Workplace carcinogens include asbestos, hydrocarbons, inorganic compounds, wood fibers, dust, leather, and heavy metal
        2. Homesite hazards may include asbestos, nearby chemical dumps and factories, and long-term exposure to air pollution
        3. Radiation exposure affects health care workers, neonates whose mothers were exposed to high levels during pregnancy, and persons exposed to nuclear explosions
    E. Lifestyle choices
        1. Tobacco and alcohol consumption have a synergistic effect
        2. Food additives (such as cyclamates, nitrites, and saccharin), obesity, and decreased dietary fiber increase the client's cancer risks
        3. Certain sexual behaviors increase the client's exposure to viruses, especially herpesvirus, type II, which increases a female client's risk of developing cervical cancer
    F. Skin factors
        1. Precancerous lesions (such as leukoplakia, certain moles, senile keratoses, cervical dysplasia, and polyps in the colon and rectum) predispose the client to skin cancer
        2. Any chronically irritated skin site or prolonged exposure to the sun can lead to cancer

ADULT NURSING

II. Assessment

A. During the health history and physical examination, consider the American Cancer Society's seven warning signs of cancer
1. Change in bowel or bladder habits
2. A sore that does not heal
3. Unusual bleeding or discharge
4. Thickening or a lump in breast or elsewhere
5. Ingestion or difficulty swallowing
6. Obvious change in a wart or mole
7. Nagging cough or hoarseness

B. Inspect the client thoroughly to detect asymmetry

C. Check the client's skin for the following
1. Ulcerations or change in lesions
2. Persistent ulceration and changes in pigmented lesions
3. Nodules (small, nodular, roughened areas with telangiectatic vessels may indicate basal cell cancer)
4. Pruritus (prevalent in Hodgkin's disease)
5. Petechiae or purpura (indicate hemorrhage)

D. Check the client's head and neck for the following
1. Leukoplakia, a precancerous lesion
2. One-sided, friable lesions that don't heal
3. Lymph node abnormalities (enlarged, hard, or fixed lymph nodes warrant further investigation)

E. Look for unilateral chest changes, such as asymmetry, dimpling, abnormal contour, and skin lesions

F. Assess the abdomen for a tumorous growth or obstruction, noting the following
1. Absent or altered bowel sounds
2. Change in contour or symmetry
3. Palpable mass or tenderness

G. Assess male genitalia
1. Prostate (by anterior rectal examination; hard, nodular, or asymmetrical posterior prostate may indicate prostatic cancer)
2. Scrotum and testes (testicular tumors occur most commonly in men ages 20 to 35)

H. Assess female genitalia, checking the cervix for cervical cancer signs
1. Precancerous lesions
2. Cyanosis
3. Ulceration or erosion, if the client is pregnant
4. Leukoplakia

III. Client teaching

A. Provide the client with a copy of the American Cancer Society's seven warning signs of cancer (see above)

B. If the client is not at high risk, recommend the following examinations
1. Physical examination every 3 years between ages 20 and 40 and a yearly examination after age 40
2. Breast examinations (female clients)
   a. Self-examination (95% of breast cancers are discovered by the client)

(1) Teach breast self-examination to girls when they start to menstruate
(2) Encourage monthly examination at the same time each month (3 to 5 days after the menstrual period ends)
(3) Advise postmenopausal women to examine their breasts on the 1st day of each month
(4) Teach the client to report asymmetry, dimpling, abnormal contour, masses, or lesions
b. Mammography (soft-tissue X-ray of the breast)
(1) A baseline X-ray should be taken between ages 35 and 40
(2) An X-ray should be taken every 1 to 2 years between ages 40 and 50 and yearly after age 50
3. Pelvic examination every 3 years until age 40, then yearly
4. Papanicolaou (Pap) smear to detect cervical cancer at age 18 (after three negative results, 1 year apart, then per physician recommendation)
5. Endometrial biopsy at menopause if client is high-risk
6. Digital rectal examination to detect rectosigmoidal or prostate cancer (recommended yearly for men over age 40)
7. Stool guaiac test yearly after age 50
8. Proctoscopic examination after age 50 (after two negative exams, 1 year apart, then every 3 to 5 years)
9. Testicular self-examination (male clients) every month to screen for testicular tumor
C. Advise a high-risk client to consult the physician about more frequent examinations

Chemotherapy

Various chemotherapeutic agents interfere with cell growth during different cell division phases (see *Chemotherapeutic agents,* page 610). These agents may be used singly or in combination, either as primary or as supplemental cancer therapy (for example, after surgery). Diligent assessment and nursing care are essential for the client undergoing chemotherapy because the drugs can have serious toxic side effects.

The following text focuses on nursing care of a client undergoing chemotherapy and having various side effects, such as skin disorders, alopecia, bone marrow depression (decrease in red blood cells, white blood cells, and thrombocytes), GI disorders (stomatitis, anorexia, nausea, vomiting, and bowel elimination changes), and renal and neurologic disorders.

Assessment

NURSING BEHAVIORS	NURSING RATIONALES
1. Assess the skin daily for hirsutism, increased pigmentation, erythema, dermatitis, urticaria, photosensitivity, jaundice, and pruritus.	**1.** Skin disorders are possible side effects of chemotherapy. Jaundice forewarns of hepatic damage.
2. Assess for hair loss.	**2.** Alopecia, a side effect of many chemotherapy agents, usually begins about 3 weeks after treatment.

Chemotherapeutic agents

DRUG	ACTION	ADVERSE REACTIONS
Alkylating agents busulfan (Myleran) carboplatin (Paraplatin) carmustine (BiCNU) chlorambucil (Leukeran) cisplatin (Platinol) cyclophosphamide (Cytoxan) dacarbazine (DTIC-Dome) ifosfamide (IFEX) lomustine (CCNU) meclorethamine (Mustargen) melphalan (Alkeran) streptozocin (Zanosar)thiotepa uracil mustard	Inhibit DNA synthesis. Active in all phases of cell cycle.	Hemorrhagic cystitis, nausea, vomiting (may be severe), bone marrow depression, pulmonary fibrosis, stomatitis, cardiac toxicity, alopecia, hypouricemia, skin rashes, renal impairment (especially with cisplatin), ototoxicity (cisplatin). Some drugs are vesicants when they infiltrate (dacarbazine, meclorethamine).
Antibiotics bleomycin (Blenoxane) dactinomycin (Cosmegen) daunorubicin (Cerubidine) doxorubicin (Adriamycin) mitomycin (Mutamycin) plicamycin (Mithracin) procarbazine (Matulane)	Block development of new DNA and RNA. Active in all phases of cell cycle.	Pulmonary fibrosis, pneumonitis, cardiac toxicity, bone marrow depression, nausea, vomiting, alopecia, stomatitis, hallucinations, confusion, hepatotoxicity, severe tissue damage with extravasation (dactinomycin, doxorubicin, mitomycin, plicamycin).
Antimetabolites cytarabine (Cytosar-U) floxuridine (FUDR) fluorouracil (Adrucil) hydroxyurea (Hydrea) mercaptopurine (Purinethol) methotrexate (Folex) thioguanine	Interfere with DNA synthesis. Work on s-phase of cell cycle.	Stomatitis, oral and GI ulcerations, nausea, vomiting, bone marrow depression, hepatotoxicity, renal impairment, pneumonitis.
Plant alkaloids vinblastine (Velban) vincristine (Oncovin)	Inhibit cell division in metaphase of cell cycle.	Central nervous system toxicity, peripheral neuropathy, paralytic ileus.
Hormones aminoglutethimide (Cytadren)	Blocks synthesis of glucocorticoids.	Bone marrow depression, hyperglycemia, impotence, gynecomastia, drowsiness, hepatitis, hot flashes, hypotension, tachycardia, adrenal insufficiency, masculinization, hirsutism, nausea, vomiting, diarrhea, hypercalcemia, skin rash, dermatitis, fever, myalgia.
estramustine phosphate sodium (Emcyt)	Alkylates (crosslinks) DNA in prostatic cancer tissue.	
flutamide (Eulexin)	Blocks androgen receptors.	
goserelin acetate (Zoladex)	Decreases secretion of FSH and LH; lowers testosterone levels in males.	
leuprolide acetate (Lupron)	Same as above.	Myocardial infarction, pulmonary embolism, edema, hot flashes.
megestrol acetate (Megace)	Alters hormonal environment in tumor tissue.	Nausea, vomiting, abdominal pain, breast sensitivity.
mitotane (Lysodren)	Selectively destroys adrenocortical tissue.	Lethargy, neurologic damage, nausea, vomiting.
tamoxifen citrate (Nolvadex)	Acts as an estrogen antagonist.	Nausea, vomiting, hot flashes, vascular thrombosis.
testolactone (Teslac)	Same as megestrol.	Edema, nausea, vomiting.
trilostane (Modrastane)	Inhibits production of glucocorticoids.	Headache, orthostatic hypertension, nausea, diarrhea.

3. Monitor erythrocyte, hematocrit (Hct), and hemoglobin(Hbg) values (Normal values: red blood cells [RBCs], 4.2 million to 5.4 million/mm^3; Hct, 40% to 48%; Hbg, 12 to 16 g/dl).

3. Decreased RBCs signal bone marrow depression, a common side effect of chemotherapy.

4. Assess the client's complaints of fatigue and headache.

4. Anemia causes increased fatigue and headache.

5. Monitor the client's white blood cell (WBC) count.

5. With bone marrow depression, leukopenia (a WBC count below 6,000/mm3) increases the client's susceptibility to infection.

6. Monitor the platelet count for thrombocytopenia (platelet count below 100,000/mm^3). Check oral mucous membranes, urine, and stools for blood. Watch for petechiae (tiny, rashlike skin hemorrhages) and ecchymoses (bruises).

6. Chemotherapy causes thrombocyte reduction and internal bleeding.

7. Observe for stomatitis.

7. Stomatitis may affect any mucous membrane, especially in the mouth. Manifestations include redness, edema, and dry, burning sensations. Having stomatitis increases the client's chances of developing secondary infection. Stomatitis causes severe discomfort. If it develops, the drug dosage may be reduced or discontinued.

8. Observe for anorexia.

8. Appetite loss may result from GI tract irritation or an unpleasant taste in the mouth.

9. Anticipate nausea and vomiting.

9. Stimulation of the medulla oblongata by the irritated GI tract causes reverse peristalsis.

10. Monitor for diarrhea and gastric ulceration and perforation.

10. Diarrhea results from irritation and damage to the rapidly regenerating GI tract mucosal cells. Black stools may indicate GI bleeding.

11. Be alert for complaints of constipation.

11. Constipation may indicate neurotoxicity. Other symptoms include abdominal tenderness, rigidity, and distention, which could indicate paralytic ileus.

12. Monitor urine output and characteristics.

12. Chemotherapy increases the potential for developing nephrotoxicity.

13. Monitor blood urea nitrogen (BUN) and creatinine levels.

13. Elevated BUN and creatinine levels suggest kidney damage.

14. Observe for urinary frequency and urgency, pain on urination, blood in urine, and renal calculi.

14. Hemorrhagic cystitis is a possible complication of chemotherapy.

15. Observe for paresthesias, decreased reflexes, gait changes, seizures, and confusion.

15. Chemotherapeutic agents derive from plants. The plant alkaloids vincristine and vinblastine are neurotoxins. Nerve damage is a side effect.

ADULT NURSING

16. Ascertain the client's pulmonary function by auscultating the lungs, checking for signs of dyspnea, and reviewing the results of chest X-rays and pulmonary function tests.

16. Pneumonitis and pulmonary fibrosis are complications of some chemotherapeutic agents.

17. Monitor the client's pulse rate.

17. Some agents are cardiotoxic, which could manifest as tachycardia.

18. Monitor for fever and chills.

18. Many chemotherapeutic agents cause this type of febrile reaction.

19. Assess the client's coping skills and emotional response to treatment.

19. Chemotherapy causes emotional distress for many clients.

Nursing diagnoses

- Impaired skin integrity related to the side effects of chemotherapy
- Sleep pattern disturbance related to pruritus
- Body image disturbance related to hair loss
- Activity intolerance related to anemia and fatigue
- Risk for infection related to a low white blood cell (WBC) count
- Risk for injury related to a low platelet count
- Altered nutrition: Less than body requirements, related to nausea and vomiting
- Diarrhea related to damaged GI mucosa from chemotherapeutic agents
- Fluid volume deficit related to vomiting and diarrhea

Planning and goals

The client will:
- be free of pruritus, infection, constipation, diarrhea, and renal and nerve damage
- adjust to an altered body image
- conserve energy and rest at frequent intervals
- experience no bleeding or other injury
- maintain weight, nutritional status, and fluid and electrolyte balance.

Implementation

NURSING BEHAVIORS

NURSING RATIONALES

1. Urge the client to keep fingernails short, to use antihistaminic lotions or colloidal baths, and to wear gloves at night.

1. These strategies decrease the risk of secondary infection with pruritus (itching) and provide relief from pruritus.

2. Administer diphenhydramine hydrochloride (Benadryl) as needed.

2. Antihistamines relieve pruritus.

3. Provide sleeping medication, if needed.

3. For many clients, the effects of pruritus seem worse at night, when fewer diversions exist. Medication helps the client sleep through the night.

4. Instruct a client taking methotrexate to avoid sunlight.

4. Methotrexate causes photosensitivity.

5. Reassure the client that hair loss is temporary.

5. Hair loss causes extreme body image alterations. Although hair usually grows back within 8 weeks, the color and texture may be changed.

ADULT NURSING

6. Provide emotional support.

6. The client needs support and an opportunity to express feelings related to an altered body image.

7. Consider applying a scalp tourniquet or an ice cap during chemotherapy treatments.

7. These implements reduce hair loss. However, their use for clients with leukemia remains controversial because they may create a reservoir for leukemic cells.

8. Encourage the client to prepare for hair loss by obtaining and using wigs, caps, or scarves.

8. Obtained before alopecia starts, cosmetic head coverings will help the client cope with an altered body image.

9. Plan client care so that it does not interfere with rest periods.

9. The nursing care plan should be organized to allow for the client's increasing fatigue.

10. Transfuse with red blood cells (RBCs), as ordered.

10. Transfusion raises the hematocrit, hemoglobin, and RBC values. However, it also increases the reaction risk.

11. Provide a diet high in protein, iron, vitamin C, B complex vitamins, and calories.

11. Nutritional iron helps prevent anemia. Vitamin C promotes iron absorption, advances healing, and improves resistance to infection. The client needs protein for normal body function and to promote healing. B complex vitamins promote metabolic functions.

12. Institute infection control measures:
• Provide protective isolation.
• Maintain aseptic technique and wash hands before and after any procedure.
• Caution the client to avoid crowds.
• Check all orifices for infection.

12. The objective is to protect the client from the environment. A client whose WBC count falls below 2,000/mm^3 risks developing a life-threatening infection. Such a client should also avoid raw vegetables, which can carry dangerous organisms. Severe leukopenia may require drug discontinuance.

13. Do not use venipuncture, parenteral injections, rectal thermometers, or other invasive procedures. Encourage the client to use a soft toothbrush or disposable tooth cleaner (Toothette), electric razor, and so forth.

13. If the client's platelet count falls below 100,000/mm^3, the risk of hemorrhage increases. All precautions must be taken to prevent bleeding.

14. Infuse thrombocytes as needed.

14. This may be the only way to stop a hemorrhage once it starts.

15. Provide a bland, soft diet and lukewarm liquids. Tell the client to avoid tart and spicy foods.

15. Bland foods and beverages are easy to digest and will minimize oral discomfort and tissue trauma if stomatitis develops. Sometimes irritation is so severe that the client must be fed by tube.

16. Prohibit commercial mouthwashes. Instead, have the client use a soft toothbrush and normal saline solution, or provide an antifungal mouthwash such as nystatin (Mycostatin). Have the client use an anesthetic mouthwash such as lidocaine (Xylocaine Viscous Solution) before meals.

16. Commercial mouthwashes may contain alcohol, an irritant to a client with stomatitis. An antifungal mouthwash helps combat *Candida* (fungus) overgrowth, which commonly accompanies chemotherapy. An anesthetic mouthwash decreases the client's discomfort, thereby enabling him to eat.

ADULT NURSING

17. Provide oral care before meals.

17. Providing oral care before meals stimulates salivary flow and creates a pleasant taste.

18. Provide small, frequent, high-protein meals or tube feedings, or total parenteral nutrition.

18. Small meals are more appetizing to the anorexic client than large ones. To meet the body's nutritional needs, foods must have high nutritional value.

19. Administer an antiemetic 30 minutes before administering chemotherapy and 30 minutes before meals.

19. An antiemetic decreases vomiting by its action on the vomiting center in the medulla oblongata, thereby allowing the client to retain foods.

20. Offer hard candy.

20. Hard candy reduces nausea.

21. Provide a laxative, stool softeners, bulk, and fluids.

21. These prevent constipation and impaction in a client receiving plant alkaloids.

22. If the client has diarrhea, clean the anal area with mild, soft soap; give the client a sitz bath; and apply A and D ointment to the irritated area.

22. These strategies promote hygiene, provide comfort, and prevent excoriation.

23. Give the client low-residue foods and beverages.

23. A low-residue diet decreases irritation and bulk in the GI tract.

24. Administer antidiarrheal medications.

24. Diphenoxylate hydrochloride (Lomotil) acts by decreasing peristalsis. Kaolin and pectin mixtures (Kaopectate) act as a protective and adsorbent.

25. Force fluids. If the client is receiving cisplatin, administer 1 to 2 liters of an I.V. solution before cisplatin and a diuretic.

25. Forcing fluids replaces fluids lost through vomiting and diarrhea, flushes the urinary tract, and helps prevent problems from cystitis and uric acid buildup.

26. Alkalinize the client's urine.

26. Cellular breakdown leads to uric acid buildup. Uric acid calculi can be prevented (partly) with an alkaline ash diet. (See *Diet considerations for clients with renal calculi,* page 589).

27. Administer allopurinol, as ordered.

27. Allopurinol inhibits uric acid production.

28. Monitor the client's urine output, review renal function tests, and weigh the client daily. Note any problems indicating nephrotoxicity and fluid overload.

28. Renal toxicity should be identified to prevent fluid volume overload and electrolyte imbalances.

29. Administer antipyretics, as ordered.

29. Antipyretics help control febrile response.

Evaluation

- The client's pruritus is relieved.
- The client copes effectively with alopecia.
- The client's erythrocyte, hematocrit, and hemoglobin values stay within normal limits.
- The client's conserved energy permits him to perform activities of daily living.
- The client remains infection free.
- The client does not hemorrhage.

ADULT NURSING

• The client maintains weight and nutritional status.
• The client's fluid and electrolyte balance remains within normal limits.
• The client maintains his normal elimination pattern.
• The client does not experience renal damage.
• The client has no nerve damage as a result of chemotherapy.

Radiation therapy

Radiation therapy makes use of electromagnetic energy waves for diagnosis (to identify internal anatomic structures) and for therapy (to control cell growth). Common diagnostic agents include X-rays and radioactive isotopes such as iodine 131 (^{131}I). Therapeutic radiation may be administered externally or internally. External-beam therapy or teletherapy is administered by megavoltage (which delivers the dose to superficial lesions) or orthovoltage (which delivers the dose to deeper body structures and spares the skin from damage). Internal administration consists of implanting radioactive elements temporarily or permanently.

Radioactive isotopes, the radiation source, occur naturally (as with radium) or synthetically (as with cobalt 60 [^{60}Co], cesium 137 [^{137}Cs], and gold 198 [^{198}Au]).

Radioactive substances emit three types of rays: alpha, beta, and gamma. Alpha rays, the least potent, cannot penetrate skin; they can be shielded by a sheet of paper. Beta rays can penetrate some tissues but can be stopped by a thin metal shield. Gamma rays, stopped only by lead shields, penetrate most tissues.

As a health care provider, you must know how to protect yourself and your clients from radiation. Consider three elements—time, distance, and shielding—when providing protection from radiation:

Time: An isotope's half-life is the time it takes for half of its emissions to decay, thereby reducing by half the risk of exposure. Because the half-lives of radioactive elements vary widely, you should know the elements being used and their half-lives. Provide competent care, quickly but responsibly, and rotate care-giving opportunities to minimize exposure. Always remember to wear a dosimeter, which measures total cumulative radiation exposure.

Distance: Your distance from the radiation source determines the degree of exposure to radiation. Radiation's intensity is measured according to the inverse square rule; for example, 2′ from the source of radiation exposure is $^1/_4$ the exposure at 1′, or $[(^1/_1) = 1, (^1/_2)^2 = ^1/_4]$. At 4′ from the source, exposure would be $^1/_{16}$ the exposure at 1′, or $(^1/_4)^2 = ^1/_{16}$. Therefore, to protect yourself when giving care to clients receiving radiation therapy, increase your distance from the radiation source whenever possible. Also, treat the client in a private room to protect other clients from radiation. (For further information, see *Distance from radiation exposure,* page 616.)

Shielding: A shield also protects you from radiation. Knowing the kinds of rays emitted from the elements in use helps you select the appropriate shield. Wear a lead-lined apron and gloves near gamma ray (most common) emissions, and store radioactive substances in lead containers.

External-beam radiation therapy

With external-beam radiation therapy, client care depends on the type and amount of radiation administered. Radiation therapy also affects rapidly dividing normal cells. Especially affected are the blood-forming organs, mucosal cells (especially in the GI tract), the bladder, the gonads, and the epithelium. Nursing care for clients with these problems is the same as for clients receiving chemotherapy. Radiation effects are usually only seen locally in the area being treated.

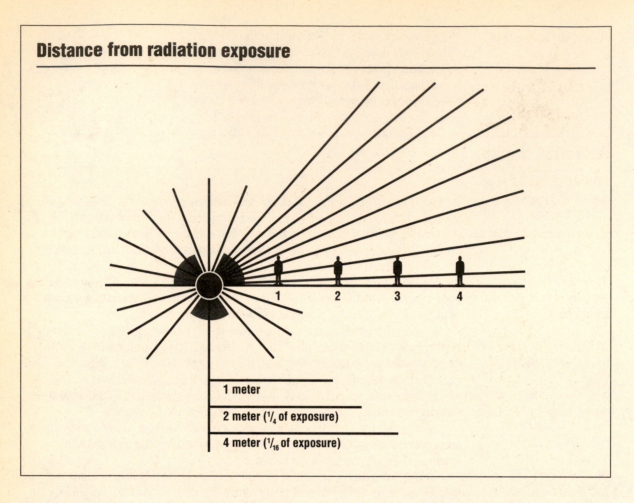

Distance from radiation exposure

1

2

3

4

1 meter

2 meter (¹/₄ of exposure)

4 meter (¹/₁₆ of exposure)

Clinical situation   Samuel Martin, age 56, is receiving a series of external beam radiation therapy treatments for a localized, nonresectable, intrathoracic lung lesion.

Assessment

NURSING BEHAVIORS

1. Observe the client's skin for erythema, pigmentation, desquamation, ulceration, sloughing, and alopecia.

2. Assess for systemic reactions similar to those caused by chemotherapeutic agents.

NURSING RATIONALES

1. Caused by radiation's action on the epithelium, pigmentation and other side effects start within 24 to 48 hours of therapy. They disappear initially but reappear in about 10 days.

2. Systemic responses occur because radiation damages the rapidly growing mucous membranes of the GI tract, bladder, and blood-forming organs.

Nursing diagnoses
- Risk for injury related to cellular damage from radiation
- Impaired skin integrity related to desquamation of tissue
- Social isolation related to the physical isolation necessary for a client with an internal implant

ADULT NURSING

Planning and goals   The client will:
- be free of injury
- have no skin ulcerations
- maintain appropriate social interaction
- feel comfortable and pain-free.

Note: Nursing implementations for radiation therapy usually include those for chemotherapy (see pages 609 to 615). The following implementations relate only to clients receiving radiation therapy.

Implementation

NURSING BEHAVIORS	NURSING RATIONALES
1. Do not remove port marks from the client's skin.	**1.** The radiotherapist places these purple marks to define the exact application site.
2. Gently clean the area between port marks with water only; do not use soaps or powder with a metal (zinc) base.	**2.** The area is sensitive. Soaps will dry skin. Anything with a metal base increases the amount of radiation absorbed.
3. Tell the client to avoid exposing the irradiated area to excessive sunlight, heat, and cold.	**3.** Exposure increases the risk of skin damage.
4. Do not apply regular tape to the client's skin. To secure a loose dressing, use hypoallergenic tape.	**4.** This will avoid unduly irritating the skin.
5. Urge the client to wear loose clothing.	**5.** This will eliminate friction over the area.
6. Advise the client to use an electric razor for shaving, if necessary.	**6.** Radiation therapy makes the skin sensitive and prone to injury.
7. Pat, don't rub, the skin.	**7.** Patting minimizes friction.
8. Check with the radiotherapist before using any ointment (usually, cornstarch, lanolin, and A and D ointment are safe).	**8.** Some ointments increase the radiation dose. The listed skin-care products will not irritate the skin.

Evaluation

- The client successfully completes radiation therapy.
- The client experiences minimal side effects.

Internal implant (Colpostat and tandem)

The following implementations pertain to a client who is receiving intracavitary radiation therapy for endometrial cancer. The client has an applicator tandem inserted in her uterus and colpostat (tubes with ovoid ends) placed in her vagina around the cervical os. Radioactive isotopes have been placed in the tandem and in the ovoids. Implants remain in place for 1 to 3 days.

Implementation

NURSING BEHAVIORS	NURSING RATIONALES
1. Ensure that the client has a private room.	**1.** This will protect other clients from the radiation.
2. Protect yourself and others by applying the principles of time, distance, and shielding.	**2.** This decreases exposure to the radiation source.

ADULT NURSING

3. Maintain the client on bed rest, with only slight head elevation.

3. Slight head elevation (not more than 20 degrees) prevents dislodgment of the isotope.

4. If the implant dislodges, retrieve it with long-handled forceps, place it in a lead container, and call the radiotherapist.

4. The first priority is to shield the client and yourself from the radiation source.

5. Before the client receives a vaginal implant, insert an indwelling urinary catheter in her bladder. Hook the catheter to straight drainage.

5. This empties the bladder, decreasing its proximity to the radiation source.

6. Decrease dietary bulk.

6. A low-bulk diet decreases the proximity of the intestines to the radiation source and prevents bowel movements that could cause the implant to dislodge.

7. Offer the client emotional support.

7. Because of radiation precautions, the client usually feels isolated.

8. Provide for sensory diversion.

8. The client may develop signs of sensory deprivation.

9. Administer an enema or laxative and irrigate the vagina, if ordered, after reaching the prescribed radiation dose and after the radiotherapist removes the implant.

9. This facilitates bowel evacuation after the client has been on a low-bulk diet. A vaginal douche may soothe irritated tissues.

Evaluation

- The client successfully completes radiation therapy, and the temporary implant is removed.
- The client is comfortable and free of injury and pain.
- The client can resume appropriate social contact.

Breast cancer

Breast cancer is the most common type of cancer in women. Self-examination uncovers most of these carcinomas; at least half of the tumors involve the upper outer quadrant. Surgery remains the treatment of choice, although controversy exists over the type of surgery. The most common procedure is the modified radical mastectomy (removal of the breast and axillary and pectoral nodes, with the pectoral muscles left intact). Radiation therapy or chemotherapy usually follows surgery, depending on the stage of the tumor and the existence of positive nodes. Lumpectomy (removal of the tumor) can be an effective surgical option for clients with small tumors and negative axillary nodes.

Clinical situation

Thelma McNab arrives at the ambulatory surgery unit (ASU) at 6 a.m. on the morning of her scheduled right modified radical mastectomy. One week ago she had a biopsy that showed a 1″ (3-cm) adenocarcinoma in the upper outer quadrant of her right breast. Since that time, she's had a full workup to check for metastasis. All tests have been negative. Her significant other, Roy Wilson, who seems attentive and concerned about her condition, accompanies her to the hospital. Ms. McNab had her preoperative teaching 3 days ago at the preadmission testing unit. She will be admitted via the ASU and will stay 3 to 4 days if she remains free of complications.

Assessment

NURSING BEHAVIORS	NURSING RATIONALES
1. While providing routine preoperative care, explore the client's feelings about surgery.	1. Women experience many fears about disfigurement, altered body image, and changed sexual role, besides fears directly related to the diagnosis.
2. Assess the client's understanding of preoperative teaching. Confirm that she has been taught arm and breathing exercises.	2. Information and instruction usually help lessen the client's anxiety. Arm exercises and deep breathing prevent postoperative complications.

Nursing diagnoses
- Fear related to the surgical procedure and cancer diagnosis
- Pain related to the postoperative status
- Body image disturbance related to loss of the breast
- Impaired skin integrity related to the incision

Planning and goals
- Ms. McNab will be free of respiratory complications and lymphedema.
- Ms. McNab will maintain full range of motion (ROM) in the affected arm.

Implementation

NURSING BEHAVIORS	NURSING RATIONALES
1. Observe the client's vital signs.	1. Any major surgery mandates these procedures to establish the client's condition.
2. Inspect the dressing for bleeding. Be sure to check under the client.	2. Bleeding should be reported to the physician immediately. Gravity may cause the blood to flow beneath the client, thereby obscuring it.
3. Ensure proper functioning of the Hemovac unit. Show the client how to empty the drain.	3. The Hemovac removes excess fluid. If it clogs, fluid builds up, stressing the suture line and providing a medium for infection. Because the drain can remain in place for about 1 week, the client will require home care instructions.
4. Identify the type and severity of the client's pain.	4. Initially, the operation causes trauma pain. Later, pain may result from nerve irritation and muscle spasm. The client may also feel a phantom breast.
5. Elevate the affected arm in an abducted position; observe for edema.	5. Transient or long-term edema can occur after removal of the lymph nodes. Arm elevation in the abducted position facilitates drainage, increases venous return, and prevents lymphedema and shoulder contracture.
6. Encourage ambulation. Have the client deep-breathe every 2 hours. Relieve pain with analgesics.	6. To prepare for discharge, the client should ambulate within the first 24 hours. Tightness of the pressure dressing and surgery-related pain increase the risk for respiratory complications.

ADULT NURSING

7. Spend time with the client, encourage her to express feelings and concerns, and provide generous emotional support.

8. Have the client's housemate participate in her care, and encourage him to communicate his love and concern.

9. Teach the client arm exercises, as follows:

• Start with simple extension and flexion of the hand, wrist, and elbow.

• Use ball squeezing as another early exercise, and continue progressive exercises, such as hair brushing, wall climbing, arm swinging, and rope pulling.

• Teach the client to continue exercises at home along with activities of daily living.

10. Before discharge, encourage the client to view her incision. Explain that once healing has occurred, the incision can be massaged with cocoa butter or cold cream.

11. Take precautions to prevent lymphedema and infection. Permit no invasive procedures on the affected arm, and give the client these instructions:

12. On discharge, offer the client a padded loose-fitting bra, and advise her to ask her physician about the "Reach to Recovery" postmastectomy program available through the local chapter of the American Cancer Society.

7. After breast removal, the client will grieve. The nurse's presence can be a source of comfort during this difficult time.

8. This reassures the client of continued nurturing.

9. These are usually progressive, beginning the first day after surgery.

• This will facilitate drainage. Other exercises can start on the 2nd and 3rd postoperative days.

• Such factors as wound healing, grafts, temperature elevation, and increased drainage may delay exercises. Consultation with the surgeon will determine when to undertake a full regimen.

• Exercises not only facilitate drainage but also prevent shoulder contracture and relieve muscle spasms.

10. Viewing the incision in the hospital and participating in self-care help the client begin to adjust to an altered body image with the support of health care professionals. A cold cream or cocoa butter massage will soften the incision.

11. These precautions help prevent long-term problems and must be continued for the rest of the client's life.
• Do not permit blood pressure checks on the affected arm.
• Wear gloves when gardening.
• Avoid all burns, including sunburn.
• Wear a thimble when sewing.
• Immediately provide care for even minor cuts and scratches.
• Whenever possible, keep the arm elevated.
• Do not wear constrictive clothing.
• Avoid undue pressure, such as from a shoulder purse.

12. Healing takes about 6 weeks, after which the client can look for a permanent prosthesis. A physician's referral is needed for "Reach to Recovery."

Evaluation

Ms. McNab:
• is free of lymphedema
• has full ROM in the affected arm
• breathes without difficulty.

Selected drugs used in adult nursing

DRUG AND USUAL ADULT DOSAGE	ACTION	NURSING CONSIDERATIONS AND COMMON SIDE EFFECTS
Common antibiotics		
Penicillins *Natural penicillin* Penicillin V potassium: 400,000 to 800,000 units (250 to 500 mg) P.O. q 6 hours	Bactericidal against many gram-positive and some gram-negative organisms; acts by preventing synthesis of the cell wall.	• Obtain culture before starting treatment. However, therapy may begin before results are available. • Check for history of *allergic reactions;* observe client for signs of *hypersensitivity,* especially with parenteral therapy. Delayed hypersensitivity may not develop for 7 days or more. • Monitor oral mucosa for signs of *candidiasis* or other *superinfection.* • May cause *nausea* and *vomiting;* if client vomits following an oral dose, check with physician. Another dosage may be ordered or the route of administration may be changed. • May cause *diarrhea;* if severe, physician may request a stool culture to check for *Clostridium difficile,* an organism that can cause *pseudomembranous colitis.* • May cause false-positive results in urine glucose tests using cupric sulfate (Clinitest or Benedict's reagent). • Food has no significant effect on oral absorption; better absorbed than penicillin G.
Synthetic penicillin Amoxicillin trihydrate: 250 to 500 mg P.O. q 8 hours	Same as above.	Same as natural penicillins, plus: • Notify physician if *rash* occurs; may or may not be an allergic reaction.
Cephalosporins Cefuroxime axetil (Ceftin): 250 mg P.O. q 12 hours Cephalexin monohydrate: 250 mg P.O. q 6 hours; higher doses (up to 4 g/day) may be needed for more severe infections	Bactericidal against many gram-positive and some gram-negative organisms; acts by preventing synthesis of the cell wall.	• Obtain culture before starting treatment. However, therapy may begin before results are available. • Check for history of *allergic reactions;* observe client for signs of *hypersensitivity,* especially with parenteral therapy. Delayed hypersensitivity may not develop for 7 days or more. • Monitor oral mucosa for signs of *candidiasis* or other *superinfection.* • May cause *nausea* and *vomiting;* if client vomits following an oral dose, check with physician. Another dosage may be ordered or the route of administration may be changed. • May cause *diarrhea;* if severe, physician may request a stool culture to check for *Clostridium difficile,* an organism that can cause *pseudomembranous colitis.* • May cause false-positive results in urine glucose tests using cupric sulfate (Clinitest or Benedict's reagent). • Food delays but does not prevent complete absorption.
Erythromycin Erythromycin: 250 to 500 mg P.O. q 6 hours	Acts on bacterial ribosomes to disrupt protein synthesis; bacteriostatic.	• Erythromycin base is not acid-stable; it must be enteric-coated or buffered to prevent destruction by stomach acid. Do not crush enteric-coated tablets. • Estolate, ethylsuccinate, and stearate forms are acid-stable. • Take with a full glass of water 1 hour before or 2 hours after meals. Enteric-coated forms may be taken with meals. • If patient experiences *nausea* and *vomiting,* physician may prescribe another drug. • May cause *diarrhea;* if severe, physician may request a stool culture to check for *Clostridium difficile,* an organism that can cause *pseudomembranous colitis.*

(continued)

ADULT NURSING

Selected drugs used in adult nursing (continued)

DRUG AND USUAL ADULT DOSAGE	ACTION	NURSING CONSIDERATIONS AND COMMON SIDE EFFECTS
Common antibiotics (continued)		
Tetracycline		
Doxycycline hyclate: 200 mg P.O. on day 1 in divided doses q 12 hours, followed by maintenance dose of 100 mg/day as a single dose or divided q 12 hours	Impairs bacterial ribosomal function; bacteriostatic.	• May cause *nausea, vomiting,* or *diarrhea.* If diarrhea is severe, physician may request a stool culture to check for *Clostridium difficile,* an organism that can cause *pseudomembranous colitis.* • Can cause false-negative results in urine test for glucose using glucose oxidase (Clinistix or Tes-Tape). • Should not be used in children who are forming their permanent teeth (usually age 8 or under) and in pregnant women because it can cause *discoloration of tooth enamel.* • Advise client to avoid sunlight, wear protective clothing, and use a sunscreen; *photosensitivity* can occur.
Aminoglycoside		
Gentamicin sulfate: dosage varies with body weight, renal function, and severity of infection; usual dose, 3 mg/kg/day I.V. in 3 equal doses q 8 hours	Acts on bacterial ribosomes to impair protein synthesis; bacteriostatic.	• Monitor renal function closely to detect *nephrotoxicity.* • Baseline and periodic audiometric tests should be performed to detect *ototoxicity.* • Monitor oral tissues for *candidiasis* and other signs of *superinfection.* • Monitor for *diarrhea, nausea,* and *vomiting;* if diarrhea is severe, physician may request a stool culture to check for *Clostridium difficile,* an organism that can cause *pseudomembranous colitis.* • Avoid concomitant administration with other ototoxic drugs (furosemide, ethacrynic acid).
Fluoroquinolone		
Ciprofloxacin: 200 to 400 mg I.V. q 12 hours, or 100 to 750 mg P.O. q 12 hours	Broad-spectrum bactericidal; inhibits deoxyribonucleic acid (DNA) replication in bacteria.	• Do not give to children under 18 years of age. • Monitor for *dizziness, headaches,* and *restlessness.* • Avoid using in clients with seizure disorders.
Sulfonamide		
Co-trimoxazole (sulfamethoxazole trimethoprim): 160 mg trimethoprim and 800 mg sulfamethoxazole P.O. q 12 hours	Bacteriostatic; used in acquired immunodeficiency (AIDS) to treat *Pneumocystis carinii* pneumonitis.	• AIDS clients are at increased risk for *hypersensitivity.* • Monitor for *blood dyscrasias, rash, fever, sore throat, nausea, vomiting,* and *diarrhea.* • Tell the client to take the drug with 8 oz of water. • Force fluids. • Advise the client to stay out of direct sunlight.
Antiprotozoal agent		
Pentamidine isethionate: 3 to 4 mg/kg I.V. or I.M. daily for 14 days; for prophylaxis, give 300 mg by inhalation every 3 to 4 weeks	May inhibit synthesis of DNA, ribonucleic acid, proteins, or phospholipids; used to treat *Pneumocystis carinii* pneumonia (PCP).	• Have client lie down during I.V. or I.M. administration. • Administer deep I.M. • Monitor client's blood pressure, blood glucose, and renal function. • Prophylaxis is used in human immunodeficiency virus (HIV)-positive clients at risk for PCP. • Administer a bronchodilator before inhalation administration to prevent bronchospasm.
Antiviral agents		
Acyclovir: 200 mg P.O. t.i.d. or q 4 hours; 5 mg/kg I.V. q 8 hours; or topical application of ointment 6 times a day for 7 days	Inhibits DNA synthesis of herpes virus; used to treat herpes simplex virus, disseminated herpes zoster, and acute varicella infections.	• Rotate injection sites when administering I.V. • Wear gloves to apply ointment. • Avoid getting ointment in eye. • Inform client that herpes can be passed to sexual partners.

Selected drugs used in adult nursing (continued)

DRUG AND USUAL ADULT DOSAGE	ACTION	NURSING CONSIDERATIONS AND COMMON SIDE EFFECTS
Antiviral agents (continued)		
Ritonavir: 600 mg P.O. b.i.d. or 7.5 ml (600 mg) of oral solution b.i.d.	Inhibits HIV replication by interfering with reverse transcriptase, an enzyme that influences DNA copying of the virus. This inhibition results in the formation of immature, noninfectious viral particles.	• Tell the client to take the drug with meals. • Oral solution can be mixed with chocolate milk to disguise taste. • Use cautiously in clients with liver disease. • Peripheral paresthesias can occur.
Saquinavir: 600 mg P.O. t.i.d.	Inhibits HIV replication by interfering with reverse transcriptase, an enzyme that influences DNA copying of the virus. This inhibition results in the formation of immature, noninfectious viral particles.	• Tell the client to take the drug within 2 hours of a meal. • Nausea and mouth ulcers may occur. • Caution the client not to take the drug with rifampin or rifabutin, either of which decreases the blood concentration of saquinavir. • Saquinavir is most effective when taken with zidovudine and zacitabine.
Zidovudine (AZT): 100 mg P.O. q 4 hours around the clock (600 mg/day); for asymptomatic clients, the drug may be taken only during the day (500 mg/day)	Inhibits replication of HIV; used to treat HIV and AIDS.	• Monitor for evidence of *blood dyscrasias.* • Provide good oral hygiene. • Encourage client to consume an adequate diet and to drink plenty of fluids.
Antitubercular agents		
Ethambutol: 15 to 25 mg/kg/day P.O.	Bacteriostatic; given as adjunctive therapy with isoniazid.	• *GI upset, peripheral neuritis,* and *optic neuritis* (leading to *decreased vision* and *color blindness*) may occur. • Administer with food. • Check client's vision monthly. Instruct client to report vision changes to physician.
Isoniazid: 5 to 10 mg/kg P.O. or I.M. as daily single dose, up to 300 mg/day	Bacteriostatic and bactericidal.	• Administer with food. • *Peripheral neuritis, hypersensitivity, liver toxicity,* and *GI distress* may occur. • Watch for *paresthesias* of hands and feet, which typically precede peripheral neuritis. As ordered, administer pyridoxine (50 mg/day) to prevent this reaction.
Pyrazinamide: 15 to 30 mg/kg P.O. daily, to a maximum daily dosage of 3 g	Bactericidal.	• *Hepatic damage* and *hyperuricemia* may occur. • Monitor hepatic and renal function.
Rifampin: 600 mg/day P.O. or I.V. as a single dose	Bactericidal.	• Administer 1 hour before or 2 hours after meals. • *GI upset, skin eruptions,* and *jaundice* may occur. • Advise client that drug colors body fluids red-orange. • Drug reduces effectiveness of oral contraceptives. Teach client to use other birth control methods. • Monitor liver and renal function.

ADULT NURSING

(continued)

Selected drugs used in adult nursing (continued)

DRUG AND USUAL ADULT DOSAGE	ACTION	NURSING CONSIDERATIONS AND COMMON SIDE EFFECTS
Antitubercular agents (continued)		
Streptomycin: 1 g I.M. daily for 2 to 3 months	Bacteriostatic and bactericidal.	• *Ototoxicity* and *renal toxicity* may occur. • Assess for tinnitus and impaired hearing. • Monitor renal function.
Antiulcer agents		
Histamine-2 (H₂) antagonists Cimetidine (Tagamet): 400 mg. P.O. b.i.d. or 800 mg h.s. Famotidine (Pepcid): 20 mg P.O. b.i.d. or 40 mg h.s. Nizatidine (Axid): 150 mg P.O. b.i.d. or 300 mg h.s. Ranitidine (Zantac): 150 mg P.O. b.i.d. or 300 mg h.s. • Separate antacid administration by at least 1 hour.	H₂ antagonists; decrease gastric acid secretions.	• Cimetidine has many interactions that can produce toxic levels of other drugs. • Elderly clients are especially prone to *confusion, bradycardia,* and *constipation.* • Check renal and hepatic functions. • Antacids impair absorption.
Prostaglandin-like Misoprostol (Cytotec): 100 to 200 mcg q.i.d.	Inhibits gastric acid secretion by synthetically mimicking prostaglandin. Used with clients on high doses of non-steroidal anti-inflammatory drugs (NSAIDs).	• Side effects include diarrhea and abdominal pain. • This drug is oxytocic—do not use in pregnancy. • Instruct client to take drug after meals and at bedtime to help decrease diarrhea.
Proton pump inhibitor Omeprazole (Prilosec): 20 mg (40 mg for gastric ulcer) daily for 4 to 8 weeks	Inhibits the acid-secreting enzyme ATPase (proton pump).	• The drug's effect lasts for about 3 weeks. Long-term effects of this amount of acid suppression are unknown. • The drug can cause nausea, diarrhea, and headache.
Protective agent Sucralfate (Carafate): 1 g P.O. q.i.d.	Forms a protective coating over the ulcer.	• Give the drug on an empty stomach about 1 hour before meals and at bedtime. • Constipation is the most common side effect. • Sucralfate may impair absorption of other drugs.
Antidiarrheal agents		
Diphenoxylate hydrochloride: 5 mg P.O. q.i.d.	Opiate; decreases GI motility and secretions.	• *Sedation, dizziness, dry mouth,* and *paralytic ileus* may occur. • *Physical dependence* may occur with long-term use.
Kaolin and pectin: 60 ml P.O. Attapulgite: 15 ml (600 mg) P.O.	Adsorbent and protective action; decreases water content of stool.	• Monitor bowel function; *constipation* can occur. • Assess fluid and electrolyte status. • Limit use to 2 days.

Selected drugs used in adult nursing *(continued)*

DRUG AND USUAL ADULT DOSAGE	ACTION	NURSING CONSIDERATIONS AND COMMON SIDE EFFECTS
Antidiarrheal agents *(continued)*		
Loperamide: 4 mg P.O. after the first loose bowel movement, followed by 2 mg after each subsequent loose bowel movement	An opiate derivative that decreases peristalsis.	• Monitor bowel function. • Caution the client to avoid driving if *drowsiness* occurs.
Laxatives		
Bisacodyl (Dulcolax): 5 to 15 mg P.O. or 10 mg P.R., as needed	Acts as an irritant in the colon, increasing motility and fluid movement by stimulating the bowel.	• Because the drug's cathartic effect does not occur for 6 to 8 hours, administer in the morning or at bedtime. • Do not give the drug within 1 hour of antacids or milk. The enteric coating will dissolve in the stomach, leading to major GI irritation.
Docusate sodium: 50 to 200 mg P.O. daily	Decreases surface tension of fecal matter so it can absorb water, softening the stool.	• May be given with another agent to increase peristalsis. • *Abdominal cramps* and *diarrhea* may occur.
Antacid		
Magnesium hydroxide plus aluminum hydroxide: 10 to 20 ml or 1 to 2 tablets after meals and at bedtime	Decreases gastric acid.	• Shake well. • Impairs absorption of many drugs; do not administer together. • Clients on sodium restrictions should use a low-sodium version. • *Constipation* (from aluminum) or *diarrhea* (from magnesium) may occur.
Antianginal agent		
Nitroglycerin: sublingual dosage, 1 tablet (0.3 mg, 0.4 mg, or 0.6 mg), may repeat q 5 minutes to a maximum of 3 doses within a 15-minute period; ointment, 0.5″ to 2″ strip; transdermal, 1 disk or pad/24 hours	Dilates coronary arteries and improves collateral circulation; used to treat ischemia.	*With oral administration:* • Instruct client to take a tablet before an activity likely to trigger angina. • Caution client to avoid alcohol when taking this drug because severe hypotension and cardiovascular collapse may occur. • Instruct client to carry tablets in a purse or jacket, and not next to the body. Tablets should be stored in a dark, tightly closed container. *With transdermal administration:* • Check client's blood pressure and watch for *postural hypotension.*
Digitalis glycosides		
Digitoxin: maintenance, 0.05 to 0.3 mg/day P.O. Digoxin: maintenance: varies with peak body store levels	Directly affects cardiac muscle; increases force of contraction and slows conduction through the SA and AV nodes, thereby slowing the heart rate.	• Take the client's apical pulse before administering the drug; if the pulse rate is below 60 beats/minute, withhold the drug and call the physician. • May cause *visual disturbances* (yellow halos). • *Nausea* and *vomiting* may be early symptoms of toxicity, especially in elderly clients. • Monitor the serum digoxin level (therapeutic range: 0.5 to 2.0 ng/ml), or the serum digitoxin level, (25-35 ng/ml). • Monitor for hypokalemia, which increases the risk of toxicity. • These drugs are used to treat congestive heart failure (CHF) and atrial arrhythmias.

(continued)

Selected drugs used in adult nursing (continued)

DRUG AND USUAL ADULT DOSAGE	ACTION	NURSING CONSIDERATIONS AND COMMON SIDE EFFECTS
Beta blockers		
Nadolol: maintenance: 40 to 240 mg daily P.O. Propranolol hydrochloride: for hypertension, 120 to 240 mg daily in divided doses b.i.d. or t.i.d.; for angina, 80 to 320 mg daily in divided doses b.i.d. to q.i.d.	Decrease blood pressure; reduce heart rate by blocking sympathetic nervous system stimulation of the heart; used for angina and hypertension.	• Do not administer unless the heart rate is at least 60 beats/minute; initially, caution the client to sit or stand slowly to prevent *fainting.* • Monitor cardiac and pulmonary function. • *Postural hypotension, heart block, fatigue, weakness, GI distress, congestive heart failure,* and *pulmonary edema* can occur.
Calcium channel blockers		
Diltiazem hydrochloride: 30 mg P.O. t.i.d. or q.i.d.; may gradually increase to 360 mg/day Verapamil hydrochloride: 80 to 120 mg t.i.d. or q.i.d.	Dilate myocardial vessels by blocking calcium ion entry to the myocardium, thereby regulating heart rate and lowering blood pressure.	• Change the client's position slowly to prevent *postural hypotension.* • If the client is taking verapamil and digoxin, monitor for *digoxin toxicity.* • Administer 1 hour before meals. • *Hypotension, headache, dizziness, flushing, nausea, constipation,* and *edema* can occur.
Diuretics		
Thiazides Chlorothiazide: 500 mg to 2 g daily P.O. in 1 or 2 doses Hydrochlorothiazide: 25 to 100 mg/day P.O.	Induce water excretion by preventing sodium reabsorption; used in CHF and hypertension.	• Monitor intake and output, weight, and serum potassium and serum sodium levels. • Encourage intake of high-potassium foods, such as bananas, apricots, and citrus fruits. • Monitor renal function. • Administer in the morning to prevent *nocturia.* • *Aplastic anemia, volume depletion, weakness, hypokalemia,* and *sodium depletion* can occur.
Loop diuretics Furosemide: 20 to 80 mg P.O. daily; 20 to 40 mg I.M. or I.V. for diuresis	Inhibits sodium and water reabsorption in loop of Henle; used to treat CHF, hypertension, and pulmonary edema and to produce diuresis.	See torsemide.
Torsemide (Demadex): for diuresis, give 10 to 20 mg P.O. or I.V. once daily; if response is inadequate, double the dosage until a response is obtained (maximum dosage is 200 mg/day). For hypertension, give 5 mg P.O. daily; increase to 10 mg if needed and tolerated; if response is still inadequate, add another antihypertensive agent	Enhances the excretion of sodium chloride, and water by an action on the ascending portion of the loop of Henle.	• Use cautiously in clients with hepatic disease with cirrhosis and ascites because sudden changes in fluid and electrolyte balance may precipitate *hepatic coma.* • Like other loop diuretics, this drug can cause *profound diuresis* and *water and electrolyte depletion.* Monitor serum electrolytes, blood pressure, and pulse rate during rapid diuresis and routinely with chronic use. • Watch for signs of *hypokalemia* (for example, muscle weakness and cramps). Clients also on digitalis have an increased risk of *digitalis toxicity* from the potassium-depleting effect. • Consult with physician and dietitian to provide a high-potassium diet. Foods rich in potassium include citrus fruits, tomatoes, bananas, dates, and apricots. • Give in a.m. to prevent nocturia. • Elderly clients are especially susceptible to *excessive diuresis,* with potential for *circulatory collapse* and *thromboembolic complications.*

Selected drugs used in adult nursing (continued)

DRUG AND USUAL ADULT DOSAGE	ACTION	NURSING CONSIDERATIONS AND COMMON SIDE EFFECTS
Diuretics (continued)		
		• Advise clients to stand slowly to prevent *dizziness,* and to limit alcohol intake and strenuous exercise in hot weather because these actions may precipitate *orthostatic hypotension.* • Advise clients to report ringing in ears immediately; it may indicate toxicity. • Remind client not to take any other nonprescription medication without first checking with the physician or pharmacist. • Rapid I.V. injection may cause *ototoxicity.*
Potassium-sparing diuretics Spironolactone: 25 to 200 mg P.O. daily	Increases sodium and water excretion and inhibits potassium excretion; used in conjunction with other diuretics to conserve potassium.	• Administer with meals. • Monitor client for evidence of *hyperkalemia.* • Teach client to avoid foods high in potassium.
Miscellaneous diuretics Acetazolamide: 250 mg P.O. 1 to 4 times a day; 5 mg/kg daily for diuresis	Carbonic anhydrase inhibitor; causes diuresis and reduces intraocular pressure; used to induce diuresis in treatment of toxicity associated with certain drugs; also used to treat glaucoma.	• Monitor client's fluid intake and output, weight, and serum potassium level.
Mannitol (Osmitrol): 50 to 100 g I.V. of 5% to 20% solution	Causes diuresis by raising osmotic pressure and preventing reabsorption of water; decreases intraocular and intracranial pressure.	• Administer with a filter and warm bottle to dissolve crystals that may form in parenteral solution. • Weigh the client daily. • Monitor his intake and output and electrolyte balance.
Antihypertensives		
Sympathetic inhibitors Clonidine hydrochloride: 0.2 to 0.6 mg/day P.O. Methyldopa: 500 mg to 2 g P.O. daily in 2 to 4 divided doses	Acts in the CNS to modify sympathetic outflow from the brain.	• Perform frequent blood studies. • Teach the client to change positions slowly. • Monitor blood pressure and pulse rate. • *Drowsiness, postural hypotension, sedation, dry mouth, constipation,* and *impotence* can occur. • Do not withdraw suddenly; rebound hypertension can occur.

(continued)

ADULT NURSING

Selected drugs used in adult nursing *(continued)*

DRUG AND USUAL ADULT DOSAGE	ACTION	NURSING CONSIDERATIONS AND COMMON SIDE EFFECTS
Antihypertensives *(continued)*		
ACE inhibitors Captopril: 25 to 50 mg P.O. b.i.d. or t.i.d. Enalapril: 10 to 40 mg P.O. daily Lisinopril: 10 to 40 mg P.O. daily	Prevent conversion of angiotensin I to angiotensin II, a powerful vasoconstrictor.	• Monitor blood pressure and pulse. • Check WBC counts periodically. • Warn the client to change positions slowly. • Check renal function. • Advise the client taking enalapril to report swelling around the face or difficulty breathing. • *Agranulocytosis, headache, dizziness, fatigue, hypotension, tachycardia, loss of taste, angioedema,* and *hyperkalemia* can occur. • Tell patient not to use salt subsitutes; most contain potassium, which can increase risk of hyperkalemia.
Anticoagulants		
Heparin: dosage and administration route depend on activated partial thromboplastin time (PTT); typical dosage is 5,000 to 10,000 units I.V. q 4 to 6 hours, or 8,000 to 10,000 units S.C. q 8 hours	Inactivates thrombin and prevents fibrinogen conversion to fibrin.	• Monitor client's activated PTT. • Do not massage the injection site. • Assess client for bleeding. • Keep protamine sulfate on hand as an antidote. • Caution client not to take over-the-counter salicylates when using this drug.
Warfarin sodium: optimal dose is established from prothrombin time (PT)/International Normalized Ratio (PT/INR) to maintain it at 2 to 3 (varies by patient and condition); dosage usually ranges from 2 to 10 mg P.O. daily	Inhibits vitamin K– dependent activation of clotting factors II, VII, IX, and X.	• Monitor client's PT. • Assess client for bleeding. • Keep vitamin K on hand to antagonize warfarin effects, if needed. • Teach client to avoid foods high in vitamin K. • Instruct client to use an electric razor and a soft toothbrush.
Skeletal muscle relaxant		
Dantrolene: gradual increase from 25 mg/day P.O. to maximum of 400 mg/day P.O.	Impairs intracellular calcium ion movement; used to decrease spasticity in skeletal muscles.	• Administer with meals. • Monitor hepatic and renal function. • Assess for *diarrhea*. • *Weakness, drowsiness, dizziness,* and *hepatitis* can occur. • Prohibit alcohol and other CNS depressants.
Anticholinergic agents		
Atropine: preoperatively, 0.4 to 0.6 mg I.M.; for bradycardia, 0.5 to 1 mg I.V. q 5 minutes, to a maximum of 2 mg	Inhibits effects of acetylcholine at muscarinic cholinergic receptors, increases heart rate, dilates pupils, and decreases GI and respiratory secretions; used to treat bradycardia and preoperatively to diminish secretions and block cardiac vagal reflexes.	• Do not give to client with narrow-angle glaucoma. • *Headache, restlessness, tachycardia, blurred vision, dry mouth,* and *urinary hesitancy* may occur. • Monitor for *tachycardia*. • Monitor urine output.

Selected drugs used in adult nursing (continued)

DRUG AND USUAL ADULT DOSAGE	ACTION	NURSING CONSIDERATIONS AND COMMON SIDE EFFECTS
Anticholinergic agents (continued)		
Benztropine: 0.5 to 6 mg/day P.O. or I.M., adjusted to meet individual requirements	Inhibits central cholinergic receptors; restores the balance of cholinergic and dopaminergic activity in the basal ganglia; used to treat Parkinson's disease.	Same as atropine, plus: • Give 30 minutes to 1 hour before meals. • Monitor for parkinsonian symptoms. • Monitor fluid intake and output. • Assess client's bowel function. • Encourage good oral hygiene. • Advise client to suck on hard sugarless candy to help relieve dry mouth. • Teach client to avoid alcohol and CNS depressants while taking this drug.
Glycopyrrolate: 1 mg P.O. b.i.d. or t.i.d.; 0.1 to 0.2 mg I.M. or I.V. q.i.d. for peptic ulcer; preoperative dosage based on body weight	Decreases secretions by inhibiting acetylcholine; used to treat bradycardia and given preoperatively to diminish secretions and block cardiac vagal reflexes.	See atropine.
Propantheline: 15 mg P.O. t.i.d. and 30 mg at bedtime	Inhibits acetylcholine effects at muscarinic cholinergic receptors (does not enter the CNS), thereby decreasing GI secretions and motility; used as an adjunct to GI disorders, such as irritable bowel syndrome.	• Do not give to client with narrow-angle glaucoma. • Monitor for *tachycardia*. • Monitor urine output. • Give 30 minutes to 1 hour before meals and at bedtime.
Trihexyphenidyl: initial dose of 1.0 mg gradually increased to maintenance dose of 5 to 15 mg/day P.O. in three divided doses	Same as benztropine.	See benztropine.
Antiparkinsonian agents (In addition to the anticholinergics *benztropine* and *trihexyphenidyl*)		
Levodopa: 0.5 to 1 g P.O. daily, given b.i.d.,t.i.d., or q.i.d.; may increase as necessary to a maximum dose of 8 g daily	Metabolized to dopamine, which replaces deficient dopamine in the basal ganglia of clients with Parkinson's disease, resulting in improved modulation of voluntary nerve impulses transmitted to motor cortex.	• Administer with meals. • *Involuntary movements, hypotension, nausea, vomiting,* and *fatigue* may occur. • Monitor complete blood count. • Monitor client for parkinsonian symptoms. • Monitor renal and hepatic function. • Tell client to change position slowly to avoid *dizziness* and *orthostatic hypotension*.

(continued)

ADULT NURSING

Selected drugs used in adult nursing (continued)

DRUG AND USUAL ADULT DOSAGE	ACTION	NURSING CONSIDERATIONS AND COMMON SIDE EFFECTS
Antiparkinsonian agents (continued)		
Levodopa-carbidopa: 3 to 6 tablets in divided doses. (Tablets contain 25 mg carbidopa and 250 mg levodopa.)	Carbidopa decreases the peripheral metabolism of levodopa to dopamine, thereby increasing the amount of levodopa available to enter the CNS.	See levodopa.
Antiemetics		
Metoclopramide: 10 mg (2 ml) I.V. or I.M.; 10 mg P.O. 30 minutes before meals and at bedtime.	Stimulates gastric motility in upper GI tract and blocks dopamine receptors in chemoreceptor trigger zone.	• Do not administer if the client has a GI obstruction. • Monitor for involuntary movements (extrapyramidal symptoms). • Tell the client to avoid activities requiring alertness; may cause *drowsiness.*
Ondansetron (Zofran): 8 mg P.O. 30 minutes before chemotherapy, followed by a second dose 8 hours after the first dose; subsequently, 8 mg q 12 hours for 1 to 2 days after completion of chemotherapy.	Blocks serotonin receptors in chemoreceptor trigger zone and on vagal nerve endings that trigger nausea and vomiting. Used to prevent nausea and vomiting caused by chemotherapy.	• This drug causes diarrhea, headache, and sedation. The client may need to take an analgesic for headache. • Watch for fluid and electrolyte depletion.
Prochlorperazine: 5 to 10 mg t.i.d. to q.i.d. P.O. or I.M., or 25 mg rectally b.i.d., or 2.5 to 10 mg I.V. p.r.n. Total I.V. dosage should not exceed 40 mg/day.	Blocks dopamine receptors in the chemoreceptor trigger zone to prevent nausea and vomiting.	• Monitor vital signs and complete blood count in patient on long-term therapy to detect *blood dyscrasias.* • Observe for extrapyramidal symptoms. • Instruct the client to change position slowly because the drug may cause *orthostatic hypotension;* to wear sunscreen and protective clothing when in sunlight because it may cause *photosensitivity;* and to avoid activities requiring alertness because it may cause *drowsiness.* • Do not administer to a client with glaucoma. The anticholinergic effects can cause *blurred vision* and may increase intraocular pressure in some clients predisposed to glaucoma. • The anticholinergic effects also can result in *dry mouth* and *constipation.* • Wash hands after touching the patch to avoid dilating the pupil. • Give by deep I.M. injection; may be painful and irritating.
Nonnarcotic analgesics and antipyretics		
Acetaminophen: 325 to 650 mg P.O. or rectally q 4 hours p.r.n. Do not exceed 4 g daily for acute therapy	Inhibits prostaglandin synthesis to decrease fever and relieve pain.	• Evaluate analgesic and antipyretic response. • Warn the client not to abuse the drug. • Overdose can be fatal if not treated immediately. • Long-term or high-dose therapy can cause *hepatic damage.*
Aspirin: 325 to 650 mg P.O. or rectally q 4 hours p.r.n.; do not exceed 4 g daily; higher doses used in arthritis	Inhibition of prostaglandins and action on hypothalamus produce analgesia, anti-inflammatory response, and antipyrexia.	• Evaluate analgesic, antipyretic, and anti-inflammatory response. • Administer with food, milk, or antacid to minimize *GI distress.* • Avoid use in clients taking anticoagulants because of the risk of *bleeding.* • High doses can cause *tinnitus.* • Can cause *GI bleeding.* Teach client signs and symptoms of GI bleeding.

Selected drugs used in adult nursing (continued)

DRUG AND USUAL ADULT DOSAGE	ACTION	NURSING CONSIDERATIONS AND COMMON SIDE EFFECTS
Nonsteroidal anti-inflammatory drugs		
Ibuprofen: nonprescription dosage, 1.2 g daily in 3 or 4 divided doses; prescription dosage, up to 3.2 g/day in 3 or 4 divided doses.	Acts as analgesic, anti-inflammatory, and antipyretic by inhibiting synthesis of prostaglandins.	• Monitor renal and hepatic function in clients receiving long-term, high-dose therapy. • Monitor for *GI bleeding*. Teach the client the signs and symptoms of GI bleeding, which can occur without warning, especially in elderly or debilitated clients or those receiving long-term, high-dose therapy. • Give with milk or meals to minimize *nausea* and reduce the risk of *ulceration*.
Ketorolac (Toradol): for single dose, 30 to 60 mg I.M. or 15 to 30 mg I.V.; for multiple doses, 15 to 30 mg I.M. or I.V. q 6 hours	Same as ibuprofen. Only NSAID that can be given I.M.	• Same as ibuprofen, plus: • The drug may cause drowsiness and dizziness. • Rotate injection site.
Narcotic analgesics		
Codeine: 15 to 60 mg P.O., I.M., or S.C. q 4 to 6 hours Meperidine: 50 to 150 mg P.O., I.M., or S.C. q 3 to 4 hours Morphine: 5 to 20 mg I.M. or S.C., 10 to 30 mg P.O., or 10 to 20 mg P.R. q 4 hours p.r.n.	Relieve mild to severe pain; act on opiate receptors in CNS to decrease pain perception and response; also suppress cough; used in pain management and as an antitussive (codeine).	• Evaluate analgesic response. • Monitor respiratory, circulatory, and bowel function. • Increase fluid and fiber intake. Administer a stool softener to overcome constipation, if needed. • Caution the client to avoid activities requiring alertness, to change positions slowly because of possible *hypotension,* and to avoid alcohol and other depressants. • These drugs can cause dependence. • May cause *respiratory depression*. Withhold the drug if the client's respiratory rate is below 12 breaths/minute or pupils are constricted. • Use with caution in head injury. • Monitor client for *urine retention*. • Commonly causes *nausea* and *vomiting*. Check with physician if severe; an antiemetic may be ordered.
Anticonvulsants		
Phenobarbital: 60 to 200 mg P.O. daily	Suppresses spread of seizure activity produced by epileptogenic foci in brain structures; also decreases excitability and raises the seizure threshold.	• Monitor vital signs. • *Blood dyscrasias, drowsiness, dizziness, fatigue,* and *"hangover"* may occur. • Use cautiously in elderly clients. • Warn client to avoid alcohol and other CNS depressants while taking this drug. • Warn client not to discontinue this drug abruptly.
Phenytoin: 300 mg P.O. daily	Limits seizure activity by affecting transport of sodium ions across cell membranes in motor cortex.	• Administer with or after meals. • Monitor complete blood count. • *Agranulocytosis, ataxia, slurred speech, diplopia, nystagmus, nausea,* and *gingival hyperplasia* may occur. • Warn client to avoid alcohol and other CNS depressants while taking this drug. • Warn client not to discontinue this drug suddenly. • Gingival hyperplasia is more common in adolescents; advise frequent dental examinations to minimize occurrence.

(continued)

ADULT NURSING

Selected drugs used in adult nursing (continued)

DRUG AND USUAL ADULT DOSAGE	ACTION	NURSING CONSIDERATIONS AND COMMON SIDE EFFECTS
Hypoglycemic agents		
Insulins Fast-acting (Regular, Semilente, Humulin R), Intermediate (Lente, NPH, Humulin N), Long-acting (Ultralente, Protamine Zinc, Humulin U): Dosage is highly variable and is based upon blood glucose concentrations.	Facilitate transport of glucose from blood into tissue for utilization as an energy source; convert glucose to glycogen for storage in the liver.	• Monitor the client's weight and blood glucose level. • Observe for signs of *hypoglycemia.* • Only regular insulin can be given I.V. • Dosage must be precise; use an insulin syringe. • Store in a cool area. • Give subcutaneously, and rotate injection sites to prevent *lipodystrophy.* • Teach the client to carry a carbohydrate source at all times. • Dosage is adjusted to achieve a blood glucose level of 80 to 140 mg/dl before meals and at h.s. In children under age 5, the blood glucose level should be 100 to 200 mg/dl.
Oral agents Chlorpropamide: 250 mg/day Glipizide: 5 mg P.O. daily; maximum daily dose is 40 mg; doses above 15 mg should be divided and given before meals. Dosage varies with extended release form.	Sulfonylureas; stimulate the pancreas to release insulin and increase peripheral tissue sensitivity to insulin.	• Administer only for type II diabetes. • The client may need insulin during periods of increased stress. • Client should monitor blood glucose carefully to detect *hypoglycemia.* • Avoid alcohol; may cause a disulfiram-like reaction (*flushing, nausea, vomiting*).
Thyroid agent		
Levothyroxine: 100 to 200 mcg P.O. daily	Replaces depleted levothyroxine (T$_4$) thyroid hormone, thus increasing all aspects of metabolism; used to treat hypothyroidism.	• Use with caution in elderly clients. • Replacement therapy is begun gradually to observe response. • Report *palpitations* or *chest pain* to the physician. • Insomnia may be one of the earliest signs of overdose. • *Overdose of hormone; nervousness, insomnia, tremor, palpitations, tachycardia,* and *angina* can occur.
Antithyroid agents		
Methimazole: 5 to 15 mg P.O. daily in 3 divided doses at 8-hour intervals Propylthiouracil: 100 to 150 mg P.O. daily in 3 divided doses at 8-hour intervals	Inhibit synthesis of thyroid hormone; propylthiouracil used preoperatively to treat thyroid storm.	• Monitor complete blood count to detect *bone marrow depression* or *agranulocytosis,* and hepatic function to detect *hepatotoxicity.* • Instruct the client to report fever and sore throat—signs of *agranulocytosis.* • Give with meals to minimize *GI upset, nausea,* and *vomiting.* • Instruct the client to avoid shellfish and cough preparations that contain iodine.
Glucocorticoids		
Cortisone acetate: dosage varies; 25 to 300 mg P.O. or I.M. daily or every other day	Anti-inflammatory and immunosuppressant; used mainly as replacement therapy in adrenal insufficiency.	• Give with milk or food; administer largest dose in the morning. • Side effects are usually dose-dependent and may include *depression, mood changes, hypertension, edema, GI ulcers, hypokalemia,* and *hyperglycemia.* • Taper dosage gradually after long-term therapy. Never discontinue abruptly; sudden withdrawal after prolonged use may be fatal. • Warn client not to discontinue the drug abruptly. • Instruct client to restrict sodium intake and to take a potassium supplement, as needed. • Monitor client's weight; observe for *edema.* • Assess for signs and symptoms of infection. • Monitor serum potassium and blood glucose levels.

Selected drugs used in adult nursing *(continued)*

DRUG AND USUAL ADULT DOSAGE	ACTION	NURSING CONSIDERATIONS AND COMMON SIDE EFFECTS
Glucocorticoids *(continued)*		
Dexamethasone: dosage and administration route (P.O., I.V., or I.M.) vary with drug salt and indication.	Anti-inflammatory and immunosuppressant; used to treat inflammatory conditions, allergic reactions, neoplasms, cerebral edema, shock, and adrenal insufficiency.	See cortisone.
Hydrocortisone: dosage and administration route (P.O., I.V., I.M. S.C., and enema) vary with drug salt and indication.	Anti-inflammatory and immunosuppressant; used mainly as replacement therapy in adrenal insufficiency.	See cortisone.
Prednisone: 2.5 to 15 mg P.O. b.i.d. to q.i.d.	Anti-inflammatory and immunosuppressant	See cortisone.
Inhaled Beclomethasone dipropionate (Beclovent; Vanceril): 2 inhalations t.i.d. or q.i.d. Triamcinolone acetonide (Azmacort): 2 inhalations t.i.d. or q.i.d.	Exert local anti-inflammatory effect in lungs. Used to decrease inflammation, which reduces severity of attack and decreases dose of bronchodilators.	• These drugs do not relieve ongoing attacks. • They can cause hoarseness and fungal overgrowth of *Candida*. Check for white patches. • Teach client to rinse mouth with water after inhaling.
Antihistamines		
Astemizole: 10 mg P.O. daily Chlorpheniramine maleate: 4 mg P.O. q 4 to 6 hours Diphenhydramine: 25 to 50 mg P.O. t.i.d. or q.i.d. at 4- to 6-hour intervals, not to exceed 300 mg in 24 hours. Or 10 to 50 mg I.M. or I.V., with maximum daily dose of 400 mg. Promethazine: 12.5 to 50 mg P.O., I.M., or P.R.	Block effects of histamine at receptor sites; can prevent allergic reactions but not reverse them; promethazine sometimes used before or after surgery for sedation and analgesia.	• Provide proper oral hygiene and sugarless gum or hard candy to prevent *dry mouth.* • May cause *drowsiness;* avoid driving and hazardous activities. • Prohibit alcohol and CNS depressants. • Administer with food. • Monitor clients on prolonged therapy for *blood dyscrasias.* • May *dry mucous membranes;* keep the client well hydrated.

(continued)

ADULT NURSING

Selected drugs used in adult nursing (continued)

DRUG AND USUAL ADULT DOSAGE	ACTION	NURSING CONSIDERATIONS AND COMMON SIDE EFFECTS
Bronchodilators		
Albuterol: 1 to 2 inhalations q 4 to 6 hours	Acts on beta$_2$-adrenergic receptors to dilate bronchial smooth muscle.	• Be sure the client understands how to use the inhaler. • Evaluate respiratory status. • *Tremor, nervousness, tachycardia,* and *nausea* can occur.
Epinephrine: 0.1 to 0.5 ml 1:1,000 I.M. or S.C.; repeat q 10 to 15 minutes	Acts on alpha- and beta-adrenergic receptors, causing vasoconstriction, bronchodilation, and cardiac stimulation.	• Monitor vital signs; observe for *tachycardia, palpitations,* or *hypertension.* • Closely monitor for relief of bronchospasm. • May cause *nervousness, tremors,* and *headache;* report these symptoms to the physician.
Salmeterol (Serevent): 2 inhalations q 12 hours	Newer beta$_2$-agonist that causes bronchodilation for up to 12 hours and helps prevent attacks while sleeping.	• Because of its long action, this drug cannot relieve an acute attack. Consequently, the client taking salmeterol also needs a more rapid acting beta$_2$-agonist. Make sure the client understands this. Misunderstanding has proved fatal to some clients.
Benzodiazepines		
Alprazolam: 0.25 to 0.5 mg P.O. t.i.d.	Exerts inhibitory action in CNS, thereby decreasing anxiety.	• Caution the client to avoid alcohol and other CNS depressants while taking this drug. • Tell him not to take over-the-counter antihistamines without consulting his physician. • Monitor the client for drowsiness, ataxia, and urine retention. • Tell the client not to stop taking the drug abruptly; instead, the physician should taper the dose.
Diazepam: 2 to 10 mg P.O. b.i.d. to q.i.d. or 2 to 10 mg I.V. or I.M., depending on indication and severity	Exerts inhibitory action in CNS. Used to treat status epilepticus, to decrease anxiety before procedures and surgery, and to relieve alcohol withdrawal symptoms and muscle spasms.	See alprazolam.
Flurazepam: 15 to 30 mg P.O. h.s.	Depresses CNS to cause sleep and sedation.	• Caution the client not to use alcohol or other CNS depressants while taking this drug. • The drug's hypnotic effect may not begin for several days. • Watch for daytime hangover effect. • Avoid prolonged use.
Lorazepam: 2 to 6 mg/day P.O. in divided doses or 2 to 4 mg h.s.	Exerts inhibitory action in CNS, thereby causing decreased anxiety and sedation.	See alprazolam.

Selected drugs used in adult nursing *(continued)*

DRUG AND USUAL ADULT DOSAGE	ACTION	NURSING CONSIDERATIONS AND COMMON SIDE EFFECTS
Antilipemics		
Cholestyramine: 4 g b.i.d. P.O. with meals; dose and frequency may vary	Binds bile salts so that more are excreted in feces, thereby lowering total cholesterol and low-density lipoprotein levels.	• The drug commonly causes constipation. Encourage the client to follow a high-fiber diet. • Monitor the client for bleeding, which may occur because of poor absorption of fat-soluble vitamins.
Gemfibrozil: 600 mg P.O. b.i.d. 30 minutes before morning and evening meal	Fibric acid derivative that lowers serum triglyceride levels.	• Monitor prothrombin time, and instruct the client to report bleeding. • Caution the client to restrict alcohol and fat intake. • Advise him that weight loss will help lower the triglyceride level.
Lovastatin: 10 to 80 mg/day P.O. in single dose or 2 divided doses	Impairs the body's ability to produce cholesterol.	• Advise the client to take the drug with meals. • Monitor the client's hepatic function. • Encourage the client to reduce his intake of dietary fat.

Part VI

ANR Post-Test

ANR Post-Test

Introduction

The National Council Licensure Examination for Registered Nurses (NCLEX-RN) is administered by state boards of nursing as part of the process used to determine whether registered nurse candidates meet licensure requirements. The examination measures a nurse's ability to practice safely and effectively as a registered nurse in an entry-level position. It is designed to test the practical application of knowledge and skills in health care situations that occur frequently in entry-level nursing practice.

American Nursing Review (ANR) has developed a post-test to assess your nursing ability, skill, and knowledge as you prepare to take or retake NCLEX-RN. This test also can be used for review by nurses returning to active practice after an absence and by those moving to a different clinical area of practice.

Since April 1994, NCLEX-RN has been administered in the United States by computer, using the computerized adaptive testing (CAT) method. The ANR post-test was written to reflect the changes made in the question format by the National Council because of the switch to CAT. (For more information on the testing method, see Part II.)

Instructions

The ANR post-test is based on the same question-and-response format used on NCLEX-RN. It has approximately the same number of questions as those received by the average nurse since CAT's introduction. You should allow about 2 hours for this test. On the actual NCLEX-RN, you will have 5 hours to complete the exam.

A hypothetical clinical situation containing essential background information, written in paragraph form, may precede some questions. The multiple-choice question that follows poses a problem to be solved. You must select the correct response from the four choices presented.

Like NCLEX-RN, the ANR post-test does not contain deliberately misleading questions. Each question has only one correct answer. Before selecting your answer, read the entire question (and clinical situation, if any) carefully to make sure you understand it. Then choose the best answer. Be aware that for some questions, all four answer choices might represent appropriate nursing behavior. However, the question will ask which behavior is *most important* or should be done *first*.

If you do not know the answer to a particular question, try to eliminate one, or preferably two, of the possible answers, and then choose the best answer from the remaining choices. Your results on this test (but not the NCLEX CAT) are based on the number of correct responses, so try to answer every question. Although doing so may mean you'll have to spend a little more time on some questions than you had intended, you'll benefit by obtaining more accurate and complete feedback on your test performance (obtained by self-grading the post-test, as discussed below).

Record your answer choices for the ANR post-test by marking your choice from the options given.

Remember to:
• read each question carefully
• choose the best answer from the four possible choices
• select only one answer for each question
• answer each question on the test.

Sample question

1. Which of the following can the nurse expect to see in a client after prolonged administration of glucocorticoids?
    1. Hypotension.
    2. Hypoglycemia.
    3. Hirsutism.
    4. Protein synthesis.

The correct answer is 3.

On the ANR post-test, the numbers 1, 2, 3, and 4 appear next to the possible answers to a question. These numbers won't appear in NCLEX-RN. They are included on the post-test to help identify the correct answer.

Post-test	NCLEX-RN
1. Atonic	Atonic
2. Dystonic	Dystonic
3. Hypotonic	Hypotonic
4. Hypertonic	Hypertonic

Using your post-test results

After you complete the ANR post-test, turn to page 652, where you'll find the answers and rationales. Carefully study the rationales for any questions you answered incorrectly. This will give you an additional opportunity to recall important nursing information. Remember—the questions on the ANR post-test, like those on NCLEX-RN, focus on practical application of nursing principles rather than recall of facts. Therefore, any studying and reviewing you do after taking the post-test should focus on the broad areas that show up as possible weaknesses on the self-grading performance profile (see page 664).

Post-Test

Questions

1. On the first postoperative day after a cholecystectomy, a client complains of pain 1 hour after receiving Demerol (meperidine) 75 mg I.M. The nurse notes that the client's position has not been changed for 2 hours. Which statement would be most appropriate for the nurse to make while turning the client?
   1. "I can't imagine why the pain medicine didn't work. I'll call the physician as soon as I leave here."
   2. "Let's turn you onto your other side. Maybe that will help."
   3. "This change in position will make you more comfortable and help the medication relieve your pain."
   4. "The physician should be here in 30 minutes. I'll have him check on you then."

2. A postpartal client observes the nurse in the nursery perform a newborn examination on her infant daughter. Later, the nurse sees the client, who is bottle-feeding, hold the infant closely and talk to her quietly as she feeds her. Which of the following would be the nurse's best response to the client's behavior?
   1. Show her how to burp the infant.
   2. Provide her with positive support.
   3. Ask if she is starting to have feelings for the infant.
   4. Show her how to stimulate the infant's sucking reflex.

3. A paranoid client refuses to eat with the other clients. The nurse finds him circling a table and staring intently at one client. Which action by the nurse would be most appropriate?
   1. Call the client by name and suggest he accompany the nurse to another area of the unit.
   2. Alert other staff members and ask the client to go with the nurse to another area of the unit.
   3. Sit down at the table and invite the client to sit at the table with the nurse.
   4. Quickly leave the room to get more help.

4. A client is scheduled for a cholecystogram. Before administering Telepaque tablets (an oral radiopaque medium) in preparation for this test, the nurse should assess the client for an allergy to which of the following?
   1. Milk and cheese.
   2. Seafood and iodine.
   3. Wheat glutens and eggs.
   4. Molds and antibiotics.

5. A boy, age 7 months, is admitted to the hospital with diarrhea and hyponatremic dehydration. His mother tells the nurse she cannot afford to buy infant formula and has been feeding him only water by bottle for the past 2 days. When monitoring the child's hydration status, the nurse should assess and document all of the following at regular intervals. Which one is most important?
   1. Body weight.
   2. Intake and output.
   3. Urine specific gravity.
   4. Anterior fontanel status.

6. A client with cervical cancer is receiving treatment with an Ernst applicator containing radiation. The intensity of radiation is estimated by using the principle of the inverse square rule. If the nurse is 4′ from the radiation source, the exposure would be:
   1. $\frac{1}{2}$ of the exposure at 1′.
   2. $\frac{1}{4}$ of the exposure at 1′.
   3. $\frac{1}{8}$ of the exposure at 1′.
   4. $\frac{1}{16}$ of the exposure at 1′.

7. When preparing to assist with a Papanicolaou (Pap) smear, the nurse should do which of the following?
   1. Ask the client what the results of her last Pap smear were.
   2. Ask the client if she has douched within the past 48 hours.
   3. Tell the client to remain very still during the procedure.
   4. Explain that the physician may do a biopsy if anything suspicious appears.

8. On the second day after undergoing a total hysterectomy for cervical cancer, a client complains of abdominal discomfort from gas pains. Which nursing measure would be most helpful in relieving the client's discomfort?
1. Helping the client to walk.
2. Repositioning the client in bed.
3. Applying an abdominal binder to the client.
4. Encouraging the client to drink plenty of fruit juice.

9. A boy, age 11, is admitted to the hospital with acute asthma. His admission orders include bed rest, I.V. fluids at 35 ml/hour, a clear liquid diet, and aminophylline 170 mg I.V. every 6 hours. Which position would be best for this client?
1. Prone, without a pillow.
2. Supine, with a pillow under the diaphragm.
3. Head elevated 30 degrees.
4. High Fowler's.

10. A client admitted to the emergency department states that she fell down a flight of stairs. On initial physical assessment, the nurse finds cuts and bruises on her face, neck, and forearms. X-rays reveal a spiral fracture of the right arm. The client seems severely anxious and upset. Once her physical needs are met, what is the most important intervention for the nurse to take?
1. Gather more information about her emotional state from family members.
2. Take steps to reduce her level of anxiety.
3. Initiate health care teaching about at-home care of her injuries and cast.
4. Have the client explain again how she got hurt.

11. A client is in the first trimester of pregnancy. During her visit to the physician's office today, the nurse is to instruct her concerning nutritional needs during pregnancy. Which of the following is most important to accomplish during this initial interview?
1. Planning a 1-week menu with the client.
2. Obtaining a diet history from the client.
3. Providing a list of nutrient requirements.
4. Emphasizing the importance of a balanced diet.

12. A client with osteoarthritis of the left hip undergoes a total left hip replacement. Postoperatively, the client develops a fine petechial rash over the chest. The nurse should suspect which condition?
1. Pneumonia.
2. Fat embolism.
3. Pulmonary embolism.
4. Antibiotic sensitivity.

13. A client is admitted to the hospital with deep second-degree burns of the arms, chest, and thighs covering 40% of total body surface area. As a result of the fluid shift that initially follows such burns, the nurse would expect which change in this client?
1. Increased urine output.
2. Increased weight.
3. Decreased pulse rate.
4. Decreased cardiac output.

14. Clients with extensive burns commonly develop stress (Curling's) ulcers. Which finding is most indicative of a stress ulcer?
1. Increased hemoglobin level.
2. Increased erythema.
3. Decreased hematocrit level.
4. Decreased abdominal girth.

15. A pregnant client at term is admitted to the hospital in early labor. She is not sure whether her membranes have ruptured, so the nurse uses nitrazine paper to test her vaginal secretions. The nurse would know the membranes have ruptured if the nitrazine paper:
1. turns olive.
2. turns yellow.
3. turns dark blue.
4. fades.

16. A client who is breast-feeding her newborn is to be discharged from the postpartum unit. She has been found to have no immunity to rubella and has orders to receive rubella vaccine on the day of discharge. What is the most important instruction for the nurse to include in the discharge plan?
    1. Practice contraception and avoid conception for at least 2 months.
    2. Discontinue breast-feeding to prevent the infant from becoming infected with the rubella virus.
    3. Avoid contact with women who are pregnant or who suspect they may be pregnant for at least 2 months.
    4. Have the infant screened for active rubella virus every 2 weeks for at least 2 months.

17. A child with acute asthma is to receive aminophylline. Immediately before and during administration of this drug, which nursing assessment is most important?
    1. Pupil size.
    2. Temperature.
    3. Apical pulse.
    4. Bilateral breath sounds.

18. Which position would be best for a client showing signs of shock?
    1. Semi-Fowler's.
    2. High Fowler's.
    3. Trendelenburg.
    4. Modified Trendelenburg.

19. A client in the manic phase of bipolar disorder invites his nurse to make love with him. Which is the BEST response for the nurse to make?
    1. Tell him no and offer a substitute activity.
    2. Ask him why he decided to ask her rather than another client.
    3. Explain that it is unethical for her to go to bed with him.
    4. Ask him how their making love would help him.

20. Which response pattern best describes Babinski's reflex?
    1. Flexion of the forearm when the biceps tendon is tapped.
    2. Extension of the leg when the patellar tendon is struck.
    3. Tremor of the foot following brisk, forcible dorsiflexion.
    4. Dorsiflexion of the great toe when the sole is scratched.

21. Which instruction should the nurse give a client who is going to have a chest tube removed?
    1. "Hyperventilate just before the tube is removed."
    2. "Inhale as the tube is being pulled out."
    3. "Take a deep breath and hold it."
    4. "Avoid the Valsalva maneuver."

22. What is the best position for a child, age 5, who is 2 hours postoperative following a tonsillectomy?
    1. On the back, with head turned to the side.
    2. On either side, with neck extended.
    3. In semi-Fowler's position, with neck hyperextended.
    4. On the abdomen, in low Fowler's position.

23. A client with heart palpitations and dizziness is referred by his family physician for outpatient mental health counseling. As counseling progresses, the nurse senses that the client has ambivalent feelings about his recent promotion to a high-level management position. How can the nurse best promote the client's ability to examine these feelings?
    1. Tell him it is normal for a person to experience upheaval when changing positions.
    2. Ask him why he is upset about such an important promotion.
    3. Have him describe in detail both his old position and his new position.
    4. Share with him the experiences others have had when they changed positions.

24. To aid respirations, the nurse should place a preterm newborn in which position?
    1. Prone.
    2. Supine.
    3. Head slightly elevated.
    4. Head slightly lowered.

25. A client has a Sengstaken-Blakemore tube in place to treat esophageal varices. Which action is most appropriate to include in the client's plan of care?
    1. Offer the client sips of water to swallow every 2 hours.
    2. Deflate the gastric balloon to prevent an upset stomach.
    3. Check pressure in the balloon by deflating and reinflating it every 4 hours.
    4. Observe for restlessness and increased respirations.

26. Which assessment finding would indicate that a client's abdominal ascites is decreasing?
    1. The amount of ankle edema remains the same.
    2. Abdominal skin becomes shinier.
    3. Urine output per void increases.
    4. The pulse rate increases over time.

27. A client has been in a psychiatric hospital for 6 months. During this time, she has been unable to meet her own hygiene and grooming needs. She spends most of her time alone and usually is nonverbal. When a staff member approaches her, she turns away. She is standing in the hall when the nurse notices a large, damp, red area on the seat of her pants. The nurse assumes the client has begun to menstruate. Which response is most appropriate for the nurse to make at this time?
    1. "You have begun your period. I want you to come into the bathroom with me."
    2. "Your pants are bloody, and you will need to go and change your clothes now."
    3. "You have started your period. Do you want me to get you some supplies?"
    4. "Did you know that you have started your period?"

28. A client's labor does not progress. After ruling out cephalopelvic disproportion, the physician orders I.V. administration of 1,000 ml normal saline with 10 units of Pitocin to run at 2 milliunits/minute. Two milliunits/minute is equivalent to how many milliliters/minute?
    1. 0.002
    2. 0.02
    3. 0.2
    4. 2.0

29. Which foods would be best for a postoperative tonsillectomy client?
    1. Toast, jelly, and ice cream.
    2. Clear soup, apple juice, and gelatin.
    3. Creamed tuna fish, root beer, and cake.
    4. Hot tea, wiener and roll, and sherbet.

30. A client is admitted to the hospital with acute urine retention caused by benign prostatic hyperplasia. An indwelling urinary catheter is inserted. After 750 ml of urine are drained, the catheter is clamped, because rapid bladder decompression can cause which condition?
    1. Dysuria.
    2. Hematuria.
    3. Oliguria.
    4. Albuminuria.

31. Which activity would best meet the diversional needs of a client who is markedly impaired with Alzheimer's disease?
    1. Playing a simple card game.
    2. Working with play dough.
    3. Singing familiar songs.
    4. Putting a puzzle together.

32. The nurse accompanies a client who is to have an intravenous pyelogram (IVP). Which reaction, if it were to occur, should the nurse report to the physician immediately?
    1. Angioedema.
    2. A feeling of warmth.
    3. Flushing of the face.
    4. Salty taste.

33. Within 48 hours after being admitted to the hospital for acute gastritis, a client seems agitated and states that he can feel bugs crawling on his body. The nurse should suspect that the client most likely is:
    1. having an acute episode of schizophrenia.
    2. in the beginning stages of delirium tremens.
    3. reacting to ingestion of an hallucinogenic substance.
    4. entering a preconvulsive state.

34. In response to the news of a plane crash, a schizophrenic client says in a flat tone of voice, "I was supposed to be on that plane. The only reason I wasn't is because the doctor took away my grounds privilege." Based on the client's statement, the nurse can infer that the client:
    1. wants to be famous.
    2. would like to fly a plane someday.
    3. is experiencing a healthy reaction to the event.
    4. may fear her own world will crash someday.

35. A client has been receiving Pitocin to aid her labor progress. The nurse caring for her notes that a contraction has remained strong for 60 seconds. Which action should the nurse take *first*?
    1. Stop the Pitocin.
    2. Notify the physician.
    3. Monitor fetal heart tones.
    4. Turn the client onto her left side.

36. A 2-year-old child, diagnosed with cystic fibrosis as an infant, is admitted to the hospital with pneumonia. She is placed in a high-humidity tent with oxygen and receives aerosol treatments followed by percussion and postural drainage four times daily. Which nursing diagnosis takes priority in planning this client's care?
    1. Altered nutrition: Less than body requirements.
    2. Altered urinary elimination.
    3. Risk for injury.
    4. Ineffective airway clearance.

37. To elicit a 2-year-old's cooperation in taking prescribed medication, the best approach by the nurse would be to say:
    1. "I have your yummy medicine for you to take now. OK?"
    2. "It's time for your medicine. Do you want to drink it from this cup or from a spoon?"
    3. "Are you ready to take your medicine now, or do you want to wait until after your bath?"
    4. "Here's your medicine. It will help you cough up those secretions so you'll feel better."

38. A client who had cataract surgery in the morning is to be discharged that afternoon. Which statement would indicate that the client understands instructions about wearing the eye shield?
    1. "I don't need to wear the eye shield after I'm discharged."
    2. "I will wear the eye shield both day and night for 3 weeks."
    3. "I will wear the eye shield at night for 1 month."
    4. "I can stop wearing the eye shield after 2 weeks."

39. When caring for a client with glaucoma who is scheduled for eye surgery, it is imperative that the nurse:
    1. not administer acetazolamide (Diamox) before the surgery.
    2. stay alert for any mydriatic medications ordered for the client.
    3. give preoperatively ordered meperidine and atropine on time.
    4. instill cycloplegic eye drops every 15 minutes for 1 hour.

40. A client, age 19, has anorexia nervosa. Laboratory results show that she has serious electrolyte imbalances. At this point, decisions about her treatment are best made by:
    1. the staff.
    2. the client.
    3. the client and treatment team.
    4. the client and her primary nurse.

41. A 2-year-old child is brought to the emergency department because she swallowed some kerosene. To detect early signs of toxicity, the nurse should make which assessment *first*?
    1. Abdominal circumference.
    2. Character of respirations.
    3. Ability to flex and hyperextend the neck.
    4. Pupillary reaction to light.

42. The nurse notes that a client takes her nortriptyline hydrochloride (Aventyl) capsules with very little water. The nurse suspects she is "cheeking" the medication. The most reliable way to validate this suspicion is to:
    1. confront the client with the suspicion.
    2. search the client's belongings and room.
    3. have a blood drug level drawn to check for therapeutic levels.
    4. engage the client in conversation immediately after she takes her medication.

43. A new mother is interested in seeing what her infant's eyes look like. Which is the most effective way for the nurse to stimulate the infant to open the eyes?
    1. Gently separate the infant's eyelids with the fingers.
    2. Stimulate the Moro response.
    3. Hold the infant in an upright position.
    4. Shine a penlight toward the infant's face.

44. A client who is taking levodopa to treat Parkinson's disease has been taught to avoid certain practices. He engages in the following practices. Which one indicates a need for further teaching?
    1. Chewing gum.
    2. Taking vitamin pills.
    3. Drinking fruit juice.
    4. Eating six small meals each day.

45. When caring for a client who has just undergone a transsphenoidal hypophysectomy, the nurse must stay *most* alert for:
    1. respiratory depression.
    2. gastric distention.
    3. cardiac arrhythmias.
    4. excessive urine output.

46. A client is admitted with a provisional diagnosis of adult-onset diabetes mellitus. During the early stages of this condition, which signs and symptoms are most likely to arise?
    1. Tachycardia, diaphoresis.
    2. Flushed face, ketonuria, abdominal pain.
    3. Headache, anuria, edema.
    4. Polyuria, thirst, weight loss.

47. A paranoid client tells the nurse that he continuously hears voices telling him to get in his car and run over people. He asks, "Can't you hear those voices, too?" Which of the following would be the most appropriate response by the nurse?
    1. "No, I can't hear the voices and soon you won't hear them either."
    2. "Let's not talk about voices. Let's take a walk."
    3. "I don't hear any voices. You seem to be upset. Tell me how you're feeling."
    4. "I'm glad you trust me enough to tell me about the voices. What are they saying to you?"

48. After a car accident, a client exhibits signs of a head injury and is admitted to the hospital for observation. The nurse sees the client take several Percodan tablets she brought from home. Which action by the nurse indicates understanding of the potential side effects of Percodan for this client?
    1. Notifying the client's physician.
    2. Raising the side rails of the client's bed.
    3. Turning off the client's TV and room lights.
    4. Monitoring the client's blood pressure every 2 hours.

49. A client is several days postoperative following a cholecystectomy. The client's blood gas results are: pH = 7.35; bicarbonate (HCO_3^-) = 30 mEq/liter; PCO_2 = 50 mm Hg; and PO_2 = 90 mm Hg. Based on these results, which intervention by the nurse is appropriate?
    1. Start the client on nasal oxygen at 2 liters/minute.
    2. Have the client turn, deep-breathe, and cough every 2 hours.
    3. Send a specimen of the client's nasogastric drainage to the lab for analysis.
    4. Obtain an order to give the client 1 ampule of sodium bicarbonate.

50. A preterm newborn is diagnosed as having respiratory distress syndrome. Which pathophysiologic problem is most clearly associated with respiratory distress syndrome?
    1. Hypocalcemia.
    2. Hypoglycemia.
    3. Inadequate synthesis of lecithin.
    4. Inadequate storage of glycogen and fat.

51. A child, age 3, is admitted to the emergency department with acute salicylate (aspirin) poisoning. Which of the following is the most crucial nursing assessment for this client?
    1. Blood pressure.
    2. Presence of petechiae.
    3. Respiratory rate and depth.
    4. Urine specific gravity.

52. A client is admitted to the emergency department after being sexually assaulted. She is accompanied by a policewoman. The nurse realizes that several important tasks should be done in sexual assault cases. Which nursing intervention should receive first priority?
    1. Assisting with medical treatment.
    2. Collecting and preparing evidence for the police.
    3. Attempting to reduce the client's anxiety from panic to a moderate level.
    4. Providing anticipatory guidance to the client about normal responses to sexual assault.

53. An Rh-negative client delivers her second child at 40 weeks' gestation. She had a rising antibody titer during pregnancy and her Coombs' test was positive. Her newborn son, of average weight for gestational age, is admitted to the normal newborn nursery for initial care. Sixteen hours after his birth, the nurse receives the following laboratory report:
    • Serum bilirubin—10 mg/100 ml
    • Coombs' test of cord blood—positive.
    Based on the above laboratory values for the newborn, which action should the nurse take first?
    1. Assess him for signs of hypoglycemia.
    2. Increase his fluid intake.
    3. Place him under the bilirubin lights.
    4. Notify his physician.

54. Which activity would be most appropriate for a client who is in a manic state?
    1. Tearing rags to make a rug.
    2. Playing a table game.
    3. Doing vigorous aerobic dancing.
    4. Reading light, entertaining stories.

55. A client is scheduled for a routine gynecologic examination by her private physician. Which action would be appropriate for the nurse who is assisting with the pelvic examination?
    1. Staying with the client throughout the examination.
    2. Instructing the client in shallow breathing to aid relaxation.
    3. Reminding the client that, should she feel embarrassed, many women have the same experience.
    4. Leaving the room after draping the client to ensure her privacy.

56. A client is receiving external beam radiation on an outpatient basis. The nurse instructs him in the care of his skin within the port marks. Which response by the client would indicate that he understands the instructions?
    1. "I will wash the area every day with soap and water."
    2. "I can use a little talcum powder to help soothe my skin."
    3. "I can use A and D Ointment if my skin becomes dry."
    4. "I will be sure to avoid washing between the marks."

57. When caring for a pregnant client with a lactose intolerance, the nurse should pay special attention to the client's need for:
    1. iron.
    2. calcium.
    3. folic acid.
    4. carbohydrates.

58. In a newborn, which sign indicates developing hydrocephalus?
    1. A pulsating anterior fontanel.
    2. Closure of the suture lines in the skull.
    3. Orthopneic positioning.
    4. "Setting sun" sign.

59. Two days after a left-eye cataract extraction, a client complains of nausea, vomiting, and seeing halos around lights. Which complication should the nurse suspect?
1. Detached retina.
2. Increased intraocular pressure.
3. Dislocated lens.
4. Corneal abrasion.

60. A client is to be discharged after a total hip replacement. Which statement indicates that the client understands the discharge instructions?
1. "I have to do special exercises several times a day."
2. "I should take frequent rides in the car to increase my activity."
3. "I should wear loose clothes so my hip movements aren't restricted.".
4. "I should walk at least 2 miles a day."

61. A client has been given the nursing diagnosis "social isolation related to fear of rejection." The nursing assessment documentation includes, "No eye contact, verbally uncommunicative, refuses to leave bedroom." Which is the best outcome criterion for determining if the goal of care for this client has been met?
1. Client performs own self-care.
2. Client smiles at nurse when nurse enters room.
3. Client remains free of hallucinations or delusions.
4. Client goes to nurses' station for medication.

62. A client with deep second-degree burns is being treated with mafenide acetate (Sulfamylon) cream. Which condition can result from use of this medication?
1. Uremia.
2. Metabolic acidosis.
3. Hypervolemia.
4. Hypotension.

63. A pregnant client is being coached by her husband during early labor. She complains of discomfort during contractions. To help his wife cope with the discomfort, which technique should the husband suggest?
1. Normal breathing.
2. Slow chest breathing.
3. Accelerated breathing.
4. Pant-blow breathing.

64. A boy with acute asthma is to receive 840 ml of I.V. fluids per day. Orders include promoting oral fluid intake. Which goal should the nurse establish for the client's oral fluid intake?
1. 250 ml/24 hours.
2. 500 ml/24 hours.
3. 750 ml/24 hours.
4. 1,000 ml/24 hours.

65. A client with second-degree burns covering 40% of her body has a nursing diagnosis of "Altered nutrition: Less than body requirements, related to large burn area and pain." She enjoys all of the following foods. Which foods would be the best choices to help her regain nutritional balance?
1. Steak and french fries.
2. Peanut butter and raisins.
3. Orange juice and carrots.
4. Corn and milk.

66. A client who has been struck by a car is being observed in the hospital for signs of injury. Present orders read:
- Vital signs q1h
- NPO for 24 hours
- Nasal O_2 at 2 liters/minute p.r.n.
- Indwelling urinary catheter to straight drainage, if needed
- 5% dextrose in 0.45% saline solution at 100 ml/hour
- Call physician for any signs of shock or increased intracranial pressure.

The nurse determines that the client is showing early signs of shock. Which action should the nurse take first?
1. Call the physician.
2. Start nasal oxygen.
3. Increase the intravenous rate.
4. Insert the urinary catheter.

67. A pediatric client is to be discharged after recovering from an acute asthmatic attack. The nurse plans to teach the child and family all of the following methods involved in managing the asthmatic client. Which one should the nurse emphasize?
1. Activity limitations.
2. Dietary restrictions.
3. Postural drainage.
4. Breathing exercises.

68. An adult client who was struck by a car has a decreased level of consciousness and exhibits other signs of increased intracranial pressure. Which position would be best for this client?
    1. Supine.
    2. Prone.
    3. Semi-Fowler's.
    4. Side-lying.

69. A gravida II, para I client is admitted to the maternity unit at 4 a.m. Five hours later, a summary report of her progress reads as follows:

TIME	DILATED	EFFACED	STATION	MEMBRANES
4 a.m.	3 cm	60%	-1	Intact
6 a.m.	5 to 6 cm	80%	0	Ruptured
8 a.m.	6 cm	80%	0	Ruptured
9 a.m.	6 cm	80%	0	Ruptured

At the same times as listed above, her contractions were as follows:

TIME	SEVERITY	INTERVAL	DURATION
4 a.m.	Moderate	q 4 to 5 minutes	30 seconds
6 a.m.	Moderate	q 4 minutes	45 seconds
8 a.m.	Moderate	q 5 to 8 minutes	35 seconds
9 a.m.	Mild	q 10 minutes	20 seconds

The above assessment data indicate dystocia. Which term best describes the type of contraction pattern?
    1. Atonic.
    2. Dystonic.
    3. Hypotonic.
    4. Hypertonic.

70. A client with increased intracranial pressure is receiving mannitol. To evaluate the effectiveness of this drug, the nurse should assess the client for which of the following?
    1. Decreased pulse rate.
    2. Decreased systolic blood pressure.
    3. Increased urine output.
    4. Increased pupillary reaction.

71. A client suffers a tension pneumothorax as a result of an injury. She is admitted to the intensive care unit from the emergency department with a sucking chest wound. A chest tube is inserted and connected to a two-bottle water-seal drainage system. Which assessment finding would indicate the development of mediastinal shift?
    1. Vomiting.
    2. Somnolence.
    3. Tachycardia.
    4. Cheyne-Stokes breathing.

72. A depressed and withdrawn client approaches the nurse, who is busy working with a social worker in the conference room. Which would be the best response by the nurse?
    1. Tell the client that the nurse will see her in 10 minutes.
    2. Tell the client she'll have to wait until the nurse and social worker are finished.
    3. Ask the client if what she wants is urgent.
    4. Ask the client how the nurse can help her.

73. When administering Pitocin, the nurse should observe for which potential side effect?
    1. Decreased pulse rate.
    2. Elevated blood pressure.
    3. Generalized rash.
    4. Increased urine output.

74. A client has been treated for cirrhosis of the liver for 3 years. Now he is hospitalized for treatment of recently diagnosed esophageal varices. Which of the following should the nurse teach the client?
    1. Eat foods quickly so they do not get cold and cause distress.
    2. Avoid straining at stool to keep venous pressure low.
    3. Decrease fluid intake to avoid ascites.
    4. Avoid exercise because it may cause bleeding of the varices.

75. Which sign would alert the nurse to possible hemorrhage in a client immediately after a tonsillectomy?
    1. Mouth breathing.
    2. Stertorous respirations.
    3. Frequent swallowing.
    4. Dark brown emesis.

76. A nurse is approached by a middle-aged male client with chronic schizophrenia. She has never seen this client before. He is unkempt and wearing a football helmet. He walks briskly up to her, puts his face close to hers, and says, "Let's screw." His affect is flat. The most reasonable inference for the nurse to make is that the client
   1. is trying to embarrass her.
   2. is asking her to relate to him.
   3. has unmet sexual needs.
   4. probably hates women.

77. The primary cause of abdominal ascites in a client with cirrhosis of the liver is:
   1. an increased vasopressin level.
   2. an increased serum sodium level.
   3. a decreased serum aldosterone level.
   4. a decreased serum albumin level.

78. A client is in acute renal failure. The nurse must assess the client carefully for which of the following potential complications?
   1. Tetany.
   2. Hypernatremia.
   3. Vascular collapse.
   4. Cardiac arrhythmias.

79. A client delivers a child spontaneously after Pitocin induction. One minute after the birth, the nurse makes the following observations of the newborn:
   • pulse—above 100 beats/minute
   • respiratory effort—good
   • active motion
   • grimace
   • body pink, extremities blue.
   Which Apgar score should the newborn receive?
   1. 4
   2. 6
   3. 8
   4. 10

80. A boy, age 4, is admitted to the hospital with acute myelogenous leukemia. He has many bruises and petechiae over his legs and arms. Which nursing measure would best prevent additional bruising?
   1. Brushing his teeth only once per day.
   2. Trimming his nails short.
   3. Handling him with the palms of the hands.
   4. Placing him in a caged crib with padded rails.

81. During admission to the pediatric unit, a 2-year-old girl clings to her blanket from home. This behavior is an example of:
   1. ritualism.
   2. negativism.
   3. dawdling.
   4. regression.

82. A client is 1 day postoperative following a transurethral resection. The client also has chronic glaucoma. Postoperative orders read:
   • Maintain continuous bladder irrigation at 100 ml/hour.
   • Belladonna and opium suppositories q4h p.r.n.
   • Pilocarpine eye drops 1% q6h in each eye.
   The client develops painful bladder spasms. Which action would be most appropriate for the nurse to take?
   1. Call the physician and question the orders.
   2. Administer the belladonna and opium suppositories.
   3. Suggest that the client try to void around the catheter.
   4. Decrease the flow rate of the continuous bladder irrigation.

83. A farmer with Alzheimer's disease is admitted to the gerontology unit. His wife asks the nurse what she should do when her husband does not recognize her. What would be the nurse's best response?
   1. Read books to him dealing with farm activities.
   2. Tell him who she is and then walk with him on the unit.
   3. Bring family pictures with her when she visits.
   4. Show him her wedding ring and remind him she is his wife.

84. When caring for a client with bulimia, the best way for the nurse to determine if she has stopped purging after meals is to:
   1. observe what she does after every meal.
   2. monitor her electrolyte lab values.
   3. weigh her before and 2 hours after each meal.
   4. not allow her to leave the unit right after meals.

85. A client who is receiving a phenothiazine medication has become restless and fidgety, and has paced the hallway continuously for the past hour. This behavior suggests that the client may be experiencing:
   1. dystonia.
   2. akathisia.
   3. parkinsonian effects.
   4. tardive dyskinesia.

86. A girl, age 12, has scoliosis with a curve greater than 40 degrees. She is admitted for treatment with halo-pelvic traction, to be followed by surgical insertion of a Harrington rod. Given her age and condition, which activity would be most appropriate for her to select during her hospitalization?
   1. Playing Monopoly with a child her age.
   2. Doing crossword puzzles.
   3. Reading a novel such as *Little Women.*
   4. Playing a card game such as "Old Maid."

87. A newborn has just been admitted to the nursery. Nursing assessment reveals all of the following findings. Which finding should the nurse consider a deviation from normal?
   1. Visible jaundice.
   2. Cyanosis of the hands and feet.
   3. Mongolian spots on the buttocks.
   4. Respiratory rate of 42 breaths/minute.

88. One month after undergoing a subtotal gastrectomy, a client complains of dizziness, sweating, and tachycardia occurring within 30 minutes after eating. These symptoms most likely result from:
   1. pernicious anemia.
   2. pyloric stenosis.
   3. dumping syndrome.
   4. a recurring ulcer.

89. Which pattern of laboratory values is most indicative of a client's recovery from acute pancreatitis?
   1. Rising serum bilirubin levels.
   2. Rising serum alkaline phosphatase levels.
   3. Decreasing serum amylase levels.
   4. Decreasing hemoglobin levels.

90. The physician prescribes benztropine mesylate (Cogentin) for a client with Parkinson's disease. After the nurse teaches the client about side effects of this drug, the client should identify which symptom as a potential side effect?
   1. Increased urine output.
   2. Blurred vision.
   3. Excessive salivation.
   4. Difficulty swallowing.

91. During a screening of first graders for the presence of sickle cell disease, a 6-year-old girl is found to be positive. Which of these assessments would support that diagnosis?
   1. She has a beefy-red tongue.
   2. She has joint nodules.
   3. She has scleral icterus.
   4. She has edema of the legs.

92. A 14-year-old boy who has a history of asthma is being seen in the physician's office. Which of these observations would indicate that his condition is worsening?
   1. He is sitting upright with his shoulders in a hunched position.
   2. He is having paroxysmal, productive coughing spells.
   3. He is breathing slowly and deeply.
   4. He is using his intercostal and diaphragmatic muscles to breathe.

93. A staff nurse on a busy surgical unit suspects that another nurse on the unit is abusing drugs. She documents her observations as follows: "When the unit was extremely busy during the evening shift of June 21, 1997, Ms. Brown could not be located on three separate occasions for 20 minutes. When she returned, her pupils were constricted and she was euphoric." The nurse's documentation of the colleague's behavior is best described as
   1. conclusive.
   2. interpretive.
   3. objective.
   4. digressive.

94. An elderly client has been taking digoxin (Lanoxin) at home for congestive heart failure. The client is admitted to the hospital because of cardiac arrhythmias. His digoxin blood level is 5.0 mg/ml. A diagnosis of digitalis toxicity is made. The nurse determines that the client has been taking the prescribed dose of digoxin as well as furosemide (Lasix). The nurse also learns that all of the following facts pertain to the client. Which one most likely caused the digitalis toxicity?
   1. He has periodic episodes of constipation.
   2. He has been taking potassium supplements.
   3. He has been overeating for the past week.
   4. Laboratory studies show renal insufficiency.

95. A client who is 28 weeks pregnant tells the nurse, "I had to have my rings cut off because my hands were so puffy." Based on this data, the nurse should seek additional information concerning the
   1. height of the fundus.
   2. fetal heart rate.
   3. presence of protein in the urine.
   4. blood level of human placental lactogen.

96. A nurse is interviewing a client who is in the second trimester of her pregnancy. Which of these questions would provide information about the client's mastery of the primary developmental task during the second trimester?
   1. "Does your baby seem to be a separate person now?"
   2. "Does your pregnancy seem real to you now?"
   3. "Have you started to prepare yourself for labor and delivery?"
   4. "Have you given your baby a name yet?"

97. A 14-year-old girl with structural scoliosis is fitted with a Milwaukee brace. Because of the brace, which of these potential nursing diagnoses should be given priority in her plan of care?
   1. Ineffective breathing pattern.
   2. Activity intolerance.
   3. Impaired skin integrity.
   4. Pain.

98. A postpartum client is planning to breast-feed. To keep the nipples in good condition for breast-feeding and to prevent infection, the nurse should include which of these measures in the client's plan of care?
   1. Washing the nipples with soap and water before each feeding.
   2. Exposing the nipples to air and sunlight for short periods of time.
   3. Using a plastic bra liner to handle leakage.
   4. Cleansing the nipples with a mild antiseptic solution.

99. A nurse is orienting a new staff nurse about the care of a client who is to have temporary internal radiation therapy for cancer of the cervix. The nurse should give the staff nurse which of these instructions about the client's care after the implantation of the radiation?
   1. "Make sure that an aluminum-lined container with long forceps is in the room at all times in case the radiation source becomes dislodged."
   2. "Collect all of the client's soiled linen in her room until it is determined that they don't contain radiation."
   3. "To minimize exposure to the radiation, pregnant staff members should plan to accomplish their direct care activities for the client in 15 minutes."
   4. "Since the client's body wastes are considered irradiated, they should be discarded down the toilet with three flushes."

100. A client who has increased intracranial pressure from a head injury is to receive mannitol (Osmitrol) intravenously. The mannitol is prescribed for which of these purposes?
   1. To restore electrolytes.
   2. To stimulate kidney function.
   3. To increase circulating blood volume.
   4. To reduce cerebral edema.

101. After a normal newborn infant is bottle-fed, the nurse should place the infant in which of these positions?
   1. Supine, with the head slightly elevated.
   2. Prone, with the head slightly lowered.
   3. Left-side lying.
   4. Right-side lying.

102. A common side effect of diphtheria, tetanus, and pertussis (DPT) vaccine given to an infant would most likely be manifested by which of these symptoms?
1. Vomiting.
2. Hematuria.
3. Sudden elevated temperature.
4. Swelling at the injection site.

103. A nurse's aide, who appears intoxicated, reports for duty on the pediatric unit. Which of these actions would be appropriate for the nurse to take initially?
1. Send the aide home to sleep it off.
2. Advise the aide to seek help from Alcoholics Anonymous.
3. Assign the aide to nonclient care tasks.
4. Discuss the aide's condition with a supervisor.

104. A client with advanced tuberculosis has been assigned to your care. Which of the following should be emphasized in your client-teaching plan?
1. Maintain a diet high in calories and low in protein.
2. Drug treatment will be intensive and of short duration.
3. Avoid physical contact with family and friends.
4. Take prescribed drugs on schedule and do not miss doses.

105. Which of the following is most effective in obtaining a postoperative client's cooperation with the treatment plan?
1. Providing adequate pain control.
2. Having thorough preoperative teaching.
3. Giving the client a sense of control.
4. Reducing unfamiliar external stimuli.

Answers and rationales

In the answers below, the question number appears in boldface type, followed by the number of the correct answer. Rationales for correct answers and, where appropriate, for incorrect options, follow. To help you evaluate your knowledge base and application of nursing behaviors, each question is classified as follows:
NP = Phase of the nursing process
CN = Client need.

1. Correct answer—3
This option promotes the client's belief in the effectiveness of the intervention, which may help potentiate its effect. Option 1 is inappropriate because the nurse should attempt nursing measures before notifying the physician. Option 2 does not suggest strongly enough that the position change will bring relief. Option 4 suggests that the nurse should wait for the physician to arrive instead of trying to relieve discomfort through nursing measures and positive suggestion.
NP: Implementation
CN: Safe, effective care environment

2. Correct answer—2
Positive reinforcement of attachment behaviors promotes such behaviors. Options 1 and 4 are inappropriate because there is no indication that the client needs help with burping or stimulating the sucking reflex. Option 3 is not appropriate at this time because the client's behavior suggests she has positive feelings; it may confuse or threaten the client.
NP: Evaluation
CN: Psychosocial integrity

3. Correct answer—2
The nurse should provide safety and take measures to defuse the potentially violent reaction between the clients. If a client shows a potential for violence, the nurse should obtain help rather than try to manage the situation alone (option 1). Option 3 would increase the risk of violence by bringing the two clients closer together. Option 4 is inappropriate because the nurse should not leave unattended a room with a potentially violent client.
NP: Implementation
CN: Psychosocial integrity

4. Correct answer—2
The nurse should check the client's history for an allergy to seafood and iodine because Telepaque tablets contain iodine. The other options are not iodine sources.
NP: Assessment
CN: Safe, effective care environment

5. Correct answer—1
Body weight provides a baseline for fluid and electrolyte replacement; the percentage of weight gained or lost is the best indicator of hydration status. Although the other options are important to monitor when assessing hydration status, weight changes are more accurate.
NP: Assessment
CN: Physiologic integrity

6. Correct answer—4
The exposure to radiation at 4′ from the source is determined by squaring ¹/₄. To receive ¹/₂ the exposure at 1′ (option 1), the nurse would have to be 1.415′ from the client; to receive ¹/₄ the exposure (option 2), the nurse would have to be 2′ from the client; to receive ¹/₈ the exposure (option 3), the nurse would have to be 2.83′ from the client.
NP: Analysis
CN: Safe, effective care environment

7. Correct answer—2
To ensure an adequate and reliable specimen, the client should not douche for 24 hours before a Pap smear. Option 1 may prove helpful later but is not necessary for this test. Options 3 and 4 are unnecessary; in addition, option 4 may cause anxiety.
NP: Implementation
CN: Safe, effective care environment

8. Correct answer—1
Walking helps restore normal peristalsis and bowel function, which helps relieve gas and the discomfort it produces. Option 2 may prove helpful but is less effective than walking. Option 3 would provide abdominal support but would not stimulate peristalsis or relieve gas pains. Drinking large amounts of fruit juice (option 4) would increase distention.
NP: Implementation
CN: Physiologic integrity

9. Correct answer—4
High Fowler's is the best choice. Even in this position, however, a child experiencing acute asthma is most comfortable leaning forward with legs tucked under (tripod position). The other options do not increase comfort during an asthma attack because the child is so short of breath.
NP: Implementation
CN: Physiologic integrity

10. Correct answer—2
Once the client's anxiety level is reduced, she will be able to cooperate with treatment and express her needs. Option 1 is inappropriate because no further information is needed for initial evaluation of the client's emotional state. The client is too anxious to accept teaching (option 3) or to give additional information (option 4).
NP: Implementation
CN: Safe, effective care environment

11. Correct answer—2
For teaching to be effective, the nurse must assess the client's usual dietary habits. The other options also are important, but should be done *after* obtaining the diet history.
NP: Assessment
CN: Health promotion and maintenance

12. Correct answer—2
Petechial rash is a sign of fat embolism—a complication that may arise after major surgery. Options 1 and 3 rarely cause such a rash. Option 4 typically causes a rash over the entire body.
NP: Assessment
CN: Physiologic integrity

13. Correct answer—4
The nurse would expect decreased cardiac output from hypovolemia. The other options describe changes opposite to those that would result from the fluid shift.
NP: Evaluation
CN: Physiologic integrity

14. Correct answer—3
A decreased hematocrit level reflects loss of red blood cells—a sign of bleeding, as in a stress ulcer. The hemoglobin level would decrease, not increase (option 1). A stress ulcer does not cause increased erythema (option 2) or decreased abdominal girth (option 4).
NP: Assessment
CN: Physiologic integrity

15. Correct answer—3
Amniotic fluid is slightly alkaline and will turn nitrazine paper blue. Options 1 and 2 would indicate intact membranes. Option 4 is incorrect because nitrazine paper does not fade.
NP: Assessment
CN: Physiologic integrity

16. Correct answer—1
The client should not become pregnant soon after being immunized because the rubella virus is teratogenic. Rubella from the vaccine is not communicable, so the client need not discontinue breast-feeding (option 2), need not avoid contact with pregnant women (option 3), and need not worry about transmitting the virus to her infant because of receiving the vaccine (option 4).
NP: Evaluation
CN: Health promotion and maintenance

17. Correct answer—3
The nurse should assess the child's apical pulse because overdose or rapid administration of aminophylline can cause cardiac arrhythmias. Aminophylline does not affect pupil size (option 1) or temperature (option 2). Although the child's breath sounds (option 4) should improve after aminophylline administration, this is not the most important assessment.
NP: Assessment
CN: Physiologic integrity

18. Correct answer—4
The modified Trendelenburg position allows full respiratory excursion by slightly elevating the head and increases venous return by elevating the feet. Full respiratory excursion is crucial to assume maximum ventilation capacity; the client is going into shock and needs all the air he can get. Options 1 and 2 promote respiratory excursion but do not improve venous return. Option 3 promotes venous return but does not aid respiratory excursion.
NP: Implementation
CN: Physiologic integrity

19. Correct answer—1
This response sets a limit and offers an alternative for the client to decrease his anxiety level. Options 2 and 4 are incorrect because they lead the client on and do not set any limits. Option 3 is incorrect because, although a reasonable response, it doesn't offer an alternative.
NP: Planning
CN: Psychosocial integrity

20. Correct answer—4
Babinski's reflex is characterized by dorsiflexion of the great toe and fanning of the other toes when the sole is stimulated. This reflex usually is absent in adults and in children over age 24 months; its presence may indicate damage to pyramidal tracts. Option 1 describes the biceps reflex. Option 2 describes the patellar reflex. Option 3 occurs with ankle clonus.
NP: Analysis
CN: Physiologic integrity

21. Correct answer—3
To prevent atmospheric air from rushing into the thoracic cavity, the nurse should instruct the client to take a deep breath and then hold it. Options 1 and 2 would allow air to enter the thoracic cavity. The Valsalva maneuver is helpful when a chest tube is removed; the nurse should not tell the client to avoid it (option 4).
NP: Implementation
CN: Physiologic integrity

22. Correct answer—2
A side-lying position with the neck extended allows secretions to drain and maintains a patent airway. The other options increase the risk of aspiration of blood, secretions, and vomitus.
NP: Implementation
CN: Physiologic integrity

23. Correct answer—3
Having the client describe the old and new positions allows him to explore his experience objectively. Options 1 and 4 minimize his experience and do not focus on his distress. Option 2 is judgmental and implies that the client should be grateful for the promotion.
NP: Planning
CN: Psychosocial integrity

24. Correct answer—3
Slightly elevating the newborn's head keeps the weight of the abdominal contents off the diaphragm and aids breathing. Option 1 would place the newborn's full weight on the chest and abdomen, compromising respiratory excursion. Option 2 would not aid respirations, unless the newborn's head is elevated and the neck extended. Option 4 would place the weight of the abdominal contents on the diaphragm, impeding respirations.
NP: Implementation
CN: Safe, effective care environment

25. Correct answer—4
Restlessness and increased respirations may indicate hemorrhage. Introducing water into the stomach (option 1) may cause metabolic alkalosis from loss of chloride or hydrogen ions. The balloon holds the tube in place and should not be deflated (option 2) until just before tube removal. The esophageal balloon controls esophageal bleeding and therefore should be kept inflated at all times; the nurse should not deflate and reinflate it periodically (option 3).
NP: Planning
CN: Safe, effective care environment

26. Correct answer—3
Increased urine output means ascitic fluid is being absorbed into the circulation and then excreted. As this fluid is absorbed, ankle edema should decrease, not remain the same (option 1), and abdominal skin should become less shiny, not shinier (option 2). With decreasing ascites, lower fluid volume would cause the pulse rate to slow, not to increase (option 4).
NP: Assessment
CN: Physiologic integrity

27. Correct answer—1
This response orients the client to reality and provides the structure the client needs to solve the immediate problem. The client is too anxious and regressed to engage in the problem solving required by options 2 and 3. Option 4 is inane because the client is unable to provide self-care as a result of severe anxiety that interferes with problem solving and prevents awareness of reality.
NP: Implementation
CN: Psychosocial integrity

28. Correct answer—3
10,000 milliunits : 1,000 ml = 2 milliunits : X ml
$$\frac{10,000}{1,000} = \frac{2}{X}$$
10,000X = 2,000
$$X = \frac{2,000}{10,000}$$
X = 0.2 ml
Each unit of Pitocin contains 1,000 milliunits. Therefore, 1,000 ml of I.V. fluid contains 10,000 milliunits (10 units) of Pitocin.
NP: Implementation
CN: Physiologic integrity

29. Correct answer—2
These foods are not irritating to the tonsil bed. The other options include solid or hard foods, which would irritate the tonsil bed.
NP: Evaluation
CN: Health promotion and maintenance

30. Correct answer—2
Rapid emptying of a distended bladder can cause shock and hemorrhage into the bladder as blood rushes to fill previously compressed blood vessels. The other options rarely occur with rapid bladder decompression.
NP: Implementation
CN: Physiologic integrity

31. Correct answer—3
Typically, the client with Alzheimer's disease responds favorably to music, especially selections that recall pleasant times and memories. The other options would give the client something to put in the mouth, which could cause choking.
NP: Implementation
CN: Psychosocial integrity

32. Correct answer—1
Angioedema is a severe allergic reaction to iodine in the dye used during an IVP; it can cause edema of the larynx and difficulty breathing. The other options are unlikely to arise as reactions to the dye.
NP: Implementation
CN: Physiologic integrity

33. Correct answer—2
The client's symptoms are consistent with early delirium tremens, which occurs 2 to 5 days after alcohol withdrawal. Gastritis is a result of increased alcohol intake; when hospitalized, the alcohol level goes to zero and the client goes into withdrawal. His symptoms are not typical of schizophrenia (option 1). A reaction to an hallucinogenic substance (option 3) would occur within minutes of ingestion. Although seizures (option 4) may occur if delirium tremens is not treated promptly, they are not likely to arise during early stages.
NP: Analysis
CN: Psychosocial integrity

34. Correct answer—4
The schizophrenic client typically communicates in a highly symbolic manner; this client's statement is a symbolic expression of her fears. The client is not sufficiently in touch with reality to express a rational or realistic desire to be famous (option 1) or to fly a plane (option 2). The schizophrenic client does not react in a healthy, reality-based manner (option 3).
NP: Analysis
CN: Psychosocial integrity

35. Correct answer—1
A contraction that remains strong for 60 seconds with no sign of letting up signals approaching tetany and could cause rupture of the uterus. Pitocin stimulates contractions and, therefore, should be stopped. The nurse also should take the actions described in the other options, but only *after* stopping the Pitocin.
NP: Implementation
CN: Physiologic integrity

36. Correct answer—4
Adequate respiratory function is essential to maintain life; a nursing diagnosis related to respiratory dysfunction takes priority over all other nursing diagnoses.
NP: Analysis
CN: Physiologic integrity

37. Correct answer—2
This option offers realistic choices to the toddler and gives the child some sense of control and autonomy. Option 1 is not realistic; the medicine probably tastes bad and the child most likely will refuse it. Option 3 gives the child an opportunity to delay taking the medicine, which is not acceptable. Although option 4 reflects a rational approach, it is not necessarily likely to make a toddler cooperate.
NP: Implementation
CN: Safe, effective care environment

38. Correct answer—3
The client should wear the eye shield at night for 1 month after surgery to guard against rubbing or hitting the eye while sleeping.
NP: Evaluation
CN: Health promotion and maintenance

39. Correct answer—2
Mydriatic agents cause pupil dilation and therefore may affect the size of the pupil desired by the surgeon during surgery. Option 1 is incorrect because acetazolamide and other carbonic anhydrase inhibitors are given preoperatively to restrict the action of the enzyme necessary to produce aqueous humor. Option 3 is incorrect because atropine is a mydriatic agent and would not be ordered preoperatively for a client with glaucoma. Option 4 is incorrect because cycloplegic eye drops also are mydriatic agents and therefore are contraindicated for this client.
NP: Implementation
CN: Physiologic integrity

40. Correct answer—1
At this point, only staff members have the knowledge base to make decisions about the client's treatment. The other options are incorrect because a client with serious electrolyte imbalances is incapable of making sound decisions about treatment.
NP: Planning
CN: Psychosocial integrity

41. Correct answer—2
If the client inhaled fumes, she might have chemical burns and chemical pneumonia; therefore, the nurse first should assess the character of her respirations. Kerosene toxicity would not cause a change in abdominal circumference (option 1). Options 3 and 4 are incorrect because inability to do neck flexion and hyperextension and absent pupillary reaction to light are late, not early, signs of kerosene toxicity. (Other late signs include dizziness, lethargy, and unconsciousness.)
NP: Assessment
CN: Physiologic integrity

42. Correct answer—4
It is difficult to produce clear speech with something in the mouth. Option 1 is likely to result in a denial and is not a reliable way to validate the nurse's suspicion. Option 2 may reveal nothing and may just make the client become more clever about hiding medication. Option 3 is incorrect because blood levels for antidepressants are not reliable.
NP: Assessment
CN: Safe, effective care environment

43. Correct answer—3
When held upright, an infant will open the eyes reflexively. Stimulation, such as by separating the eyelids (option 1), induces the blink reflex, which causes the eyes to close. Option 2 also causes the eyes to close. Option 4 is incorrect because infants are sensitive to light and will frown and close their eyes if a bright light is flashed into them.
NP: Implementation
CN: Physiologic integrity

44. Correct answer—2
A client receiving levodopa should avoid vitamin pills and foods high in vitamin B_6 because they reverse the effects of the drug. Option 1 helps remind the client to swallow and helps prevent drooling. Option 3 provides a good source of fluid. Option 4 may be helpful for this client because eating small meals is less tiresome than eating large meals.
NP: Evaluation
CN: Health promotion and maintenance

45. Correct answer—4
Pituitary gland removal may lead to signs of diabetes insipidus by decreasing production of antidiuretic hormone (ADH). With insufficient ADH production, the client may lose up to 15 liters/day of urine and may be at risk for severe dehydration. Although the nurse also must assess for respiratory depression (option 1), gastric distention (option 2), and cardiac arrhythmias (option 3), these changes are less significant than excessive urine output in a client recovering from a transsphenoidal hypophysectomy.
NP: Assessment
CN: Physiologic integrity

46. Correct answer—4
Polyuria, thirst, and weight loss (from inadequate carbohydrate metabolism) are classic early findings in diabetes mellitus. Option 1 lists signs of hypoglycemia. The findings listed in options 2 and 3 do not occur in early diabetes.
NP: Assessment
CN: Physiologic integrity

47. Correct answer—3
This response points out reality and encourages the client to express his feelings. Option 1 gives false reassurance. Option 2 does not allow a therapeutic exchange. Option 4 reinforces the client's psychosis.
NP: Implementation
CN: Psychosocial integrity

48. Correct answer—1
For a client with a head injury, use of any central nervous system (CNS) depressant is potentially dangerous and must be reported to the physician. Option 2 does not address this danger. Option 3 is unnecessary. Option 4 may be important but does not address the risks of CNS depressant use in this client.
NP: Implementation
CN: Physiologic integrity

49. Correct answer—2
The client's blood gas results indicate postoperative hypoventilation and atelectasis; vigorous ventilation, as from deep breathing, can correct these problems. Administering oxygen (option 1) is not helpful because the client is hypoventilating, not hypoxic. Analysis of gastric secretions (option 3) will not help correct the client's respiratory problems. Sodium bicarbonate administration (option 4) is not indicated because the blood gases do not indicate respiratory acidosis.
NP: Implementation
CN: Physiologic integrity

50. Correct answer—3
Lecithin is a surfactant that is necessary for alveolar stability, lung expansion, and adequate respiration. The other options ultimately may lead to metabolic imbalances, but are not directly related to newborn respiratory distress syndrome.
NP: Analysis
CN: Physiologic integrity

51. Correct answer—3
Hyperventilation is the most common sign of salicylate overdose. Assessing blood pressure (option 1) and urine specific gravity (option 4) would not initially yield crucial information for this client. Petechiae (option 2) may occur with chronic, but not acute, salicylate poisoning.
NP: Assessment
CN: Physiologic integrity

52. Correct answer—3
Reducing anxiety will help the client participate in medical, forensic, and legal follow-up activities. Option 1 should be done as soon as the client's anxiety decreases below the panic level. Option 2 does not take high priority. Option 4 is of little use until the client's anxiety level decreases.
NP: Implementation
CN: Psychosocial integrity

53. Correct answer—4
In a newborn less than 24 hours old, the laboratory values reported indicate clinical hemolytic disease. The nurse should notify the physician, who will determine further management. Options 1 and 2 are appropriate but do not take precedence over notifying the physician. Option 3 may be indicated but requires a physician's order.
NP: Implementation
CN: Physiologic integrity

54. Correct answer—1
During a manic state, the client has severe anxiety; the broad muscle activity involved in tearing rags will help drain off excess energy. Option 2 requires concentration and problem solving—abilities a manic client lacks. Option 3 is highly stimulating and could exhaust the client. Option 4 requires too much concentration for this client.
NP: Implementation
CN: Psychosocial integrity

55. Correct answer—1
Staying with the client during the examination offers the most support. Option 2 is inappropriate because deep, not shallow, breathing usually aids relaxation. Option 3 is too general and does not acknowledge the client's individuality. Option 4 is inappropriate because the nurse should always remain in the room during a pelvic examination.
NP: Implementation
CN: Safe, effective care environment

56. Correct answer—3
Although skin care instructions may vary among facilities, most permit use of A & D Ointment and baby oil to ease drying and desquamation. Port marks must be retained because they guide the radiation therapist. Within the port marks, skin is red, tender, and dry and should not be washed; soap may erase marks and contribute to dry skin.
NP: Evaluation
CN: Safe, effective care environment

57. Correct answer—2
A client with a lactose intolerance may have a calcium deficiency, from difficulty digesting milk and dairy products. The other options are not diminished in clients with lactose intolerance.
NP: Planning
CN: Health promotion and maintenance

58. Correct answer—4
"Setting sun" sign (downward deviation of the eyes, so that the sclera is visible above each iris) is a classic sign of hydrocephalus. A pulsating anterior fontanel (option 1) is normal. Swelling cranial contents causes suture lines to widen, not close (option 2). Orthopneic positioning (option 3) is not related to hydrocephalus.
NP: Assessment
CN: Physiologic integrity

59. Correct answer—2
Nausea, vomiting, seeing halos around lights, and pain are signs of increased intraocular pressure. The client's symptoms do not suggest the other options.
NP: Assessment
CN: Physiologic integrity

60. Correct answer—1
After a total hip replacement, the client must do specially designed exercises to help regain muscle strength. Riding in a car (option 2) should be discouraged because it may cause injury or dislocation of the prosthesis. The client need not wear loose clothes (option 3) because most ordinary clothes do not restrict movement. Walking 2 miles a day (option 4) is excessive; the client should walk for short distances only to start, then increase the distance gradually.
NP: Evaluation
CN: Health promotion and maintenance

61. Correct answer—4
The best outcome criterion would be the client leaving her room and going to the nurses' station for medication. Option 1 does not suggest a decrease in social isolation. Option 2 is a positive sign but is not as definitive as leaving the room. Option 3 is an inappropriate outcome criterion because no evidence suggests this client is hallucinating or delusional.
NP: Evaluation
CN: Psychosocial integrity

62. Correct answer—2
Mafenide acetate can cause metabolic acidosis, rash, and increased respirations. The other options have not been identified as potential side effects. The drug may cause hypovolemia, not hypervolemia (option 3).
NP: Evaluation
CN: Physiologic integrity

63. Correct answer—2
Slow, rhythmic chest breathing is the most relaxing and requires the least concentration of the learned breathing techniques. Option 1 would not provide relief. Options 3 and 4 should be reserved for later stages of labor.
NP: Evaluation
CN: Safe, effective care environment

64. Correct answer—4
The nurse should establish a minimum goal of 1,000 ml/24 hours to liquify respiratory secretions and replace fluid lost via the lungs from increased respirations. The other options are inadequate for this client.
NP: Planning
CN: Physiologic integrity

65. Correct answer—2
Peanut butter provides protein and fat, while raisins provide iron. Option 1 provides adequate nutrients but too much fat. Options 3 and 4 do not provide adequate protein or iron.
NP: Planning
CN: Physiologic integrity

66. Correct answer—2
Shock causes tissue hypoxia. The first action should be to start nasal oxygen to promote tissue oxygenation. Option 1 is appropriate after oxygen therapy is initiated. Before implementing option 3, the nurse would need further data. Option 4 is important, but does not take precedence over starting oxygen.
NP: Implementation
CN: Physiologic integrity

67. Correct answer—4
Breathing exercises help establish normal breathing patterns, strengthen the respiratory muscles, and remove mucus from the lungs. The physician may or may not order options 1 or 2. Option 3 is used to manage an acute attack; it is not a preventive measure.
NP: Planning
CN: Physiologic integrity

68. Correct answer—3
Semi-Fowler's is the best position for this client because it promotes venous drainage and uses gravity to decrease cerebral edema. The other options do not take advantage of gravity to decrease cerebral edema.
NP: Implementation
CN: Physiologic integrity

69. Correct answer—3
Hypotonic contractions are irregular and poor in quality; they commonly occur during the active phase of stage one of labor. An atonic pattern (option 1) is characterized by lack of tone. In a dystonic pattern (option 2), contractions are painful, ineffective, and asymmetrical. In a hypertonic pattern (option 4), contractions are strong, painful, and uncoordinated.
NP: Assessment
CN: Physiologic integrity

70. Correct answer—3
An osmotic diuretic, mannitol increases urine output. The other options are not side effects of mannitol.
NP: Evaluation
CN: Physiologic integrity

71. Correct answer—3
Tachycardia and arrhythmias should alert the nurse to the onset of mediastinal shift. The other options are not signs of mediastinal shift.
NP: Assessment
CN: Physiologic integrity

72. Correct answer—4
The client is attempting to interact with the nurse, who should not squander this opportunity for therapeutic intervention. The other options are not therapeutic responses because a depressed client cannot problem solve and is capable of following only simple directions.
NP: Implementation
CN: Psychosocial integrity

73. Correct answer—2
Pitocin causes vasoconstriction, resulting in hypertension. Option 1 is incorrect because Pitocin is associated with an increased pulse rate (tachycardia). The drug does not cause a rash (option 3). Option 4 is incorrect because the drug's antidiuretic effect may decrease urine output.
NP: Assessment
CN: Physiologic integrity

74. Correct answer—2
Straining during a bowel movement raises venous pressure and could cause rupture of the varices. Eating quickly (option 1) could irritate the varices; the client should eat slowly and chew foods well. Option 3 is incorrect because the client does not have ascites. Option 4 is incorrect because exercise is not contraindicated unless the varices are bleeding.
NP: Implementation
CN: Physiologic integrity

75. Correct answer—3
Blood trickling down the throat stimulates the swallowing reflex; therefore, frequent swallowing indicates bleeding. Option 1 is common after a tonsillectomy. Option 2 is also a common post-tonsillectomy finding and results from moderate edema of the nasopharynx. Option 4 indicates old blood swallowed during surgery.
NP: Assessment
CN: Physiologic integrity

76. Correct answer—2
A client with chronic mental illness has severe anxiety and thought disorganization. Unable to communicate clearly, his statements are symbolic communications. Before considering the other options, the nurse would need more information.
NP: Analysis
CN: Psychosocial integrity

77. Correct answer—4
With a decrease in serum albumin, hydrostatic pressure of the blood pushes fluid and electrolytes into the extracellular space, thus causing ascites. An increased vasopressin level (option 1) contributes to fluid retention but does not cause ascites. An increased serum sodium level (option 2) leads to fluid retention but is not the primary cause of ascites. In cirrhosis, the serum aldosterone level increases, not decreases (option 3).
NP: Assessment
CN: Physiologic integrity

78. Correct answer—4
An elevated serum potassium level (hyperkalemia) is common in acute renal failure and puts the client at risk for cardiac arrhythmias. Option 1 results from a below-normal serum calcium level (hypocalcemia); although hypocalcemia may occur in acute renal failure, it does not cause signs or symptoms because the acidosis that occurs with renal failure keeps more calcium in an ionized form. Option 2 is not a complication of acute renal failure because damaged renal tubules cannot conserve sodium; therefore, sodium excretion increases, causing a normal or below-normal serum sodium level. Option 3 suggests shock, which has not been identified as a complication of acute renal failure.
NP: Assessment
CN: Physiologic integrity

79. Correct answer—3
The newborn receives a score of 2 for a pulse above 100 beats/minute, 2 for good respiratory effort, 2 for active motion, 1 for pink body and blue extremities, and 1 for a grimace. Added together, these scores result in an Apgar score of 8. Options 1 and 2 are too low; option 4 is too high.
NP: Analysis
CN: Physiologic integrity

80. Correct answer—3
Handling the child with the palms will prevent further bruising (which results from a decreased platelet count). The client's teeth should be brushed more than once a day (option 1) to prevent gum infection. Trimming his nails short (option 2) may cause bleeding. A 4-year-old child probably would object to being placed in a crib (option 4).
NP: Implementation
CN: Physiologic integrity

81. Correct answer—1
During the toddler stage, the child begins to develop autonomy and needs rituals and specific objects to gain a sense of consistency and order. Option 2 is typical toddler behavior—saying no to everything and doing nothing, which has nothing to do with clinging to her blanket. Option 3 is also characteristic toddler behavior and has nothing to do with clinging to her blanket. Option 4 is age-appropriate; clinging to a ritual is not regressive behavior.
NP: Analysis
CN: Psychosocial integrity

82. Correct answer—1
Although belladonna decreases bladder spasms when given with opium, it is contraindicated in the presence of glaucoma because its anticholinergic effect would increase intraocular pressure. Therefore, the nurse should question the physician's orders. Option 2 is incorrect because belladonna is contraindicated in glaucoma. If the urinary catheter is functioning properly, urine will drain through it from the bladder; therefore, voiding around the catheter (option 3) should not be possible. Option 4 would not relieve the spasms.
NP: Implementation
CN: Physiologic integrity

83. Correct answer—2
This action orients the client directly and meets his need for diversional activity. Before the client's wife can interact with him further, such as by reading books to him (option 1) or showing him family pictures (option 3), the client needs to be oriented to her. Showing him her wedding ring (option 4) would provide only an indirect reference to her identity; this client needs direct orientation.
NP: Implementation
CN: Psychosocial integrity

84. Correct answer—2
Lab values are valid and reliable indicators of the client's electrolyte status and would be altered by purging. No client can be watched every minute after every meal (option 1). Weighing her (option 3) would not determine accurately if she is still purging. Restricting her movement (option 4) would not be therapeutic; she could always find a way to get rid of food while on the unit.
NP: Assessment
CN: Safe, effective care environment

85. Correct answer—2
The client's behavior suggests akathisia—a side effect of phenothiazines. Dystonia (option 1) would manifest as excessive salivation, difficulty speaking, and involuntary movements of the face, neck, arms, and legs. Parkinsonian effects (option 3) include a shuffling gait, hand tremors, drooling, rigidity, and loose arm movements. Tardive dyskinesia (option 4) is characterized by odd facial and tongue movements, difficulty swallowing, and a stiff neck.
NP: Analysis
CN: Physiologic integrity

86. Correct answer—1
Children in this age range have a strong interest in competitive games, which provide the socializing so important to children in this age group. Solitary activities, such as doing crossword puzzles (option 2) and reading (option 3), are less desirable than those that encourage socialization. Playing "Old Maid" (option 4) is appropriate for much younger children.
NP: Planning
CN: Psychosocial integrity

87. Correct answer—1
Jaundice during the first 24 hours after birth is always considered pathologic. The other options are considered normal in the newborn.
NP: Assessment
CN: Physiologic integrity

88. Correct answer—3
Dumping syndrome is the rapid emptying of gastric contents into the small intestine, causing a decrease in circulating blood volume and a blood glucose elevation. The resulting insulin oversecretion leads to hypoglycemia, which may manifest as dizziness, sweating, and tachycardia. Pernicious anemia (option 1) would not cause the client's symptoms. Pyloric stenosis (option 2) would cause projectile vomiting. A recurring ulcer (option 4) would result in pain.
NP: Analysis
CN: Physiologic integrity

89. Correct answer—3
Serum amylase is a major indicator of pancreatic function; decreasing levels indicate resolution of inflammation. Option 1 is associated with biliary tract disease; option 2, with hypoparathyroidism and bone and liver disease. Option 4 would reflect anemia or a dietary deficiency.
NP: Analysis
CN: Physiologic integrity

90. Correct answer—2
Like other anticholinergic drugs, Cogentin can cause blurred vision. The drug may lead to urine retention; it does not cause increased urine output (option 1). Excessive salivation (option 3) and difficulty swallowing (option 4) are symptoms of Parkinson's disease, not side effects of Cogentin.
NP: Assessment
CN: Physiologic integrity

91. Correct answer—3
Frequently, the first signs of sickle cell disease are lack of appetite, irritability, and an increased susceptibility to infection. The child might be small for age and gain weight slowly. The mucous membranes are pale, and scleral icterus is evident. Option 1 is a sign of scarlet fever. Option 2 is seen in rheumatic fever. Option 4 is a sign of cardiac or renal disease or water overload, not sickle cell anemia.
NP: Assessment
CN: Physiologic integrity

92. Correct answer—1
During an acute attack of asthma, older children tend to sit upright with their shoulders in a hunched-over position, with hands on the bed or chair and arms braced to facilitate the use of accessory muscles of respiration. Option 2 is incorrect because an asthmatic episode begins with a hacking, paroxysmal, nonproductive cough caused by bronchial edema. Option 3 is incorrect because the child with a severe attack is short of breath and tries to breathe more deeply. The expiratory phase becomes prolonged and is accompanied by wheezing. Option 4 is incorrect because intercostal and diaphragmatic muscles are normally used for breathing.
NP: Assessment
CN: Physiologic integrity

93. Correct answer—3
The documentation objectively describes the nurse's observations of her colleague. It does not draw conclusions (option 1), interpret the colleague's behavior (option 2), or digress from the topic of concern.
NP: Assessment
CN: Safe, effective care environment

94. Correct answer—4
About 80% to 90% of digoxin is excreted by the kidneys. If the kidneys are not functioning properly, large amounts of the drug are not eliminated, which can cause digitalis toxicity. Option 1 is incorrect because diarrhea (not constipation) may be a side effect of the drug. Option 2 is incorrect because potassium supplements are frequently prescribed with furosemide to prevent digitalis toxicity. Option 3 is incorrect because excessive food intake for 1 week would not cause digitalis toxicity.
NP: Analysis
CN: Physiologic integrity

95. Correct answer—3
The client is reporting symptoms that suggest pregnancy-induced hypertension. Therefore, her urine should be checked for the presence of protein. Fundal height (option 1), fetal heart rate (option 2), and presence of human placental lactogen in maternal blood (option 4) have lower priorities in assessing this client.
NP: Analysis
CN: Health promotion and maintenance

96. Correct answer—1
The main developmental task of the second trimester is to recognize the fetus as a separate being. Accepting the pregnancy (option 2) is the major task of the first trimester, and preparing for childbirth (option 3) is the main task of the third trimester. Selecting a name for the baby (option 4) is begun during pregnancy, but a definite decision is made after birth.
NP: Assessment
CN: Health promotion and maintenance

97. Correct answer—3
Impaired skin integrity related to the corrective device is the nursing diagnosis that should be given priority. The goal is to prevent skin irritation and breakdown. Other potential nursing diagnoses related to the brace in this condition include *Risk for injury* and *Body image disturbance*. Options 1, 2, and 4 are incorrect.
NP: Analysis
CN: Safe, effective care environment

98. Correct answer—2
Exposing the nipples to air and sunlight will help toughen them. Soap (option 1) and antiseptics (option 4) should not be used on the nipples because they remove protective oils that keep nipples supple. Plastic bra liners (option 3) are not recommended because they retain moisture against the nipples.
NP: Planning
CN: Health promotion and maintenance

99. Correct answer—2
Soiled linens should be kept in the client's room until radiation monitoring determines that they do not contain a source of radiation that has become dislodged from the site of placement. Options 1, 3, and 4 are incorrect. The container should be lined with lead (not aluminum). Persons under age 18 and those who are pregnant or lactating should not visit or care for a client who has internal radiation. Body excreta are not irradiated, so no special precautions (aside from standard precautions) are required for their disposal.
NP: Implementation
CN: Safe, effective care environment

100. Correct answer—4
Mannitol, an osmotic diuretic, is prescribed to reduce increased intracranial pressure, which will then reduce cerebral edema. Options 1, 2, and 3 are incorrect. Many diuretics put the client at risk for electrolyte imbalance. Although mannitol is sometimes used to prevent or treat the oliguric phase of acute renal failure, no evidence in the question indicates that the client has that problem. A diuretic will tend to reduce blood volume rather than increase it.
NP: Planning
CN: Physiologic integrity

101. Correct answer—4
The right-side lying position permits the feeding to flow toward the lower end of the stomach and any swallowed air to rise. Options 1, 2, and 3 are, therefore, incorrect.
NP: Implementation
CN: Safe, effective care environment

102. Correct answer—4
With inactivated antigens, such as DTP, side effects are most likely to occur within a few hours or days of administration and are usually limited to local tenderness, erythema, and swelling at the injection site; low grade fever; and behavior changes. Options 1, 2, and 3 are incorrect.
NP: Evaluation
CN: Physiologic integrity

103. Correct answer—4
Chemically impaired staff members place clients at risk for harm and the employing agency at risk for liability for negligent actions. Therefore, the nurse's supervisor should be informed about the situation and should help verify perceptions and clarify procedures. Sending the aide home (option 1) is not the best action initially. The supervisor should first be consulted. More information should be obtained before referring the aide to Alcoholics Anonymous (option 2). Assigning the aide to nonclient care tasks (option 3), such as sterilizing equipment, could harm clients or the aide and also would foster denial of the problem.
NP: Implementation
CN: Safe, effective care environment

104. Correct answer—4
Combination antitubercular drugs inhibit the ability of the bacillus to reproduce. Therapeutic blood levels of the drugs must be maintained to kill the TB bacillus and avoid development of a drug-resistant strain. Adherence to the treatment plan is vital to success. Option 1 is incorrect because clients with TB are commonly debilitated and require a well-rounded diet, not a low-protein diet. Option 2 is incorrect because successful treatment of TB requires drug therapy for at least 6 to 12 months. Option 3 is incorrect because physical contact is not prohibited, as long as proper infection-control procedures, especially covering the mouth when coughing, are followed.
NP: Evaluation
CN: Health promotion and maintenance

105. Correct answer—2
Knowing what to expect is the most effective way to allay fear and reduce anxiety. A client who is well informed can anticipate what is likely to take place postoperatively and cooperate in the care. Providing adequate pain control (option 1) is important to maintain comfort but not as important as knowledge in securing cooperation. Giving the client a sense of control (option 3) is not realistic while the client is in the post-anesthesia recovery area or intensive care unit. Reducing unfamiliar external stimuli (option 4) is not always possible and would have little effect on promoting a client's cooperation.
NP: Implementation
CN: Safe, effective care environment

Post-test self-diagnostic profile

QUESTION NUMBER																												TOTALS
Test-taking skills																												
1. Misread question																												
2. Missed important point																												
3. Forgot fact or concept																												
4. Applied wrong fact or concept																												
5. Drew wrong conclusion																												
6. Incorrectly evaluated distractors																												
7. Mistakenly indicated wrong answer																												
8. Read into question																												
9. Guessed wrong																												
10. Misunderstood question																												
Client need																												
1. Safe, effective care environment																												
2. Physiologic integrity																												
3. Psychosocial integrity																												
4. Health promotion and maintenance																												
Nursing process																												
1. Assessing																												
2. Analyzing																												
3. Planning																												
4. Implementing																												
5. Evaluating																												

Part VII

Appendices, references, and index

Part VII

Appendices, references, and index

Appendix 1: Normal values for common laboratory tests

ELECTROLYTE LEVELS
Sodium: 135 to 145 mEq/L
Potassium: 3.5 to 5 mEq/L
Calcium: 4.5 to 5.8 mEq/L or 9 to 10.5 mg/dl

ARTERIAL BLOOD GAS LEVELS
pH: 7.35 to 7.45
Pao_2: 80 to 100 mm Hg
$Paco_2$: 35 to 45 mm Hg
Serum bicarbonate: 21 to 29 mEq/L
Oxygen saturation: 95% to 100%

COMPLETE BLOOD COUNT
Red blood cell count: 4.2 to 6 million/mm^3
Hemoglobin level: 12 to 18 g/dl
White blood cell count: 5,000 to 10,000/mm^3
Platelet count: 150,000 to 400,000/mm^3
Erythrocyte sedimentation rate: 1 to 20 mm/ hour
Prothrombin time: 11 to 12.5 seconds
Partial thromboplastin time: 30 to 40 seconds

OTHER BLOOD TESTS
Fasting plasma glucose test: 80 to 120 mg/dl
Serum cholesterol level: 150 to 250 mg/dl

RENAL FUNCTION TESTS
Blood urea nitrogen level: 8 to 20 mg/dl
Creatinine level: 0.8 to 1.5 mg/dl

LIVER FUNCTION TESTS
Total protein: 6 to 8 g/dl
Albumin-globulin ratio: Albumin—3.5 to 5.5 g/dl; Globulin—2.5 to 3.5 g/dl; Ratio—1.5:1 to 2.5:1
ALT (formerly SGPT): 5 to 35 U/ml
AST (formerly SGOT): 5 to 40 U/ml
Lactate dehydrogenase: 200 to 450 U/ml
Alkaline phosphatase: 1.5 to 4 Bodansky units or 3 to 13 King-Armstrong units
Serum bilirubin: Less than 1 mg/dl
Prothrombin time: 11 to 12.5 seconds or 100%
Clotting time: 6 to 17 minutes
Partial thromboplastin time: 30 to 40 seconds

Appendix 2: NANDA taxonomy of nursing diagnoses

The currently accepted classification system for nursing diagnoses is that of the North American Nursing Diagnosis Association (NANDA), as shown in *NANDA Nursing Diagnoses: Definitions and Classification 1997-1998*. It is organized around nine human response patterns: exchanging, communicating, relating, valuing, choosing, moving, perceiving, knowing, and feeling.

The complete taxonomic structure is listed here. The series of numbers before each diagnosis is its classification number, used to determine the placement of the diagnosis within the taxonomy. The number of digits delineates the level of abstraction of the nursing diagnosis (more specific diagnoses are assigned longer numbers).

Pattern 1. Exchanging (Mutual giving and receiving)

1.1.2.1	Altered nutrition: More than body requirements
1.1.2.2	Altered nutrition: Less than body requirements
1.1.2.3	Altered nutrition: Risk for more than body requirements
1.2.1.1	Risk for infection
1.2.2.1	Risk for altered body temperature
1.2.2.2	Hypothermia
1.2.2.3	Hyperthermia
1.2.2.4	Ineffective thermoregulation
1.2.3.1	Dysreflexia
1.3.1.1	Constipation
1.3.1.1.1	Perceived constipation
1.3.1.1.2	Colonic constipation
1.3.1.2	Diarrhea
1.3.1.3	Bowel incontinence
1.3.2	Altered urinary elimination
1.3.2.1.1	Stress incontinence
1.3.2.1.2	Reflex incontinence
1.3.2.1.3	Urge incontinence
1.3.2.1.4	Functional incontinence
1.3.2.1.5	Total incontinence
1.3.2.2	Urinary retention
1.4.1.1	Altered (specify type) tissue perfusion (renal, cerebral, cardiopulmonary, gastrointestinal, peripheral)
1.4.1.2.1	Fluid volume excess
1.4.1.2.2.1	Fluid volume deficit
1.4.1.2.2.2	Risk for fluid volume deficit
1.4.2.1	Decreased cardiac output
1.5.1.1	Impaired gas exchange
1.5.1.2	Ineffective airway clearance
1.5.1.3	Ineffective breathing pattern
1.5.1.3.1	Inability to sustain spontaneous ventilation
1.5.1.3.2	Dysfunctional ventilatory weaning response (DVWR)
1.6.1	Risk for injury
1.6.1.1	Risk for suffocation
1.6.1.2	Risk for poisoning
1.6.1.3	Risk for trauma
1.6.1.4	Risk for aspiration
1.6.1.5	Risk for disuse syndrome
1.6.2	Altered protection
1.6.2.1	Impaired tissue integrity
1.6.2.1.1	Altered oral mucous membrane
1.6.2.1.2.1	Impaired skin integrity
1.6.2.1.2.2	Risk for impaired skin integrity
1.7.1	Decreased adaptive capacity: Intracranial
1.8	Energy field disturbance

Pattern 2. Communicating (Sending messages)

2.1.1.1	Impaired verbal communication

Pattern 3. Relating (Establishing bonds)

3.1.1	Impaired social interaction
3.1.2	Social isolation
3.1.3	Risk for loneliness
3.2.1	Altered role performance
3.2.1.1.1	Altered parenting
3.2.1.1.2	Risk for altered parenting
3.2.1.1.2.1	Risk for altered parent, infant, or child attachment
3.2.1.2.1	Sexual dysfunction
3.2.2	Altered family processes
3.2.2.1	Caregiver role strain
3.2.2.2	Risk for caregiver role strain
3.2.2.3.1	Altered family process: Alcoholism
3.2.3.1	Parental role conflict
3.3	Altered sexuality patterns

Pattern 4. Valuing (Assigning relative worth)

4.1.1	Spiritual distress (distress of the human spirit)
4.2	Potential for enhanced spiritual well-being

Pattern 5. Choosing (Selecting alternatives)

5.1.1.1	Ineffective individual coping
5.1.1.1.1	Impaired adjustment
5.1.1.1.2	Defensive coping
5.1.1.1.3	Ineffective denial
5.1.2.1.1	Ineffective family coping: Disabling
5.1.2.1.2	Ineffective family coping: Compromised
5.1.2.2	Family coping: Potential for growth
5.1.3.1	Potential for enhanced community coping
5.1.3.2	Ineffective community coping
5.2.1	Ineffective management of therapeutic regimen (individuals)
5.2.1.1	Noncompliance (specify)
5.2.2	Ineffective management of therapeutic regimen: Families

(continued)

Appendix 2: NANDA taxonomy of nursing diagnoses *(continued)*

Pattern 5. Choosing (Selecting alternatives)*(continued)*

5.2.3	Ineffective management of therapeutic regimen: Community
5.2.4	Effective management of therapeutic regimen: Individual
5.3.1.1	Decisional conflict (specify)
5.4	Health-seeking behaviors (specify)

Pattern 6. Moving (Involving activity)

6.1.1.1	Impaired physical mobility
6.1.1.1.1	Risk for peripheral neurovascular dysfunction
6.1.1.1.2	Risk for perioperative positioning injury
6.1.1.2	Activity intolerance
6.1.1.2.1	Fatigue
6.1.1.3	Risk for activity intolerance
6.2.1	Sleep pattern disturbance
6.3.1.1	Diversional activity deficit
6.4.1.1	Impaired home maintenance management
6.4.2	Altered health maintenance
6.5.1	Feeding self-care deficit
6.5.1.1	Impaired swallowing
6.5.1.2	Ineffective breast-feeding
6.5.1.2.1	Interrupted breast-feeding
6.5.1.3	Effective breast-feeding
6.5.1.4	Ineffective infant feeding pattern
6.5.2	Bathing or hygiene self-care deficit
6.5.3	Dressing or grooming self-care deficit
6.5.4	Toileting self-care deficit
6.6	Altered growth and development
6.7	Relocation stress syndrome
6.8.1	Risk for disorganized infant behavior
6.8.2	Disorganized infant behavior
6.8.3	Potential for enhanced organized infant behavior

Pattern 7. Perceiving (Receiving information)

7.1.1	Body image disturbance
7.1.2	Self-esteem disturbance
7.1.2.1	Chronic low self-esteem
7.1.2.2	Situational low self-esteem
7.1.3	Personal identity disturbance
7.2	Sensory or perceptual alterations (specify visual, auditory, kinesthetic, gustatory, tactile, olfactory)
7.2.1.1	Unilateral neglect
7.3.1	Hopelessness
7.3.2	Powerlessness

Pattern 8. Knowing (Associating meaning with information)

8.1.1	Knowledge deficit (specify)
8.2.1	Impaired environmental interpretation syndrome
8.2.2	Acute confusion
8.2.3	Chronic confusion
8.3	Altered thought processes
8.3.1	Impaired memory

Pattern 9. Feeling (Being subjectively aware of information)

9.1.1	Pain
9.1.1.1	Chronic pain
9.2.1.1	Dysfunctional grieving
9.2.1.2	Anticipatory grieving
9.2.2	Risk for violence: Self-directed or directed at others
9.2.2.1	Risk for self-mutilation
9.2.3	Post-trauma response
9.2.3.1	Rape-trauma syndrome
9.2.3.1.1	Rape-trauma syndrome: Compound reaction
9.2.3.1.2	Rape-trauma syndrome: Silent reaction
9.3.1	Anxiety
9.3.2	Fear

Appendix 3: Drug administration rights, calculations, and equivalents

Drug administration rights

When administering any drug, remember to use the five rights:

1. right client   2. right drug   3. right dose   4. right route   5. right time

Calculations

To calculate the number of doses in a specified amount of medicine:

$$\text{Number of doses} = \frac{\text{Total amount}}{\text{Size of dose}}$$

To calculate the size of each dose, given a specified amount of medication and the number of doses it contains:

$$\text{Size of dose} = \frac{\text{Total amount}}{\text{Number of doses}}$$

To calculate the amount of a medicine, given the number of doses it contains and the size of each dose:

$$\text{Total amount} = \text{Number of doses} \times \text{size of dose}$$

Short formula for determining rate of I.V. solution infusion:

$$\frac{\text{Volume of solution}}{\text{Time interval in minutes}} \times \text{Drop factor} = \text{Drops/minute}$$

Equivalents

Metric weight equivalents	Conversions	Metric volume equivalents
1 kg = 1,000 g	1 oz = 30 g	1 L = 1,000 ml
1 g = 1,000 mg	1 lb = 453.6 g	1 dl = 100 ml
1 mg = 0.001 g	2.2 lb = 1 kg	
1 mcg or µg = 0.001 mg		

Liquid measures	Household	=	Apothecaries'	=	Metric	
	1 teaspoonful	=	1 fluidram	=	4 or 5	ml‡
	1 tablespoonful	=	4 fluidrams	=	15 or 16	ml
	2 tablespoonfuls	=	1 fluid ounce	=	30	ml
	1 measuring cupful	=	8 fluid ounces	=	240	ml
	1 pint	=	16 fluid ounces	=	500	ml
	1 quart	=	32 fluid ounces	=	1,000	ml

‡Although the fluidram is about 4 ml, in prescriptions it is considered equivalent to the teaspoon (which is 5 ml).

Temperature conversion	Celsius to Fahrenheit	Fahrenheit to Celsius
	$(°C \times {}^9/_5) + 32 = °F$	$(°F - 32) \times {}^5/_9 = °C$

Appendix 4: State boards of nursing

Candidates for the NCLEX-RN must make an appointment to take the test by calling an approved test center. Contact your state board of nursing for more information.

STATE BOARDS OF NURSING

Alabama
Alabama Board of Nursing
P.O. Box 303900
Montgomery, AL 36130-3900
(334) 242-4060

Alaska
Alaska Board of Nursing
Dept. of Comm. & Econ. Development
Div. of Occupational Licensing
3601 "C" St., Suite 722
Anchorage, AK 99503
(907) 269-8161

American Samoa
American Samoa Health Services
Regulatory Board
LBJ Tropical Medical Center
Pago Pago, AS 96799
(684) 633-1222

Arizona
Arizona State Board of Nursing
1651 E. Morten Ave.
Suite 150
Phoenix, AZ 85020
(602) 255-5092

Arkansas
Arkansas State Board of Nursing
University Tower Bldg.
1123 S. University Ave.
Suite 800
Little Rock, AR 72204
(501) 686-2700

California
California Board of Registered
Nursing
P.O. Box 944210
Sacramento, CA 94244
(916) 322-3350

Colorado
Colorado Board of Nursing
1560 Broadway
Suite 670
Denver, CO 80202
(303) 894-2430

Connecticut
Connecticut Board of Examiners for
Nursing
Dept. of Public Health
410 Capital Ave., MS#13ADJ
Hartford, CT 06134
(860) 509-7624

Delaware
Delaware Board of Nursing
Cannon Bldg., Suite 203
P.O. Box 1401
Dover, DE 19903
(302) 739-4522

District of Columbia
District of Columbia Board of Nursing
614 H St., NW
Washington, DC 20001
(202) 727-7468

Florida
Florida Board of Nursing
4080 Woodcock Dr., Suite 202
Jacksonville, FL 32207
(904) 858-6940

Georgia
Georgia Board of Nursing
166 Pryor St. SW
Atlanta, GA 30303
(404) 656-3943

Guam
Guam Board of Nurse Examiners
P.O. Box 2816
Agana, GU 96910
(671) 475-0251

Hawaii
Hawaii Board of Nursing
Professional and Vocational Licensing
Div.
Box 3469
Honolulu, HI 96801
(808) 586-2695

Idaho
Idaho Board of Nursing
P.O. Box 83720
Boise, ID 83720
(208) 334-3110

Illinois
Dept. of Professional Regulation
James R. Thompson Center
100 W. Randolph, Suite 9-300
Chicago, IL 60601
(312) 814-2715

Indiana
Indiana State Board of Nursing
402 W. Washington St., Suite 041
Indianapolis, IN 46204
(317) 232-2960

Iowa
Iowa Board of Nursing
State Capital Complex
1223 E. Court Ave.
Des Moines, IA 50319
(515) 281-3255

Kansas
Kansas State Board of Nursing
Landan State Office Bldg.
900 S.W. Jackson, Suite 551-S
Topeka, KS 66612-1230
(913) 296-4929

Kentucky
Kentucky Board of Nursing
312 Whittington Pkwy.
Suite 300
Louisville, KY 40222
(502) 329-7000

Louisiana
Louisiana State Board of Nursing
3510 N. Causeway Blvd., Suite 501
Metairie, LA 70002
(504) 838-5332

Maine
Maine Board of Nursing
State House Station 158
Augusta, ME 04333
(207) 287-1133

Maryland
Maryland Board of Nursing
4140 Patterson Ave.
Baltimore, MD 21215
(410) 764-5124

Massachusetts
Massachusetts Board of Registration in Nursing
Leverett Saltonstall Bldg.
100 Cambridge St.
Rm. 1519
Boston, MA 02202
(617) 727-9961

Michigan
Michigan State Board of Nursing
CIS/Office of Health Services
611 W. Ottowa St., 4th Floor
Lansing, MI 48933
(517) 373-9102

Minnesota
Minnesota Board of Nursing
2829 University Ave. SE
Suite 500
Minneapolis, MN 55414-3253
(612) 617-2270

(continued)

Appendix 4: State boards of nursing (continued)

Mississippi
Mississippi Board of Nursing
239 N. Lamar St., Suite 401
Jackson, MS 39201
(601) 359-6170

Missouri
Missouri State Board of Nursing
P.O. Box 656
Jefferson City, MO 65102
(573) 751-0681

Montana
Montana State Board of Nursing
111 N. Jackson
P.O. Box 200513
Helena, MT 59620
(406) 444-2071

Nebraska
Dept. of Health and Human Ser-
    vices Regulation and Licensure
Credentialing Division - Nursing/
    Nursing Support Section
P.O. Box 94986
Lincoln, NE 68509-4986
(402) 471-4376

Nevada
Nevada State Board of Nursing
1755 E. Plumb Lane, Suite 260
Reno, NV 89502
(702) 786-2778

New Hampshire
New Hampshire Board of Nursing
6 Hazen Dr.
Concord, NH 03301
(603) 271-2323

New Jersey
New Jersey Board of Nursing
P.O. Box 45010
Newark, NJ 07101
(201) 504-6586

New Mexico
Board of Nursing
4206 Louisiana Blvd. NE
Suite A
Albuquerque, NM 87109
(505) 841-8340

New York
New York State Board of Nursing
Cultural Education Center
Rm. 3023
Albany, NY 12230
(518) 474-3845

North Carolina
North Carolina Board of Nursing
3724 National Dr.
Raleigh, NC 27602
(919) 782-3211

North Dakota
North Dakota Board of Nursing
919 S. 7th St.
Suite 504
Bismarck, ND 58504
(701) 328-9777

Ohio
Ohio Board of Nursing
77 S. High St., 17th Floor
Columbus, OH 43266-0316
(614) 466-3947

Oklahoma
Oklahoma Board of Nursing
2915 N. Classen Blvd.
Suite 524
Oklahoma City, OK 73106
(405) 525-2076

Oregon
Oregon State Board of Nursing
800 N.E. Oregon St., Box 25
Portland, OR 97232
(503) 731-4745

Pennsylvania
Pennsylvania State Board of Nursing
Box 2649
Harrisburg, PA 17105
(717) 783-7142

Puerto Rico
Commonwealth of Puerto Rico Board
    of Nurse Examiners
Call Box 10200
Santurce, PR 00908
(787) 725-8161

Rhode Island
Rhode Island Board of Nurse Registra-
    tion and Nursing Education
Cannon Health Bldg.
3 Capital Hill, Rm. 104
Providence, RI 02908
(401) 277-2827

South Carolina
South Carolina State Board of Nursing
P.O. Box 12367
Columbia, SC 29211-2367
(803) 896-4550

South Dakota
South Dakota Board of Nursing
3307 S. Lincoln Ave.
Sioux Falls, SD 57105
(605) 367-5940

Tennessee
Tennessee State Board of Nursing
425 Fifth Ave. North
First Floor - Cordell Hull Building
Nashville, TN 37247-1010
(615) 532-5166

Texas
Texas Board of Nurse Examiners
P.O. Box 430
Austin, TX 78767
(512) 305-7400

Utah
Utah State Board of Nursing
Div. of Occupational and Profes-
    sional Licensing
P.O. Box 45805
Salt Lake City, UT 84145
(801) 530-6628

Vermont
Vermont State Board of Nursing
109 State St.
Montpelier, VT 05609-1106
(802) 828-2396

Virginia
Virginia Board of Nursing
6606 Broad St., 4th Floor
Richmond, VA 23230
(804) 662-9909

Virgin Islands
Virgin Islands Board of Nurse Licen-
    sure
P.O. Box 4247
Veterans Drive Station
St. Thomas, VI 00803
(809) 776-7397

Washington
Washington State Nursing Care
    Quality Assurance Commission
Dept. of Health
P.O. Box 47864
Olympia, WA 98504
(360) 753-2686

West Virginia
West Virginia State Board of Exam-
    iners for Registered Professional
    Nurses
101 Dee Dr.
Charleston, WV 25311
(304) 558-3596

Wisconsin
Wisconsin Department of Regula-
    tion and Licensing
1400 E. Washington Ave.
P.O. Box 8935
Madison, WI 53708-8935
(608) 266-2112

Wyoming
Wyoming State Board of Nursing
2020 Carey Ave., Suite 110
Cheyenne, WY 82002
(307) 777-7601

Appendix 5: Canadian licensing examination dates and registered nurses' associations by province

In Canada, licensing examinations are administered by each province's licensing body through the Canadian Nurses Association Testing Service, 50 The Driveway, Ottawa, Ontario K2P 1E2; (613) 237-2133. Given four times annually, the tests are traditionally held on Wednesdays and Thursdays during the 3rd week of January, the 1st week of June and August, and the 2nd week of October. Test dates through 1999 are:

>1997: January 22-23, June 4-5, August 6-7, October 8-9
>1998: January 21, June 3, August 5, October 14
>1999 (tentative): January 20, June 9, August 4, October 13

The following is a list of registered nurses' associations by province:

Alberta
Registrar
Alberta Association of Registered Nurses
11620 - 168th Street
Edmonton, AB T5M 4A6

British Columbia
Director of Regulatory Services
Registered Nurses Association of British Columbia
2855 Arbutus Street
Vancouver, BC V6J 3Y8

Manitoba
Registrar
Manitoba Association of Registered Nurses
647 Broadway Avenue
Winnipeg, MB R3C 0X2

New Brunswick
Registrar
Nurses Association of New Brunswick
165 Regent Street
Fredericton, NB E3B 3W5

Newfoundland
Registrar
Association of Registered Nurses of Newfoundland
55 Military Road
P.O. Box 6116
St. John's, NF A1C 5X8

Northwest Territories
Executive Director/Registrar
Northwest Territories Registered Nurses
  Association
P.O. Box 2757
Yellowknife, NT X1A 2R1

Nova Scotia
Registrar
Registered Nurses Association of Nova Scotia
Suite 104, 120 Eileen Stubbs Avenue
Dartmouth, NS B3B, 1Y1

Ontario
Director, Registration
College of Nurses of Ontario
101 Davenport Road
Toronto, ON M5R 3P1

Prince Edward Island
Executive Director/Registrar
Association of Nurses of Prince Edward Island
17 Pownal Street, P.O. Box 1838
Charlottetown, PEI C1A 7N5

Québec
Directrice des services de l'admission à la
  profession
Ordre des infirmières et infirmiers du Québec
4200 ouest, boulevard Dorchester
Montréal, PQ H3Z 1V4

Saskatchewan
Registrar
Saskatchewan Registered Nurses Association
2066 Retallack Street
Regina, SK S4T 2K2

Yukon
Executive Director
Yukon Registered Nurses Association
P.O. Box 5371
Whitehorse, YK Y1A 4Z2

Appendix 6: ANA Code for Nurses

The *Code for Nurses* is based on a belief about the nature of individuals, nursing, health, and society. Nursing encompasses the protection, promotion, and restoration of health; the prevention of illness; and the alleviation of suffering in the care of clients, including individuals, families, groups, and communities. The statements of the *Code* and their interpretation provide guidance for conduct and relationships in carrying out nursing responsibilities consistent with the ethical obligations of the profession and with high quality in nursing care.

1. The nurse provides services with respect for human dignity and the uniqueness of the client, unrestricted by considerations of social or economic status, personal attributes, or the nature of health problems.

2. The nurse safeguards the client's right to privacy by judiciously protecting information of a confidential nature.

3. The nurse acts to safeguard the client and the public when health care and safety are affected by the incompetent, unethical, or illegal practice of any person.

4. The nurse assumes responsibility and accountability for individual nursing judgments and actions.

5. The nurse maintains competence in nursing.

6. The nurse exercises informed judgment and uses individual competence and qualifications as criteria in seeking consultation, accepting responsibilities, and delegating nursing activities to others.

7. The nurse participates in activities that contribute to the ongoing development of the profession's body of knowledge.

8. The nurse participates in the profession's efforts to implement and improve standards of nursing.

9. The nurse participates in the profession's efforts to establish and maintain conditions of employment conducive to high-quality nursing care.

10. The nurse participates in the profession's efforts to protect the public from misinformation and misrepresentation and to maintain the integrity of nursing.

11. The nurse collaborates with members of the health professions and other citizens in promoting community and national efforts to meet the health needs of the public.

Reprinted with permission from *Code for Nurses with Interpretive Statements*, 1985, American Nurses Association, Kansas City, MO.

References

GENERAL

Carpenito, L.J. *Nursing Diagnoses,* 6th ed. Philadelphia: J.B. Lippincott Co., 1995.

Mathewson-Kuhn, M. *Pharmacotherapeutics: A Nursing Process Approach,* 3rd ed. Philadelphia: F.A. Davis, 1993.

McCance, K.L., and Heuther, S.E. *Pathophysiology: The Biologic Basis for Disease in Adults and Children.* St. Louis: Mosby-Year Book, Inc., 1994.

Nursing97 Drug Handbook. Springhouse, Pa.: Springhouse Corp., 1997.

Price, S.A., and Wilson, L.M. *Pathophysiology: Clinical Concepts of Disease Processes.* St. Louis: Mosby-Year Book, Inc., 1996.

MENTAL HEALTH NURSING

Burgess, A.W. *Psychiatric Nursing in the 21st Century—Preparing for Primary Mental Health Care.* East Norwalk, Conn.: Appleton & Lange, 1996.

Diagnostic and Statistical Manual of Mental Disorders, 4th ed. (DSM-IV). Washington, D.C.: American Psychiatric Association, 1994.

Rawlings, R.D. *Clinical Manual of Psychiatric Nursing.* St. Louis: Mosby-Year Book, Inc., 1993.

Stuart, G., and Surdeen, S. *Principles and Practice of Psychiatric Nursing,* 5th ed. St. Louis: Mosby-Year Book, Inc., 1994.

Townsend, M.C. *Drug Guide for Psychiatric Nursing,* 2nd ed. Philadelphia: F.A. Davis, 1995.

Varcaris, E.M. *Foundations of Psychiatric Mental Health Nursing,* 2nd ed. Philadelphia: W.B. Saunders Co., 1994.

Wilson, B., et al. *Nurses Drug Guide 1997.* East Norwalk, Conn.: Appleton & Lange, 1997.

MATERNAL-NEWBORN NURSING

Bobak, I.M., and Lowdermilk, D.L., *Maternity Nursing,* 4th ed. St. Louis: Mosby-Year Book, Inc., 1995.

Novak, W., and Broom B., *Ingals' Maternal and Child Health Nursing,* 8th ed. St. Louis: Mosby-Year Book, Inc., 1994.

Olds, S., et al. *Maternal-Newborn Nursing,* 5th ed. Redwood City, Calif.: Addison-Wesley Publishing Co., 1996.

CHILD NURSING

Jackson, D.B., and Saunders, R. *Child Health Nursing: A Comprehensive Approach.* Philadelphia: J.B. Lippincott Co., 1993.

Nelson, W.E., et al. *Nelson Textbook of Pediatrics,* 15th ed. Philadelphia: W.B. Saunders, 1996.

Rudolph, A.M., et al. *Rudolph's Pediatrics,* 20th ed. East Norwalk, Conn.: Appleton & Lange, 1996.

Wilson, B., et al. *Nurses Drug Guide 1997.* East Norwalk, Conn.: Appleton & Lange, 1997.

Wong, D.L. *Waley and Wong's Essentials of Pediatric Nursing,* 5th ed. St. Louis: Mosby-Year Book, Inc., 1997.

Wong, D.L. *Waley and Wong's Nursing Care of Infants and Children,* 5th ed. St. Louis: Mosby-Year Book, Inc., 1995.

ADULT NURSING

Anastasi, J.K., and Rivera, J. "Understanding Prophylactic Therapy for HIV Infections," *AJN* 2:36-41, February 1994.

Ignatavicius, D.D., et al. *Medical-Surgical Nursing: A Nursing Process Approach,* 2nd ed. Philadelphia: W.B. Saunders Co., 1995.

Long, B.C., et al. *Medical-Surgical Nursing,* 3rd ed. St. Louis: Mosby-Year Book, Inc., 1993.

Phipps, W.J., et al. *Medical-Surgical Nursing: Concepts and Clinical Practice,* 5th ed. St. Louis: Mosby-Year Book, Inc., 1995.

Polaski, A.L., and Tatro, S.E. *Luckman's Core Principles and Practice of Medical-Surgical Nursing.* Philadelphia: W.B. Saunders Co., 1996.

ReJohnson, J. "Caring for the Woman Who's Had a Mastectomy," *AJN* 5:25-31, May 1994.

Smeltzer, S.C., and Bare, B. *Brunner and Suddarth's Textbook of Medical-Surgical Nursing,* 8th ed. Philadelphia: Lippincott-Raven, Inc., 1996.

Thompson, J.M., et al. *Mosby's Clinical Nursing,* 3rd ed. St. Louis: Mosby-Year Book, Inc., 1993.

Index

i refers to an illustration; *t* refers to a table.

i refers to an illustration; *t* refers to a table.

i refers to an illustration; *t* refers to a table.

i refers to an illustration; *t* refers to a table.

i refers to an illustration; *t* refers to a table.

i refers to an illustration; *t* refers to a table.

i refers to an illustration; *t* refers to a table.

i refers to an illustration; *t* refers to a table.

ANR Practice Disk for NCLEX-RN

The ANR practice disk for NCLEX-RN (inside back cover) includes two 75-item tests in the latest NCLEX-RN computer format. These 150 questions do not duplicate test items from the book's pretest or post-test. When taking the tests on disk, you'll use the same keyboard functions and screen layout as those used in the actual NCLEX-RN computerized adaptive test (CAT).

You can take either test repeatedly, with a random selection of questions each time. The program provides the correct answer and rationale after each question (learning mode) and a performance appraisal at the end of the test (proficiency mode). Furthermore, the program allows you to select questions by clinical area, nursing process step, or client need category. This unique feature allows you to review any weak areas identified in the performance appraisal.

To install the tests on your hard drive
If you are using Windows 3.X or Windows 95:
• Start Windows and insert disk.
• In Program Manager, choose File (for Windows 95, click Start button); then select Run.
• Type A:wininstl.exe (where A: is the letter of your floppy drive) and click OK.
• To start program from Windows, double-click on the NCLEX-RN icon. For Windows 95, select NCLEX-RN from the program list.

If you are using DOS:
• Insert disk.
• At the C:\> prompt, type A: (where A: is the letter of your floppy drive) and press Enter. Then type Install and press Enter.
• To start program from DOS, at the C:\> prompt, type CD\sprn and press Enter. Then type ANR and press Enter.

To take the tests directly from a $3^1/_2''$ floppy drive (in DOS)
• Insert the disk in the floppy drive.
• Type the drive letter (A: or B:), and press Enter. Type cd sprn and press Enter.
• Type ANR and press Enter.

For software support: Call 1-732-469-6060.